Synopsis and Atlas of Lever's Histopathology of the Skin

Synopsis and Atlas of Lever's Histopathology of the Skin

David Elder, M.B., Ch.B., F.R.C.P.A.
Professor and Associate Director
Division of Anatomic Pathology
Department of Pathology and Laboratory Medicine
University of Pennsylvania School of Medicine
Philadelphia, Pennsylvania

Rosalie Elenitsas, M.D.
Assistant Professor
Department of Dermatology
University of Pennsylvania School of Medicine
Associate Director of Dermatopathology
Department of Dermatology
Hospital of the University of Pennsylvania
Philadelphia, Pennsylvania

Michael Ioffreda, M.D.
Assistant Professor
Department of Dermatology
Hospital of the University
of Pennsylvania
Philadelphia, Pennsylvania

Bernett Johnson, Jr., M.D.
Professor
Departments of Dermatology and Pathology
University of Pennsylvania School of Medicine
Vice-Chairman
Department of Dermatology
Hospital of the University of Pennsylvania
Philadelphia, Pennsylvania

Jeffrey J. Miller, M.D.
Assistant Professor
Department of Dermatology
The Milton S. Hershey Medical Center
Hershey, Pennsylvania

O. Fred Miller III, M.D.
Director
Division of Dermatology
Department of Medicine
Geisinger Medical Center
Danville, Pennsylvania

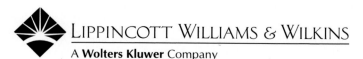
LIPPINCOTT WILLIAMS & WILKINS
A **Wolters Kluwer** Company
Philadelphia • Baltimore • New York • London
Buenos Aires • Hong Kong • Sydney • Tokyo

Acquisitions Editor: Beth Barry
Developmental Editor: Ellen DiFrancesco
Manufacturing Manager: Dennis Teston
Production Manager: Cassie Moore
Production Editor: Rosemary Palumbo
Cover Designer: Double R Design, Inc.
Indexer: Phyllis Manner
Compositor: Maryland Composition Co., Inc.

Printed and bound in China

9 8 7 6 5 4 3 2

Library of Congress Cataloging-in-Publication Data

Synopsis and atlas of Lever's histopathology of the skin   /   David E.
   Elder . . . [et al.].
       p.   cm.
    Includes bibliographical references and index.
    ISBN 0-397-58420-2
    1. Skin—Histopathology.   2. Skin—Histopathology—Atlases.   I.
 Elder, David E.   II. Lever, Walter F. (Walter Frederick), 1909–   III.
 Lever's histopathology of the skin.
 RL95 .S96   1999
 616.5′07—dc21
                                                            98-27635
                                                               CIP

Care has been taken to confirm the accuracy of the information presented and to describe generally accepted practices. However, the authors, editors, and publisher are not responsible for errors or omissions or for any consequences from application of the information in this book and make no warranty, expressed or implied, with respect to the contents of the publication.

The authors, editors, and publisher have exerted every effort to ensure that drug selection and dosage set forth in this text are in accordance with current recommendations and practice at the time of publication. However, in view of ongoing research, changes in government regulations, and the constant flow of information relating to drug therapy and drug reactions, the reader is urged to check the package insert for each drug for any change in indications and dosage and for added warnings and precautions. This is particularly important when the recommended agent is a new or infrequently employed drug.

Some drugs and medical devices presented in this publication have Food and Drug Administration (FDA) clearance for limited use in restricted research settings. It is the responsibility of the health care provider to ascertain the FDA status of each drug or device planned for use in their clinical practice.

Contents

Preface

As defined by its title, this volume has been planned and executed as a synopsis and atlas of *Lever's Histopathology of the Skin*. The histopathology of the skin, or dermatopathology, is an important subspecialty discipline of both dermatology and pathology, sharing the language and concepts of each of these major specialties. Comprehensive texts of dermatopathology are typically large and ponderous (both in literary style and in physical weight). These heavy texts serve as excellent references to the literature and provide comprehensive descriptions of a majority of the known classified diseases. However, the knowledge they contain is excessive, in many cases, for readers who may be studying for a nonspecialty board examination, or certainly for residents in the early period of learning their discipline. A more synoptic text can fill this gap by providing information that is selected to provide a framework for future learning, as well as a first step toward the development of basic diagnostic skills in the subject.

The synopsis presented in this book has been literally derived and shortened from the original text published as the eighth edition of *Lever's Histopathology of the Skin* in 1997. Accordingly, we as editors acknowledge a debt of gratitude to the contributors to that edition, who are listed in the Acknowledgments of this book. In a few instances, we have used photomicrographs that were contributed by others to the eighth edition, and in these cases we have specifically acknowledged the contributor in the figure legends. Most of the color photomicrographs in this volume have been painstakingly prepared to ensure consistency by Michael Ioffreda. The case material used for these photomicrographs has been taken almost exclusively from cases seen by the Penn Cutaneous Pathology Section of the Department of Dermatology at the Hospital of the University of Pennsylvania, selected by Bernett Johnson, Rosalie Elenitsas, and Michael Ioffreda. Some of the material has been taken from the Course in Dermatopathology offered annually under the direction of Drs. Elenitsas and Johnson. Some additional cases have been identified from the files of the Section of Surgical Pathology at the Hospital of the University of Pennsylvania. Other new material in this volume includes an excellent series of clinical photographs of fine quality derived for the most part from the collections of our father-and-son colleagues, O. Fred Miller and Jeffrey J. Miller. These clinical images, which represent the gross pathology of the diseases, will no doubt be especially useful to those who may not be in regular contact with patients suffering from a large variety of common and uncommon skin diseases.

Traditionally, dermatopathology texts have been organized according to a classification of diseases by a combination of pathophysiologic and clinicopathologic criteria. As discussed in more detail in the Introduction, this approach may serve well as a compendium of multiple disease characteristics, but it does not truly parallel the way in which common reaction patterns may present in histopathological material. These reaction patterns often appear similar in different diseases, which may therefore be difficult or impossible to distinguish from one another in a histology preparation. As a result, the reader of a traditional text will often have difficulty building a histological differential diagnosis because the histological lookalikes are covered in different chapters of the text. In this volume, the subject matter is organized according to the major patterns and cell types that may be involved in the morphological expression of various disease entities in different levels of the skin and subcutaneous tissues. This organization should facilitate an understanding of the way in which different diseases may induce similar reaction patterns in the skin, and should aid in developing a more comprehensive differential diagnosis for a given case.

In selecting the materials to be covered in this volume, we have attempted to provide at least one important example of essentially all of the possible reaction patterns in the skin. For those diseases considered prototypic of particular reaction patterns, we have provided brief synopses of clinical aspects and histopathology. We have also attempted to illustrate the major entities in the differential diagnosis of the prototypes, usually with an associated text synopsis. In this manner, we have attempted to cover most of the important dermatological diseases (for example, those that might be covered in a board review course for dermatology residents) in one or more sections of the book. Of course, the book is not intended to provide coverage as comprehensive or exhaustive as that in the heavy texts.

This book is directed to all students of dermatopathology, including perhaps some medical students, but in particular pathology and dermatology residents and practicing dermatologists and pathologists. In addition, this book could benefit those family practitioners who do skin biopsies and would like to have a better understanding of the pathology reports that they receive from their laboratories. The particular contributions of this book to the educational experience or diagnostic armamentarium of its readers should include an appreciation for the relationships between clinical and microscopic morphology of the common diseases of the skin, and for the manner in which different diseases may present with similar reaction patterns and thus simulate one another. This should result in an enhanced understanding of the process of differential diagnosis development for unknown skin lesions, and thus in greater diagnostic accuracy.

David Elder
Philadelphia, Pennsylvania
June 1998

Acknowledgments

This synopsis has been prepared in part from the eighth edition of *Lever's Histopathology of the Skin*. Accordingly, we wish to acknowledge the contributors to that edition for their part in the development of the material that we have presented here in a considerably edited form. If any errors are present in this material, however, they are not attributable to these individuals, but to us.

In addition to the contributors listed alphabetically below, we wish to acknowledge first and foremost the contributions of the founding author of this text, Walter Lever, M.D., and of his spouse and collaborator, Gundula Schaumberg-Lever, M.D.

Others to whom we are grateful for assistance in the preparation of this volume include many colleagues who have supported our effort, either in the form of helpful discussion, or by the provision of materials used in the book. Several colleagues have graciously provided materials from their collections to complete our work. These include our staff colleagues and the residents and fellows at Penn and Geisinger. We thank them for their helpful contributions.

Contributors to the eighth edition of *Lever's Histopathology of the Skin*:

Edward Abell, M.D.
Zsolt Argenyi, M.D.
Raymond L. Barnhill, M.D.
Martin M. Black, M.D., F.R.C.Path.
Walter H.C. Burgdorf, M.D.
Klaus J. Busam, M.D.
Eduardo Calonje, M.D., Dip.R.C.Path.
Wallace H. Clark, Jr., M.D.
Lisa M. Cohen, M.D.
Félix Contreras, M.D.
Jacinto Convit, M.D.
A. Neil Crowson, M.D.
David Elder, M.B., Ch.B., F.R.C.P.A.
Rosalie Elenitsas, M.D.
Robert J. Friedman, M.D., M.Sc.(Med.)
Thomas D. Griffin, M.D.
Allan C. Halpern, M.D.
Terence J. Harrist, M.D.
John L.M. Hawk, M.D.
Peter J. Heenan, M.B., B.S., F.R.C.Path., F.R.C.P.A.
Edward R. Heilman, M.D.
Paul Honig, M.D.
Thomas Horn, M.D.
Michael Ioffreda, M.D.
Christine Jaworsky, M.D.

Bernett Johnson Jr., M.D.
Waine C. Johnson, M.D.
Hideko Kamino, M.D.
Gary R. Kantor, M.D.
Nigel Kirkham, M.D., F.R.C.Path.
Philip E. LeBoit, M.D.
B. Jack Longley, M.D.
Sebastian Lucas, F.R.C.Path.
Timothy H. McCalmont, M.D.
N. Scott McNutt, M.D.
Cynthia Magro, M.D.
John Maize, M.D.
John Metcalf, M.D.
Martin Mihm, Jr., M.D.
Abelardo Moreno, M.D.
George F. Murphy, M.D.
Neal Penneys, M.D., Ph.D.
Bruce D. Ragsdale, M.D.
Richard J. Reed, M.D.
Philip E. Shapiro, M.D
Debra Karp Skopicki, M.D.
Neil P. Smith, M.D.
Richard L. Spielvogel, M.D.
Sonia Touissant, M.D.
Patricia Van Belle, D.S.N
Edward Wilson-Jones, M.D.

Introduction

In this work, it is our goal to provide the reader with an expanded introduction to the concept of diagnosis of cutaneous disease by pattern analysis. This concept was developed by others in a body of work spanning more than 30 years, and was adapted by us in an introductory form in the eighth edition of *Lever's Histopathology of the Skin* (1). As we stated in that chapter, the diagnosis of disease concerns the ability to classify disorders into categories that predict clinically important attributes such as prognosis or response to therapy. This permits the planning of appropriate interventions for particular patients. A complete understanding of this process would involve mastery of the stages of disease, the mechanisms of changes in morphology over time, and the molecular, cellular, gross clinical, and epidemiological reasons for the differences among diseases. However, in practice, many diseases are successfully diagnosed using only a few of their distinguishing features or diagnostic attributes.

As there are hundreds of diseases, each potentially with scores of diagnostic attributes, it is evident that an efficient strategy must be employed to enable diagnoses to be considered, dismissed, or retained for further consideration. Observation of an experienced dermatopathologist reveals a rapidity of accurate diagnosis that precludes the simultaneous consideration of more than a few variables. The process of diagnosis by an experienced observer is quite different from that employed by the novice, and is based on the rapid recognition of combinations or patterns of criteria (2,3). Just as the recognition of an old friend occurs by a process that does not require the serial enumeration of particular facial features, this process of pattern recognition occurs almost instantly, and is based on broad parameters that do not, at least initially, require detailed evaluation.

In clinical medicine, patterns may present as combinations of symptoms and signs, or even of laboratory values; in dermatopathology, the most predictive diagnostic patterns are recognized through the scanning lens of the microscope, or even before microscopy, as the microscopist holds the slide up to the light to evaluate its profile and distribution of colors. Occasionally, a specific diagnosis can be made during this initial stage of pattern recognition, by a process of gestalt, or instant recognition, but this should be tempered with a subsequent moment of healthy analytical scrutiny. More often, the scanning magnification pattern suggests a small list of possible diagnoses, or a differential diagnosis. Then, features that are more readily recognized at higher magnification may be employed to differentiate among the possibilities. Put in the language of science, the scanning magnification pattern suggests a series of hypotheses, which are then tested by additional observations (2). The tests may be observations made at higher magnification, the results of special studies such as immunohistochemistry, or external findings such as the clinical appearance of the patient, or the results of laboratory investigations. For example, a broad plaque-like configuration of small blue dots near the dermal-epidermal junction could represent a lichenoid dermatitis, or a lichenoid actinic keratosis. At higher magnification, the blue dots are confirmed to be lymphocytes, and one might seek evidence of parakeratosis, atypical keratinocytes, and plasma cells in the lesion, a combination that would rule out lichen planus and establish a diagnosis of actinic keratosis.

Most diagnoses in dermatopathology are established either by the "gestalt" method, or by the process of hypothesis generation and testing (differential diagnosis and investigation) just described. In both cases, the basis of the methods is the identification of simple patterns recognizable with the scanning lens that suggest a manageably short list of differential diagnostic considerations. This pattern recognition method was first developed in a series of lectures given in Boston by the late Wallace H. Clark (4), and has been refined since for inflammatory skin disease by Ackerman (5), for inflammatory and neoplastic skin disease by Mihm (6), and most recently by Murphy (7). The latter authors have published texts based more or less extensively on the pattern classification.

In the work on which this book is based, the classification of diseases was organized based upon traditional lines, in which diseases were discussed on the basis of pathogenesis (mechanisms) or etiology as well as upon reaction patterns. This classification has the significant advantage of placing disorders such as infections in a common relationship to one another, facilitating the description of their many common attributes. From a histopathological point of view, however, the novice must learn that some infections, such as syphilis, can resemble disorders as disparate as psoriasis, lichen planus, a cutaneous lymphoma, or a granulomatous dermatitis.

Because there are a limited number of reaction patterns in the skin, morphological simulants of disparate disease processes are common in the skin, as elsewhere. For this reason, classification methods based on patterns and those based on pathogenesis are only loosely compatible with each other. An observer who is studying an unknown case has only the morphological patterns under consideration. Only when the diagnosis is known can the pathogenesis of the disease be well understood. Thus, it is difficult to use a book based on pathogenic classification as a guide to the diagnosis of an unknown case. To partially circumvent this problem, this book presents a pattern-based classification of cutaneous pathology based on location in the skin, reaction patterns, and, where applicable, cell type. This classification has been based on original lecture notes prepared by Wallace H. Clark, Jr., M.D., in 1965 (with permission), and on the published works cited above, especially those of Hood, Kwan, Mihm, and Horn (6).

The classification is first presented in outline form and is redundant, in that a particular disease entity may appear under several entries because of the morphological heterogeneity of disease processes, which are often based on evolutionary or involutionary morphological changes as a disease waxes and wanes. Within each morphological category, one or more disorders considered to be prototypic of that category are described and illustrated. For example, lichen planus is the prototypic lichenoid dermatitis. The prototypic member of each category is emphasized in detailed descriptions, because such entities constitute the descriptive standard in a given category, and they are also the standard against which other entities are evaluated. For example, drug eruptions may adopt any of a number of morphologies as reflected by their appearance in the lichenoid category, and also in the psoriasiform, perivascular, and bullous categories as well as elsewhere. A "naked" epithelioid cell granuloma may suggest sarcoidosis, the prototypic epithelioid cell granuloma, while the presence of lymphocytes and necrosis in addition to granulomas might suggest tuberculosis, plasma cells might suggest syphilis, and neuritis might suggest leprosy.

After discussion of the prototypic entity in each category, a list of differential diagnostic possibilities is presented. The order of presentation of particular entities in any given position in this list reflects the authors' opinion of the relative frequency of the entities in the list, as encountered in a typical dermatopathology practice. For example, lichenoid drug eruption may be more common than lichen planus in most hospital-based practices. Some of these differential diagnostic possibilities are discussed in more detail because of their importance as diseases in their own right. For example, Spitz nevi are discussed in the section that contains nodular melanoma, and keratoacanthomas are discussed along with squamous cell carcinomas. The classification outlines may be used as the basis of an algorithmic approach to differential diagnosis, or as a guide to the descriptions in other books, including the eighth edition of *Lever's Histopathology of the Skin*. For example, a psoriasiform dermatitis with plasma cells may represent syphilis or mycosis fungoides, whose descriptions can be found in Chapters 22 and 32, respectively, of the eighth edition of *Lever's Histopathology of the Skin*. Terms such as psoriasiform and lichenoid are defined briefly, so that the reader may review more specific criteria for the distinctions among morphological simulants. This system of hypothesis generating and testing should lead not only to more efficiency in the evaluation and diagnosis of unknown cases, but should also facilitate the development of pattern recognition skills as more subtle diagnostic clues are absorbed into the diagnostic repertoire to allow for "tempered gestalt" diagnosis in an increasing percentage of cases.

This book is intended as a guide to differential diagnosis but should not be construed as an infallible diagnostic tool. Diagnosis should be based not only on the diagnostic considerations presented here, but also on those discussed elsewhere in the literature, all considered in a clinical and epidemiological context appropriate to the individual patient.

REFERENCES

1. Elder DE, Elenitsas R, Johnson, BL Jr., Jaworsky C, Ioffreda M. Algorithmic classification of skin disease for differential diagnosis. In: Elder DE, Elenitsas R, Jaworsky C, Johnson BL Jr., eds. *Lever's histopathology of the skin*, 8th ed. Philadelphia: Lippincott–Raven Publishers, 1997:61.
2. Sackett DL, Haynes RB, Guyatt GH, et al. *Clinical epidemiology. A basic science for clinical medicine.* 2nd ed. Boston: Little, Brown and Company, 1991.
3. Foucar E. Diagnostic decision-making in surgical pathology. In: Weidner N. *Diagnosis of the difficult case.*
4. Reed RJ, Clark WH Jr. Pathophysiologic reactions of the skin. In: Fitzpatrick TB, ed. *Dermatology in general medicine.* New York: McGraw-Hill, 1971:192.
5. Ackerman AB. *Histologic diagnosis of inflammatory skin diseases. A method by pattern analysis.* Philadelphia: Lea & Febiger, 1978.
6. Hood AF, Kwan TH, Mihm MC, Horn TD. *Primer of dermatopathology.* Boston: Little, Brown and Company, 1993.
7. Murphy GF. *Dermatopathology.* Philadelphia: WB Saunders, 1995.

In this atlas, the cutaneous diseases are listed in morphological categories based on their location in the skin, their architectural patterns, and their cytology. The list of diseases in each morphological category serves as a differential diagnosis for unknown disorders that present with the attributes of that category. The diseases are listed in rough order of their expected frequency in an average dermatopathology practice. In this atlas, representative disorders in each category are briefly described and illustrated. More detailed discussions of most of these and the other lesions in the lists can be found in the parent volume, *Lever's Histopathology of the Skin,* eighth edition.

Synopsis and Atlas of Lever's Histopathology of the Skin

I

Disorders Mostly Limited to the Epidermis and Stratum Corneum

The stratum corneum is usually arranged in a delicate meshlike or "basket-weave" pattern. It may be shed (exfoliation) or thickened (hyperkeratosis) with or without retention of nuclei (parakeratosis or orthokeratosis, respectively). The granular layer may be normal, increased (hypergranulosis), or reduced (hypogranulosis). Alterations in the stratum corneum usually result from inflammatory or neoplastic changes that affect the whole epidermis and, more often than not, the superficial dermis. Only a few conditions, mentioned in this section, show pathology mostly or entirely limited to the stratum corneum.

IA. HYPERKERATOSIS WITH HYPOGRANULOSIS

The stratum corneum is thickened, and the granular cell layer is absent or thinned.

IA1. No Inflammation

The dermis contains only the normal scattered perivascular lymphocytes, and there is no epidermal spongiosis or exocytosis. *Ichthyosis vulgaris* is the prototype.

Ichthyosis Vulgaris

CLINICAL SUMMARY. Ichthyosis vulgaris (1), which is inherited in an autosomal dominant fashion, is a common disorder. The skin shows scales that on the extensor surfaces of the extremities are large and adherent, resembling fish scales, and elsewhere are small. The flexural creases are spared.

HISTOPATHOLOGY. The characteristic finding is the association of moderate hyperkeratosis with a thin or absent granular layer. The hyperkeratosis often extends into the hair follicles, resulting in large keratotic follicular plugs. The dermis is normal.

1

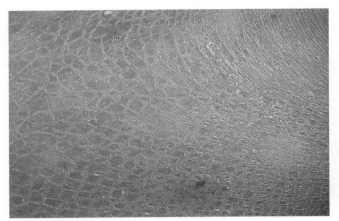

Clin. Fig. IA1

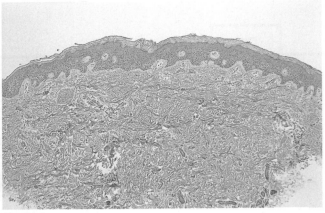

Fig. IA1.a

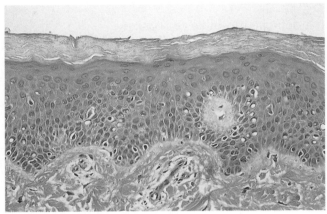

Fig. IA1.b

Clin. Fig. IA1. *Ichthyosis vulgaris (autosomal dominant).* Noninflammatory fishlike scales are clinically evident on the thigh in a middle-aged man with a strong family history of ichthyosis vulgaris.

Fig. IA1.a. *Ichthyosis vulgaris, low power.* At this power, the epidermis appears normal, except for uniform thickening of the stratum corneum.

Fig. IA1.b. *Ichthyosis vulgaris, high power.* The stratum corneum contains no parakeratotic nuclei, constituting orthokeratosis. The granular layer is diminished or, as here, completely absent.

IB. HYPERKERATOSIS WITH NORMAL OR HYPERGRANULOSIS

The stratum corneum is thickened, the granular cell layer is normal or thickened, and the dermis shows only sparse perivascular lymphocytes. There is no epidermal spongiosis or exocytosis.

1. No Inflammation
2. Scant Inflammation

IB1. No Inflammation

There is hyperkeratosis, and the upper dermis contains only sparse perivascular lymphocytes.

X-linked Ichthyosis

CLINICAL SUMMARY.   X-linked ichthyosis (1) is recessively inherited. About 90% of cases are caused by gene deletion. It is only rarely present at birth. Although female heterozygotes are frequently affected, males have a more severe form of the disorder. The thickness of the adherent scales in- creases during childhood. In contrast to ichthyosis vulgaris, the flexural creases may be involved.

HISTOPATHOLOGY.   There is hyperkeratosis. The granular layer is normal or slightly thickened but not thinned as in dominant ichthyosis vulgaris. The epidermis may be slightly thickened.

Epidermolytic Hyperkeratosis

CLINICAL SUMMARY.   This rather striking histologic reaction pattern is also known as *granular degeneration of the epidermis.* It is seen in some linear epidermal nevi and in bullous congenital ichthyosiform erythroderma. It is also seen as a reaction pattern in Grover's disease, and the same pattern is commonly observed as an incidental finding, when it may be referred to as "focal acantholytic dyskeratosis (2)."

HISTOPATHOLOGY.   The salient histologic features are perinuclear vacuolization of the cells in the stratum spinosum and in the stratum granulosum, irregular cellular boundaries peripheral to the vacuolization, an increased number of irregularly shaped large keratohyaline granules, and compact hyperkeratosis in the stratum corneum.

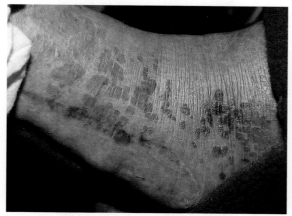

Clin. Fig. IB1.a

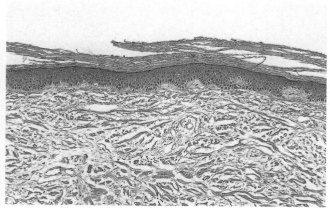

Fig. IB1.a

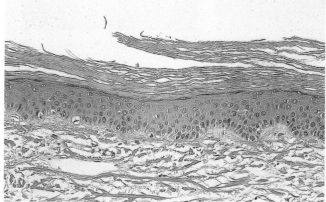

Fig. IB1.b

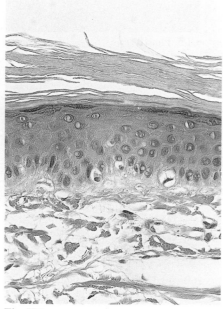

Fig. IB1.c

Clin. Fig. IB1.a. *X-linked ichthyosis.* Large "dirty" scales on the ankle are characteristic.

Fig. IB1.a. *X-linked ichthyosis.* At scanning power, the epidermis appears normal, except for uniform thickening of the stratum corneum.

Fig. IB1.b. *X-linked ichthyosis, medium power.* The thickened stratum corneum contains no parakeratotic nuclei, constituting orthokeratosis.

Fig. IB1.c. *X-linked ichthyosis, high power.* A normal granular layer is present.

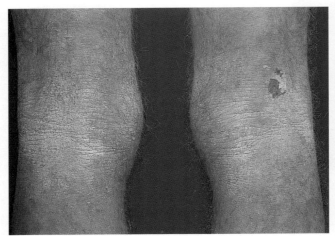

Clin. Fig. IB1.b

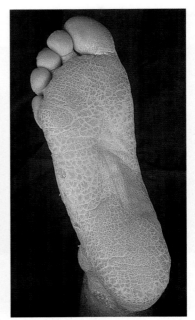

Clin. Fig. IB1.c

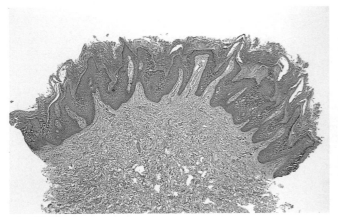

Fig. IB1.d

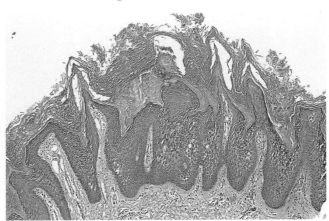

Fig. IB1.e

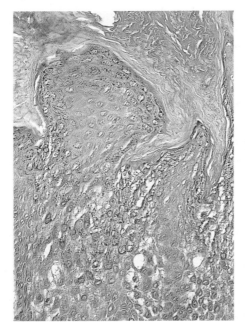

Fig. IB1.f

Clin. Fig. IB1.b. *Epidermolytic hyperkeratosis in bullous congenital ichthyosiform erythroderma.* Popliteal flexures are involved with keratotic, almost verrucous, malodorous scale. Erosions appear in sites of bullae.

Clin. Fig. IB1.c. *Bullous congenital ichthyosiform erythroderma.* The sole of the same patient's foot shows characteristic symptomatic yellow keratoderma. The patient's son shares this autosomal dominant condition.

Fig. IB1.d. *Epidermolytic hyperkeratosis, low power.* The epidermis is thickened and there is papillomatosis (these changes are not usually seen in focal acantholytic dyskeratoses). There is compact hyperkeratosis in the stratum corneum.

Fig. IB1.e. *Epidermolytic hyperkeratosis, medium power.* The epidermis shows vacuolated keratinocytes with large keratohyaline granules. There is compact hyperkeratosis in the stratum corneum.

Fig. IB1.f. *Epidermolytic hyperkeratosis, high power.* There is orthokeratotic hyperkeratosis. The epidermis shows vacuolated keratinocytes with large keratohyaline granules. The keratohyaline granules are irregular and cell borders are ill-defined.

Conditions to consider in the differential diagnosis:

   lamellar ichthyosis
   X-linked ichthyosis
   epidermolytic hyperkeratosis
   epidermolytic acanthoma
   oculocutaneous tyrosinosis (tyrosinemia)
   acanthosis nigricans
   large-cell acanthoma
   hyperkeratosis lenticularis perstans (Flegel's disease)

IB2. Scant Inflammation

There is hyperkeratosis, and lymphocytes are minimally increased around the superficial plexus. There may be a few neutrophils in the stratum corneum.

Lichen Amyloidosis and Macular Amyloidosis

CLINICAL SUMMARY.   Lichen amyloidosis (3) and macular amyloidosis are best considered as different manifestations of the same disease process. Lichen amyloidosis is characterized by closely set, discrete, brown-red, pruritic, often some-what scaly papules and plaques that are most commonly located on the legs, especially the shins. The plaques often have verrucous surfaces and then resemble hypertrophic lichen planus or lichen simplex chronicus. It is assumed by some that the pruritus leads to damage of keratinocytes by scratching and to subsequent production of amyloid.

HISTOPATHOLOGY.   Lichen and macular amyloidoses show deposits of amyloid that are limited to the papillary dermis. Most of the amyloid is situated within the dermal papillae. Although the deposits usually are smaller in macular amyloidosis than in lichen amyloidosis, differentiation of the two on the basis of the amount of amyloid is not possible. The two conditions actually differ only in the appearance of the epidermis, which is hyperplastic and hyperkeratotic in lichen amyloidosis. Occasionally, the amount of amyloid in macular amyloidosis is so small that it is missed, even when special stains are used on frozen sections. In such instances, more than one biopsy may be necessary to confirm the diagnosis.

Conditions to consider in the differential diagnosis:

   dermatophytosis
   lichen amyloidosis and macular amyloidosis

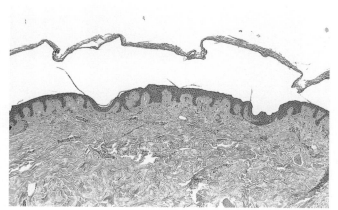

Fig. IB2.a

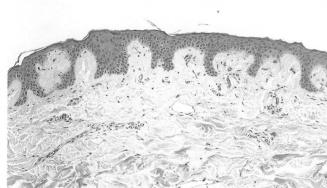

Fig. IB2.b

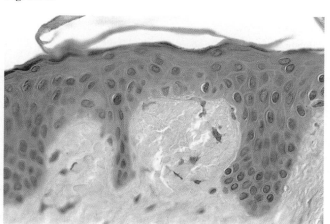

Fig. IB2.c

Fig. IB2.a. *Macular amyloidosis, low power.* At scanning magnification, there is slight hyperkeratosis with minimal inflammation.

Fig. IB2.b. *Macular amyloidosis, medium power.* At this power, the epidermis appears normal, except for slight uniform acanthosis. Subtle deposits of pink amorphous material (amyloid) are seen in dermal papillae.

Fig. IB2.c. *Macular amyloidosis, high power.* There is orthokeratotic hyperkeratosis. The granular layer is normal. There are deposits of amyloid filling the papillary dermis.

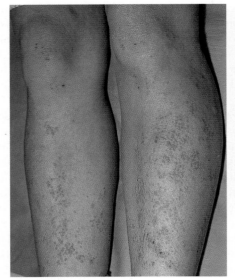

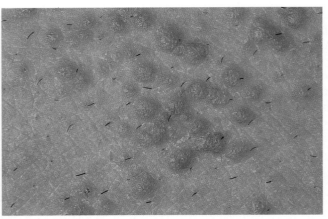

Clin. Fig. IB2.b

Clin. Fig. IB2.a

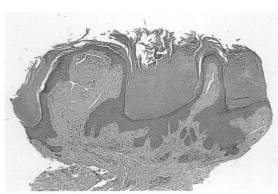

Fig. IB2.d

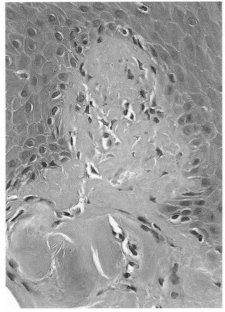

Fig. IB2.e

Clin. Fig. IB2.a. *Lichen amyloidosis.* This patient presented with pruritic papules on the pretibial areas.

Clin. Fig. IB2.b. Pigmented discrete papules result from deposition of amyloid derived from keratinocytes.

Fig. IB2.d. *Lichen amyloidosis, low power.* In contrast to macular amyloidosis, lichen amyloidosis reveals irregular acanthosis, papillomatosis, and hyperkeratosis. The papillary dermis is expanded and there is a mild perivascular inflammatory infiltrate.

Fig. IB2.e. *Lichen amyloidosis, high power.* At higher magnification, the amorphous deposits of amyloid are seen in the papillary dermis associated with pigment-laden macrophages.

IC. HYPERKERATOSIS WITH PARAKERATOSIS

The stratum corneum is thickened, the granular cell layer is reduced, and there is parakeratosis. The dermis may show only sparse perivascular lymphocytes, although some of the conditions listed here in other instances may show more substantial inflammation. There is no epidermal spongiosis or exocytosis. Most examples of dermatoses associated with parakeratosis have significant inflammation in the dermis (see sections IIIA–E). Some neoplastic disorders (e.g., actinic keratoses) present with parakeratosis, usually also associated with epidermal thickening, and inflammation in the dermis (see section IIA).

IC1. Scant or No Inflammation

Lymphocytes are minimally increased around the superficial plexus. There may be a few lymphocytes and/or neutrophils in the stratum corneum. *Dermatophytosis* is prototypic (4). However, many examples of dermatophytosis have significant inflammation, simulating one or another of the superficial inflammatory dermatoses (see Chapter III).

Dermatophytosis

CLINICAL SUMMARY.   Fungal infections of seven anatomic regions are commonly recognized: tinea capitis (including tinea favosa or favus of the scalp), tinea barbae, tinea faciei, tinea corporis (including tinea imbricata), tinea cruris, tinea of the hands and feet, and tinea unguium. Tinea corporis may be caused by any dermatophyte, but by far the most common

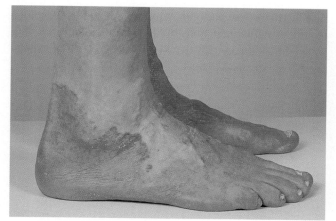

Clin. Fig. IC1

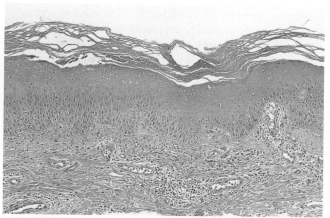

Fig. IC1.a

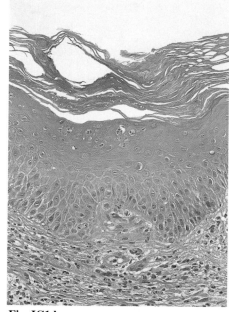

Fig. IC1.b

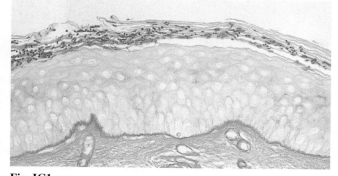

Fig. IC1.c

Clin. Fig. IC1. *Tinea pedis.* A leading edge of scale and erythema in a moccasin distribution characterizes this infection, most commonly caused by the dermatophyte *Trichophyton rubrum.*

Fig. IC1.a. *Dermatophytosis, medium power.* At this magnification, the epidermis may appear normal, slightly thickened as here, spongiotic, and/or psoriasiform. There is slight uniform thickening of the stratum corneum.

Fig. IC1.b. *Dermatophytosis, high power.* At high magnification, there is mixed orthokeratotic hyperkeratosis often sandwiched above a layer of parakeratosis and with focal collections of neutrophils. The granular layer is normal.

Fig. IC1.c. *Dermatophytosis, high power—periodic acid–Schiff (PAS) stain for fungi.* A PAS stain highlights fungal hyphae in the stratum corneum. These are likely to be most numerous in areas away from the collections of neutrophils.

cause in the United States is *Trichophyton rubrum*, followed by *Microsporum canis* and *Trichophyton mentagrophytes*. In *T. rubrum* infection there are large patches showing central clearing and a polycyclic scaling border, which may be quite narrow and threadlike.

HISTOPATHOLOGY. Fungi may present as filamentous hyphae, arthrospores, yeast forms, or pseudohyphae. Hyphae are threadlike structures that may be septate or nonseptate. Arthrospores are spores formed by fragmentation of septate hyphae at the septum, usually appearing as rounded, boxlike, or short cylindrical forms. Yeasts are single-celled forms that appear as round, elongated, or ovoid bodies; they grow by budding, and their progeny may adhere to each other and form elongated chains called pseudohyphae. If fungi are present in the horny layer, they usually are "sandwiched" between two zones of cornified cells, the upper being orthokeratotic and the lower consisting partially of parakeratotic cells. This "sandwich sign" should prompt the performance of a stain for fungi for verification. The presence of neutrophils in the stratum corneum is another valuable diagnostic clue. In the absence of demonstrable fungi, the histologic picture of fungal infections of the glabrous skin is not diagnostic. Depending on the degree of reaction of the skin to the

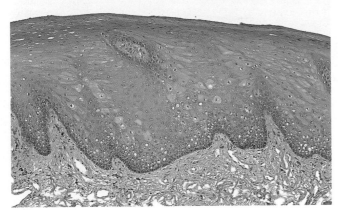

Clin. Fig. ID1.a

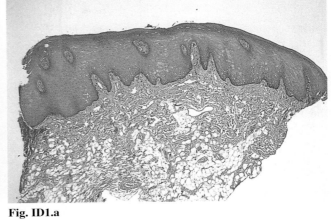

Fig. ID1.a

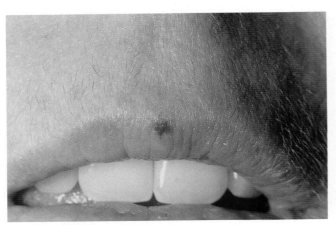

Fig. ID1.b

Clin. Fig. ID1.a. *Labial melanotic macule.* A benign acquired macule with irregular borders and uniform brown pigmentation developed near the vermilion border in a middle-aged woman. Melanoma is considered in the differential diagnosis.

Fig. ID1.a. *Labial lentigo, low power.* At this magnification, the epidermis may appear completely normal, unless the difference in melanin pigment content between the lesion and the adjacent skin can be appreciated. Often, however, there is slight acanthosis, as in this example. There may be patchy lymphocytes and melanophages in the papillary dermis or inflammatory cells may be completely absent, as seen here.

Fig. ID1.b. *Labial lentigo, high power.* There is increased melanin pigment in basal keratinocytes. Melanocytes may be slightly increased, but there is no contiguous melanocytic proliferation, as in nevi and melanomas. A few melanophages are present in the papillary dermis.

presence of fungi, there may be histologic features of an acute, a subacute, or a chronic spongiotic dermatitis.

Conditions to consider in the differential diagnosis:

dermatophytosis
scurvy
vitamin A deficiency
pellagra (niacin deficiency)
Hartnup disease
acrokeratosis neoplastica (Bazex syndrome)
epidermal dysmaturation (cytotoxic
  chemotherapy–variable keratin alterations)
epidermolytic hyperkeratosis
epidermal nevi
porokeratotic eccrine duct nevus
cutaneous horn
oral leukoplakia
leukoplakia of the vulva
syphilis cornee/keratoderma punctatum

ID. LOCALIZED OR DIFFUSE HYPERPIGMENTATIONS

Increased melanin pigment is present in basal keratinocytes, without melanocytic proliferation.

1. No Inflammation
2. Scant Inflammation

ID1. No Inflammation

The upper dermis contains only sparse perivascular lymphocytes. *Mucosal melanotic macule (melanosis)* is the prototype (5).

Mucosal Melanotic Macules

CLINICAL SUMMARY.   These benign lesions present as a pigmented patch on a mucous membrane. Common locations include the vermilion border of the lower lip, the oral cavity, the vulva, and, less often, the penis. The lesions may be synonymously referred to as "mucosal lentigo" or "mucosal melanotic macule." In the common location on the vulva ("vulvar lentigo"), this process may present as a broad, irregular, and asymmetric patch of brown to blue-black hyperpigmentation, resembling a melanoma. The lesions are entirely macular, unlike most invasive melanomas. The so-called labial lentigo ("labial melanotic macule"), a hyperpigmented macule of the lower lip, is uniformly pigmented brown, usually completely macular, and usually less than 6 mm in diameter.

HISTOPATHOLOGY.   At first glance, a biopsy specimen may appear normal. The findings include mild acanthosis without elongation of rete ridges and hyperpigmentation of basal keratinocytes, recognized in comparison with surrounding epithelium, with scattered melanophages in the dermis. Although melanocytes may be normal in number, in most instances the number is slightly increased. Because of this slight increase in the number of melanocytes, the term "genital lentiginosis" has recently been proposed for these lesions. Although these lesions may simulate melanoma clinically, histologically there is no contiguous melanocytic proliferation and no significant atypia. Occasionally, especially in the penile and vulvar lesions, there are prominent dendrites of melanocytes ramifying among the hyperpigmented keratinocytes. There may be associated mild keratinocytic hyperplasia, and patchy lymphocytes with scattered melanophages in the papillary dermis may account for the blue-black color that may simulate melanoma clinically.

Ephelids (Freckles)

CLINICAL SUMMARY.   Freckles, or ephelids, are small brown macules scattered over skin exposed to the sun. Exposure to the sun deepens the pigmentation of freckles, in contrast to lentigo simplex, whose already deep pigment does not change. Freckles, simple lentigines, and solar lentigines are difficult to distinguish from one another clinically and are considered together in most clinical and epidemiologic studies. Taken together, these lesions constitute a significant risk factor for the development of melanoma.

HISTOPATHOLOGY.   Freckles show hyperpigmentation of the basal cell layer, but in contrast to lentigo simplex, there is no elongation of the rete ridges and, by definition, no obvious increase in the concentration of melanocytes. In fact, in epidermal spreads of freckled skin, the number of dopa-positive melanocytes within the freckles may appear decreased compared with the adjacent epidermis. However, the melanocytes that are present may be larger and may show more numerous and longer dendritic processes than the melanocytes of the surrounding epidermis.

Conditions to consider in the differential diagnosis:

simple ephelis
mucosal melanotic macules
cafe au lait macule
actinic lentigo
pigmented actinic keratosis
melasma
Becker's nevus
congenital diffuse melanosis
reticulated hyperpigmentations
Addison's disease
alkaptonuric ochronosis
hemochromatosis

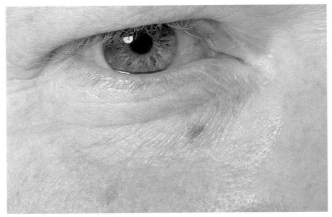

Clin. Fig. ID1.b

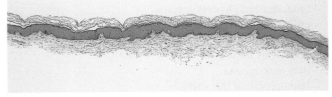

Fig. ID1.c

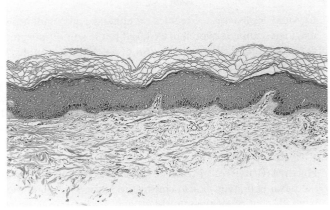

Fig. ID1.d

Clin. Fig. ID1.b. *Ephelis.* Fair-complected male has prominent brown macule that darkens in sunlight.

Fig. ID1.c. *Ephelis, low power.* At this magnification, the epidermis may appear completely normal, unless the difference in melanin pigment content between the lesion and the adjacent skin can be appreciated.

Fig. ID1.d. *Ephelis, medium power.* There is increased melanin pigment in basal keratinocytes. Melanocytes are not increased in number.

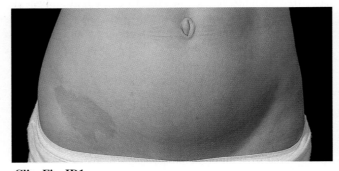

Clin. Fig. ID1.c

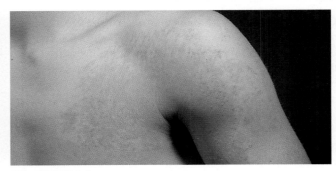

Clin. Fig. ID1.d

Clin. Fig. ID1.c. *Cafe au lait macule.* Evenly tan-colored macules can be seen in normal individuals. Multiple cafe au lait changes raise suspicion for neurofibromatosis.

Clin. Fig. ID1.d. *Becker's nevus.* A teenaged boy acquired an enlarging tan macule with scalloped borders on his shoulder and chest. Hypertrichosis may develop.

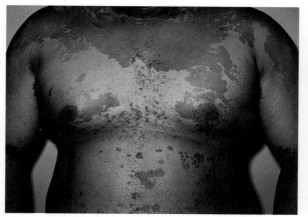

Clin. Fig. ID2

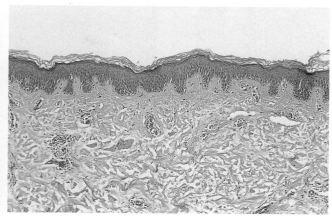

Fig. ID2.a

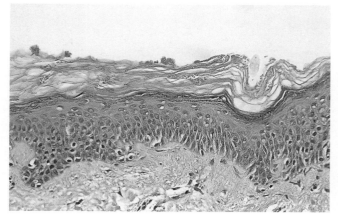

Fig. ID2.b

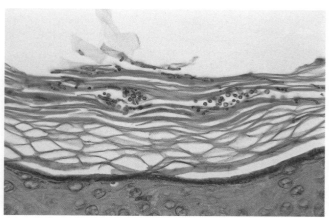

Fig. ID2.c

Clin. Fig. ID2. *Pityriasis versicolor.* Hyperpigmented patches, commonly as here present on the trunk, have "furfuraceous" scale with gentle scraping. Potassium hydroxide examination in this case demonstrated abundant hyphae and spores. The clinical differential diagnosis for this case would include vitiligo.

Fig. ID2.a. *Pityriasis versicolor, low power.* The epidermis may appear completely normal at scanning magnification. There may be a few perivascular lymphocytes in the papillary dermis or these may be absent.

Fig. ID2.b. *Pityriasis versicolor, medium power.* Upon closer inspection, one can identify a hyperkeratotic stratum corneum, containing organisms.

Fig. ID2.c. *Pityriasis versicolor, high power.* The stratum corneum contains abundant yeasts. Hyphae are present in addition, and the classic "spaghetti and meatballs" appearance results.

ID2. Scant Inflammation

Lymphocytes are minimally increased around the superficial plexus. There may be a few lymphocytes and/or neutrophils in the stratum corneum. Melanophages may be present in the papillary dermis. *Pityriasis (tinea) versicolor* is the prototype (6).

Pityriasis (Tinea) Versicolor

CLINICAL SUMMARY. The frequently used term "tinea versicolor" is not accurate because the causative organism, *Malassezia furfur*, is not a dermatophyte. Pityriasis versicolor usually affects the upper trunk, where there are multi-

ple pink to brown papules that may appear hyper- or hypopigmented. On gentle scraping, the surface of the discolored areas is finely scaled.

HISTOPATHOLOGY. In contrast to other fungal infections of the glabrous skin, the horny layer in lesions of pityriasis versicolor contains abundant amounts of fungal elements, which can often be visualized in sections stained with hematoxylin-eosin as faintly basophilic structures. *Malassezia (Pityrosporum)* is present as a combination of both hyphae and spores, often referred to as "spaghetti and meatballs." The inflammatory response in pityriasis versicolor is usually

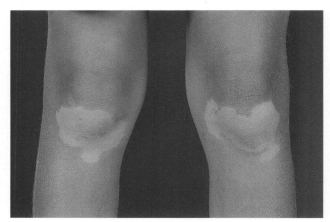

Clin. Fig. IE1

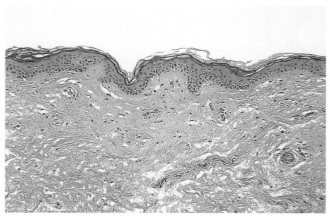

Fig. IE1.a

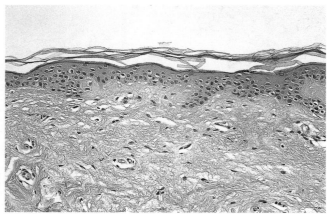

Fig. IE1.b

Clin. Fig. IE1. *Vitiligo.* Acquired depigmented well-demarcated patches often appear with striking symmetry.

Fig. IE1.a. *Vitiligo, low power.* The epidermis may appear completely normal at scanning magnification, unless it is appreciated that melanin pigment is reduced compared with surrounding skin.

Fig. IE1.b. *Vitiligo, high power.* At high magnification, a careful search reveals the absence of melanocytes from the basal lamina region.

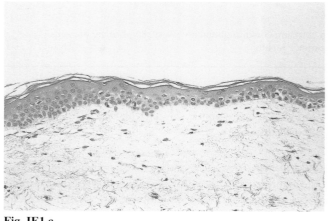

Fig. IE1.c

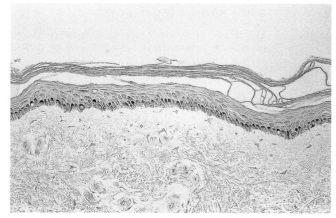

Fig. IE1.d

Fig. IE1.c. *Vitiligo, Fontana stain, medium power.* A Fontana stain reveals the absence of melanin pigment in basal layer keratinocytes, changes typical of vitiligo.

Fig. IE1.d. *Vitiligo, Fontana stain, medium power.* In contrast, in a biopsy of normal skin, the Fontana stain highlights the melanin pigment that stains black in the basal layer keratinocytes.

minimal, although there may occasionally be slight hyperkeratosis, slight spongiosis, or a minimal superficial perivascular lymphocytic infiltrate.

Conditions to consider in the differential diagnosis:

pityriasis (tinea) versicolor
lichen amyloidosis
postinflammatory hyperpigmentation
erythema dyschromicum perstans
pretibial pigmented patches in diabetes

IE. LOCALIZED OR DIFFUSE HYPOPIGMENTATIONS

Melanin pigment is reduced in basal keratinocytes, with (vitiligo) or without (early stages of chemical depigmentation) a reduction in the number of melanocytes.

IE1. With or Without Slight Inflammation

Lymphocytes may be minimally increased around the dermal–epidermal junction, as in the active phase of vitiligo, or may be absent, as in albinism. *Vitiligo* is the prototype (7).

Vitiligo

CLINICAL SUMMARY.   Vitiligo is an acquired, disfiguring, patchy, total loss of skin pigment. Stable patches often have an irregular border but are sharply demarcated from the surrounding skin. In expanding lesions, there may rarely be a slight rim of erythema at the border and a thin zone of transitory partial depigmentation.

HISTOPATHOLOGY.   The central process in vitiligo is the destruction of melanocytes at the dermal–epidermal junction. With silver stains or the dopa reaction, well-established lesions of vitiligo are totally devoid of melanocytes. The periphery of expanding lesions that are hypopigmented rather than completely depigmented still show a few dopa-positive melanocytes and some melanin granules in the basal layer. In the outer border of patches of vitiligo, melanocytes are often prominent and demonstrate long dendritic processes filled with melanin granules. Rarely, a superficial perivascular and somewhat lichenoid mononuclear cell infiltrate with vacuolar change is observed at the border of the depigmented areas.

Conditions to consider in the differential diagnosis:

vitiligo
chemical depigmentation
idiopathic guttate hypomelanosis
albinism
tinea versicolor
piebaldism
Chediak–Higashi syndrome
hypopigmented mycosis fungoides

REFERENCES

1. Frost P, Van Scott EJ. Ichthyosiform dermatoses. *Arch Dermatol* 1966;94:113.
2. Ackerman AB. Focal acantholytic dyskeratosis. *Arch Dermatol* 1972;106:702.
3. Jambrosic J, From L, Hanna W. Lichen amyloidosus. *Am J Dermatopathol* 1984;6:151.
4. Kwon-Chung KJ, Bennett JE. Dermatophytosis. In: Kwon-Chung KJ, Bennett JE, eds. *Medical mycology*. Philadelphia: Lea & Febiger, 1992:105.
5. Maize JC. Mucosal melanosis. *Dermatol Clin* 1988;6:283.
6. Galadari I, el Komy M, Mousa A, et al. Tinea versicolor: histologic and ultrastructural investigation of pigmentary changes. *Int J Dermatol* 1992;31:253.
7. Fisher AA. Differential diagnosis of idiopathic vitiligo. Part III. Occupational leukoderma. *Cutis* 1994;53:278.

Localized Superficial Epidermal or Melanocytic Proliferations

Localized superficial epithelial and melanocytic proliferations may be reactive but are often neoplastic. The epidermis (keratinocytes) may proliferate without extension into the dermis, may extend into the dermis, and may be squamous or basaloid. Melanocytes within the epidermis may proliferate with or without cytologic atypia (nevi, dysplastic nevi, melanoma *in situ*), in a proliferative epidermis (superficial spreading melanoma *in situ*, Spitz nevi), or an atrophic epidermis (lentigo maligna); they can also extend into the dermis as proliferative infiltrates [invasive melanoma with or without vertical growth phase (VGP)]. There may be an associated variably cellular, often mixed inflammatory infiltrate, or inflammation may be essentially absent.

IIA. LOCALIZED IRREGULAR THICKENING OF THE EPIDERMIS

Localized irregular epidermal proliferations are usually neoplastic.

1. Localized Epidermal Proliferations
2. Superficial Melanocytic Proliferations

IIA1. Localized Epidermal Proliferations

The epidermis is thickened secondary to a localized proliferation of keratinocytes (acanthosis). The proliferation can be cytologically atypical, as in squamous cell carcinoma *in situ*, or bland, as in eccrine poroma. It may be papillary, as in seborrheic keratoses and verrucae, or highly irregular, as in pseudoepitheliomatous hyperplasia. Actinic keratosis and squamous cell carcinoma are prototypic examples. Clearcell acanthoma may also be included in this category or may mimic an inflammatory condition.

Actinic Keratosis

CLINICAL SUMMARY. Actinic keratoses (1) are usually seen as multiple lesions in sun-exposed areas of the skin in fair-complected persons in or past midlife. Usually, the lesions measure less than 1 cm in diameter. They are erythematous, are often covered by adherent scales, and are barely palpable except in their hypertrophic form.

HISTOPATHOLOGY. Five types of actinic keratosis can be recognized histologically: hypertrophic, atrophic, bowenoid,

acantholytic, and pigmented. In the *hypertrophic type*, hyperkeratosis is pronounced and is intermingled with areas of parakeratosis. The epidermis is thickened in most areas and shows irregular downward proliferation that is limited to the uppermost dermis and does not represent frank invasion. Keratinocytes in the stratum malpighii show a loss of polarity and thus a disorderly arrangement. Some of these cells show crowding, pleomorphism, and atypicality of their nuclei, which appear large, irregular, and hyperchromatic; some of the cells are dyskeratotic or apoptotic. In contrast to the epidermal keratinocytes, the cells of the hair follicles and eccrine ducts that penetrate the epidermis within actinic keratoses retain their normal appearance and keratinize normally, giving rise to the characteristic alternating columns of hyperkeratosis and orthokeratosis.

Atrophic actinic keratoses lack the hypertrophic epidermal proliferation seen in the hypertrophic type, bowenoid keratoses are characterized by high-grade atypia that approaches full thickness, acantholytic keratoses show dyshesion of lesional cells that may simulate a glandular pattern, and pigmented keratoses resemble any of the other forms but contain increased melanin pigment.

In all five types of actinic keratosis, the upper dermis usually shows a fairly dense, chronic, inflammatory infiltrate composed predominantly of lymphoid cells but often also containing plasma cells. The upper dermis usually shows solar or basophilic degeneration.

Eccrine Poroma

CLINICAL SUMMARY. Eccrine poroma (2) is a fairly common solitary tumor, found most commonly on the sole or the sides of the foot and next in frequency on the hands and fingers. It may also appear in other areas of the skin, such as the neck, chest, and nose. Eccrine poroma generally arises in middle-aged persons. The tumor has a rather firm consistency, is raised and often slightly pedunculated, is asymptomatic, and usually measures less than 2 cm in diameter. In *eccrine poromatosis*, more than 100 papules are observed on the palms and soles.

HISTOPATHOLOGY. In its typical form, eccrine poroma arises within the lower portion of the epidermis, from where it extends downward into the dermis as tumor masses that often consist of broad anastomosing bands. The tumor cells are smaller than squamous cells, have a uniform cuboidal appearance and a round deeply basophilic nucleus, and are connected by intercellular bridges. They show no tendency to keratinize within the tumor, except on the surface. Although the border between tumor formations and the stroma is sharp, tumor cells located at the periphery show no palisading. As a characteristic feature, the tumor cells contain significant amounts of glycogen, usually in an uneven distribution. In most but not all eccrine poromas, narrow ductal lumina and occasionally cystic spaces are found within the tumor, lined by an eosinophilic, periodic acid–Schiff- (PAS)

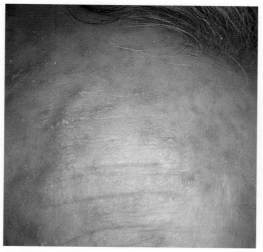

Clin. Fig. IIA1.a

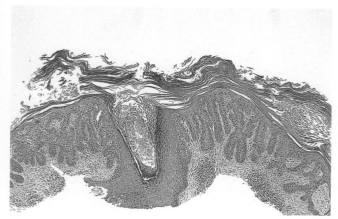

Fig. IIA1.a

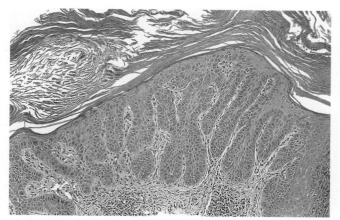

Fig. IIA1.b

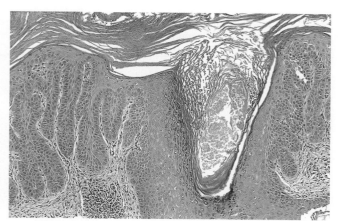

Fig. IIA1.c

Clin. Fig. IIA1.a. *Actinic keratosis*. Scaly erythematous macules and papules with a "sandpaper" texture appear commonly on face and dorsal hands, areas subject to chronic sun exposure.

Fig. IIA1.a. *Hypertrophic actinic keratosis, low power*. There is hyperkeratosis alternating with parakeratosis and irregular thickening of the epithelium. In the dermis, there are patchy lymphocytes and plasma cells.

Fig. IIA1.b. *Hypertrophic actinic keratosis, medium power*. The normal epidermal maturation pattern is disturbed, with increased thickness of the basal layer.

Fig. IIA1.c. *Hypertrophic actinic keratosis, high power*. Basal keratinocytes show attributes of dysplasia or *in situ* malignancy—nuclear crowding, enlargement, hyperchromatism, and pleomorphism. Note the orthokeratotic column above the hyperplastic follicular infundibulum in the center of the image.

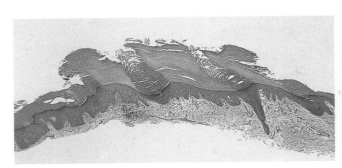
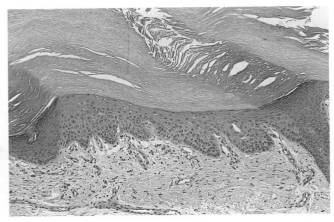

Fig. IIA1.d   **Fig. IIA1.e**

Fig. IIA1.d. *Bowenoid actinic keratosis, low power*. This lesion demonstrates striking alternating columns of hyperkeratosis and parakeratosis. The epithelium is irregularly thickened.

Fig. IIA1.e. *Bowenoid actinic keratosis, low power*. Columns of orthokeratotic keratin extend above the hyperplastic epithelium of skin adnexa (sweat ducts in this instance). Parakeratotic keratin extends above the full-thickness dysplastic epithelium.

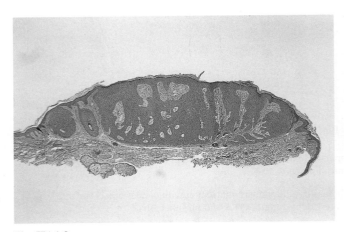
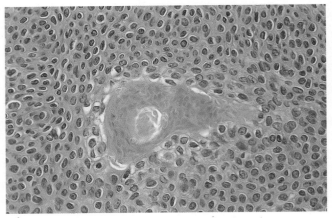

Fig. IIA1.f   **Fig. IIA1.g**

Fig. IIA1.f. *Eccrine poroma, scanning magnification*. There is a well-defined epidermal proliferation that is sharply circumscribed from the adjacent skin.

Fig. IIA1.g. *Eccrine poroma, high magnification*. At higher magnifications this lesion is composed of uniform bland-appearing epithelial cells associated with formation of small ducts that are filled with amorphous material.

positive, diastase-resistant cuticle similar to that lining the lumina of eccrine sweat ducts and by a single row of luminal cells.

Squamous Cell Carcinoma In Situ (Bowen's Disease)

CLINICAL SUMMARY.   Bowen's disease usually consists of a solitary lesion manifested as a slowly enlarging erythematous patch of sharp but irregular outline within which there are generally areas of scaling and crusting. It may occur on exposed or on unexposed skin and in pigmented or poorly pigmented skin. It may be caused on exposed skin by exposure to the sun and on unexposed skin by the ingestion of arsenic.

HISTOPATHOLOGY.   Bowen's disease (3) is an intraepidermal squamous cell carcinoma also referred to as squamous cell carcinoma *in situ*. When full-thickness atypia is present in an actinic keratosis, the term squamous cell carcinoma *in situ* may also appropriately be applied. The *bowenoid type* of actinic keratosis is histologically indistinguishable from Bowen's disease. As in Bowen's disease, there is within the epidermis considerable disorder in the arrangement of the nuclei and clumping of nuclei and dyskeratosis. The epidermis is acanthotic and the cells lie in complete disorder, resulting in a "windblown" appearance. Many cells are highly atypical, with large hyperchromatic nuclei and, frequently, multiple clustered nuclei. The horny layer is usually thickened and consists largely of parakeratotic cells with atypical hyper-

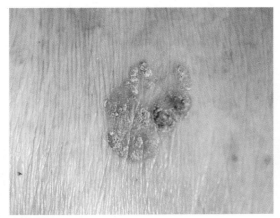

Clin. Fig. IIA1.b

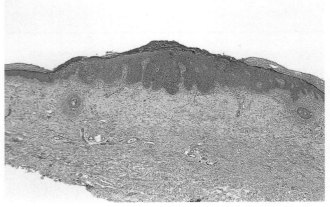

Fig. IIA1.h

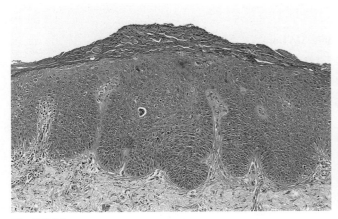

Fig. IIA1.i

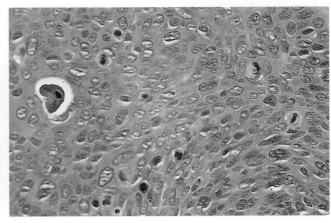

Fig. IIA1.j

Clin. Fig. IIA1.b. *Squamous cell carcinoma* in situ. A slightly elevated, scaly, flesh-colored plaque of long duration. Although Bowen's disease is seen commonly on the head and neck, it can arise on sun-protected skin as well. (Photo by William K. Witmer, Department of Dermatology, University of Pennsylvania.)

Fig. IIA1.h. *Squamous cell carcinoma* in situ, *scanning power.* The epidermis appears irregularly thickened with hyperkeratosis. In the dermis, there is a dense inflammatory infiltrate and solar elastosis.

Fig. IIA1.i. *Squamous cell carcinoma* in situ, *medium power.* The normal maturation pattern of keratinocytic epithelium is disturbed, imparting a "windblown" look to the neoplastic epithelium. There is a parakeratotic scale.

Fig. IIA1.j. *Squamous cell carcinoma* in situ, *high power.* The lesional cells exhibit nuclear attributes of malignancy—enlargement, hyperchromatism, pleomorphism, and dyskeratosis.

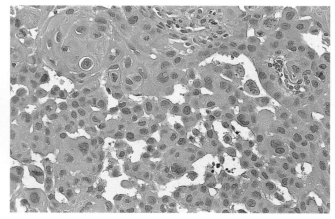

Fig. IIA1.k

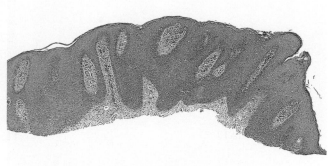

Fig. IIA1.l

Fig. IIA1.k. *Squamous cell carcinoma in situ with acantholysis, low power*. This relatively well-circumscribed acanthotic epithelial proliferation shows clear spaces in the mid and lower epidermal layers.

Fig. IIA1.l. *Squamous cell carcinoma in situ with acantholysis, high power*. Acantholysis is seen within the spinous layer. The presence of cytologic atypia is essential in differentiating this lesion from other acantholytic disorders.

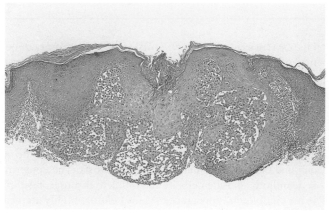

Clin. Fig. IIA1.c

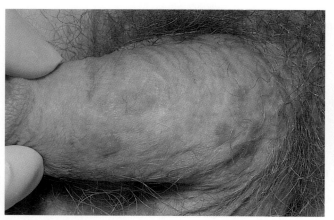

Fig. IIA1.m

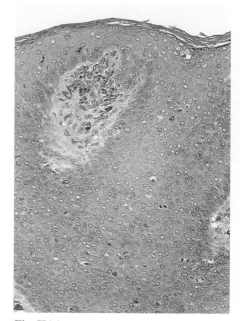

Fig. IIA1.n

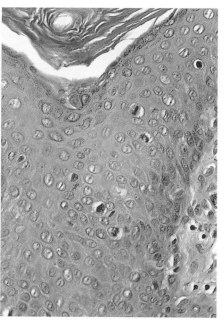

Fig. IIA1.o

Clin. Fig. IIA1.c. *Bowenoid papulosis*. A middle-aged man presented with a long-standing history of asymptomatic reddish-brown papules.

Fig. IIA1.m. *Bowenoid papulosis, low power*. There is mildly irregular epidermal thickening, and hyperpigmentation.

Fig. IIA1.n. *Bowenoid papulosis, medium power*. Focally, one can identify perinuclear vacuolization similar to what is seen in common condylomata.

Fig. IIA1.o. *Bowenoid papulosis, high power*. In contrast to condyloma acuminatum, bowenoid papulosis reveals nuclear atypia and numerous mitotic figures.

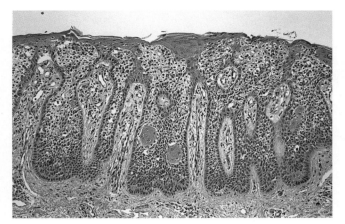

Fig. IIA1.p. *Clear-cell squamous cell carcinoma* in situ, *medium power.* In this variant, the atypical keratinocytes show an abundance of clear cytoplasm. Frequently, there is sparing of basal-layer keratinocytes. Identification of keratinocyte atypia is crucial in distinguishing this lesion from a clear-cell acanthoma.

chromatic nuclei. In contrast to actinic keratoses where the adnexal epithelium is hyperplastic, the infiltrate of atypical cells in Bowen's disease frequently extends into follicular infundibula and causes replacement of the follicular epithelium by atypical cells down to the entrance of the sebaceous duct. In a small percentage of cases of Bowen's disease (about 3% to 5%), an invasive squamous cell carcinoma develops.

Bowenoid Papulosis

See Figs. IIA1.m–IIA1.o.

Clear-Cell Squamous Cell Carcinoma In Situ

See Fig. IIA1.p.

Clear-Cell Acanthoma

CLINICAL SUMMARY.   This not uncommon tumor (4) typically occurs as a solitary lesion on the legs as a slowly grow-

ing, sharply delineated, red nodule or plaque 1 to 2 cm in diameter covered with a thin crust and exuding some moisture. A collarette is often seen at the periphery. The lesion appears "stuck on," like a seborrheic keratosis, and is vascular, like a granuloma pyogenicum.

HISTOPATHOLOGY.   Within a sharply demarcated area of the epidermis, the epidermal cells, with the exception of those of the basal cell layer, appear strikingly clear and slightly enlarged. Their nuclei appear normal. Staining with PAS reaction reveals large amounts of glycogen within the cells. The rete ridges are elongated and may be intertwined. The surface is parakeratotic with few or no granular cells. The acrosyringia and acrotrichia within the tumor retain their normal stainability. A conspicuous feature in most lesions is the presence throughout the epidermis of numerous neutrophils, many with fragmentation of their nuclei, often forming microabscesses in the parakeratotic horny layer. Slight spongiosis is present between the clear cells. Dilated capillaries are seen in the elongated papillae and often also in the dermis underlying the tumor. In addition, there is a mild to moderately severe lymphoid infiltrate in the dermis. Some clear-cell acanthomas appear papillomatous, with the configuration of a seborrheic keratosis.

Conditions to consider in the differential diagnosis:
No cytologic atypia:

    seborrheic keratosis
    verrucae
    dermatosis papulosa nigra
    stucco keratosis
    large-cell acanthoma
    clear-cell acanthoma
    epidermal nevi
    eccrine poroma

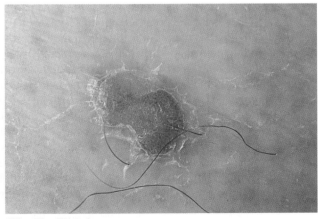

Clin. Fig. IIA1.d

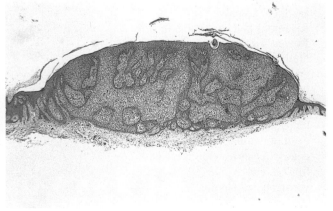

Fig. IIA1.q

Clin. Fig. IIA1.d. *Clear-cell acanthoma.* An elderly man developed an asymptomatic benign erythematous eroded papule with a collarette of scale on the calf. Differential diagnosis includes amelanotic melanoma, squamous cell carcinoma, and eccrine poroma.

Fig. IIA1.q. *Clear-cell acanthoma, scanning power.* There is a zone of epidermal hyperplasia with mild hyper-keratosis. This pale-staining epithelial neoplasm is sharply demarcated from the adjacent normal epidermis. *(continues)*

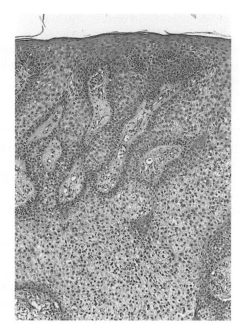

Fig. IIA1.r

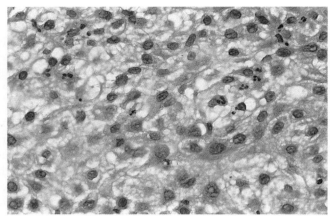

Fig. IIA1.s

Fig. IIA1.r. *Clear-cell acanthoma, medium power.* The lesion is composed of pale-staining bland-appearing keratinocytes. The cells are pale because of an abundance of glycogen.

Fig. IIA1.s. *Clear-cell acanthoma, high power.* Upon close inspection, neutrophils can be seen throughout this lesion; they may also accumulate in the overlying stratum corneum.

---

hidroacanthoma simplex
oral white sponge nevus
leukoedema of the oral mucosa
verrucous hyperplasia of oral mucosa (oral florid
  papillomatosis)
With cytologic atypia:
  actinic keratosis
  arsenical keratosis
  squamous cell carcinoma *in situ*
  Bowen's disease
  erythroplasia of Queyrat
  erythroplakia of the oral mucosa
  bowenoid papulosis
Pseudoepitheliomatous hyperplasia:
  halogenodermas
  deep fungal infections
  epidermis above granular cell tumor
  Spitz nevus
  verrucous melanoma

IIA2. Superficial Melanocytic Proliferations

The epidermis may be thickened (acanthosis) and is associated with a proliferation of single or nested melanocytic cells. The proliferation can be malignant, as in superficial spreading melanoma, or benign, as in nevi. These are the prototypes.

Superficial Melanocytic Nevi and Melanomas

CLINICAL SUMMARY. Melanocytic nevi (5) vary considerably in their clinical appearance. Five clinical types can be recognized: (a) flat lesions, which are for the most part histologically junctional nevi, and compound nevi, which include (b) slightly elevated lesions often with raised centers and flat peripheries, many of which are histologically dysplastic nevi; (c) dome-shaped lesions; (d) papillomatous lesions; and (e) pedunculated lesions. The first two types are usually pigmented and are superficial at the histologic level (confined to the epidermis and papillary dermis); the latter three may or may not be pigmented and may involve the reticular dermis. Most small, flat lesions represent either a lentigo simplex or a junctional nevus; flat lesions or lesions with flat peripheries greater than 5 mm in diameter with irregular indefinite borders and pigment variegation are clinically dysplastic nevi.

Melanomas are neoplastic proliferations of cytologically malignant melanocytes. Two major steps or phases of melanoma development can be distinguished. The first is the radial growth phase (RGP), which presents clinically as an irregular patch or plaque of variegated pigmentation. Histologically, in this step the melanomas may be *in situ* or microinvasive but are nontumorigenic (they do not form a mass in the dermis). In the next step, the vertical growth phase (VGP), a clinically evident tumor mass is formed, often within the confines of an antecedent RGP, constituting a tumor within a plaque. The RGP plaque is seen histologically at the edges of the VGP tumor as a lateral or horizontal component. Three major clinicopathologic types of RGP *in situ* or microinvasive melanoma are recognized: superficial spreading, lentigo maligna, and acral lentiginous types. A fourth type of melanoma is defined by the lack of a discernible adjacent RGP component. This is termed nodular melanoma and is discussed in section VIB3.

HISTOPATHOLOGY. Melanocytic nevi are defined and recognized by the presence of nevus cells that, even though they are melanocytes, differ from ordinary melanocytes by being arranged at least partially in clusters or "nests," by having a tendency toward rounded rather than dendritic cell shape, and by a propensity to retain pigment in their cytoplasm rather than to transfer it to neighboring keratinocytes. Although a histologic subdivision of nevi into junctional, compound, and intradermal nevi is generally accepted, it should be realized that these are transitional stages in the "life cycle" of nevi, which start out as junctional nevi and, after having become intradermal nevi, undergo involution. The lentigo simplex is regarded as an early or evolving form of melanocytic nevus. It has the clinical appearance of a small lenticulate or lens-shaped pigmented spot (hence the term "lentigo") and is characterized histologically by the presence of single melanocytes arranged in contiguity about elongated rete ridges. The lack of nests at the histologic level distinguishes a lentigo from a nevus. The lentiginous pattern is seen in the common lentiginous junctional nevus, in which nevus cells in nests are present in combination with the "lentiginous pattern" just described. Dysplastic nevi also exhibit a lentiginous architecture, but they are larger (greater than 4 to 5 mm in histologic section diameter) and there is cytologic atypia affecting randomly scattered nevus cells.

The lentiginous pattern of proliferation is also seen in the "lentiginous" forms of melanoma, in which in contrast to nevi, the lesional cells are uniformly atypical and the pattern is less well organized than in nevi, often with haphazard proliferation of keratinocytes resulting in irregular thickening and thinning of the epidermis. In the most common form of melanoma, the superficial spreading type, the pattern of proliferation is termed "pagetoid," with lesional cells extending singly and in groups up into the keratinocytic epithelium, which as in lentiginous melanomas tends to be irregularly thickened and thinned. Some degree of pagetoid proliferation, often slight, is usually present in the lentiginous melanomas as well, and pagetoid proliferation may also be seen on occasion in benign nevi, especially Spitz nevi (see section IID2), and pigmented spindle cell nevi (see below).

Junctional nevi, including dysplastic nevi, may exhibit an irregularly thickened epidermis but more often tend to have regularly elongated rete ridges and are discussed in a later section (see section IIC1). The pigmented spindle cell nevus of Reed is a lesion that often has a rather irregularly thickened rete pattern and is discussed here as a prototype. *In situ* or microinvasive melanomas of the superficial spreading and acral lentiginous types also tend to have an irregularly thickened and thinned epidermis. The former is discussed in the section on pagetoid proliferations (see section IID2), and the latter is discussed below.

Pigmented Spindle Cell Nevus

CLINICAL SUMMARY. The pigmented spindle cell nevus (6), first described by Richard Reed, may be regarded as a variant of the classical Spitz nevus. The lesions are usually 3 to 6 mm in diameter, deeply pigmented, and either flat or slightly raised dome-shaped lesions. Most patients are young adults, and the most common location is on the lower extremities. Because of the heavy pigment and the history of sudden appearance, a clinical diagnosis of melanoma is often suspected clinically. The lesions are generally stable after a relatively sudden appearance and a short-lived period of growth.

HISTOPATHOLOGY. The lesion is characterized by its relatively small size and its symmetry and by a proliferation of uniform, narrow, elongated, spindle-shaped, often heavily pigmented melanocytes at the dermal–epidermal junction. The epidermis tends to be irregularly thickened, and there is hyperkeratosis often with conspicuous melanin pigment in the stratum corneum. The nests of spindle cells are vertically oriented and tend to blend with adjacent keratinocytes rather than forming clefts as in Spitz nevi. Kamino bodies may be present as in Spitz nevi. In the papillary dermis, the nevus cells lie in a compact cluster pattern, pushing the connective tissue aside. Involvement of the reticular dermis, common in Spitz nevi, is unusual in pigmented spindle cell nevi. Some lesions may show upward epidermal extension of junctional nests of melanocytes or of single cells in a "pagetoid pattern." In contrast to superficial spreading melanomas, pigmented spindle cell nevi are smaller, symmetric, and show sharply demarcated lateral margins. The tumor cells appear strikingly uniform from side to side. If lesional cells descend into the papillary dermis, they mature along nevus lines in pigmented spindle cell nevi, in contrast to melanomas. Mitoses may be present in the epidermis in either lesion, but are uncommon in the dermis in pigmented spindle cell nevi. Abnormal mitoses are very uncommon.

Acral Lentiginous Melanoma

CLINICAL SUMMARY. Acral lentiginous melanoma occurs on the hairless skin of the palms and soles, and in the ungual and periungual regions. The soles are the most common site (7). In groups such as Asians, Hispanics, Polynesians, and African-Americans, for whom the overall incidence of melanoma is low, most melanomas are of the acral type.

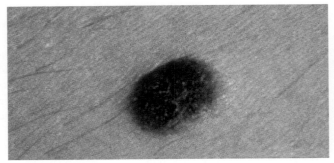

Clin. Fig. IIA2.a

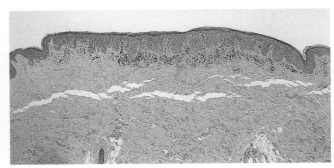

Fig. IIA2.a

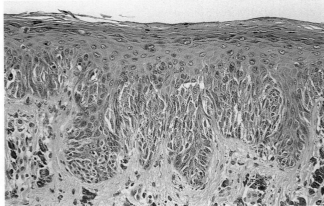

Fig. IIA2.b

Fig. IIA2.c

Clin. Fig. IIA2.a. *Pigmented spindle cell nevus.* A well-circumscribed, symmetric, small, uniformly pigmented lesion that appeared rapidly on the thigh of a young woman but then remained stable. The dark blue-black color differs from the pink or tan color of most classic Spitz nevi and may suggest the possibility of melanoma clinically. (Photo by W. Witmer, Dept. of Dermatology, University of Pennsylvania.)

Fig. IIA2.a. *Pigmented spindle cell nevus, low power.* These lesions may be entirely within the epidermis (junctional) or they may be compound. In the latter case, they tend to be confined to the papillary dermis. In this scanning magnification, the lesion is well circumscribed; there is an abundance of brown pigment, both within the thickened epidermal layer and within the superficial dermis.

Fig. IIA2.b. *Pigmented spindle cell nevus, medium power.* At higher magnification this nevus is composed of a proliferation of single and nested uniform melanocytes that contain an abundance of melanin pigment. The nests tend to blend with the surrounding keratinocytes in contrast to the clefting artifact that characterizes classic Spitz nevi.

Fig. IIA2.c. *Pigmented spindle cell nevus, high power.* The melanocytes are spindled in form and frequently oriented perpendicular to the skin surface. The keratinocytes and the stratum corneum also contain an abundance of melanin pigment, and there are numerous melanophages in the superficial dermis.

However, the absolute incidence of acral melanoma in these groups is similar to that in whites, who have a much higher overall incidence of melanoma. These considerations suggest that different etiologic factors, probably not involving sunlight, are operative in acral than in other sites. Although the survival rate of patients with acral melanomas in most series is poor, this is probably a result of their typically advanced microstage and/or stage at diagnosis.

Clinically, *in situ* or microinvasive acral lentiginous melanoma shows uneven pigmentation with an irregular, often indefinite, border. The soles of the feet are most commonly involved. If the tumor is situated in the nail matrix, the nail and nail bed may show a longitudinal pigmented band, and the pigment may extend onto the nail fold (Hutchinson's sign). Tumorigenic vertical growth may be heralded by the onset of a nodule, with development of ulceration. However, some acral melanomas may be deeply invasive while remaining quite flat, because the thick stratum corneum acts as a barrier to exophytic growth.

HISTOPATHOLOGY. The lesions are termed "lentiginous" because most lesional cells are single and located near the dermal–epidermal junction, especially at the periphery of the lesion. Usually, however, some tumor cells can be found in the upper layers of the epidermis, especially near areas of invasion in the centers of the lesions. The histologic picture differs from that of lentigo maligna, because of irregular acanthosis, the lack of elastosis in the dermis, and the fre-

quently dendritic character of the lesional cells. Early *in situ* or microinvasive lesions may show, especially at the periphery, a deceptively benign histologic picture consisting of an increase in basal melanocytes and hyperpigmentation with only focal atypia of the melanocytes. However, in the centers of the lesions, uniform severe cytologic atypia is usually readily evident. There may be a lichenoid lymphocytic infiltrate that may largely obscure the dermal–epidermal junction, and in some cases this may be so dense as to simulate an inflammatory process. In most lesions, both spindle-shaped and rounded tumor cells are observed, and in many cases, pigmented dendritic cells are prominent. Pigmentation is often pronounced, resulting in the presence of melanophages in the upper dermis and of large aggregates of melanin in the broad stratum corneum. As in lentigo maligna, when tumorigenic VGP is present, it is often of the spindle cell type and not uncommonly desmoplastic and/or neurotropic. In other instances, the invasive and tumorigenic cells in the dermis may be deceptively differentiated along nevus lines.

Conditions to consider in the differential diagnosis:

junctional nevi
recurrent melanocytic nevi
pigmented spindle cell nevi
junctional and superficial compound Spitz nevi
compound or dermal nevi, papillomatous
junctional or superficial compound dysplastic nevi

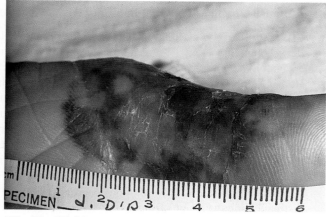

Clin. Fig. IIA2.b

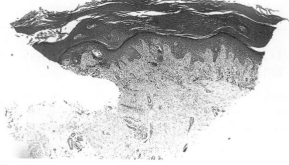

Fig. IIA2.d

Clin. Fig. IIA2.b. *Acral lentiginous melanoma.* There is an irregular patch of variegated hyperpigmentation in acral skin, including shades of tan, brown, gray-white, red, and blue-black. Although much of this lesion represents the nontumorigenic radial growth phase, there was an invasive component that extended into the reticular dermis to a depth of 1.4 mm. (Photo by W. Witmer, Dept. of Dermatology, University of Pennsylvania.)

Fig. IIA2.d. *Acral lentiginous melanoma, low power.* This punch biopsy of acral skin is from a large lesion of the type illustrated above. A thickened stratum corneum is typical of this site. There is a melanocytic proliferation within the epidermis associated with moderate inflammation in the superficial dermis. *(continues)*

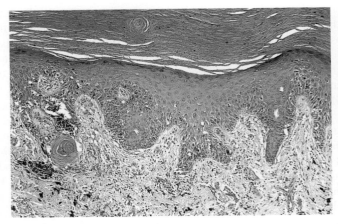

Fig. IIA2.e

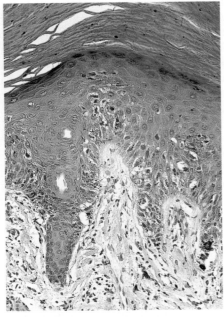

Fig. IIA2.f

Fig. IIA2.e. *Acral lentiginous melanoma, medium power.* Within the epidermis there is a disorganized proliferation of predominantly single but focally clustered heavily pigmented melanocytic cells. Orderly nests are not present in this proliferation. Within the superficial dermis there is moderate lymphocytic infiltrate and numerous melanophages.

Fig. IIA2.f. *Acral lentiginous melanoma, high power.* Higher magnification reveals that the proliferation is almost exclusively of single atypical often dendritic melanocytes in the basal cell zone, with a few in the spinous layer as well.

---

in situ or microinvasive melanoma, superficial
   spreading type
in situ or microinvasive melanoma, acral lentiginous
   type

IIB. LOCALIZED LESIONS WITH THINNING OF THE EPIDERMIS

A thinned epidermis is characteristic of aged or chronically sun-damaged skin. The epidermis is thinned secondary to diminished number and to decreased size of keratinocytes.

1. With Melanocytic Proliferation
2. Without Melanocytic Proliferation

IIB1. With Melanocytic Proliferation

The epidermis is thinned (atrophic) and there is proliferation of single or small groups of atypical melanocytes, resulting in the localization of melanocytes in contiguity with one another, in the basal layer of the epidermis. *Lentigo maligna* is a prototypic example.

Lentigo Maligna Melanoma, In Situ *or Microinvasive*

CLINICAL SUMMARY. Lentigo maligna melanoma (LMM) (8) accounts for about 10% of all melanomas and typically occurs on the chronically exposed cutaneous surfaces of the elderly, most commonly on the face. The lesion evolves slowly over many years, starting as an unevenly pigmented macule that gradually extends peripherally and may attain a diameter of several centimeters. It has an irregular border and, as long as it remains *in situ* or microinvasive, is not indurated. The color is variegated, ranging from light brown to brown, with dark brown, black, or gray-white flecks. Fine reticulated lines are usually also present and are helpful in distinguishing the lesions from actinic lentigines.

HISTOPATHOLOGY. Although the earliest stages may be subtle, fully evolved lentigo maligna is characterized by contiguous proliferation of lesional melanocytes, occurring in an atrophic flattened epidermis. This epidermal architectural pattern is in contrast to superficial spreading melanoma (SSM), where it is irregularly thickened and thinned, or to actinic lentigines and dysplastic nevi, where there is elongation of the rete. Cytologically, the lesional cells tend to be elongated and spindle shaped. Their nuclei are atypical, being enlarged, hyperchromatic, and pleomorphic. This atypia is "uniform" (i.e., present in most lesional cells), in contrast to dysplastic nevi. Frequently, atypical melanocytes extend along the basal cell layer of hair follicles, often for a considerable distance and frequently extending to the base of a shave biopsy specimen. There is usually some upward pagetoid extension of atypical melanocytes. Although single cells predominate, some nesting of melanocytes in the basal layer may be observed. The atypical melanocytes within the nests usually retain their spindle shape, and they often "hang down" like raindrops from the interface. The upper dermis, which almost always shows severe elastotic solar degeneration, contains numerous melanophages

and a rather pronounced, often bandlike, inflammatory infiltrate. Microinvasion may be demonstrated in these areas of dermal inflammation.

The differential diagnosis of LMM includes lentiginous junctional nevi and dysplastic nevi and actinic lentigines. These lesions are characterized by lentiginous elongation of rete ridges (see section IIC) in contrast to the solar atrophy that characterizes the epidermis in LMM. Junctional nevi exhibit little or no cytologic atypia, and dysplastic nevi exhibit mild to moderate random atypia, in contrast to the uniform moderate to severe atypia that characterizes most examples of LMM.

Conditions to consider in the differential diagnosis:
melanoma *in situ* (lentigo maligna type)
actinic lentigo (atrophic lesions)

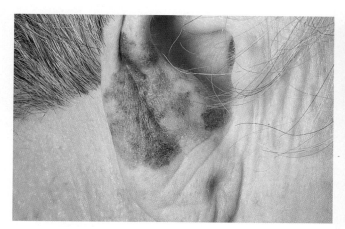

Clin. Fig. IIB1.a

Clin. Fig. IIB1.b

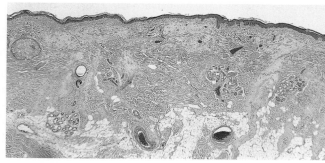

Fig. IIB1.a

Clin. Fig. IIB1.a. *Lentigo maligna.* An elderly woman had a many year history of an enlarging macule on the ear, with varying shades of brown and irregular borders.

Clin. Fig. IIB1.b. *Lentigo maligna melanoma.* A long-standing enlarging lesion on the temple region shows variegated colors, large size, a papular component, and irregular borders.

Fig. IIB1.a. *Lentigo maligna, low power.* At scanning magnification the lesion is very broad and poorly circumscribed, the epidermis is atrophic, and many areas show a flattened rete ridge architecture. *(continues)*

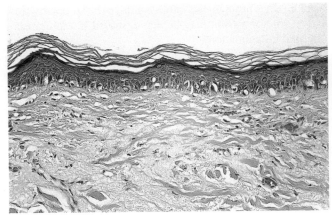

Fig. IIB1.b

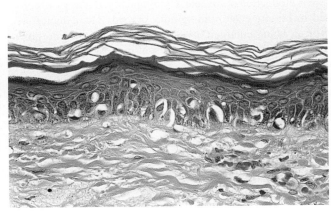

Fig. IIB1.c

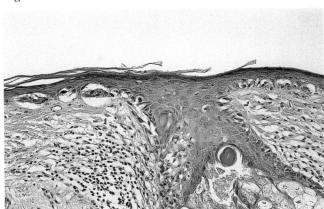

Fig. IIB1.d

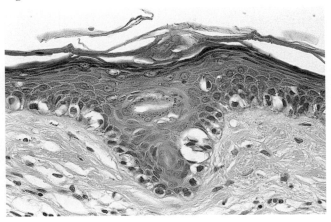

Fig. IIB1.e

Fig. IIB1.b. *Lentigo maligna, medium power.* In the basal cell zone, there is a lentiginous proliferation of predominantly single uniformly atypical melanocytes that focally grow in a confluent or contiguous manner. The underlying dermis reveals a broad zone of solar elastosis.

Fig. IIB1.c. *Lentigo maligna, high power.* Higher magnification reveals enlarged, hyperchromatic, and irregular nuclei of most lesional melanocytic cells ("uniform cytologic atypia").

Fig. IIB1.d,e. *Lentigo maligna, medium power.* This atypical melanocytic proliferation may extend along follicular epithelium and eccrine epithelium.

IIB2. Without Melanocytic Proliferation

The epidermis is thinned without proliferation of keratinocytes or melanocytes. Each melanocyte is separated from the next by several keratinocytes. Atrophic actinic keratosis and porokeratosis are prototypic examples.

Atrophic Actinic Keratosis

Atrophic actinic keratoses lack the hypertrophic epidermal proliferation seen in the hypertrophic type (see also section IIA1).

Porokeratosis

CLINICAL SUMMARY.   Porokeratosis (9) is characterized by a distinct peripheral keratotic ridge that corresponds histolog-

ically to the cornoid lamella. Although five different forms can be distinguished, *disseminated superficial actinic porokeratosis* is by far the most common type. The lesions often are most pronounced in sun-exposed areas and may be exacerbated by exposure to the sun. They present as small patches surrounded only by a narrow, slightly raised, hyperkeratotic ridge without a distinct furrow.

HISTOPATHOLOGY.   The peripheral, raised, hyperkeratotic ridge shows a keratin-filled invagination of the epidermis. In the prototypic *plaque type* of porokeratosis, the invagination extends deeply downward at an angle, the apex of which points away from the central portion of the lesion. In the center of this keratin-filled invagination rises a parakeratotic column, the so-called cornoid lamella, representing the most characteristic feature of porokeratosis of Mibelli. In the epi-

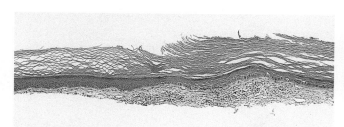

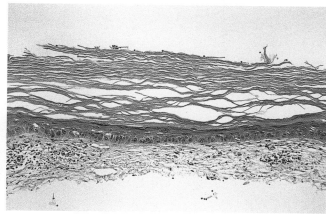

Fig. IIB2.a   **Fig. IIB2.b**

Fig. IIB2.a. *Atrophic actinic keratosis, low power.* There is hyperkeratosis with patchy parakeratosis. The underlying epidermis is thin.

Fig. IIB2.b. *Atrophic actinic keratosis, medium power.* There is slight atypia of basal keratinocytes, with patchy to bandlike lymphocytes usually with plasma cells in the papillary dermis and actinic elastosis.

---

dermis beneath the parakeratotic column, the keratinocytes are irregularly arranged, and some cells possess an eosinophilic cytoplasm as a result of premature keratinization. Usually, no granular layer is found at the site at which the parakeratotic column arises, but elsewhere the keratin-filled invagination of the epidermis has a well-developed granular layer. The histologic changes in disseminated superficial actinic porokeratosis are similar but less pronounced, the central invagination being rather shallow.

Conditions to consider in the differential diagnosis:
    atrophic actinic keratosis
    porokeratosis

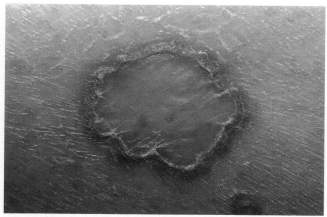

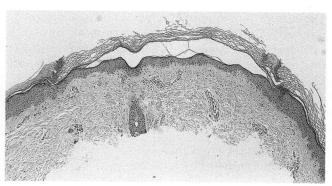

Clin. Fig. IIB2   **Fig. IIB2.c**

Clin. Fig. IIB2. *Disseminated superficial actinic porokeratosis.* Illustrated here are two of many oval plaques and papules with slightly raised keratotic rims and atrophic centers that developed on sun-exposed legs.

Fig. IIB.2.c. *Porokeratosis, low power.* On each end of this shave biopsy specimen there are two cornoid lamellae that can be seen at scanning magnification as discrete foci of parakeratosis. Parakeratotic columns lean toward the center of the lesion. *(continues)*

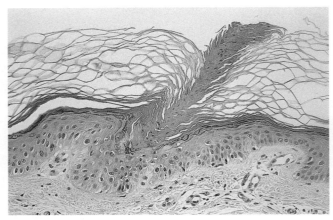

Fig. IIB2.d

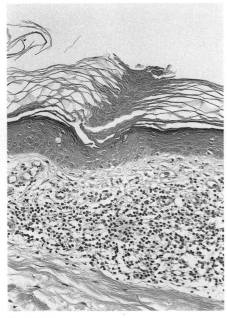

Fig. IIB2.e

Fig. IIB.2.d. *Porokeratosis, high power.* The cornoid lamella is characterized by a well-defined stack of parakeratotic keratin that overlies an invagination of the epidermis. Beneath the parakeratotic column there is focal loss of the granular cell layer and dyskeratosis.

Fig. IIB.2.e. *Porokeratosis, medium power.* Porokeratosis may be associated with a patchy to bandlike lichenoid mononuclear cell infiltrate in the superficial dermis.

IIC. LOCALIZED LESIONS WITH ELONGATED RETE RIDGES

Elongation of the rete ridges without melanocytic proliferation is termed "psoriasiform hyperplasia" because this pattern is seen in psoriasis. Elongated rete with melanocytic proliferation and predominance of single cells over nests is termed a "lentiginous" pattern. This pattern may be seen in lentiginous junctional and compound nevi, in dysplastic nevi and in the "lentiginous" melanomas. However, in melanomas, the epidermal rete pattern is more often irregularly thickened and thinned than regularly elongated.

1. With Melanocytic Proliferation
2. Without Melanocytic Proliferation

IIC1. With Melanocytic Proliferation

The epidermal rete ridges are elongated, and within these rete ridges there is melanocytic proliferation. *Actinic lentigo*, *lentigo simplex*, *lentiginous junctional nevus*, and *dysplastic nevus* are prototypic.

Actinic Lentigo

CLINICAL SUMMARY. Lentigines are macular hyperpigmentations in which the number of epidermal melanocytes is increased histologically, but the nests of melanocytes that define nevus cells are not present. In actinic lentigo, which arises most frequently in older adults, there are usually multiple lesions with a predilection to areas of sun exposure. They are relatively large compared with simple lentigines (usually about 5 mm, but with some lesions greater than 1 cm) and are rather asymmetric and poorly circumscribed macules that are variably pigmented in shades of brown, usually without black. When the asymmetry and pigmentary variegation are more prominent, biopsy may be necessary to distinguish these lesions from lentigo maligna.

HISTOPATHOLOGY. The findings include, in a relatively large lesion, slight or moderate elongation of the rete ridges, with an obvious increase in the amount of melanin in both the melanocytes and the basal keratinocytes and often with the presence of melanophages in the upper dermis. In some instances, melanin is also present in the upper layers of the epidermis and stratum corneum. Melanocytes may not obvi-

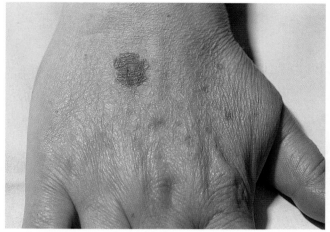

Clin. Fig. IIC1.a

Clin. Fig. IIC1.a. *Actinic lentigo.* A 1-cm rather irregular patch of slightly variegated hyperpigmentation in a background of chronic solar damage.

Fig. IIC1.a. *Actinic lentigo, low power.* At scanning magnification there is uniform elongation of rete ridges with hyperpigmentation. Significant inflammation is not present.

Fig. IIC1.b. *Actinic lentigo, medium power.* Melanocytes are slightly increased in number, but in contrast to lentigo maligna, the rete ridges are elongated and there is no contiguous proliferation of uniformly atypical melanocytes.

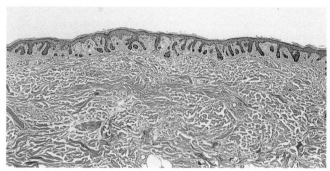

Fig. IIC1.a

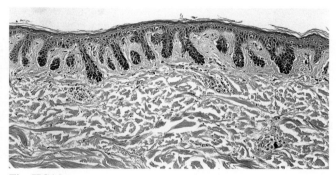

Fig. IIC1.b

ously be increased in number, but careful quantitative studies have shown them to be increased.

Lentigo Simplex

CLINICAL SUMMARY. Lentigines are macular hyperpigmentations in which histologically the number of epidermal melanocytes is increased but the nests of melanocytes that define nevus cells are not present. In lentigo simplex, which arises most frequently in childhood, there are usually only a few scattered lesions without predilection to areas of sun exposure. They are small (usually 2 to 3 mm), symmetric, and well-circumscribed macules that are evenly pigmented but vary individually from brown to black. The definition is a histologic one, and clinically, lentigo simplex is indistinguishable from a junctional nevus.

HISTOPATHOLOGY. In a small lesion (usually 2 to 3 mm or less in diameter), the findings include a slight or moderate elongation of the rete ridges, an increase in the concentration of melanocytes in the basal layer, an increase in the amount

of melanin in both the melanocytes and the basal keratinocytes, and the presence of melanophages in the upper dermis. In some instances, melanin is also present in the upper layers of the epidermis and stratum corneum. Because of the existence of these transitional forms, the lentigo simplex is regarded as a form of evolving melanocytic nevus.

Lentiginous Junctional Nevus

CLINICAL SUMMARY. The term "lentigo" derives from a clinical appearance of a small lenticulate or lens-shaped pigmented spot. The prototype of the lentiginous pattern is seen in the lentigo simplex, which is regarded as an early or evolving form of melanocytic nevus. In lesions otherwise clinically characteristic of lentigo simplex, small nests of nevus cells may be present at the epidermal–dermal junction, especially at the lowest pole of rete ridges. These lesions then combine features of a lentigo simplex and a junctional nevus (lentiginous junctional nevus, or "jentigo"). If nevus cells are also present in the dermis but there is a junctional component that extends beyond the dermal component, the

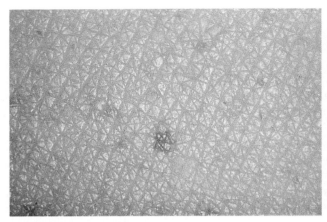

Clin. Fig. IIC1.b

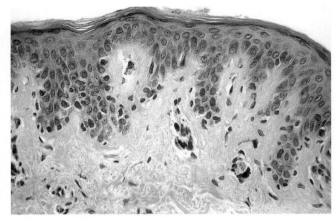

Fig. IIC1.c

Clin. Fig. IIC1.b. *Lentigo simplex.* A 2- to 3-mm uniform patch of brown or dark brown to black hyperpigmentation in normal or sun-damaged skin.

Fig. IIC1.c. *Lentigo simplex, medium power.* In contrast to actinic lentigo, melanocytes are obviously increased at the dermal–epidermal junction and are at least focally contiguous with one another. In contrast to a dysplastic nevus or a lentigo maligna, the lesion is small and there is no significant cytologic atypia.

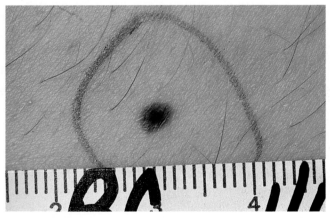

Clin. Fig. IIC1.c

Clin. Fig. IIC1.c. *Lentiginous junctional nevus.* A 2- to 5-mm uniform patch of brown or dark brown to black hyperpigmentation.

Fig. IIC1.d. *Lentiginous junctional nevus, low power.* Scanning magnification reveals a small melanocytic lesion confined to the epidermis. There is elongation of rete ridges and a very sparse superficial lymphocytic infiltrate.

Fig. IIC1.e. *Lentiginous junctional nevus, medium power.* Higher magnification reveals a lentiginous proliferation of single and nested melanocytes along the dermal–epidermal junction. The nests are located predominantly at the tips of rete ridges. Atypia of melanocytes is not seen.

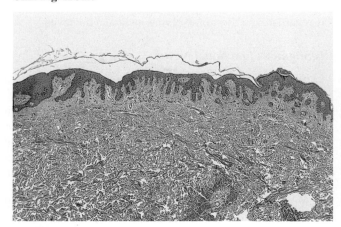

Fig. IIC1.d

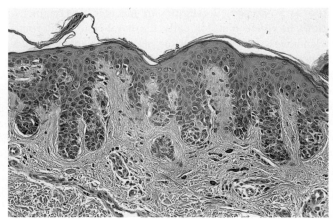

Fig. IIC1.e

term "lentiginous compound nevus" may be used. Lentiginous junctional and compound nevi are typically in the range of 2 to 5 mm; lesions larger than 5 mm are often dysplastic nevi.

HISTOPATHOLOGY. Although the term "lentigo" is originally of clinical derivation, it has taken on a histologic connotation defined by the presence of single melanocytes arranged in contiguity about elongated rete ridges, as in lentigo simplex. The lack of nests at the histologic level distinguishes a lentigo from a nevus. In a *lentiginous junctional nevus*, nevus cells lie in well-circumscribed nests either entirely within the lower epidermis or bulging downward into the dermis but still in contact with the epidermis. In addition, varying numbers of diffusely arranged single nevus cells are seen in the lowermost epidermis, especially in the basal cell layer. The rete ridges tend to be uniformly elongated, completing the lentiginous pattern. Dysplastic nevi also exhibit a lentiginous architecture, but they are larger (greater than 4 to 5 mm in histologic section) and there is cytologic atypia affecting randomly scattered nevus cells. Lesions smaller than 4 mm that exhibit lentiginous architecture and cytologic atypia are occasionally encountered. We sign these lesions out descriptively, with a note that additional evaluation of the patient may be indicated to rule out the possibilities of other clinically atypical nevi or of a family or personal history of melanoma. If these or other risk factors for melanoma are found, then periodic surveillance of the patient may be indicated, depending on the magnitude of the risk as judged clinically.

Nevus Spilus

CLINICAL SUMMARY. The *speckled lentiginous nevus*, or *nevus spilus*, consists of a light-brown patch or band present from the time of birth that in childhood becomes dotted with small dark-brown macules.

HISTOPATHOLOGY. The light-brown patch or band shows basal hyperpigmentation of keratinocytes similar to a cafe au lait macule. The speckled areas show junctional nests of nevus cells at the lowest poles of some of the rete ridges and diffuse junctional activity and dermal aggregates of nevus cells, similar to a lentigo simplex.

Junctional or Superficial Compound Dysplastic Nevi

CLINICAL SUMMARY. Dysplastic nevi (10) form, clinically and histologically, a continuum extending from a common nevus to a superficial spreading melanoma. They may be located anywhere on the body, but are most common on the trunk. A clinically dysplastic nevus is defined by (a) the presence of a macular component either as the entire lesion or surrounding a papular center; (b) a large size, exceeding 5 mm; (c) an irregular or ill-defined fuzzy border; and (d) irregular pigmentation within the lesion.

HISTOPATHOLOGY. Architectural features include a lentiginous pattern of elongation of the rete ridges with an increase in the number of melanocytes. The latter are arranged as single cells and in nests whose long axes tend to lie parallel to the epidermal surface and that tend to form "bridges" be-

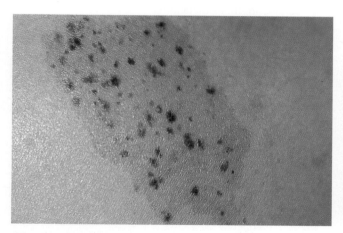

Clin. Fig. IIC1.d

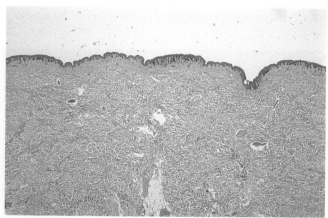

Fig. IIC1.f

Clin. Fig. IIC1.d. *Nevus spilus.* This usually congenital lesion presents as a light-brown patch in which speckled brown macules appear in childhood.

Fig. IIC1.f. *Nevus spilus, low power.* Scanning magnification may seem to show only a single small melanocytic lesion confined to the epidermis or to the epidermis and papillary dermis. Depending on the size of the biopsy (which may be submitted to rule out melanoma), there may be more than one of these small lesions. Between the lesions, the epidermis is hyperpigmented, but this may not be apparent histologically unless the normal skin at the edge of the lesion is included for comparison. *(continues)*

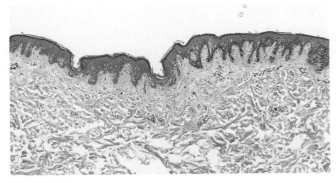

Fig. IIC1.g

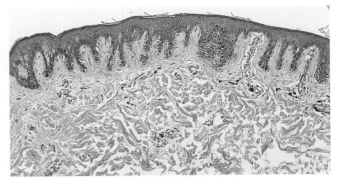

Fig. IIC1.h

Fig. IIC1.g. *Nevus spilus, medium power.* In the focal lesions, there is elongation of rete ridges and a very sparse superficial lymphocytic infiltrate. The appearances are identical to a lentiginous nevus.

Fig. IIC1.h. *Nevus spilus, high power.* Higher magnification reveals a lentiginous proliferation of single and nested melanocytes along the dermal–epidermal junction. Atypia of melanocytes is not seen.

tween adjacent retia. The melanocytes in the junctional nests are frequently spindle shaped, but they may be large and epithelioid with abundant cytoplasm containing fine dusty melanin particles. If the lesion is compound, nests of melanocytes in the papillary dermis show evidence of maturation with descent into the dermis. In these compound dysplastic nevi, the intraepidermal component extends by definition beyond the lateral border of the dermal component, forming a "shoulder" to the lesion histologically and a "targetlike" or "fried-egg" pattern clinically. A patchy lymphocytic infiltrate is present in the dermis. Pagetoid extension of melanocytes into the epidermis is absent or slight and is limited to the lowermost layers. Cytologically, in addition to the lentiginous melanocytic hyperplasia, melanocytic nuclear atypia is required for the diagnosis, characterized by irregu-

larly shaped, large, hyperchromatic nuclei in some melanocytes. Most atypical melanocytes lie singly or in small groups, and the atypia involves only some lesional cells ("random" cytologic atypia). Focal extension of atypical-appearing melanocytes into the lower spinous layer may occur, but if this is prominent, transformation into melanoma *in situ* may have occurred.

Conditions to consider in the differential diagnosis:

    lentigo simplex
    nevus spilus
    lentiginous junctional nevus
    junctional nevus
    dysplastic nevus
    acral lentiginous melanoma
    mucosal lentiginous melanoma

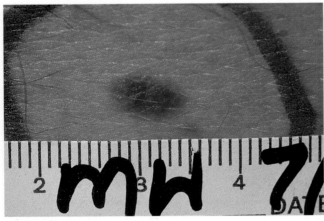

Clin. Fig. IIC1.e

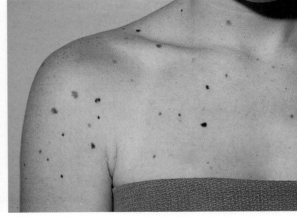

Clin. Fig. IIC1.f

Clin. Fig. IIC1.e. *Dysplastic nevus.* This pigmented lesion fulfills criteria for a dysplastic nevus: macule with indefinite edge, size >5 mm, irregular border, and irregular pigmentation.

Clin. Fig. IIC1.f. *Dysplastic nevi.* This young patient has been followed since childhood. She developed multiple dysplastic nevi around the age of puberty, and since this picture was taken she has developed several primary melanomas, all in the curable nontumorigenic or radial growth phase stage of evolution.

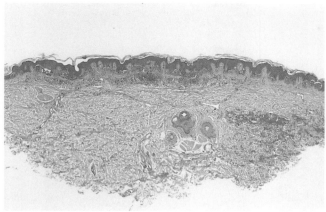

Fig. IIC1.i

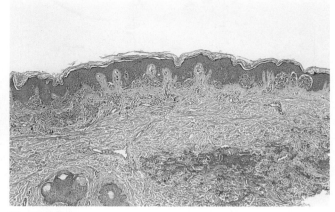

Fig. IIC1.j

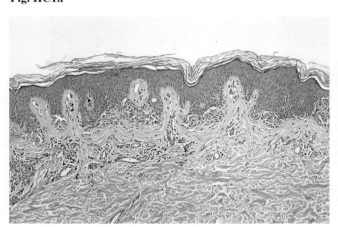

Fig. IIC1.k

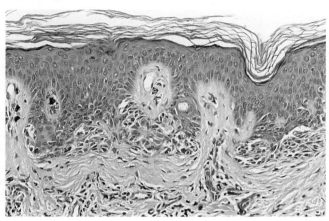

Fig. IIC1.l

Fig. IIC1.i. *Compound dysplastic nevus, low power.* At scanning magnification there is a broad compound nevus. Near the center of the lesion the nevus is compound with both an epidermal and dermal component. The "shoulders" at the periphery of the lesion are composed only of a junctional component.

Fig. IIC1.j. *Compound dysplastic nevus, low power.* The epidermal rete ridges are uniformly elongated. Nests of melanocytes form "bridges" between these elongated rete. The dermal component of the lesion is at the left of this image, and the junctional component extends to the right, forming the "shoulder."

Fig. IIC1.k. *Compound dysplastic nevus, medium power.* The intraepidermal component is composed of single and nested melanocytes which may show bridging from one rete to the next. The dermis reveals a sparse lymphocytic infiltrate, often with prominent small vessels, and with a sprinkling of melanophages in this example.

Fig. IIC1.l. *Compound dysplastic nevus, medium power.* Beneath the nests of lesional cells, there is lamellar fibroplasia characterized by zones of eosinophilic collagen and spindle cells resembling fibroblasts oriented parallel to the rete epithelium. *(continues)*

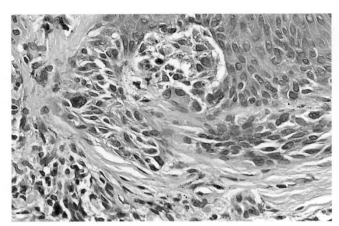

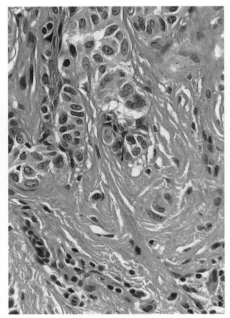

Fig. IIC1.m   **Fig. IIC1.n**

Fig. IIC1.m. *Compound dysplastic nevus, high power.* At high magnification, the majority of the lesional cells are bland in appearance but there are randomly scattered cells which show mild nuclear atypia, characterized by enlargement, irregularity, and hyperchromatism involving a minority of the lesional cell nuclei. Some of the spindle cells in the lamellar fibroplasia contain melanin, suggesting that they are of melanocytic rather than fibroblastic origin.

Fig. IIC1.n. *Compound dysplastic nevus, high power.* In another example, several of the lesional cell nuclei are moderately enlarged and hyperchromatic. However, the majority of the nuclei are not atypical. This constitutes "random" cytologic atypia. In the dermis, there is eosinophilic fibroplasia, which differs from lamellar fibroplasia in that the collagen does not contain lamellated spindle cells (see Fig. IIC1.l).

IIC2. Without Melanocytic Proliferation

The epidermis is thickened (acanthotic). Melanocytes are normal as are keratinocytes. The only change is acanthosis. *Epidermal nevi* are prototypic (11). The differential diagnosis includes *acanthosis nigricans*.

Epidermal Nevus

CLINICAL FEATURES. Epidermal nevi, or verrucous nevi, may be either localized or systematized. In the *localized type*, which is present usually but not invariably at birth, only one linear lesion is present, often referred to as *nevus unius lateris*. It consists of closely set, papillomatous, hyperkeratotic papules. In the *systematized type*, papillomatous hyperkeratotic papules often in a linear configuration are present as many lesions. These lesions are often linear in a parallel arrangement, particularly on the trunk. The term *ichthyosis hystrix* is occasionally used, perhaps unnecessarily, for instances of extensive bilateral lesions. Linear epidermal nevi may occasionally be associated with skeletal deformities and central nervous system deficiencies, such as mental retardation, epilepsy, and neural deafness, and, rarely, with basal or squamous cell carcinoma.

HISTOPATHOLOGY. Nearly all cases of the localized type of linear epidermal nevus and some cases of the systematized type show the histologic picture of a benign papilloma. One observes considerable hyperkeratosis, papillomatosis, and acanthosis with elongation of the rete ridges resembling seborrheic keratosis. In other instances, papillomatosis may be inconspicuous and orthokeratotic hyperkeratosis may be the major finding.

Seborrheic Keratosis

See Figs. IIC2.d and IIC2.e.

Acanthosis Nigricans

CLINICAL SUMMARY. There are eight types of acanthosis nigricans: malignant (12), benign inherited, obesity-associated and syndromic, which are often associated with insulin resistance syndromes (13), acral, unilateral, drug induced, and mixed. Clinically, acanthosis nigricans presents papillomatous brown patches, predominantly in the intertriginous areas such as the axillae, the neck, and the genital and submammary regions. In extensive cases of the malignant type, mucosal surfaces, such as the mouth, the vulva, and the palpebral conjunctivae, may be involved. In the acral type, there is velvety hyperpigmentation of the dorsa of the hands and feet.

HISTOPATHOLOGY. The lesions show hyperkeratosis and papillomatosis but only slight irregular acanthosis and usually no hyperpigmentation. Thus, the term *acanthosis nigricans* has little histologic justification. In a typical lesion, the dermal papillae project upward as fingerlike projections. The valleys between the papillae show mild to moderate acanthosis and are filled with keratotic material. Horn pseudocysts can occur in some cases. The epidermis at the tips of the papillae and often also on the sides of the protruding papillae appears thinned. Slight hyperpigmentation of the basal layer is demonstrated with silver nitrate staining in some cases but not in others. The brown color of the lesions is caused more by hyperkeratosis than by melanin.

Conditions to consider in the differential diagnosis:

    epidermal nevi
    psoriasis
    lichen simplex chronicus
    acanthosis nigricans
    actinic lentigo

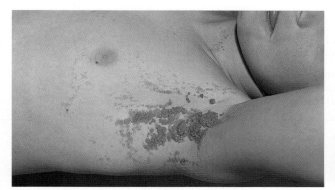

Clin. Fig. IIC2.a

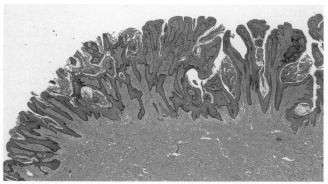

Fig. IIC2.a

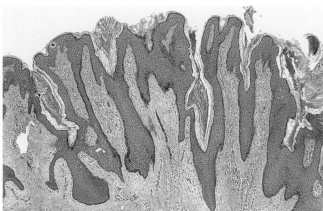

Fig. IIC2.b

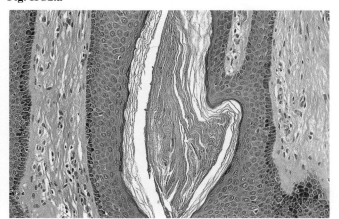

Fig. IIC2.c

Clin. Fig. IIC2.a. *Epidermal nevus.* This child had a linear arrangement of brown warty papules coalescing into plaques. He had no skeletal, ocular, or central nervous system involvement.

Fig. IIC2.a. *Epidermal nevus, low power.* At scanning magnification, epidermal nevi show papillomatosis and hyperkeratosis. The underlying dermis is essentially unremarkable.

Fig. IIC2.b. *Epidermal nevus, medium power.* The epidermis shows varying degrees of acanthosis and papillomatosis with hyperkeratosis. Frequently there is pseudohorn cyst formation resembling a seborrheic keratosis.

Fig. IIC2.c. *Epidermal nevus, high power.* Epidermal maturation is essentially normal. Pigment is variable. The papillary dermis may show fibroplasia with little or no inflammation.

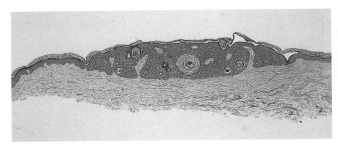

Fig. IIC2.d

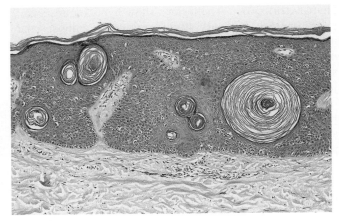

Fig. IIC2.e

Fig. IIC2.d. *Seborrheic keratosis, low power.* Compared with epidermal nevi, seborrheic keratoses tend to be more sharply circumscribed lesions that lie above the plane of the adjacent epidermal surface.

Fig. IIC2.e. *Seborrheic keratosis, medium power.* Seborrheic keratoses are composed of basaloid cells that show squamous differentiation only near the surface. In an epidermal nevus, the pattern of normal keratinocytic maturation from a single basal layer is more closely maintained (see Figs. IIC2.b and IIC2.c).

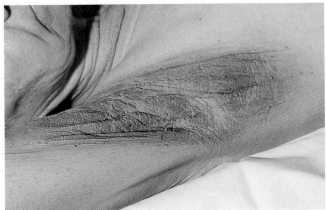

Clin. Fig. IIC2.b

Clin. Fig. IIC2.b. *Acanthosis nigricans.* An elderly woman had an explosive development of velvety hyperpigmented plaques in the intertriginous areas. She had metastatic endometrial carcinoma.

Fig. IIC2.f. *Acanthosis nigricans, medium power.* There is papillomatosis with prominent hyperkeratosis that is predominantly orthokeratotic.

Fig. IIC2.g. *Acanthosis nigricans, high power.* In contrast to a seborrheic keratosis, acanthosis nigricans fails to reveal significant acanthosis of the epidermis.

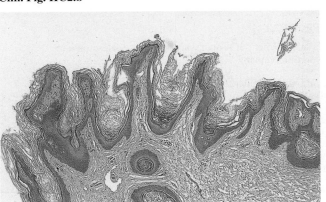

Fig. IIC2.f

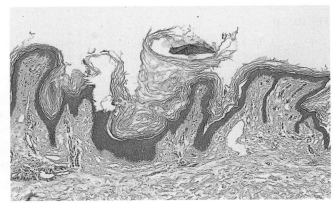

Fig. IIC2.g

IID. LOCALIZED LESIONS WITH PAGETOID EPITHELIAL PROLIFERATION

A neoplastic proliferation of one cell type distributed as single cells or nests within a benign epithelium is termed "pagetoid" after Paget's disease of the breast (mammary carcinoma cells proliferating in skin of the nipple).

1. Keratinocytic Proliferations
2. Melanocytic Proliferations
3. Glandular Epithelial Proliferations
4. Lymphoid Proliferations

IID1. Keratinocytic Proliferations

The epidermis has atypical keratinocytes scattered within mature epithelium at all or multiple levels; there is loss of normal maturation. Mitoses are increased and there may be individual cell necrosis. *Pagetoid squamous cell carcinoma in situ* is a prototypic example.

Pagetoid Squamous Cell Carcinoma In Situ

An occasional finding in squamous cell carcinoma *in situ* [Bowen's disease (3)] is vacuolization of the cells, especially in the upper portion of the epidermis. Also, in exceptional cases, multiple nests of atypical cells are scattered through a normal epidermis, sometimes with sparing of the basal cell layer (see also section IIA1).

Clonal Seborrheic Keratosis

In the clonal, or nesting, type of seborrheic keratosis, well-defined nests of cells are located within the epidermis (14). In some instances, the nests resemble foci of basal cell epithelioma because the nuclei appear small and dark-staining and intercellular bridges are seen in only a few areas. In other instances of clonal seborrheic keratosis, the nests are composed of fairly large cells showing distinct intercellular bridges, with the nests separated from one another by strands of cells exhibiting small dark nuclei.

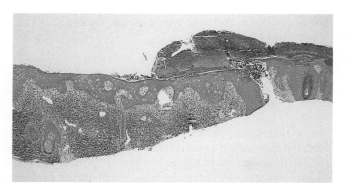

Fig. IID1.a

Fig. IID1.a. *Pagetoid squamous cell carcinoma* in situ, *low power.* The epidermis is irregularly thickened and thinned, with effaced rete ridges, and a parakeratotic scale crust. There is a dense band-like lymphoplasmacytic infiltrate in the dermis.

Fig. IID1.b. *Pagetoid squamous cell carcinoma* in situ, *medium power.* Large pale cells are present among more compact eosinophilic keratinocytes.

Fig. IID1.c. *Pagetoid squamous cell carcinoma* in situ, *high power.* At high magnification, a search for desmosomes usually reveals their presence between the neoplastic cells and their less atypical neighbors, establishing the diagnosis of squamous cell carcinoma *in situ* and ruling out melanoma and Paget's disease.

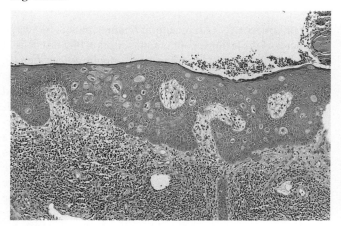

Fig. IID1.b

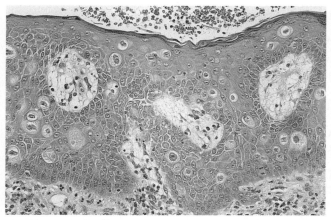

Fig. IID1.c

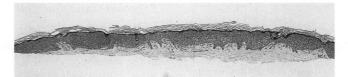

Fig. IID1.d

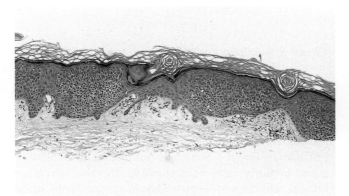

Fig. IID1.e

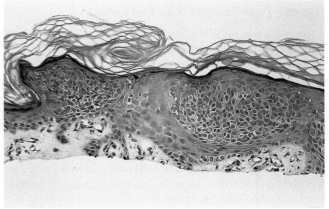

Fig. IID1.f

Fig. IID1.d. *Clonal seborrheic keratosis, low power.* In contrast to a squamous cell carcinoma *in situ*, this lesion shows uniform acanthosis of the epidermis with a predominantly basket-weave stratum corneum.

Fig. IID1.e. *Clonal seborrheic keratosis, medium power.* Within a thickened epidermal layer there are "clones" composed of aggregates of bland-appearing epithelial cells clustered within the epidermis.

Fig. IID1.f. *Clonal seborrheic keratosis, medium power.* Lack of cytologic atypia, mitotic figures, and an atypical parakeratotic scale help differentiate this lesion from a squamous cell carcinoma *in situ* with a clonal pattern.

Conditions to consider in the differential diagnosis:

   pagetoid squamous cell carcinoma *in situ*
   clonal seborrheic keratosis
   intraepithelial epithelioma (Borst-Jadassohn)

IID2. Melanocytic Proliferations

Atypical melanocytes are seen at all levels within the otherwise mature but often hyperplastic epidermis. *Melanoma in situ or microinvasive (superficial spreading type)* is prototypic (15). Pigmented spindle cell nevus (6) is an important differential.

Melanoma In Situ *or Microinvasive, Superficial Spreading Type*

CLINICAL SUMMARY. The lesions may occur on exposed skin but are more commonly found on intermittently exposed skin and are rare on unexposed skin. The most frequently involved sites are the upper back, especially in men, and the lower legs in women. The lesions are slightly or definitely elevated, with palpable borders and irregular partly arciform outlines. There is often variation in color that includes not only tan, brown, and black but also pink, blue, and gray. Gray-white areas may be observed at sites of sponta-

neous regression. Microinvasion may be clinically inapparent, but the onset of tumorigenic vertical growth is indicated by the development of a papule followed by nodularity and sometimes also ulceration, the latter usually being a late feature.

HISTOPATHOLOGY. Architectural features include the large diameter of the lesions, poor circumscription (the last cells at the edge of the lesion are often small, single, and scattered), and asymmetry (one half of the lesion does not mirror the other half). The epidermis is irregularly thickened and thinned with distortion of the rete ridge pattern. Rather uniformly rounded large melanocytes are present near the dermal–epidermal junction and usually are also scattered in a pagetoid pattern throughout the epidermis. The large cells lie in nests and singly. The nests tend to vary a good deal in size and shape. Dermal melanophages and a dermal infiltrate are usually present, except in some strictly *in situ* lesions. The lymphocytic infiltrate is typically dense and bandlike, especially in invasive lesions. Cytologically, the lesional cells are rather uniform and have atypical hyperchromatic nuclei and abundant cytoplasm containing varying amounts of melanin that often consist of small dusty particles. This "uniform cytologic atypia" is of considerable diagnostic importance and contrasts with the random atypia of dysplastic nevi. Distinc-

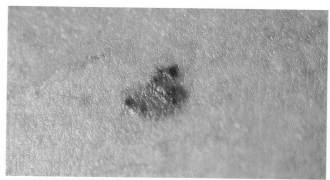

Clin. Fig. IID2.a

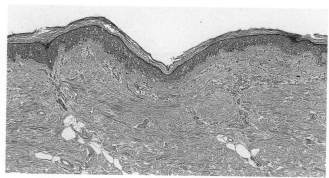

Fig. IID2.a

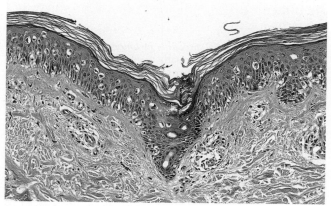

Fig. IID2.b

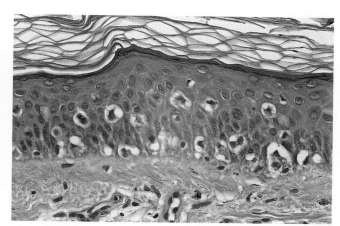

Fig. IID2.c

Clin. Fig. IID2.a. *Melanoma* in situ, *superficial spreading type.* A slowly enlarging pigmented lesion on the chest of a middle-aged man. The asymmetric irregular notched border, color variegation, and size raise suspicion for melanoma.

Fig. IID2.a. *Superficial spreading melanoma* in situ, *medium power.* There is a broad and poorly circumscribed lesion characterized by an increased number of uniformly enlarged melanocytes in the epidermis. Strictly *in situ* lesions such as this may have little or no dermal inflammation.

Fig. IID2.b. *Superficial spreading melanoma* in situ, *medium power.* The cells have a uniform appearance ("uniform cytologic atypia").

Fig. IID2.c. *Superficial spreading melanoma* in situ, *high power.* Cytologic atypia, characterized here by nuclear enlargement, hyperchromatism, and irregularity, may be moderate, as here, or severe.

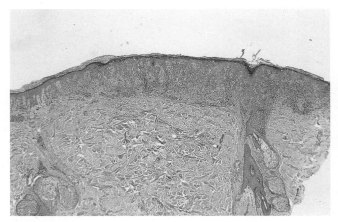

Fig. IID2.d

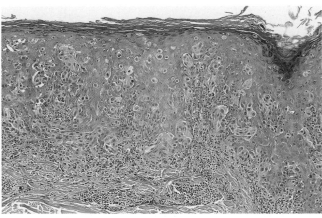

Fig. IID2.e

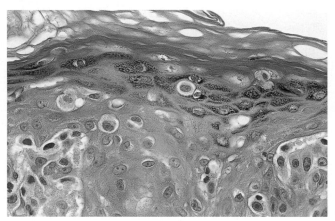

Fig. IID2.f

Fig. IID2.d. *Superficial spreading melanoma, microinvasive, low power.* The epidermis is irregularly thickened with distortion of the rete ridge pattern. There is a perivascular to diffuse lymphocytic infiltrate in the papillary dermis.

Fig. IID2.e. *Superficial spreading melanoma, microinvasive, medium power.* Enlarged epithelioid melanocytes are scattered in a "pagetoid" or "buckshot scatter" pattern among keratinocytes. A few lesional cells are seen in the papillary dermis, constituting microinvasion.

Fig. IID2.f. *Superficial spreading melanoma, microinvasive, high power.* The lesional cells are large, with abundant cytoplasm and, often, finely divided cytoplasmic melanin pigment. Their nuclei are uniformly enlarged, somewhat hyperchromatic, and have prominent nucleoli.

tion from a dysplastic nevus is based on greater size, asymmetry, and cellularity, the presence of high-level and extensive pagetoid proliferation or of contiguous basilar proliferation of uniformly atypical cells, the presence of moderate to severe and uniform cytologic atypia, and the presence of lesional cell mitoses in some melanomas.

Recurrent Nevus (Pseudomelanoma)

CLINICAL SUMMARY.   Recurrence of a nevus may show clinical hyperpigmentation that on biopsy may exhibit histologic changes suggestive of melanoma (16). The recurrence may follow incomplete removal of a nevus, particularly by a shave biopsy or electrodesiccation, or the nevus may apparently have been completely excised. The pigmentation in recurrent nevi is confined to the region of the scar and typically presents within a few weeks of the surgical procedure. After this rapid appearance, the pigment is stable. In contrast, recurrent melanoma does not respect the border of the scar and extends over time into the adjacent skin. Paradoxically, recurrent melanoma occurs more slowly, over months or years, but progresses inexorably.

HISTOPATHOLOGY.   Although most recurrent nevi are not

atypical, in a few instances they contain slightly atypical melanocyte, both singly and in nests, arranged mainly along the epidermal–dermal junction but occasionally also extending into the upper dermis and also extending up into the epidermis in a pagetoid pattern. Deep remnants of the nevus may be seen in the reticular dermis beneath the scar. A lymphocytic infiltrate with melanophages may be observed in the upper dermis. Distinction from melanoma may be difficult without a pertinent history. However, the presence of fibrosis in the upper dermis and often of remnants of a melanocytic nevus beneath the zone of fibrosis and the sharp lateral demarcation usually make a correct diagnosis possible. As is true clinically, the recurrent nevus is confined to the epidermis above the scar, whereas recurrent melanoma may extend into the adjacent epidermis.

Junctional Spitz Nevus with Pagetoid Proliferation

Although most Spitz nevi are compound nevi that involve the reticular dermis (discussed in section VIB3), junctional examples are also not uncommonly observed, especially in young children but also in adults. The differential diagnosis of melanoma should always be considered and multiple histologic attributes should be evaluated including size, symmetry,

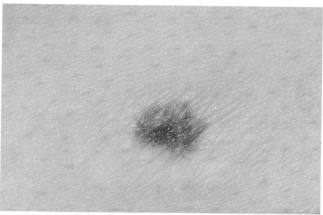

Clin. Fig. IID2.b

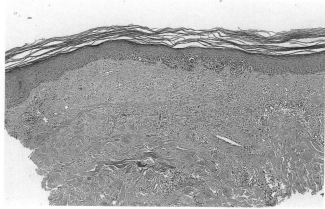

Fig. IID2.g

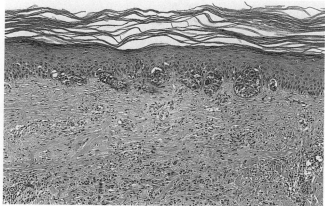

Fig. IID2.h

Clin. Fig. IID2.b. *Recurrent melanocytic nevus.* Dark-brown macule with irregular borders recurred in the surgical site of a previously shave biopsied dysplastic nevus in a teen-aged girl.

Fig. IID2.g. *Recurrent nevus phenomenon, low power.* At scanning magnification, one can see a flattened rete ridge architecture, a feature that is a clue to previous trauma or biopsy. There is a proliferation of melanocytes in the epidermis that does not extend beyond the lateral border of the scar.

Fig. IID2.h. *Recurrent nevus phenomenon, medium power.* At the dermal–epidermal interface there is a lentiginous proliferation of single and nested heavily pigmented melanocytes that overlie a zone of scar tissue in the superficial dermis. The lesional cells may be large with enlarged nuclei and prominent nucleoli, single cells may be prominent, and there may be cells extending above the dermal–epidermal junction. These features taken together may suggest melanoma, but the proliferation does not extend beyond the lateral border of scar.

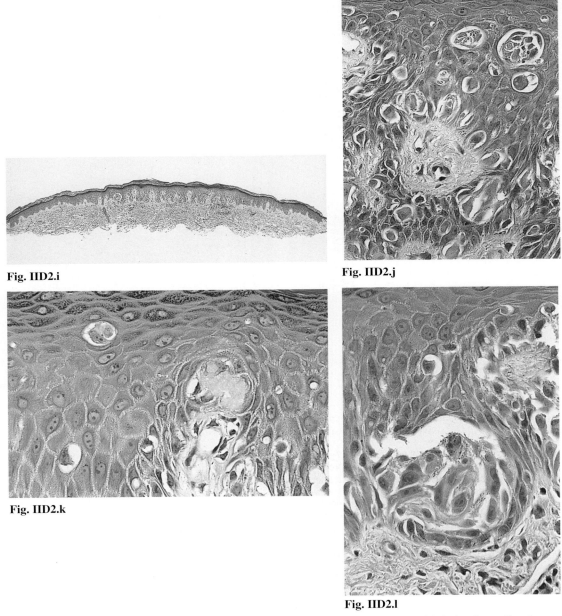

Fig. IID2.i

Fig. IID2.j

Fig. IID2.k

Fig. IID2.l

Fig. IID2.i. *Junctional Spitz nevus, low power.* In contrast to malignant melanoma, this lesion is small and symmetric.

Fig. IID2.j. *Junctional Spitz nevus, high power.* Pagetoid proliferation of melanocytes is not uncommon in Spitz nevi, especially in young patients. Clefting artifact between the nests of Spitz nevus cells and the adjacent keratinocytes is a characteristic feature.

Fig. IID2.k. *Junctional Spitz nevus, high power.* Globoid eosinophilic globules (Kamino bodies) are characteristic of classic Spitz nevi, especially when confluent as here. They also may occasionally be seen in melanomas.

Fig. IID2.l. *Junctional Spitz nevus, high power.* The Spitz nevus is composed of large nevoid melanocytes with abundant amphophilic cytoplasm and large nuclei with prominent eosinophilic nucleoli.

the age of the patient, the presence of eosinophilic globules (Kamino bodies, depicted in Figure IID2.i), and predominance of nests or single cells. Occasionally in adults, pagetoid proliferation of Spitz nevus cells in the epidermis may be seen.

Conditions to consider in the differential diagnosis:

> melanoma *in situ* (superficial spreading type)
> pigmented spindle cell nevus
> recurrent melanocytic nevus (pseudomelanoma)
> certain Spitz nevi with pagetoid proliferation
> certain acral nevi with pagetoid proliferation

IID3. Glandular Epithelial Proliferations

Atypical large clear cells with glandular differentiation (mucin production, lumen formation) proliferate in a normally maturing epidermis. *Paget's disease (mammary or extramammary)* is a prototypic example (17).

Paget's Disease

CLINICAL SUMMARY.   The cutaneous lesion in Paget's disease of the breast begins either on the nipple or the areola of the breast and extends slowly to the surrounding skin. It is always unilateral and consists of a sharply defined slightly infiltrated area of erythema showing scaling, oozing, and crusting. There may or may not be ulceration or retraction of the nipple. The cutaneous lesion is nearly always associated with underlying mammary carcinoma. Extramammary Paget's disease, which usually occurs in genital skin in either sex, is similar in its clinical appearance but is not usually associated with an underlying carcinoma.

HISTOPATHOLOGY.   In early lesions of Paget's disease of the breast, the epidermis usually shows only a few scattered Paget cells. They are large rounded cells that are devoid of intercellular bridges and contain a large nucleus and ample cytoplasm. The cytoplasm of these cells stains much lighter than that of the adjacent squamous cells. As the number of Paget cells increases, they compress the squamous cells to such an extent that the latter may merely form a network, the meshes of which are filled with Paget cells lying singly and in groups. In particular, one often observes flattened basal cells lying between Paget cells and the underlying dermis. Although Paget cells do not as a rule invade the dermis from the epidermis, they may be seen extending from the epidermis into the epithelium of hair follicles.

Conditions to consider in the differential diagnosis:

> Paget's disease (mammary or extramammary)
> superficial spreading melanoma
> pagetoid squamous cell carcinoma *in situ*
> pagetoid reticulosis

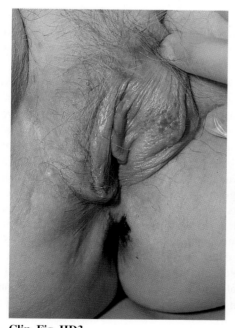

Clin. Fig. IID3

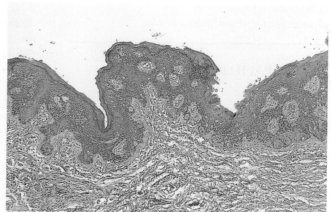

Fig. IID3.a

Clin. Fig. IID3. *Extramammary Paget's disease.* This elderly woman presented with a 1-year history of an erythematous plaque with scattered erosions on the left labium majus. Workup for underlying malignancy was negative.

Fig. IID3.a. *Extramammary Paget's disease, low power.* The epidermis may appear normal or irregularly thickened, as seen here. Even at scanning magnification, large pale cells may be appreciable among otherwise mature keratinocytes. *(continues)*

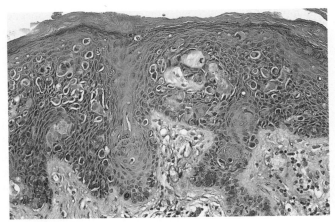

Fig. IID3.b

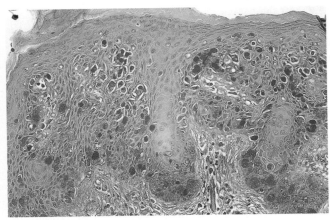

Fig. IID3.c

Fig. IID3.b. *Extramammary Paget's disease, medium power.* The large neoplastic cells have pale cytoplasm, sometimes with obvious mucin vacuoles. Their nuclei tend to be enlarged and hyperchromatic, often with prominent nucleoli.

Fig. IID3.c. *Extramammary Paget's disease, medium power.* A PAS stain highlights the glycoprotein constituents of the intracellular mucin contained in the lesional cells, accentuating the "pagetoid pattern" of neoplastic cells scattered among benign epithelial cells.

IID4. Lymphoid Proliferations

Atypical large clear lymphoid cells proliferate in a normally maturing epidermis.

Conditions to consider in the differential diagnosis:

    pagetoid reticulosis
    localized (Woringer-Kolopp)
    disseminated (Ketron-Goodman)
    Paget's disease (mammary or extramammary)
    superficial spreading melanoma
    pagetoid squamous cell carcinoma *in situ*

IIE. LOCALIZED PAPILLOMATOUS EPITHELIAL LESIONS

A "papilla" may be likened to a "finger" of stroma with a few blood vessels, collagen fibers, and fibroblasts, covered by a "glove" of epithelium, which may be reactive or neoplastic, benign or malignant.

1. With Viral Cytopathic Effects
2. No Viral Cytopathic Effect

IIE1. With Viral Cytopathic Effects

The epidermis is acanthotic with vacuolated cells (koilocytes), the granular cell layer is usually thickened with enlarged keratohyaline granules, and there is parakeratosis in tall columns overlying the thickened epidermis. Large inclusions are seen in molluscum contagiosum. Verruca vulgaris and molluscum contagiosum are prototypic.

Verruca Vulgaris

CLINICAL SUMMARY. Verrucae vulgares are circumscribed, firm, elevated papules with papillomatous ("verrucous") hyperkeratotic surfaces. They occur singly or in groups, most commonly on the dorsal aspects of the fingers and hands.

HISTOPATHOLOGY. Verruca vulgaris is characterized by acanthosis, papillomatosis, and hyperkeratosis. The rete ridges are elongated and, at the periphery of the verruca, are often bent inward so that they appear to point radially toward the center (arborization). The characteristic features that distinguish verruca vulgaris from other papillomas are foci of vacuolated cells located in the upper stratum malpighii and in the granular layer, referred to as koilocytotic cells, vertical tiers of parakeratotic cells, and foci of clumped keratohyaline granules. These three changes are quite pronounced in young verrucae vulgares. The koilocytes possess small, round, deeply basophilic nuclei surrounded by a clear halo and pale-staining cytoplasm. The vertical tiers of parakeratotic cells are often located at the crests of papillomatous elevations of the rete malpighii overlying a focus of vacuolated cells.

Verruca Plana

CLINICAL SUMMARY. Verrucae planae are slightly elevated, flat, smooth papules that may be hyperpigmented and affect the face and the dorsa of the hands most commonly. In rare instances, there is extensive involvement, with lesions also on the extremities and trunk.

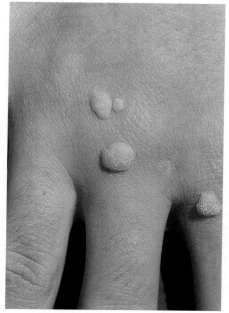

Clin. Fig. IIE1.a

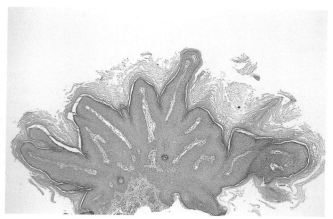

Fig. IIE1.a

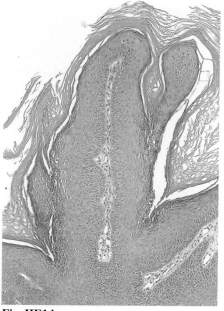

Fig. IIE1.b

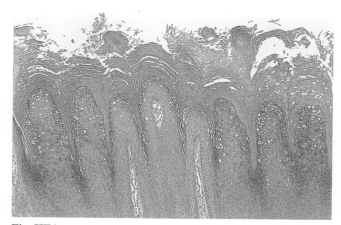

Fig. IIE1.c

Clin. Fig. IIE1.a. *Verruca vulgaris.* Multiple grouped, well-circumscribed, flesh-colored papules appear on a child's hand.

Fig. IIE1.a. *Verruca vulgaris, low power.* Elongated rete ridges at the periphery of the lesion often appear to point inward toward the center.

Fig. IIE1.b. *Verruca vulgaris, medium power.* Vertical tiers of parakeratotic cells are often located at the crests of papillomatous elevations of the rete malpighii.

Fig. IIE1.c. *Verruca vulgaris, medium power.* Although no granular cells are seen overlying the papillomatous crests, they are increased in number and size in the intervening valleys and contain heavy irregular clumps of keratohyaline granules. *(continues)*

Fig. IIE1.d. *Verruca vulgaris, high power.* The virally altered cells, termed koilocytes, possess small, round, deeply basophilic nuclei surrounded by a clear halo and pale-staining cytoplasm.

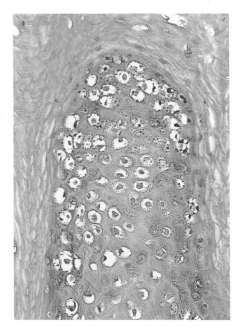

HISTOPATHOLOGY. Verrucae planae show hyperkeratosis and acanthosis but, unlike verrucae vulgares, have no papillomatosis, only slight elongation of the rete ridges, and no areas of parakeratosis. In the upper stratum malpighii, includ-

ing the granular layer, there is diffuse vacuolization of the cells, some of which are enlarged to about twice their normal size. The nuclei of the vacuolated cells lie at the centers of the cells, and some of them appear deeply basophilic. The granular layer is uniformly thickened, and the stratum corneum has a pronounced basket-weave appearance resulting from vacuolization of the horny cells. The dermis appears normal.

Deep Palmoplantar Warts (Myrmecia)

CLINICAL SUMMARY. Deep palmoplantar warts can be tender and occasionally swollen and red. Although they may be multiple, they do not coalesce as do mosaic warts, which are verrucae vulgares. Deep palmoplantar warts occur not only on the palms and soles but also on the lateral aspects and tips of the fingers and toes. Unlike superficial mosaic-type palmoplantar warts, deep palmoplantar warts usually are covered with a thick callus. When the callus is removed with a scalpel, the wart becomes apparent.

HISTOPATHOLOGY. Whereas superficial mosaic-type palmoplantar warts have a histologic appearance analogous to that of verruca vulgaris and represent human papilloma virus types 2 or 4, deep palmoplantar warts represent human papilloma virus type 1. These lesions, also known as myrmecia ("anthill") or inclusion warts, are characterized by abundant keratohyalin, which differs from normal keratohyalin by be-

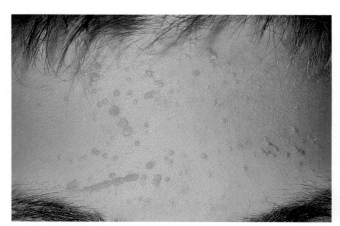

Clin. Fig. IIE1.b

Clin. Fig. IIE1.b. *Verruca plana.* Multiple, smooth, discrete, flesh-colored papules appear on a child's forehead. Linear arrangement of papules appear in traumatized areas (Koebnerization).

Fig. IIE1.e. *Verruca plana, low power.* There is irregular acanthosis with a thickened stratum corneum.

Fig. IIE1.f. *Verruca plana, high power.* There is prominent viral cytopathic effect affecting keratinocytes, including vacuolization, enlargement, and nuclear basophilia, with a prominent granular layer.

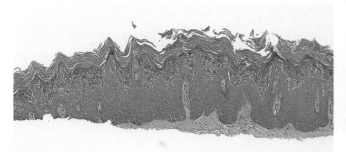

Fig. IIE1.e

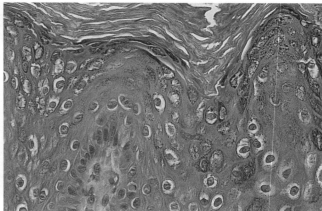

Fig. IIE1.f

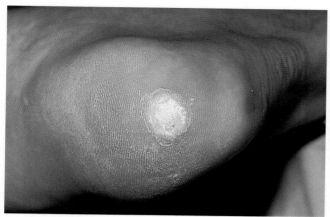

Clin. Fig. IIE1.c

Clin. Fig. IIE1.c. *Plantar wart.* A slightly tender rather ill-defined hyperkeratotic nodule on the plantar skin. (Photo by W. Witmer, Dept. of Dermatology, University of Pennsylvania.)

Fig. IIE1.g. *Deep plantar wart (myrmecia), low power.* There is papillomatosis and thickening of the epidermis with a thickened stratum corneum.

Fig. IIE1.h. *Deep plantar wart (myrmecia), high power.* There are large, irregularly shaped, homogeneous "inclusion bodies" in the cytoplasm of virally affected keratinocytes in the upper stratum spinosum.

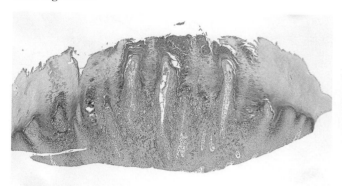

Fig. IIE1.g

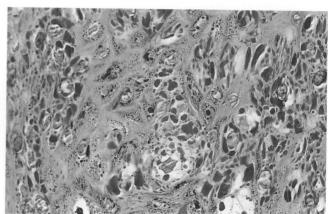

Fig. IIE1.h

ing eosinophilic. Starting in the lower epidermis, the cytoplasm of many cells contains numerous eosinophilic granules, which enlarge in the upper stratum malpighii and coalesce to form large, irregularly shaped, homogeneous "inclusion bodies." In addition to the large intracytoplasmic eosinophilic inclusion bodies, some cells in the upper stratum spinosum with vacuolated nuclei contain a small intranuclear eosinophilic inclusion body. It is round and of about the same size as the nucleolus, which, however, is basophilic. Both the intranuclear eosinophilic inclusion body and the basophilic nucleolus disappear as the vacuolated nucleus changes into a smaller deeply basophilic structure.

Condyloma Acuminatum

CLINICAL SUMMARY. Condylomata acuminata, or anogenital warts, can occur on the penis, on the female genitals, and in the anal region (18). Condylomata of the skin consist of fairly soft, verrucous papules that occasionally coalesce into cauliflower-like masses. Condylomata are flatter on mucosal surfaces.

HISTOPATHOLOGY. The stratum corneum is only slightly thickened. Lesions located on mucosal surfaces show parakeratosis. The stratum malpighii shows papillomatosis and

considerable acanthosis, with thickening and elongation of the rete ridges. Mitotic figures may be present. Usually, invasive squamous cell carcinoma can be ruled out because the epithelial cells show an orderly arrangement and the border between the epithelial proliferations and the dermis is sharp. The most characteristic feature, important for the diagnosis, is the presence of areas in which the epithelial cells show distinct perinuclear vacuolization. These vacuolated epithelial cells are relatively large and possess hyperchromatic round nuclei resembling the nuclei seen in the upper portion of the epidermis in verrucae vulgares. It must be kept in mind, however, that vacuolization is a normal occurrence in the upper portions of all mucosal surfaces, so that vacuolization in condylomata acuminata can be regarded as being possibly of viral genesis only if it extends into the deeper portions of the stratum malpighii. Koilocytotic ("raisin") nuclei, double nuclei, and apoptotic keratinocytes may be present but are often less prominent than in uterine cervical lesions.

Molluscum Contagiosum

CLINICAL SUMMARY. Molluscum contagiosum (19) occurs most frequently in the pediatric age group and consists of a variable number of small, discrete, waxy, skin-colored, delled, dome-shaped papules, usually 2 to 4 mm in size. In

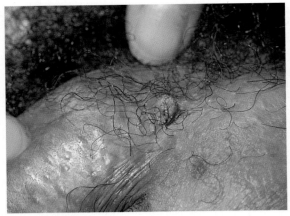

Clin. Fig. IIE1.d

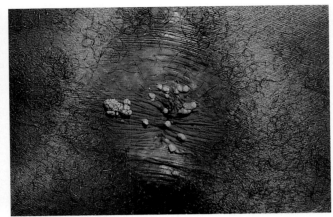

Clin. Fig. IIE1.e

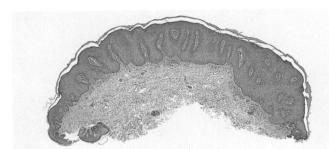

Fig. IIE1.i

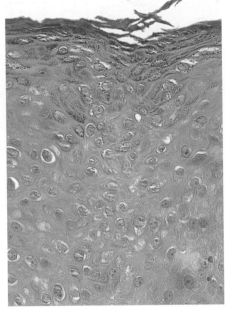

Fig. IIE1.j

Clin. Fig. IIE1.d. *Condyloma acuminatum.* A pedunculated papilloma at the base of the penis.

Clin. Fig. IIE1.e. *Condyloma acuminatum.* Multiple papillomas are seen in the anal area of this human immuno-deficiency virus-positive patient.

Fig. IIE1.i. *Condyloma acuminatum, low power.* There is thickening of the epidermis with rounded thickened rete ridges, with little or no thickening of the stratum corneum. There may be focal areas of parakeratosis.

Fig. IIE1.j. *Condyloma acuminatum, high power.* There are koilocytotic changes of virally affected keratinocytes, including hypergranulosis, perinuclear vacuoles, and irregular nuclear membranes.

adults, molluscum contagiosum is primarily a sexually transmitted disease. In immunocompetent patients, the lesions involute spontaneously. During involution, there may be mild inflammation and tenderness. In the setting of immunosuppression, such as in human immunodeficiency virus infection, molluscum contagiosum can attain considerable size and be widely disseminated.

HISTOPATHOLOGY. The epidermis is acanthotic, and many epidermal cells contain large intracytoplasmic inclusion bodies—the so-called molluscum bodies. These first appear as single, minute, ovoid eosinophilic structures in the lower cells of the stratum malpighii at a level one or two layers above the basal cell layer. As infected cells move toward the surface, the molluscum bodies increase in size, and in the upper layers of the epidermis they displace and compress the nucleus so that it appears as a thin crescent at the periphery

of the cell. At the level of the granular layer, the staining reaction of the molluscum bodies changes from eosinophilic to basophilic. In the horny layer, basophilic molluscum bodies measuring up to 35 mm in diameter lie enmeshed in a network of eosinophilic horny fibers. In the center of the lesion, the stratum corneum ultimately disintegrates, releasing the molluscum bodies and forming a central crater.

Parapox Virus Infections (Milker's Nodules, Orf)

CLINICAL SUMMARY. Milker's nodules, orf, and bovine papular stomatitis pox are clinically identical in humans and are induced by indistinguishable parapox viruses. Milker's nodules are acquired from udders infected with pseudocowpox or paravaccinia (parapox). This disease is called bovine papular stomatitis pox when the source of the infection is calves with oral sores. Orf (ecthyma contagiosum) is ac-

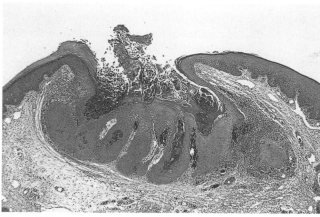

Clin. Fig. IIE1.f

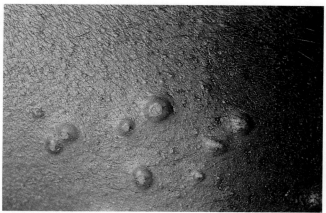

Fig. IIE1.k

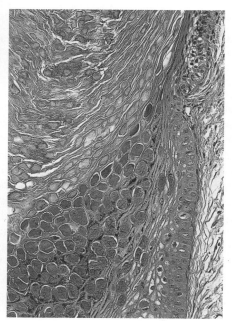

Fig. IIE1.l

Clin. Fig. IIE1.f. *Molluscum contagiosum.* Multiple umbilicated papules in a human immunodeficiency virus-positive patient contained intracellular inclusions (molluscum bodies) on molluscum prep.

Fig. IIE1.k. *Molluscum contagiosum, low power.* Molluscum contagiosum frequently shows an invagination of hyperplastic epithelium.

Fig. IIE1.l. *Molluscum contagiosum, high power.* The keratinocytes that are infected with this pox virus show large eosinophilic cytoplasmic inclusions, called "molluscum bodies."

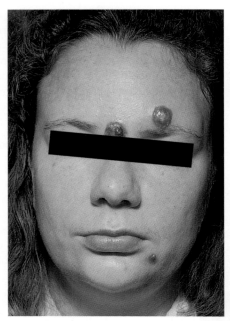

Clin. Fig. IIE1.g

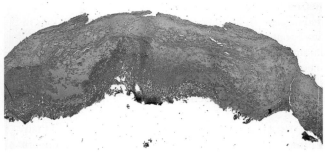

Fig. IIE1.m

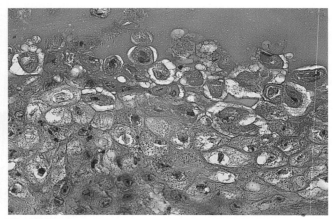

Fig. IIE1.n

Clin. Fig. IIE1.g. *Orf.* Multiple painful erythematous nodules developed gradually in a farmer who fed goats. Examination of goats' mouths by a veterinarian identified the source of the virus.

Fig. IIE1.m. *Orf, low power.* The top of a papillomatous lesion with an overlying scale crust.

Fig. IIE1.n. *Orf, high power.* The lesional keratinocytes are swollen, with occasional intracytoplasmic eosinophilic inclusions.

---

quired from infected sheep or goats with crusted lesions on the lips and in the mouth. After an incubation period of 3 to 7 days, parapox virus infections produce one to three (rarely more) painful lesions measuring 1 to 2 cm in diameter on the fingers or occasionally elsewhere as a result of autoinoculation. During a period of approximately 6 weeks, they pass through six clinical stages, each lasting about 1 week: (a) the maculopapular stage; (b) the target stage, during which the lesions have red centers, white rings, and red halos; (c) the acute weeping stage; (d) the nodular stage, which shows hard nontender nodules; (e) the papillomatous stage, in which the nodules have irregular surfaces; and (f) the regressive stage, during which the lesions involute without scarring.

HISTOPATHOLOGY. During the maculopapular and target stages, there is vacuolization of cells in the upper third of the stratum malpighii, leading to multilocular vesicles. Eosinophilic inclusion bodies are in the cytoplasm of vacuolated epidermal cells, a distinguishing feature from herpes virus infections. Intranuclear eosinophilic inclusion bodies are also present in some cases. During the target stage, vacuolated epidermal cells with inclusion bodies are only in the

surrounding white ring. The epidermis shows elongation of the rete ridges, and the dermis contains many newly formed dilated capillaries and a mononuclear infiltrate. In the acute weeping stage, the epidermis is necrotic throughout. A massive infiltrate of mononuclear cells extends throughout the dermis. In the later stages, the epidermis shows acanthosis with fingerlike downward projections, and the dermis shows vasodilatation and chronic inflammation, followed by resolution.

Conditions to consider in the differential diagnosis:

> verruca vulgaris
> orf
> condyloma acuminatum
> molluscum contagiosum
> bowenoid papulosis

IIE2. Without Viral Cytopathic Effect

The epidermis proliferates focally. The cells may be basophilic or "basaloid" in type (seborrheic keratoses). There may be increased stratum corneum and elongation of the dermal papillae (squamous papilloma) or there may be basilar keratinocytic atypia (actinic keratosis). Seborrheic keratosis is a prototypic example.

Seborrheic Keratosis

CLINICAL SUMMARY.   Seborrheic keratoses (20) are very common lesions, which are sometimes single but often multiple. They usually occur during middle age, mainly on the trunk and face but also on the extremities, with the exception of the palms and soles. They are sharply demarcated, brownish in color, and slightly raised, so that they often look as if they are stuck on the surface of the skin. Most have a verrucous surface, which has a soft friable consistency. Some, however, have a smooth surface but characteristically show keratotic plugs. Although most lesions measure only a few millimeters in diameter, a lesion may occasionally reach a size of several centimeters. Some may become inflamed.

HISTOPATHOLOGY.   Seven types are generally recognized: irritated, adenoid or reticulated, plane, clonal, melanoacanthoma, inverted follicular keratosis, and benign squamous keratosis. Often more than one type is found in the same lesion. All have hyperkeratosis, acanthosis, and papillomatosis in common. The acanthosis in most instances is due entirely to upward extension of the tumor. Thus, the lower border of the tumor is even and generally lies on a straight line that may be drawn from the normal epidermis at one end of the tumor to the normal epidermis at the other end. Two types of cells

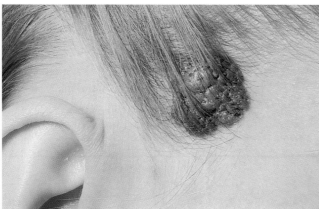

Clin. Fig. IIE2

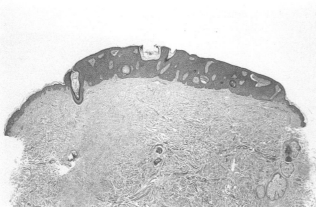

Fig. IIE2.a

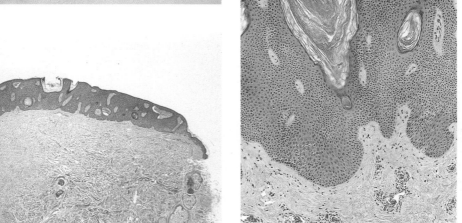

Fig. IIE2.b

Clin. Fig. IIE2. *Seborrheic keratosis.* A middle-aged woman developed a pigmented "stuck-on" papule with a "waxy" feel. Keratin-filled ostia help to distinguish this common lesion. A slightly scaly surface can be accentuated by rubbing or light scratching of the lesion.

Fig. IIE2.a. *Seborrheic keratosis, low power.* The tumor extends upward above a line drawn through the normal epidermis on each side. Keratin tunnels ("horn cysts") containing whorls of keratin are a prominent feature. This lesion was removed as a full-thickness excision because it was clinically diagnosed as melanoma.

Fig. IIE2.b. *Seborrheic keratosis, medium power.* The lesion is composed predominantly of basaloid cells, with squamous differentiation beneath the stratum corneum.

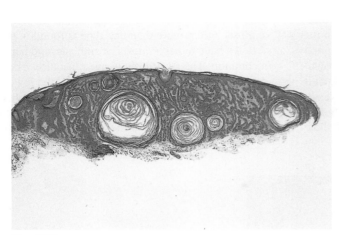

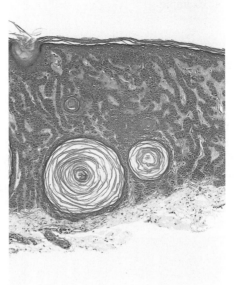

Fig. IIE2.c   **Fig. IIE2.d**

Fig. IIE2.c. *Reticulated seborrheic keratosis, low power.* The lesion is composed of anastomosing cords of cells in a reticulated or "adenoid" pattern, with scattered "horn cysts."

Fig. IIE2.d. *Reticulated seborrheic keratosis, medium power.* The cells in the cords show basaloid and squamous differentiation. In this example, there is moderate melanin pigment in the basaloid cells.

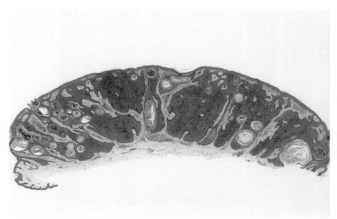

Fig. IIE2.e. *Pigmented seborrheic keratosis, low power.* The lesion contains abundant brown melanin pigment, simulating a nodular melanoma clinically.

Fig. IIE2.f. *Pigmented seborrheic keratosis, medium power.* The pigment is located mainly in the basaloid cells. It is produced by melanocytes that populate the lesion.

Fig. IIE2.e

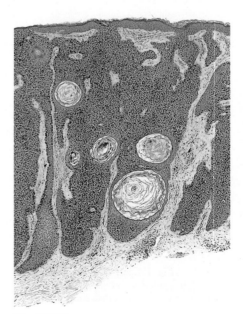

Fig. IIE2.f

are usually seen in the acanthotic epidermis; basaloid cells, which resemble the cells found normally in the basal layer of the epidermis, tend to predominate over squamous cells.

Conditions to consider in the differential diagnosis:

seborrheic keratosis
acanthosis nigricans
confluent and reticulated papillomatosis
actinic keratosis, hypertrophic
nonspecific squamous papilloma
epithelial nevus/epidermal nevus
hyperkeratosis of the nipple and areola
verruciform xanthoma
verrucous melanoma

IIF. IRREGULAR PROLIFERATIONS EXTENDING INTO THE SUPERFICIAL DERMIS

Irregular or asymmetric proliferations of keratinocytes extending into the dermis are usually neoplastic. The differential diagnosis includes reactive pseudoepitheliomatous hyperplasia, which may be seen around chronic ulcers or in association with other inflammatory conditions (see section VIB1).

1. Squamous Differentiation
2. Basaloid Differentiation

IIF1. Squamous Differentiation

The epidermis is irregularly thickened, the maturation is abnormal, and there may be keratinocytic atypia (squamous cell carcinoma). The proliferation is often associated with a thick parakeratotic scale. *Superficial squamous cell carcinoma* is a prototypic example.

Inverted Follicular Keratosis

See Figs. IIF1.d and IIF1.e.

Conditions to consider in the differential diagnosis:

lichen simplex chronicus
squamous cell carcinoma, superficial
keratoacanthoma
prurigo nodularis
actinic prurigo
inverted follicular keratosis
verrucous carcinoma
of oral mucosa

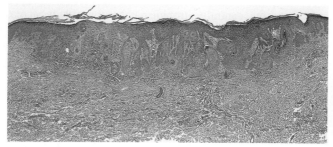

Fig. IIF1.a

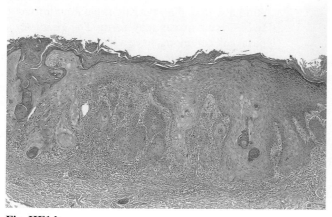

Fig. IIF1.b

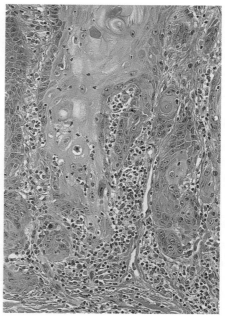

Fig. IIF1.c

Fig. IIF1.a. *Squamous cell carcinoma, invasive, low power.* Endophytic proliferative lobules of atypical epithelium, which are associated with a patchy lymphocytic infiltrate, arise from the base of the epidermis.

Fig. IIF1.b. *Squamous cell carcinoma, invasive, medium power.* The haphazardly oriented lobules are of varying shapes and sizes and show an infiltrative growth pattern within the dermis.

Fig. IIF1.c. *Squamous cell carcinoma, invasive, high power.* At higher magnification, formation of squamous pearls, whorled aggregates of parakeratin within the epithelial islands, and the atypical keratinocytes may show a spectrum of cytologic atypia from mild to severe.

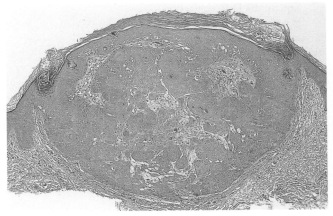

Fig. IIF1.d

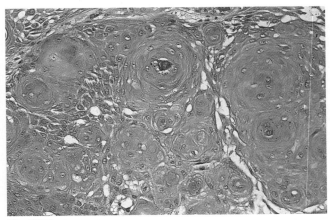

Fig. IIF1.e

Fig. IIF1.d. *Inverted follicular keratosis, low power.* This epithelial neoplasm arises from the epidermis and shows an endophytic lobulated architecture with a symmetric profile and a regular border. The epithelial proliferation is embedded in a fibrotic stroma and is sharply separated from the adjacent reticular dermal collagen.

Fig. IIF1.e. *Inverted follicular keratosis, high power.* Keratin-filled cystic structures may be seen within the epithelial proliferation, and squamous eddies as depicted here are a characteristic feature of an inverted follicular keratosis.

of genitoanal region (giant condyloma of Buschke and Lowenstein)
of plantar skin (epithelioma cuniculatum)
pseudoepitheliomatous hyperplasia
deep fungal infection
halogenoderma
chronic ulcers
granular cell tumor
Spitz nevus
verrucous melanoma

IIF2. Basaloid Differentiation

The proliferation is of basal cells from the epidermis, extending into the dermis. The epidermis can be thickened, normal, or atrophic. Basal cell carcinoma is a prototypic example.

Basal Cell Carcinoma

CLINICAL SUMMARY. Five clinical types of basal cell carcinoma occur. *Noduloulcerative basal cell carcinoma* begins as a small waxy nodule that often shows a few small telangiectatic vessels on its surface. The nodule usually increases slowly in size and often undergoes central ulceration surrounded by a pearly rolled border. This represents the so-called rodent ulcer. *Pigmented basal cell carcinoma* differs from the noduloulcerative type only by the brown pigmentation of the lesion. *Morphealike or fibrosing basal cell carcinoma* manifests itself as a solitary, flat, or slightly depressed, indurated, ill defined, smooth, yellowish plaque. This type has a high incidence of local recurrence. *Superficial basal cell carcinoma* consists of one or several erythematous, scal-

ing, centrally atrophic patches that slowly increase in size by peripheral extension and are surrounded, at least in part, by a fine, threadlike, pearly border. The patches usually show small areas of superficial ulceration and crusting. *Fibroepithelioma* presents as a raised, moderately firm, slightly pedunculated, reddish nodule resembling a fibroma.

HISTOPATHOLOGY. In the common clinically *noduloulcerative* and histologically *solid* type of basal cell carcinoma, nodular masses of basaloid cells extend into the dermis in relation to a delicate, specialized, somewhat myxoid tumor stroma with a characteristic separation artifact between the two. Cystic spaces may form. The characteristic cells of basal cell carcinoma have a large, oval, or elongated nucleus and relatively little cytoplasm. The nuclei resemble those of epidermal basal cells but differ by having a larger ratio of nucleus to cytoplasm and by lacking intercellular bridges. Although most basal cell carcinomas appear well demarcated, some show an infiltrative growth into the reticular dermis. These latter are now widely recognized as a distinct histologic subtype (infiltrating basal cell carcinoma).

Superficial basal cell carcinoma shows buds and irregular proliferations of peripherally palisaded basaloid cells attached to the undersurface of the epidermis and penetrating only slightly into the dermis. The overlying epidermis is usually atrophic. Fibroblasts, often in a fairly large number, are arranged around the tumor cell proliferations. In addition, a mild or moderate amount of a nonspecific chronic inflammatory infiltrate is present in the upper dermis.

In *fibroepithelioma*, long, thin, branching, anastomosing strands of basal cell carcinoma are embedded in a fibrous stroma. Many strands are connected to the surface epidermis. Here and there, small groups of dark-staining cells showing a

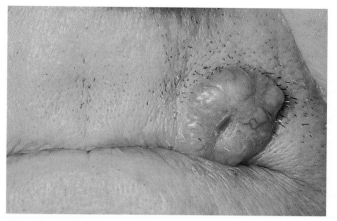

Clin. Fig. IIF2.a.

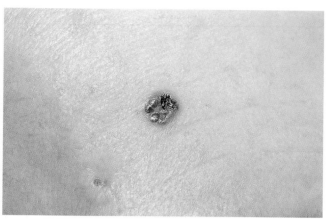

Clin. Fig. IIF2.b

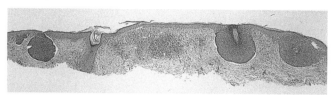

Fig. IIF2.a

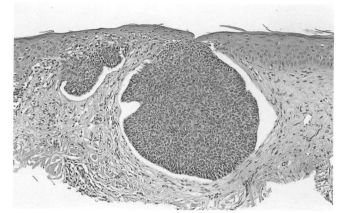

Fig. IIF2.b

Clin. Fig. IIF2.a. *Noduloulcerative basal cell carcinoma.* The rolled pearly borders with telangiectases and central ulceration typify basal cell carcinoma, the most common skin malignancy.

Clin. Fig. IIF2.b. *Pigmented basal cell carcinoma.* An elderly man developed a forehead papule with a pigmented rolled border and central concavity.

Fig. IIF2.a. *Superficial "multicentric" basal cell carcinoma, low power.* Irregular masses of basophilic cells extend from the epidermis into the dermis.

Fig. IIF2.b. *Superficial "multicentric" basal cell carcinoma, medium power.* The cells at the periphery of the tumor masses are palisaded, and there is a cleft between them and the characteristic delicate collagenous stroma.

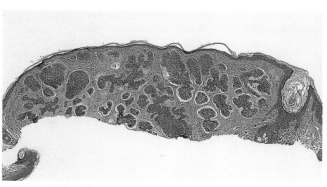

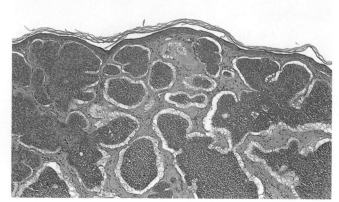

Fig. IIF2.c. *Nodular basal cell carcinoma, low power.* Nodular aggregates of atypical basaloid cells associated with cleft formation arise from the base of the epithelium.

Fig. IIF2.d. *Nodular basal cell carcinoma, medium power.* Bluish mucinous material is seen in the cleft. The stroma of basal cell carcinomas may be fibrotic, as seen here, or may be loose with an abundance of mucinous material.

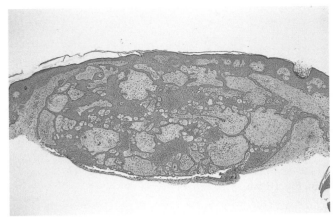

Fig. IIF2.e

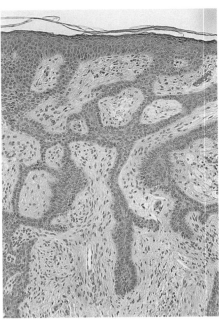

Fig. IIF2.e. *Fibroepithelioma of Pinkus, low power.* This variant of basal cell carcinoma shows numerous thin anastomosing strands of epithelial cells that arise from the base of the epidermis.

Fig. IIF2.f. *Fibroepithelioma of Pinkus, medium power.* These epithelial strands form small basaloid buds with peripheral palisading. The stroma is hypercellular and fibrotic.

Fig. IIF2.f

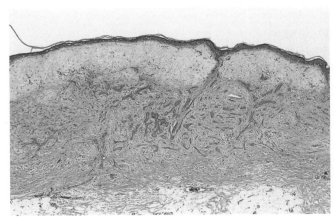

Fig. IIF2.g

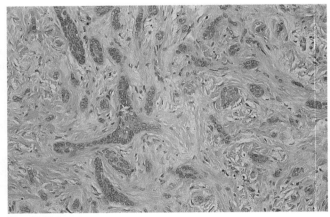

Fig. IIF2.h

Fig. IIF2.g. *Morpheaform basal cell carcinoma, low power.* This aggressive variant of basal cell carcinoma is composed of numerous small islands of basal cell carcinoma that generally infiltrate into the reticular dermis.

Fig. IIF2.h. *Morpheaform basal cell carcinoma, high power.* At higher magnification, this lesion is composed of very small islands of atypical basaloid cells that are embedded in a fibrotic stroma.

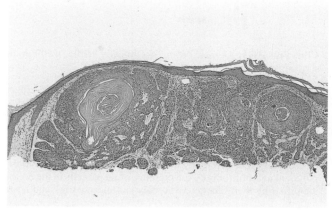

Fig. IIF2.i

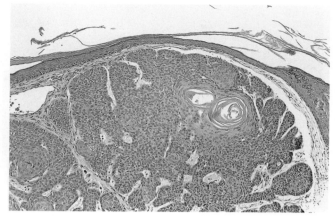

Fig. IIF2.j

Fig. IIF2.i. *Keratinizing basal cell carcinoma, low power.* Basal cell carcinoma may show foci of keratinization within the lobules of atypical basaloid cells.

Fig. IIF2.j. *Keratinizing basal cell carcinoma, medium power.* These areas of keratinization may resemble horn cysts or keratin pearls. If a lesion is partially biopsied, this finding may cause confusion between the basal cell carcinoma and squamous cell carcinoma.

palisade arrangement of the peripheral cell layer may be seen along the epithelial strands, like buds on a branch. Usually, the tumor is quite superficial and is well demarcated at its lower border. Fibroepithelioma combines features of the intra-canalicular fibroadenoma of the breast, the reticulated type of seborrheic keratosis, and superficial basal cell carcinoma.

Conditions to consider in the differential diagnosis:

basal cell carcinoma, superficial types

IIG. SUPERFICIAL POLYPOID LESIONS

A polyp consists of a "finger" of stroma covered by a "glove" of epithelium. It is to be distinguished from a papilloma, which shows elongated papillae.

1. Melanocytic Lesions
2. Spindle Cell and Stromal Lesions

IIG1. Melanocytic Lesions

The polyp contains mature nevus cells in a compound nevus or atypical melanocytes in a polypoid melanoma. *Polypoid dermal and compound nevi* are prototypic (5).

Polypoid Dermal and Compound Nevi

A compound nevus possesses features of both a junctional and an intradermal nevus (see also section IIA2). Nevus cell nests are present in the epidermis and in the dermis. Nevus cells in the upper, middle, and lower dermis may present characteristic morphologic variations called *types A, B,* and *C,* respectively. Usually, the type A nevus cells in the upper dermis are cuboidal and show abundant cytoplasm containing varying amounts of melanin granules. Type B cells are distinctly smaller than type A cells, display less cytoplasm and less melanin, and generally lie in well-defined aggregates. Type C nevus cells in the lower dermis tend to resemble fibroblasts or Schwann cells, because they are usually elongated and have spindle-shaped nuclei. If dermal nevus cells are confined to the papillary dermis, they often retain a discrete or "pushing" border with the stroma. However, nevus cells that enter the reticular dermis tend to disperse among collagen fiber bundles as single cells or attenuated single files of cells. This pattern of infiltration of the dermis differs from that in melanomas, where groups of cells tend to dissect and displace the collagen bundles in a more "expansive" pattern. Lesions where nevus cells extend into the lower reticular dermis and the subcutaneous fat, or are located within nerves, hair follicles, sweat ducts, and sebaceous glands, may be termed "congenital pattern nevi." Intradermal nevi show essentially no junctional activity. The upper dermis contains nests and cords of nevus cells similar to those described above. Occasional intradermal nevi are devoid of nevus cell nests in the upper dermis and contain only spindle-shaped nevus cells embedded in abundant loosely arranged collagenous tissue. These nevi may be referred to as neural nevi.

Conditions to consider in the differential diagnosis:

polypoid dermal and compound nevi
polypoid melanoma (see also section VIB3)

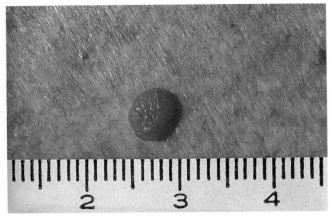

Clin. Fig. IIG1. *Dermal nevus.* A clinically stable, well-circumscribed, symmetric, flesh-colored papule.

Fig. IIG1.a. *Polypoid dermal nevus, low power.* In this tangentially sectioned example, the intradermal location of the dermal nevus cells and the polypoid character of the lesion are readily apparent.

Fig. IIG1.b. *Polypoid dermal nevus, medium power.* The polypoid dermal nevus is differentiated from a fibroepithelial polyp or a polypoid neurofibroma by the presence of nevus cells in the dermis, identified by their characteristic cuboidal morphology and nested pattern.

Clin. Fig. IIG1

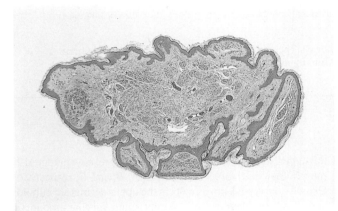

Fig. IIG1.a

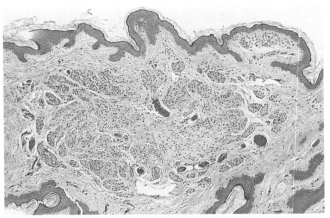

Fig. IIG1.b

IIG2. Spindle Cell and Stromal Lesions

The polyp contains stromal cells of types that may be seen in the dermis, including fibroblasts, fat cells, or schwannian cells. *Neurofibroma* is a prototypic example (21).

Neurofibroma

CLINICAL SUMMARY. Extraneural sporadic cutaneous neurofibromas (the common sporadic neurofibromas) are soft, polypoid, skin-colored or slightly tan, and small (rarely larger than a centimeter in diameter). They usually arise in adulthood. The identification of as many as four small cutaneous neurofibromas in a single patient, in the absence of other confirmatory findings, would not qualify as stigmata of neurofibromatosis.

HISTOPATHOLOGY. Most sporadic neurofibromas are faintly eosinophilic and are circumscribed but not encapsulated: They are extraneural. Thin spindle cells with elongated wavy nuclei are regularly spaced among thin, wavy, collagenous strands. The strands are either closely spaced (homogeneous pattern) or loosely spaced in a clear matrix (loose pattern). The two patterns are often intermixed in a single lesion. The regular spacing of adnexa is preserved in

cutaneous neurofibromas. Entrapped small nerves occasionally are enlarged and hypercellular. The differentiation from a neurotized nevus may be difficult in routinely stained sections, but distinction may be possible if a few type A or B nevus cells are present in addition to the spindle cells or with an immunohistochemical stain for myelin basic protein, which is positive only in neurofibromas.

Fibroepithelial Polyp

CLINICAL SUMMARY. Fibroepithelial polyps, also called "soft fibromas," "acrochordons," or "cutaneous tags," occur as three types: (a) multiple, small, furrowed papules, especially on the neck and in the axillae, generally only 1 to 2 mm long; (b) single or multiple filiform smooth growths in varying locations, about 2 mm wide and 5 mm long; and (c) solitary baglike pedunculated growths, usually about 1 cm in diameter but occasionally much larger, seen most commonly on the lower trunk. There may be associations with diabetes and acromegaly.

HISTOPATHOLOGY. The multiple small furrowed papules usually show papillomatosis, hyperkeratosis, and regular acanthosis and occasionally also horn cysts within their acanthotic epidermis. Thus, there is often considerable re-

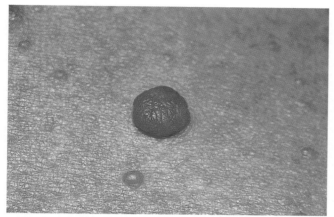

Clin. Fig. IIG2.a

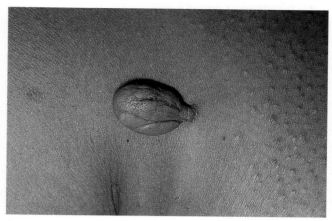

Clin. Fig. IIG2.b

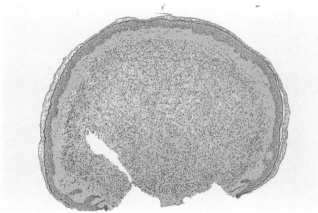

Fig. IIG2.a

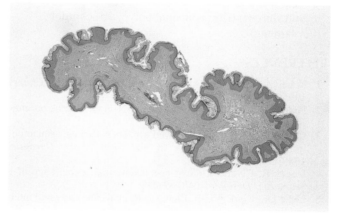

Fig. IIG2.c

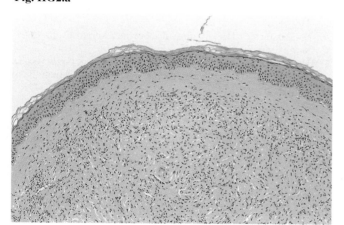

Fig. IIG2.b

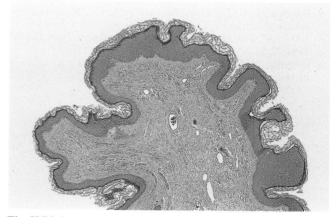

Fig. IIG2.d

Clin. Fig. IIG2.a. *Neurofibroma.* Patient with neurofibromatosis presented with a classical sign—multiple, soft, flesh-colored papules and nodules on the trunk.

Fig. IIG2.a. *Neurofibroma, low power.* At scanning magnification, this polypoid lesion shows an essentially normal epidermis. Within the dermis there is a uniformly symmetric proliferation of spindled cells.

Fig. IIG2.b. *Neurofibroma, medium power.* At higher magnification, these small spindled cells are wavy and bland in appearance and are embedded in an eosinophilic matrix.

Clin. Fig. IIG2.b. *Soft fibroma.* A traumatized pedunculated papule along the bra line.

Fig. IIG2.c. *Fibroepithelial polyp, low power.* At scanning magnification, this polypoid lesion may resemble both a nevus and a neurofibroma. However, upon closer inspection, neither nevus cells nor wavy neural cells are seen within the stroma of this lesion.

Fig. IIG2.d. *Fibroepithelial polyp, medium power.* The core of this lesion is composed of well-vascularized connective tissue and the lesion is surfaced by slightly acanthotic and papillomatous epithelium.

semblance to a pedunculated seborrheic keratosis. The common filiform smooth growths show slight to moderate acanthosis and occasionally mild papillomatosis. The connective tissue stalk is composed of loose collagen fibers and often contains numerous dilated capillaries filled with erythrocytes. Nevus cells are found in many filiform growths, indicating that some of them represent involuting melanocytic nevi. The baglike soft fibromas generally show a flattened epidermis overlying loosely arranged collagen fibers and mature fat cells in the center. In some instances, the dermis is quite thin, so that the fat cells compose a significant portion of the tumor, which may then be regarded as a lipofibroma.

Conditions to consider in the differential diagnosis:

> neurofibroma
> neurotized nevus
> soft fibroma (fibroepithelial polyp, acrochordon, skin tag)

REFERENCES

1. Sober AJ, Burstein JM. Precursors to skin cancer. *Cancer* 1995;75:645.
2. Penneys NS, Ackerman AB, Indgin SN, et al. Eccrine poroma. *Br J Dermatol* 1970;82:613.
3. Callen JP, Headington J. Bowen's and non-Bowen's squamous intraepidermal neoplasia of the skin. *Arch Dermatol* 1980;116:422.
4. Degos R, Civatte J. Clear-cell acanthoma: experience of 8 years. *Br J Dermatol* 1970;83:248.
5. Elder DE, Clark WH Jr, Elenitsas R, et al. The early and intermediate precursor lesions of tumor progression in the melanocytic system: common acquired nevi and atypical (dysplastic) nevi. *Semin Diagn Pathol* 1993;10:18.
6. Barnhill RL, Barnhill MA, Berwick M, Mihm MC Jr. The histologic spectrum of pigmented spindle cell nevus: a review of 120 cases with emphasis on atypical variants. *Hum Pathol* 1991;22:52.
7. Coleman WP III, Loria PR, Reed RJ, et al. Acral lentiginous melanoma. *Arch Dermatol* 1980;116:773.
8. Clark WH Jr, Mihm MC Jr. Lentigo maligna and lentigo-maligna melanoma. *Am J Pathol* 1969;55:39.
9. Schwarz T, Seiser A, Gschnait F. Disseminated superficial actinic porokeratosis. *J Am Acad Dermatol* 1984;11:724.
10. De Wit PEJ, Vant Hof-Grootenboer B, Ruiter DJ, et al. Validity of the histopathological criteria used for diagnosing dysplastic nevi. *Eur J Cancer* 1993;29A:831.
11. Su WPD. Histopathologic varieties of epidermal nevus. *Am J Dermatopathol* 1982;4:161.
12. Wilgenbus K, Lentner A, Kuckelkorn R, et al. Further evidence that acanthosis nigricans maligna is linked to enhanced secretion by the tumour of transforming growth factor alpha. *Arch Dermatol Res* 1992;284:266.
13. Cruz PD, Hud JA. Excess insulin binding to insulin-like growth factor receptors: proposed mechanism for acanthosis nigricans. *J Invest Dermatol* 1992;98:82S.
14. Okun MF, Edelstein LM. Clonal seborrheic keratosis. In: Okun MF, Edelstein LM, eds. *Gross and microscopic pathology of the skin.* Vol. 2. Boston: Dermatopathology Foundation Press, 1976:576.
15. Elder DE, Murphy GF. Malignant tumors: melanomas and related lesions. In: Elder DE, Murphy GF, eds. *Melanocytic tumors of the skin.* Washington, DC: Armed Forces Institute of Pathology, 1991:103.
16. Park HK, Leonard DM, Arrington JH III, et al. Recurrent melanocytic nevi: clinical and histologic review of 175 cases. *J Am Acad Dermatol* 1987;17:285.
17. Raiten K, Paniago-Pereira C, Ackerman AB. Pagetoid Bowen's disease vs. extramammary Paget's disease. *J Dermatol Surg Oncol* 1976;2:24.
18. Rock B, Shah KV, Farmer ER. A morphologic, pathologic, and virologic study of anogenital warts in men. *Arch Dermatol* 1992;127:495.
19. Forghani B, Oshiro LS, Chan CS, et al. Direct detection of molluscum contagiosum virus in clinical specimens by in situ hybridization using biotinylated probe. *Mol Cell Probes* 1992;6:67.
20. Sanderson KF. The structure of seborrheic keratoses. *Br J Dermatol* 1968;80:588
21. Harkin JC, Reed RJ. *Tumors of the peripheral nervous system.* 2nd series, Fasc. 3. Washington, DC: Armed Forces Institute of Pathology, 1969.

Disorders of the Superficial Cutaneous Reactive Unit

The epidermis, papillary dermis, and superficial capillary–venular plexus react together in many dermatologic conditions and have been termed the "superficial cutaneous reactive unit" by Wallace H. Clark, Jr. (unpublished data). Many dermatoses are associated with infiltrates of lymphocytes with or without other cell types around the superficial vessels. The epidermis in pathologic conditions can be thinned (atrophic), thickened (acanthosis), edematous (spongiosis), and/or infiltrated (exocytosis). The epidermis may proliferate in response to chronic irritation or infection (bacterial, yeast, deep fungal, or viral). The epidermis may proliferate in response to dermatologic conditions (psoriasis, atopic dermatitis, prurigo). The papillary dermis and superficial vascular plexus may have a variety of inflammatory cells, can be edematous, may have increased ground substance (hyaluronic acid), and may be sclerotic or homogenized.

IIIA. SUPERFICIAL PERIVASCULAR DERMATITIS

Many dermatoses are associated with infiltrates of lymphocytes with or without other cell types around the vessels of the superficial capillary–venular plexus. The vessel walls may be quite unremarkable, or there may be slight to moderate endothelial swelling. Eosinophilic change ("fibrinoid necrosis"), a hallmark of true vasculitis, is not seen. The term "lymphocytic vasculitis" may encompass some of the conditions mentioned here, but is of doubtful validity in the absence of vessel wall damage. The epidermis is variable in its thickness, amount, and type of exocytotic cell, and the integrity of the basal cell zone (liquefaction degeneration). In some of the entities listed here, the perivascular infiltrate may involve the mid and deep vessels in some cases. These conditions are also listed in Chapter V.

1. Superficial Perivascular Dermatitis, Mostly Lymphocytes
1a. Superficial Perivascular Dermatitis with Eosinophils
1b. Superficial Perivascular Dermatitis with Neutrophils
1c. Superficial Perivascular Dermatitis with Plasma Cells
1d. Superficial Perivascular Dermatitis with Extravasated Red Cells
1e. Superficial Perivascular Dermatitis, Melanophages Prominent

2. Superficial Perivascular Dermatitis, Mast Cells Predominant

IIIA1. Superficial Perivascular Dermatitis, Mostly Lymphocytes

Lymphocytes are seen around the superficial vascular plexus. Other cell types are rare or absent.

Viral Exanthem

CLINICAL SUMMARY. Five groups of viruses can affect the skin or the adjoining mucous surfaces: (a) the herpesvirus group, including herpes simplex types 1 and 2 and the varicella-zoster virus, which are DNA-containing organisms that

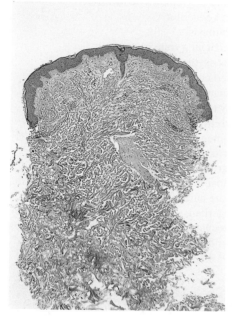

Fig. IIIA1.a

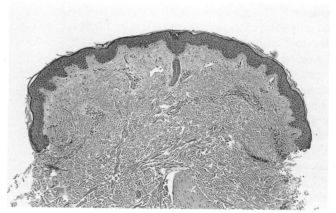

Fig. IIIA1.b

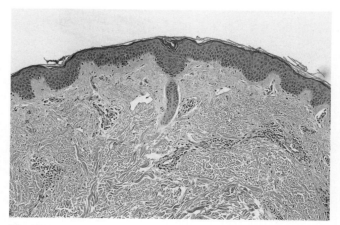

Fig. IIIA1.c

Fig. IIIA1.a. *Morbilliform viral exanthem, low power.* There is an inflammatory infiltrate around dermal vessels in the reticular dermis.

Fig. IIIA1.b. *Morbilliform viral exanthem, medium power.* A thin keratin scale overlies an evenly acanthotic epidermis. There is vascular ectasia in the upper reticular dermis.

Fig. IIIA1.c. *Morbilliform viral exanthem, high power.* A lymphocytic inflammatory infiltrate is seen around the dermal vessels. Superficial telangiectasia is well defined. The epidermis is focally acanthotic and does not show atypia.

multiply within the nucleus of the host cell; (b) the poxvirus group, including smallpox, milker's nodules, orf, and molluscum contagiosum, which are DNA-containing agents that multiply within the cytoplasm; (c) the papovavirus group, including the various types of verrucae, which contain DNA and replicate in the nucleus; (d) the picornavirus group, including coxsackievirus group A, causing hand-foot-and-mouth disease, which contain RNA rather than DNA in their nucleoids; and (e) retroviruses, including human immunodeficiency virus (HIV), the cause of acquired immunodeficiency syndrome (AIDS). Primary HIV infection may be associated with both an exanthem and an enanthem, which are histologically nondescript. The array of skin lesions associated with HIV is generally a consequence of eventual immunosuppression.

HISTOPATHOLOGY.   There is no unique histology of HIV infection in the skin. Primary exanthems of HIV show nonspecific lymphocytoid infiltrates with mild epidermal changes, primarily spongiosis (1). Seborrheic dermatitis in patients with AIDS may show nonspecific changes, including spotty keratinocytic necrosis, leukoexocytosis, and plasma cells in a superficial perivascular infiltrate (2). A "papular eruption" may exhibit nonspecific perivascular eosinophils with mild folliculitis, although epithelioid cell granulomas have also been reported (3). An "interface dermatitis" shows, as the name implies, vacuolar alteration of the basal cell layer, scattered necrotic keratinocytes, and a superficial perivascular lymphohistiocytic infiltrate. The vacuolar alteration and number of necrotic keratinocytes tend to be more pronounced than in drug eruptions. Biopsies of AIDS-related eruptions are often nonspecific.

Tinea Versicolor

See Fig. IIIA1.d.

Lupus Erythematosus, Acute

See Figs. IIIA1.e–IIIA1.g.

Guttate Parapsoriasis

See Figs. IIIA1.h–IIIA1.j.

Conditions to consider in the differential diagnosis:
    morbilliform viral exanthem
    papular acrodermatitis (Gianotti–Crosti)
    stasis dermatitis
    pityriasis lichenoides et varioliformis acuta (PLEVA),
        early
    Jessner's lymphocytic infiltrate
    tinea versicolor
    candidiasis
    superficial gyrate erythemas
    lupus erythematosus, acute
    mixed connective tissue disease
    dermatomyositis
    early herpes simplex, zoster
    morbilliform drug eruption
    cytomegalovirus inclusion disease
    polymorphous drug eruption
    progressive pigmented purpura
    parapsoriasis, small plaque type (digitate dermatosis)
    guttate parapsoriasis
    Langerhans cell histiocytosis (early lesions)
    mucocutaneous lymph node syndrome (Kawasaki disease)
    secondary syphilis

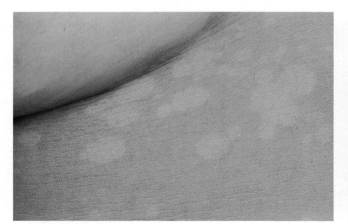

Clin. Fig. IIIA1.a

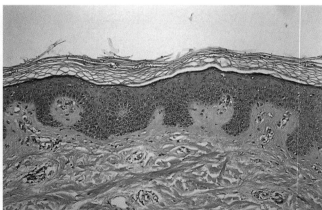

Fig. IIIA1.d

Clin. Fig. IIIA1.a. *Tinea versicolor.* Macular areas of hypopigmentation on the upper trunk. On gentle scraping, the surface of the discolored areas shows a fine scale.

Fig. IIIA1.d. *Tinea versicolor, medium power.* In the hyperkeratotic stratum corneum there are basophilic staining hyphae and spores. The epidermis is acanthotic with basal layer pigmentation and a sparse lymphocytic infiltrate.

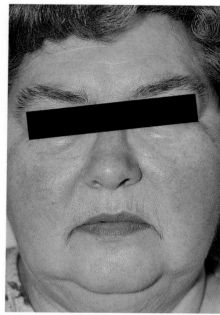

Clin. Fig. IIIA1.b

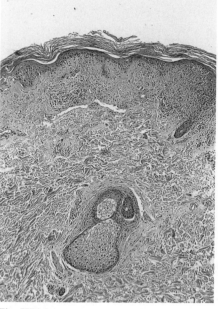

Fig. IIIA1.e

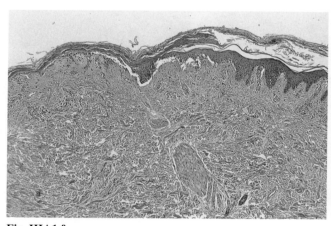

Fig. IIIA1.f

Fig. IIIA1.g

Clin. Fig. IIIA1.b. *Lupus erythematosus, acute*. A photosensitive woman presented with edematous malar erythema. Lack of papules and pustules helps to distinguish lupus from rosacea.

Fig. IIIA1.e. *Lupus erythematosus, acute, low power*. There is hyperkeratosis with a focally acanthotic epidermis and dermal–epidermal separation. There is an infiltrate around dermal vessels seen in the reticular dermis.

Fig. IIIA1.f. *Lupus erythematosus, acute, medium power*. A separation is seen at the dermal–epidermal interface with an overlying hyperkeratotic scale. The inflammatory infiltrate in the dermis is lymphocytic.

Fig. IIIA1.g. *Lupus erythematosus, acute, medium power*. A lichenoid inflammatory infiltrate obscures the dermal–epidermal interface. The inflammatory cells are exocytotic to the alternatingly acanthotic, atrophic epidermis.

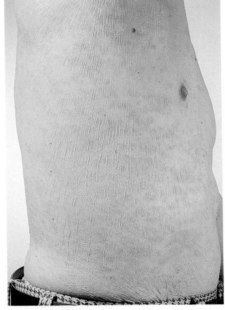

Clin. Fig. IIIA1.c

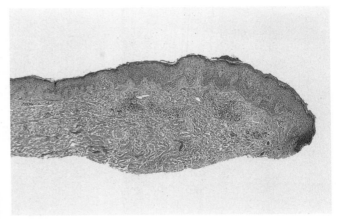

Fig. IIIA1.h

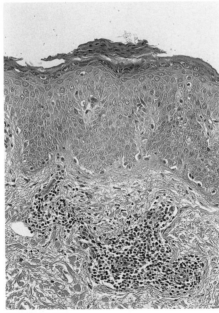

Fig. IIIA1.i

Fig. IIIA1.j

Clin. Fig. IIIA1.c. *Parapsoriasis.* Brown finely scaled macular fingerlike morphology with atrophy characterizes the benign digitate variant.

Fig. IIIA1.h. *Guttate parapsoriasis, low power.* There is a focal parakeratotic scale overlying an acanthotic epidermis. In the dermis there is a dense infiltrate around superficial dermal vessels in a localized area.

Fig. IIIA1.i. *Guttate parapsoriasis, medium power.* A parakeratotic scale overlies an acanthotic epidermis in which there is sparse exocytosis and mild spongiosis. There is a dense inflammatory cell infiltrate around dermal vessels.

Fig. IIIA1.j. *Guttate parapsoriasis, high power.* There is a dense infiltrate of mononuclear cells around the dermal vessels.

IIIA1a. Superficial Perivascular Dermatitis with Eosinophils

In addition to lymphocytes, eosinophils are present in varying numbers, with both a perivascular and interstitial distribution.

Morbilliform Drug Eruption

CLINICAL SUMMARY. Virtually any drug may be associated with a morbilliform eruption; the nonspecific clinical and histologic changes make definitive implication of a specific agent difficult (4). The most common class of medications causing morbilliform eruptions is antibacterial antibiotics.

The morbilliform rash consists of fine blanching papules, which appear suddenly, are symmetric, and often are brightly erythematous in white patients.

HISTOPATHOLOGY. The typical morbilliform drug eruption displays a variable, often sparse, mainly perivascular infiltrate of lymphocytes and eosinophils. Eosinophils may be absent. Some vacuolization of the dermal–epidermal junction with few apoptotic epidermal cells may be observed, but not to the degree typical of erythema multiforme or toxic epidermal necrolysis. There is a variable degree of urticarial edema (allergic urticarial eruption, see below). Distinction of morbilliform drug eruption from viral exanthem in the ab-

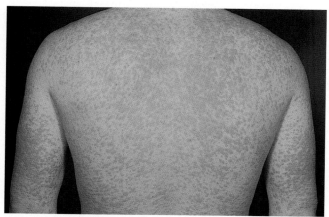

Clin. Fig. IIIA1a.a

Fig. IIIA1a.a

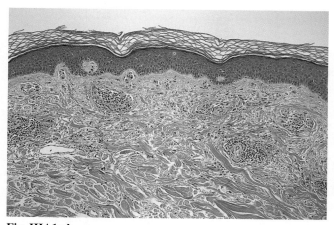

Fig. IIIA1a.b

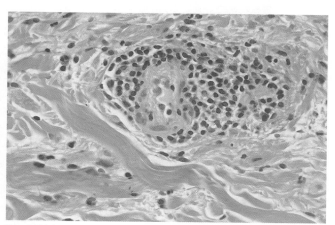

Fig. IIIA1a.c

Clin. Fig. IIIA1a.a. *Morbilliform exanthem (drug).* A teenaged boy abruptly developed a blanchable erythematous maculopapular exanthem with areas of confluence after several days of ampicillin therapy for a sore throat.

Fig. IIIA1a.a. *Allergic urticarial reaction, low power.* There is an orthokeratotic scale overlying an evenly acanthotic epidermis. The dermis shows a dense perivascular inflammatory infiltrate.

Fig. IIIA1a.b. *Allergic urticarial reaction, medium power.* There is an orthokeratotic scale overlying an evenly acanthotic epidermis. The papillary dermis is edematous with a dense infiltrate around thick-walled dermal vessels.

Fig. IIIA1a.c. *Allergic urticarial reaction, high power.* There is an inflammatory infiltrate around the dermal vessels composed of lymphocytes and eosinophils.

sence of eosinophils is generally not possible. More than occasional dyskeratotic epidermal cells should prompt consideration of erythema multiforme, toxic epidermal necrolysis, or fixed drug eruption.

Allergic Urticarial Reaction (Morbilliform Drug Eruption)

See Figs. IIIA1a.a–IIIA1a.c.

Urticaria

CLINICAL SUMMARY.   Urticaria is characterized by the presence of transient recurrent wheals, which are raised, and erythematous areas of edema usually accompanied by itching. When large wheals occur, in which the edema extends to the subcutaneous tissue, the process is referred to as an-

gioedema. Acute episodes of urticaria generally last only several hours. When episodes of urticaria last up to 24 hours and recur over a period of at least 6 weeks, the condition is considered chronic urticaria. Urticaria and angioedema may occur simultaneously, in which case the affliction tends to have a chronic course. In approximately 15% to 25% of patients with urticaria, an eliciting stimulus or underlying predisposing condition can be identified, including soluble antigens in foods, drugs, insect venom, and contact allergens; physical stimuli such as pressure, vibration, solar radiation, and cold temperature; occult infections and malignancies, and some hereditary syndromes.

HISTOPATHOLOGY.   In acute urticaria, one observes interstitial dermal edema, dilated venules with endothelial swelling, and a paucity of inflammatory cells. In chronic urticaria, in-

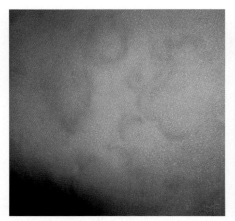

Clin. Fig. IIIA1a.b

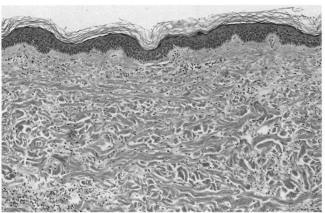

Fig. IIIA1a.d

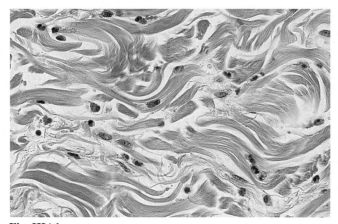

Fig. IIIA1a.e

Clin. Fig. IIIA1a.b. *Urticaria.* Large edematous plaques with central clearing and geographic configuration are typical of urticaria.

Fig. IIIA1a.d. *Urticaria, low power.* Sparse superficial perivascular and interstitial inflammatory infiltrate and separation of collagen bundles by edema fluid. (R. Barnhill and K. Busam)

Fig. IIIA1a.e. *Urticaria, high power.* Interstitial infiltrate of eosinophils, neutrophils and lymphocytes. (R. Barnhill and K. Busam)

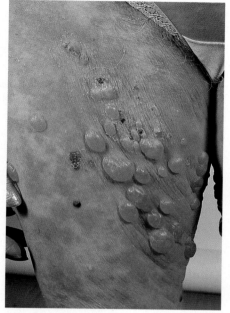

Clin. Fig. IIIA1a.c

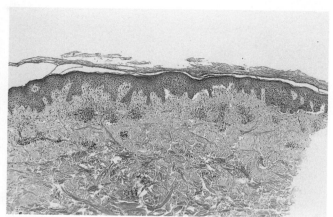

Fig. IIIA1a.f

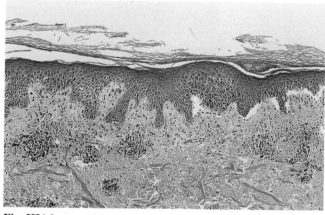

Fig. IIIA1a.g

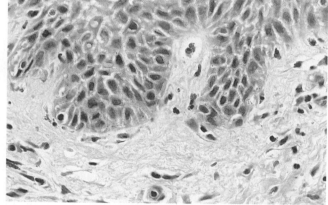

Fig. IIIA1a.h

Clin. Fig. IIIA1a.c. *Bullous pemphigoid, urticarial and early bullous phases.* Urticarial plaques on the thigh evolved into tense bullae.

Fig. IIIA1a.f. *Urticarial bullous pemphigoid, low power.* The features seen are those of an orthokeratotic scale overlying an epidermis that is acanthotic. There is edema of the papillary dermis with early dermal–epidermal separation. A perivascular infiltrate is seen around dermal vessels.

Fig. IIIA1a.g. *Urticarial bullous pemphigoid, medium power.* There is papillary dermal edema with dermal–epidermal separation and a diffuse and perivascular infiltrate of lymphocytes and eosinophils.

Fig. IIIA1a.h. *Urticarial bullous pemphigoid, high power.* The epidermis is spongiotic and in the edematous papillary dermis is an infiltrate of eosinophils and lymphocytes. Several eosinophils are exocytotic to the overlying spongiotic epidermis.

---

terstitial dermal edema and a perivascular and interstitial mixed-cell infiltrate with variable numbers of lymphocytes, eosinophils, and neutrophils are present. In angioedema, the edema and infiltrate extend into the subcutaneous tissue. In hereditary angioedema, there is subcutaneous and submucosal edema without infiltrating inflammatory cells.

Urticarial Bullous Pemphigoid

See Figs. IIIA1a.f–IIIA1a.h.

Conditions to consider in the differential diagnosis:
arthropod bite reaction
allergic urticarial reaction (drug)
bullous pemphigoid, urticarial phase

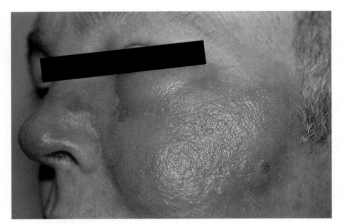

Clin. Fig. IIIA1b

Clin. Fig. IIIA1b. *Erysipelas*. This patient, a 51-year-old man, had fever, chills, and an expanding sharply marginated erythematous edematous plaque on the cheek.

Fig. IIIA1b.a. *Cellulitis, low power*. The dermis shows marked edema with separation of collagen bundles and a diffuse cellular infiltrate.

Fig. IIIA1b.b. *Cellulitis, medium power*. There is marked papillary dermal and reticular dermal edema and a diffuse infiltrate of lymphocytes and neutrophils and fragmented neutrophils.

Fig. IIIA1b.c. *Cellulitis, medium power*. In an edematous dermis that shows fragmentation of collagen, there is an infiltrate of lymphocytes with plasma cells and neutrophils.

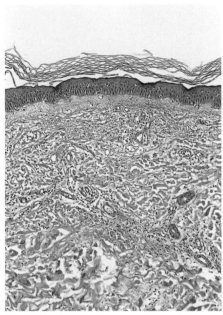

Fig. IIIA1b.a

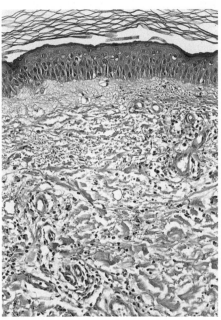

Fig. IIIA1b.b

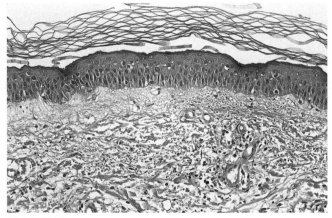

Fig. IIIA1b.c

urticaria
erythema toxicum neonatorum
Well's syndrome
mastocytosis/telangiectasia eruptiva macularis perstans
angiolymphoid hyperplasia with eosinophilia
Kimura's disease
Langerhans cell histiocytosis (early lesions)

IIIA1b. Superficial Perivascular Dermatitis with Neutrophils

In addition to lymphocytes, neutrophils are present in varying numbers, with both a perivascular and interstitial distribution. *Cellulitis and erysipelas* are prototypic (see also section VC2).

Erysipelas

CLINICAL SUMMARY. Erysipelas is an acute superficial cellulitis of the skin caused by group A streptococci (5). It is characterized by the presence of a well-demarcated, slightly indurated, dusky red area with an advancing palpable border. In some patients, erysipelas has a tendency to recur periodically in the same areas. In the early antibiotic era, the incidence of erysipelas appeared to be on the decline and most cases occurred on the face. More recently, however, there appears to be an increase in the incidence, and facial sites are now less common, whereas erysipelas of the legs is predominant. Potential complications in patients with poor resistance or after inadequate therapy may include abscess formation, spreading necrosis of the soft tissue, infrequently necrotizing fasciitis, and septicemia. Erysipelas is usually produced by nonnephritogenic and nonrheumatogenic strains of streptococci.

HISTOPATHOLOGY. The dermis shows marked edema and dilatation of the lymphatics and capillaries. There is a diffuse infiltrate, composed chiefly of neutrophils, that extends throughout the dermis and occasionally into the subcutaneous fat. It shows a loose arrangement around dilated blood and lymph vessels. This pattern may be descriptively termed "cellulitis" and is not diagnostic of erysipelas per se. In erysipelas, streptococci may be found in the tissue and within lymphatics in sections stained with the Giemsa or Gram stain.

Erysipelas/Cellulitis

See Figs. IIIA1b.a–IIIA1b.c.
Conditions to consider in the differential diagnosis:
cellulitis
erysipelas

IIIA1c. Superficial Perivascular Dermatitis with Plasma Cells

Plasma cells are seen around the dermal vessels and in the interstitium. They are most often admixed with lymphocytes. *Secondary syphilis* is the prototype.

Secondary Syphilis

CLINICAL SUMMARY. Secondary syphilis (6) is typically characterized by a generalized eruption comprised of brown-red macules and papules, papulosquamous lesions resembling guttate psoriasis, and, rarely, pustules. Lesions may be follicular based, annular, or serpiginous, particularly in recurrent attacks. Other skin signs include alopecia and condylomata lata, the latter comprising broad, raised, gray, confluent papular lesions arising in anogenital areas, pitted hyperkeratotic palmoplantar papules termed "syphilis cornee," and, in rare severe cases, ulcerating lesions that define "lues maligna." Some patients develop mucous patches composed of multiple shallow, painless ulcers.

HISTOPATHOLOGY. The two fundamental pathologic changes in syphilis are swelling and proliferation of endothelial cells, and a predominantly perivascular infiltrate composed of lymphoid cells and often plasma cells. In late secondary and tertiary syphilis, there are also granulomatous infiltrates of epithelioid histiocytes and giant cells. Biopsies generally reveal varying degrees of psoriasiform hyperplasia of the epidermis with variable spongiosis and basilar vacuolar alteration. Exocytosis of lymphocytes, spongiform pustulation, and parakeratosis also may be observed, with or without intracorneal neutrophilic abscesses. Scattered necrotic keratinocytes may be observed. The dermal changes include variable papillary dermal edema and a perivascular and/or periadnexal infiltrate that usually includes plasma cells and may be lymphocyte predominant, lymphohistiocytic, histiocytic predominant, or frankly granulomatous, and that is of greatest intensity in the papillary dermis and extends as loose perivascular aggregates into the reticular dermis. Vascular changes such as endothelial swelling and mural edema accompany the angiocentric infiltrates in about half of the cases. A silver stain shows the presence of spirochetes in about a third of the cases, mainly within the epidermis and less commonly around the blood vessels of the superficial plexus. Lesions of condylomata lata show all of the aforementioned changes observed in macular, papular, and papulosquamous lesions, but more florid epithelial hyperplasia and intraepithelial microabscess formation are observed. A silver stain shows numerous treponemes. In addition to small sarcoidal granulomata in papular lesions of early secondary syphilis, late secondary syphilis may show extensive lymphoplasmacellular and histiocytic infiltrates resembling nodular tertiary syphilis (see Figs. IIIA1c.a and IIIA1c.b).

Kaposi's Sarcoma, Patch Stage

See Figs. IIIA1c.d and IIIA1c.e.
Conditions to consider in the differential diagnosis:
secondary syphilis
arthropod bite reaction
Kaposi's sarcoma, nonspecific patch stage
actinic keratoses and Bowen's disease
Zoon's plasma cell balanitis circumscripta
erythroplasia of Queyrat

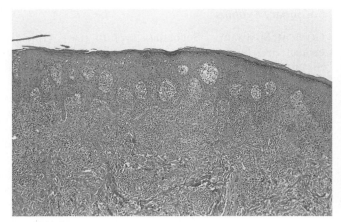

Fig. IIIA1c.a

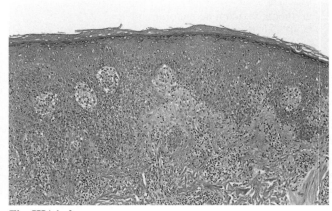

Fig. IIIA1c.b

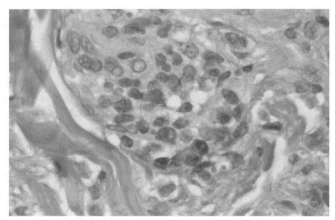

Fig. IIIA1c.c

Fig. IIIA1c.a. *Secondary syphilis, low power.* There is a thin keratin scale overlying an acanthotic epidermis. The papillary dermis is edematous. There is an infiltrate at the dermal–epidermal interface and around the superficial dermal vessels.

Fig. IIIA1c.b. *Secondary syphilis, medium power.* Marked exocytosis of mononuclear cells into an acanthotic epidermis. The papillary dermis is edematous and there is a dense collection of cells about dermal vessels.

Fig. IIIA1c.c. *Secondary syphilis, high power.* The inflammatory infiltrate in the dermis is composed of plasma cells, lymphocytes, and histiocytes.

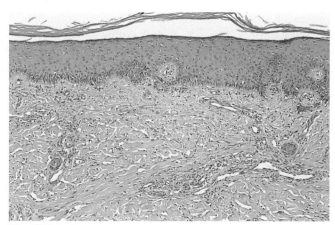

Fig. IIIA1c.d

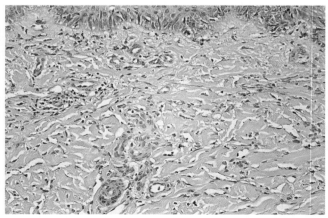

Fig. IIIA1c.e

Fig. IIIA1c.d. *Kaposi's sarcoma, patch stage, medium power.* The epidermis is effaced and shows basal layer pigmentation. In the dermis there is hemorrhage with a scattered mononuclear cell infiltrate around thin-walled blood vessels.

Fig. IIIA1c.e. *Kaposi's sarcoma, patch stage, medium power.* The dermis shows ill-defined, jagged, thin-walled vessels with hemorrhage and a mononuclear cell infiltrate. *(continues)*

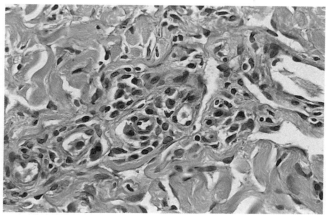

Fig. IIIA1c.f

Fig. IIIA1c.f. *Kaposi's sarcoma, patch stage, high power.* The infiltrate around the dermal vessels includes lymphocytes and plasma cells.

IIIA1d. Superficial Perivascular Dermatitis with Extravasated Red Cells

A perivascular lymphocytic infiltrate is associated with extravasation of lymphocytes without fibrinoid necrosis of vessels. *Pityriasis rosea* and PLEVA are prototypic.

Pityriasis Rosea

CLINICAL SUMMARY. Pityriasis rosea (7) is a self-limited dermatitis lasting from 4 to 7 weeks. It frequently starts with the larger herald patch followed by a disseminated eruption. The lesions, found chiefly on the trunk, neck, and proximal extremities, consist of round to oval salmon-colored patches following the lines of cleavage and showing peripherally attached, thin, cigarette paper-like scales. Several typical and atypical clinical variants have been described, including papular, vesicular, urticarial, purpuric, and recurrent forms.

HISTOPATHOLOGY. The patches of the disseminated eruption show a superficial perivascular infiltrate in the dermis that consists predominantly of lymphocytes, with occasional eosinophils and histiocytes. Lymphocytes extend into the epidermis (exocytosis), where there are spongiosis, intracellular edema, mild to moderate acanthosis, areas of decreased or absent granular layer, and focal parakeratosis with or without plasma cells. Intraepidermal spongiotic vesicles and a few necrotic keratinocytes are found in some cases. A common feature is the presence of extravasated erythrocytes in the papillary dermis, which sometimes extends into the overlying epidermis. Occasionally, multinucleated keratinocytes can be seen in the affected epidermis. Late lesions from the disseminated eruption are more likely to have a psoriasiform or lichen planus-like appearance and a relatively increased

number of eosinophils in the inflammatory infiltrate (see Figs. IIIA1d.a–IIIA1d.c).

Pityriasis Lichenoides

CLINICAL SUMMARY. Pityriasis lichenoides is an uncommon cutaneous eruption usually classified in two forms that differ in severity. The milder form, called *pityriasis lichenoides chronica*, is characterized by recurrent crops of brown-red papules 4 to 10 mm in size, mainly on the trunk and extremities, that are covered with a scale and generally involute within 3 to 6 weeks with postinflammatory pigmentary changes. The more severe form, called *PLEVA* or *Mucha–Habermann disease*, consists of a fairly extensive eruption present mainly on the trunk and proximal extremities. It is characterized by erythematous papules that develop into papulonecrotic, occasionally hemorrhagic, or vesiculopustular lesions that resolve within a few weeks, usually with little or no scarring (see also section VB2).

HISTOPATHOLOGY. In pityriasis lichenoides chronica, there is a superficial perivascular infiltrate composed of lymphocytes that extend into the epidermis, where there is vacuolar alteration of the basal layer, mild spongiosis, a few necrotic keratinocytes, and confluent parakeratosis. Melanophages and small numbers of extravasated erythrocytes are commonly seen in the papillary dermis. In PLEVA, the more severe form, the perivascular (predominantly lymphocytic) infiltrate is dense in the papillary dermis and extends into the reticular dermis in a wedge-shaped pattern. The infiltrate obscures the dermal–epidermal junction with pronounced vacuolar alteration of the basal layer, marked exocytosis of lymphocytes and erythrocytes, and intercellular and intracellular edema leading to a variable degree of epidermal necrosis. Ultimately, erosion or even ulceration may occur. The overlying cornified layer shows parakeratosis and a scaly crust with neutrophils in the more severe cases. Variable degrees of papillary dermal edema, endothelial swelling, and extravasated erythrocytes are seen in most cases (see Figs. IIIA1d.d–IIIA1d.e).

Pigmented Purpuric Dermatosis

CLINICAL SUMMARY. Although several variants of purpura pigmentosa chronica have been described, they are all closely related and often cannot be reliably distinguished on clinical and histologic grounds. Clinically, the primary lesion consists of discrete puncta often limited to the lower extremities. Gradually, telangiectatic puncta appear as a result of capillary dilatation and pigmentation as a result of hemosiderin deposits. In some cases, the findings may mimic those of stasis. Not infrequently, clinical signs of inflammation are present, such as erythema, papules, scaling, and lichenification. There are no systemic symptoms related to this disease process.

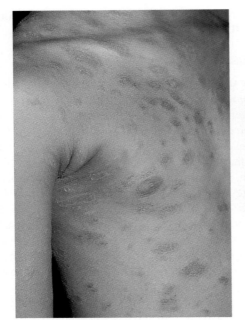

Clin. Fig. IIIA1d.a

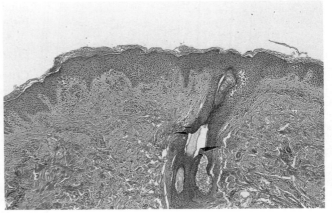

Fig. IIIA1d.a

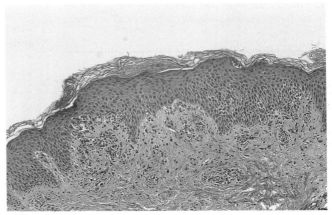

Fig. IIIA1d.b

Clin. Fig. IIIA1d.a. *Pityriasis rosea.* Oval brown patches following the lines of cleavage that may show peripheral thin scales.

Fig. IIIA1d.a. *Pityriasis rosea, low power.* There is an ortho- and parakeratotic scale overlying an epidermis that is acanthotic and spongiotic. The papillary dermis is edematous and contains an infiltrate of lymphocytes and red blood cells. This inflammatory infiltrate is seen around dermal vessels.

Fig. IIIA1d.b. *Pityriasis rosea, medium power.* The dermal papillae are widened, edematous, and contain an infiltrate of lymphocytes and red blood cells.

Fig. IIIA1d.c. *Pityriasis rosea, high power.* The edematous papillary dermis is hemorrhagic. There is exocytosis of mononuclear cells and red blood cells into the acanthotic spongiotic epidermis. The ortho- and parakeratotic scale forms characteristic small mounds of parakeratosis.

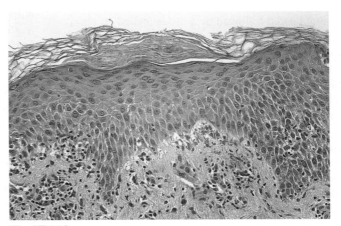

Fig. IIIA1d.c

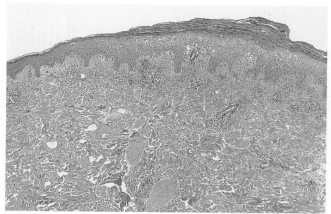

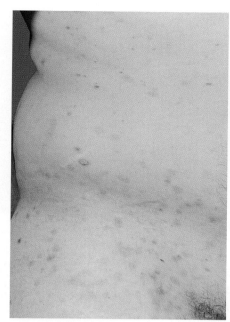

Fig. IIIA1d.d

Clin. Fig. IIIA1d.b

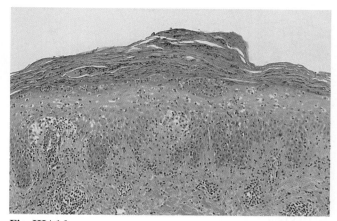

Fig. IIIA1d.e

Clin. Fig. IIIA1d.b. *Pityriasis lichenoides et varioliformis acuta (PLEVA).* Erythematous papules and papu-lonecrotic lesions developed suddenly on the trunk of a young man.

Fig. IIIA1d.d. *Pityriasis lichenoides et varioliformis acuta (PLEVA), low power.* Lichenoid inflammatory pattern with a superficial and mid dermal perivascular inflammatory infiltrate. (H. Kamino and S. Toussaint)

Fig. IIIA.1d.e. *Pityriasis lichenoides et varioliformis acuta (PLEVA), medium power.* Closer view reveals lichenoid inflammation with an infiltrate of lymphocytes, extravasated erythrocytes, irregular acanthosis, pallor of the upper layers of the epidermis, spongiosis, necrotic keratinocytes, and confluent mounds of parakeratosis with plasma, neutrophils, and lymphocytes. (H. Kamino and S. Toussaint)

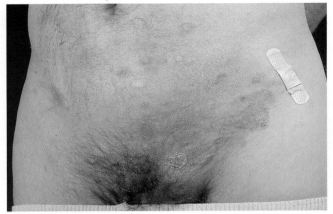

Clin. Fig. IIIA1d.c

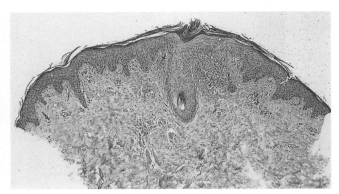

Fig. IIIA1d.f

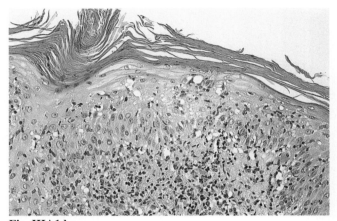

Fig. IIIA1d.g

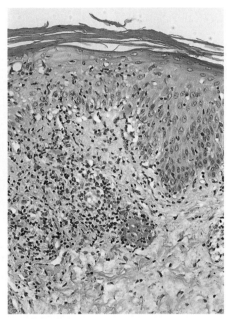

Fig. IIIA1d.h

Clin. Fig. IIIA1d.c. *Pityriasis lichenoides chronica.* A 29-year-old man gave an 8-month history of asymptomatic dully erythematous macules and papules with light scale on the trunk and extremities.

Fig. IIIA1d.f. *Pityriasis lichenoides chronica, low power.* A focal lesion characterized by hyperkeratosis and a lichenoid inflammatory infiltrate.

Fig. IIIA1d.g. *Pityriasis lichenoides chronica, medium power.* There is hyperkeratosis without the scale-crust or frank necrosis that may be seen in lesions of pityriasis lichenoides et varioliformis acuta (PLEVA).

Fig. IIIA1d.h. *Pityriasis lichenoides chronica, high power.* There is vacuolar alteration of the basal layer, with mild spongiosis and a few necrotic keratinocytes in the epidermis. In addition to lymphocytes, a few extravasated erythrocytes are present in the papillary dermis.

HISTOPATHOLOGY. The basic process is a lymphocytic perivascular infiltrate limited to the papillary dermis. In some instances, the infiltrate may assume a bandlike or lichenoid pattern and may involve the reticular dermis in a perivascular distribution. Evidence of vascular damage may be present. The extent of vascular injury is usually mild and insufficient to justify the term "vasculitis," commonly consisting only of endothelial cell swelling and dermal hemorrhage. Extravasated red blood cells are usually found in the vicinity of the capillaries. In old lesions, the capillaries often show dilatation of their lumen and proliferation of their endothelium. Extravasated red blood cells may no longer be

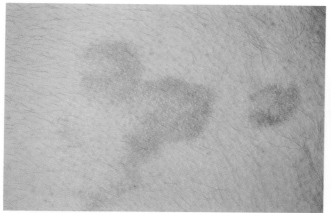

Clin. Fig. IIIA1d.d

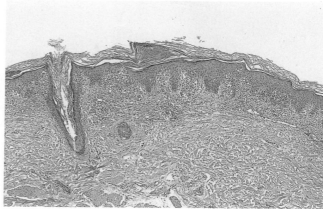

Fig. IIIA1d.i

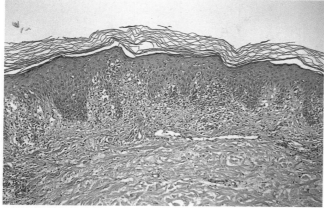

Fig. IIIA1d.j

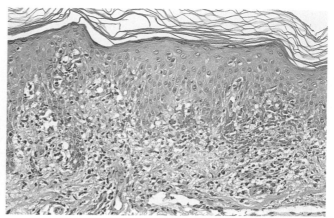

Fig. IIIA1d.k

Clin. Fig. IIIA1d.d. *Pigmented purpuric dermatosis (Gougerot–Blum).* A 15-year-old boy developed asymptomatic nonblanching orange-brown and erythematous lichenoid papules on the lower extremities.

Fig. IIIA1d.i. *Pigmented purpuric dermatosis, low power.* An ortho- and parakeratotic scale are present overlying an acanthotic epidermis. There is an inflammatory infiltrate in the papillary dermis. Hemorrhage is seen within the papillary dermis.

Fig. IIIA1d.j. *Pigmented purpuric dermatosis, medium power.* The papillary dermis shows hemorrhage and a mononuclear cell infiltrate. There is superficial telangiectasia.

Fig. IIIA1d.k. *Pigmented purpuric dermatosis, high power.* The epidermis is acanthotic and shows exocytosis of lymphocytes and red blood cells. There is significant hemorrhage in the papillary dermis.

present, but one frequently finds hemosiderin, in varying amounts. The inflammatory infiltrate is less pronounced than in the early stage.

Conditions to consider in the differential diagnosis:

pityriasis rosea
lupus erythematosus, subacute
lupus erythematosus, acute
postinflammatory hyperpigmentation
stasis dermatitis
Kaposi's sarcoma, patch stage
PLEVA
pityriasis lichenoides chronica
pigmented purpuric dermatoses (Gougerot–Blum)

IIIA1e. Superficial Perivascular Dermatitis, Melanophages Prominent

There is a perivascular infiltrate of lymphocytes, with an admixture of pigment-laden melanophages, indicative of prior damage to the basal layer and "pigmentary incontinence." Some degree of residual interface damage may also be evident. *Postinflammatory hyperpigmentation* is a prototype.

Postinflammatory Hyperpigmentation

CLINICAL SUMMARY. Postinflammatory hyperpigmentation may follow any dermatitis that affects the dermal–epidermal junction and results in release of melanin pigment from basal

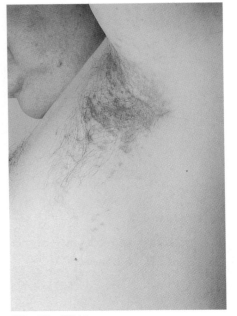

Clin. Fig. IIIA1e

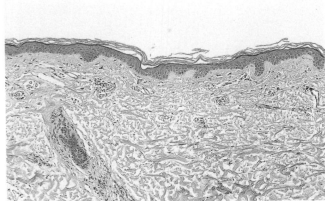

Fig. IIIA1e.a

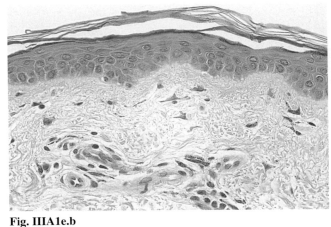

Fig. IIIA1e.b

Fig. IIIA1e.c

Clin. Fig. IIIA1e. *Postinflammatory hyperpigmentation.* A 77-year-old man presented with macular brown changes in sites of previous lichen planus.

Fig. IIIA1e.a. *Postinflammatory hyperpigmentation, low power.* The dermis is edematous and there is an inflammatory infiltrate of lymphocytes and melanophages.

Fig. IIIA1e.b. *Postinflammatory hyperpigmentation, high power.* There is an orthokeratotic scale overlying an epidermis that shows distinct patchy basal layer pigmentation. In the dermis there are melanophages containing brown pigment granules. Around the dermal vessels is a mononuclear cell infiltrate.

Fig. IIIA1e.c. *Postinflammatory hyperpigmentation, high power.* The edematous papillary dermis shows melanophage pigmentation with mononuclear cells around the dermal vessels. Scattered apoptotic cells are present, indicative of a low-grade process resulting in release of pigment from damaged keratinocytes.

---

keratinocytes into the dermis. Lichenoid dermatoses such as lichen planus, vacuolar dermatoses such as discoid lupus, or apoptotic/cytotoxic dermatoses such as erythema multiforme or fixed drug eruptions may all result in this reaction pattern. Lesions are sometimes biopsied to rule out melanoma. If features diagnostic of a specific underlying dermatosis are lacking in the biopsy, the descriptive diagnosis of postinflammatory hyperpigmentation may be all that can be made.

HISTOPATHOLOGY. Sections show the phenomena of pigmentary incontinence. Melanin pigment deposited in the dermis is taken up by melanophages. These are large cells with abundant cytoplasm stuffed with pigment and with plump nuclei having open chromatin and sometimes a small nucleolus.

Conditions to consider in the differential diagnosis:

postinflammatory hyperpigmentation
postchemotherapy hyperpigmentation

chlorpromazine pigmentation
amyloidosis

IIIA2. Superficial Perivascular Dermatitis, Mast Cells Predominant

Mast cells are the main infiltrating cells seen in the dermis. Lymphocytes are also present, and there may be a few eosinophils. *Urticaria pigmentosa* is the example.

Urticaria Pigmentosa

CLINICAL SUMMARY. Urticaria pigmentosa (8) can be divided into four forms: urticaria pigmentosa arising in infancy or early childhood without significant systemic lesions, urticaria pigmentosa arising in adolescence or adult life without significant systemic lesions, systemic mast cell disease, and mast cell leukemia. Five types of cutaneous lesions are seen. The maculopapular type, which is the most common, consists usually of dozens or even hundreds of small brown lesions that urticate on stroking; a second type exhibits multiple brown nodules or plaques and, on stroking, shows urtication and occasionally blister formation. A third type, seen almost exclusively in infants, is characterized by a usually solitary large cutaneous nodule, which on stroking often shows not only urtication but also large bullae. The fourth type, the diffuse erythrodermic type, always starts in early infancy and shows generalized brownish-red soft infiltration of the skin, with urtication on stroking. The fifth type, telangiectasia macularis eruptiva perstans (TMEP), which

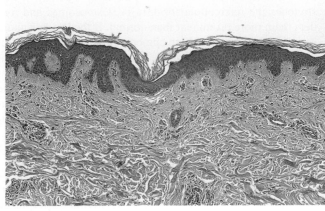

Clin. Fig. IIIA2.a

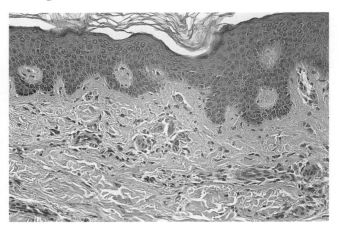

Clin. Fig. IIIA2.b

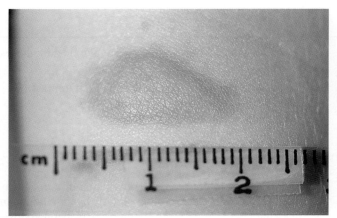

Fig. IIIA2.a

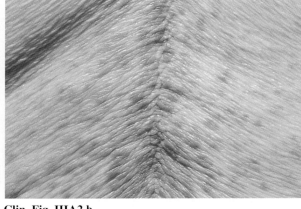

Fig. IIIA2.b

Clin. Fig. IIIA2.a. *Urticaria pigmentosa, nodular* type. A 2 year old had a recurrently erythematous and "swollen" solitary 2-cm yellow-brown nodule on the volar forearm.

Clin. Fig. IIIA2.b. *Telangiectasia macularis eruptive perstans.* A 78-year-old woman with 2-year history of telangiectatic erythematous blanching macules on the trunk, neck, and thighs. Darier's sign (urtication after stroking) was positive.

Fig. IIIA2.a. *Adult mast cell disease (TMEP), low power.* The epidermis is acanthotic with distinct basal layer pigmentation. There is a perivascular infiltrate of mononuclear cells around dermal vessels.

Fig. IIIA2.b. *Adult mast cell disease, medium power.* The epidermis is acanthotic with basal layer pigmentation. There is, in the dermis, a diffuse and perivascular infiltrate of lymphocytes and mast cells. *(continues)*

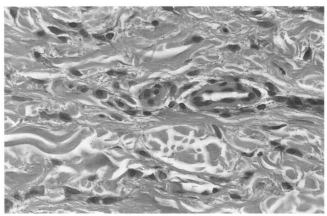

Fig. IIIA2.c

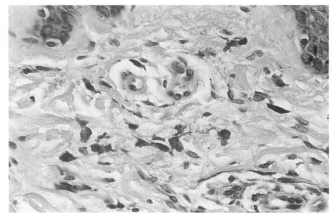

Fig. IIIA2.d

Fig. IIIA2.c. *Adult mast cell disease, high power.* Mast cells are seen around the thick-walled dermal vessels.

Fig. IIIA2.d. *Adult mast cell disease, high power, Giemsa stain.* Large mast cells containing metachromatic granules are seen in the dermis and around dermal vessels.

usually occurs in adults, consists of an extensive eruption of brownish-red macules showing fine telangiectasias, with little or no urtication on stroking.

HISTOPATHOLOGY. In all five types of lesions, the histologic picture shows an infiltrate composed chiefly of mast cells, which are characterized by the presence of metachromatic granules in their cytoplasm. These granules can be visualized with a Giemsa or toluidine blue stain or with the naphthol AS-D chloroacetate esterase reaction (Leder stain). In the maculopapular type and in telangiectasia macularis eruptiva perstans, the mast cells are limited to the upper third of the dermis and are generally located around capillaries. In some mast cells, the nuclei may be round or oval, but in most, they are spindle shaped. The diagnosis may be missed unless special staining is used. In cases with multiple nodules or plaques or with a solitary large nodule, the mast cells lie closely packed in tumorlike aggregates and the infiltrate may extend into the subcutaneous fat. In the diffuse erythrodermic type, there is a dense bandlike infiltrate of mast cells in the upper dermis. Eosinophils may be present in small numbers in all types of urticaria pigmentosa with the exception of TMEP, in which eosinophils are generally absent because of the small numbers of mast cells within the lesions.

Conditions to consider in the differential diagnosis:

urticaria pigmentosa, nodular type
TMEP, adult mast cell disease

IIIB. SUPERFICIAL DERMATITIS WITH SPONGIOSIS (SPONGIOTIC DERMATITIS)

Spongiotic dermatitis is characterized by intercellular edema in the epidermis. In mild or early lesions, the intercellular space is increased with stretching of desmosomes, but the integrity of the epithelium is intact. In more severe spongiotic conditions, there is separation of keratinocytes to form spaces (vesicles). For this reason, the spongiotic dermatoses are also listed in Chapter IV.

1. Spongiotic Dermatitis, Lymphocytes Predominant
1a. Spongiotic Dermatitis, with Eosinophils
1b. Spongiotic Dermatitis, with Plasma Cells
1c. Spongiotic Dermatitis, with Neutrophils

Acute Spongiotic Dermatitis

In acute spongiotic dermatitis (9), the stratum corneum is normal in a very early lesion, but is slightly hyperkeratotic in a somewhat later lesion. If the lesion persists, parakeratosis develops as it evolves further. The epidermal keratinocytes are partially separated by intercellular edema, which stretches the intercellular bridges or desmosomes and renders them more prominent than normal. If the lesion is more severe, the desmosomal attachments rupture and intercellular spaces appear, usually in the spinous layer, forming spongiotic vesicles. Lymphocytes and occasionally larger Langerhans histiocytes are present in the spaces and in the edematous epidermis. In addition, there is a loose perivascular infiltrate around the vessels of the superficial capillary–venular plexus.

Subacute Spongiotic Dermatitis

In subacute spongiotic dermatitis, after several days of a persistent spongiotic lesion, there is epithelial hyperplasia, which tends to elongate the rete ridges in a pattern that is termed "psoriasiform." Unlike in psoriasis, the suprapapillary plates of keratinocytes are not thinned; in fact, they tend to be somewhat thickened. The etiology of the process is made apparent by the presence of spongiotic changes in the epidermis similar to those described above, although vesicle formation is often minimal. A similar perivascular infiltrate is present in the superficial dermis. Because the pattern of subacute spongiotic dermatitis is predominantly psoriasiform, these conditions are also discussed in section IIID.

Chronic Spongiotic Dermatitis

In chronic spongiotic dermatitis, there is prominent hyperkeratosis and parakeratosis. Spongiosis is usually present but may be quite inconspicuous in a given biopsy. Psoriasiform hyperplasia is prominent and when florid and complex may border on pseudoepitheliomatous hyperplasia. A perivascular lymphocytic infiltrate is present and may include an admixture of histiocytes and even plasma cells, depending on the etiology of the condition. There is often a distinctive pattern of increased collagen fibers arranged vertically between the elongated rete ridges. This papillary dermis sclerosis may be attributable to chronic rubbing or scratching of the lesions, resulting in the condition termed lichen simplex chronicus, which may have as its underlying basis any of the chronic pruritic dermatoses.

The disorders listed below all tend to follow the course listed above, from an acute to a subacute to a chronic spongiotic dermatitis, if the condition persists, and depending on associated factors, such as the severity of the condition, the effects of treatment, and the effects of added irritants, including the presence or thickening of excoriations as a result of chronic rubbing and scratching. The differential diagnosis suggested by a given biopsy specimen may vary to some extent as discussed below, depending, for example, on the admixture of cell types such as eosinophils or plasma cells and on the patterns of hyperkeratosis and parakeratosis, of psoriasiform epidermal hyperplasia, and of papillary dermis sclerosis. However, it is often difficult or impossible to distinguish among the various etiologic categories of spongiotic dermatitis in a given biopsy. Although a biopsy may be of value to rule out other competing possibilities, such as lymphoma, and may tend to favor one or another of the possibilities listed in the differential diagnosis tables, the exact classification of these disorders usually depends on clinicopathologic correlation.

IIIB1. Spongiotic Dermatitis, Lymphocytes Predominant

There is marked intercellular edema (spongiosis) within the epidermis. In the dermis, perivascular lymphocytes are predominant. *Nummular dermatitis* is prototypic.

Nummular Dermatitis (Eczema)

CLINICAL SUMMARY. The eruption is characterized by pruritic, coin-shaped (nummular), erythematous, scaly, crusted plaques. The lesions tend to develop on the extensor surfaces of the extremities.

HISTOPATHOLOGY. Nummular dermatitis is the prototype of subacute spongiotic dermatitis. There is mild to moderate spongiosis, usually without vesiculation, and a superficial perivascular infiltrate composed of lymphocytes, histio-

cytes, and occasional eosinophils. The epidermis is moderately acanthotic and parakeratotic. The stratum corneum contains aggregates of coagulated plasma and scattered neutrophils, forming a crust. Mild papillary dermal edema and vascular dilatation may be present.

Eczematous Dermatitis

Conditions to consider in the differential diagnosis:

    eczematous dermatitis
    atopic dermatitis
    allergic contact dermatitis
    photoallergic drug eruption
    irritant contact dermatitis
    nummular eczema
    dyshidrotic dermatitis
    parapsoriasis, small plaque type (digitate dermatosis)
    polymorphous light eruption
    lichen striatus
    chronic actinic dermatitis (actinic reticuloid)
    actinic prurigo, early lesions
    "id" reaction
    seborrheic dermatitis
    stasis dermatitis
    erythroderma
    miliaria
    pityriasis rosea
    Sezary syndrome
    papular acrodermatitis (Gianotti–Crosti)

IIIB1a. Spongiotic Dermatitis, with Eosinophils

There is marked intercellular edema (spongiosis) within the epidermis. In the dermis, lymphocytes are predominant. Eosinophils can be found in most examples of atopy and allergic contact dermatitis and are numerous in incontinentia pigmenti. *Allergic contact dermatitis* is the prototype.

Allergic Contact Dermatitis

CLINICAL SUMMARY. The prototype of acute spongiotic dermatitis is allergic contact dermatitis, for example, that secondary to exposure to poison ivy. Usually between 24 and 72 hours after exposure to the antigen, the patient develops pruritic, edematous, erythematous papules and plaques and, in some cases, vesicles. Linear papules and vesicles are common in allergic contact dermatitis to poison ivy, reflecting the points of contact between the plant and the skin.

HISTOPATHOLOGY. Early lesions are an acute spongiotic dermatitis. If vesicles develop, they may contain clusters of Langerhans cells. Eosinophils may be present in the dermal infiltrate and within areas of spongiosis. In patients with con-

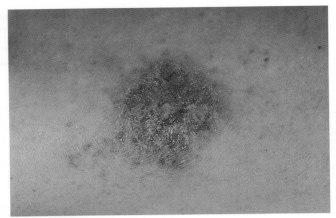

Clin. Fig. IIIB1

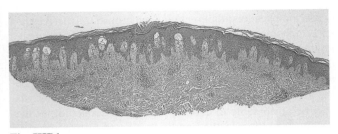

Fig. IIIB1.a

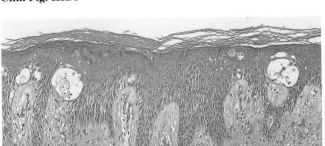

Fig. IIIB1.b

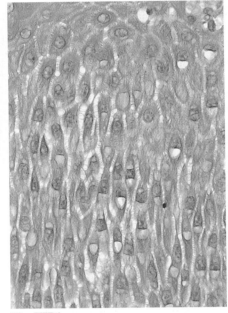

Fig. IIIB1.c

Clin. Fig. IIIB1. *Nummular eczema.* A crusted coin-shaped plaque with serous exudate on the extensor surface of the lower extremity typifies this pruritic episodic condition.

Fig. IIIB1.a. *Subacute spongiotic dermatitis, low power.* There is a keratotic scale overlying an acanthotic epidermis. In the dermis there is a perivascular mononuclear cell infiltrate.

Fig. IIIB1.b. *Subacute spongiotic dermatitis, medium power.* The epidermis is acanthotic and spongiotic. The papillary dermis shows an infiltrate of lymphocytes around superficial dermal vessels.

Fig. IIIB1.c. *Subacute spongiotic dermatitis, high power.* The epidermal keratinocytes are partially separated by edema (spongiosis), stretching the intercellular desmosomes.

tinued exposure to the antigen, the biopsy may show a subacute or later a chronic spongiotic dermatitis, often lichen simplex chronicus due to rubbing.

Conditions to consider in the differential diagnosis:

spongiotic (eczematous) dermatitis
atopic dermatitis

allergic contact dermatitis
photoallergic drug eruption
incontinentia pigmenti, vesicular stage
eczematous nevus (Meyerson's nevus)
erythema gyratum repens
scabies
erythema toxicum neonatorum

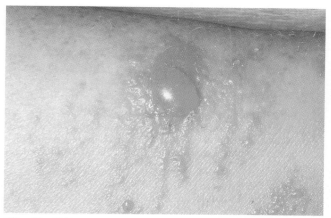

Clin. Fig. IIIB1a.a

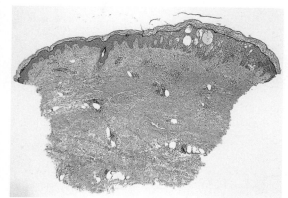

Fig. IIIB1a.a

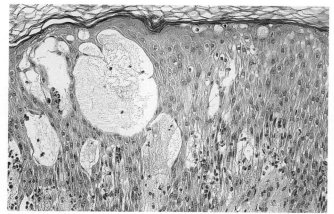

Fig. IIIB1a.b

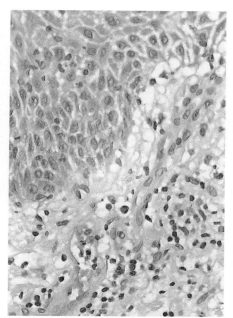

Fig. IIIB1a.c

Clin. Fig. IIIB1a.a. *Allergic contact dermatitis.* Vesicles and bullae developed on volar forearm after application of perfume.

Fig. IIIB1a.a. *Acute allergic contact dermatitis, low power.* The stratum corneum consists of normal basket-weave keratin, indicative of an acute disorder that has not had time to elicit alterations in the pattern of keratinization. The epidermis is thickened by spongiosis and exocytosis, with prominent vesicle formation. A dense infiltrate of mononuclear cells is seen around dermal vessels.

Fig. IIIB1a.b. *Acute allergic contact dermatitis, high power.* Tense spongiotic vesicles are formed by the confluence of spongiotic intercellular edema.

Fig. IIIB1a.c. *Acute allergic contact dermatitis, high power.* The papillary dermis is edematous and contains a diffuse infiltrate of lymphocytes and eosinophils.

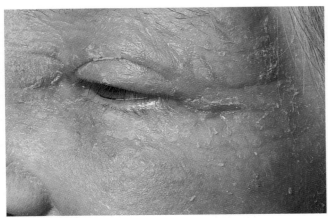

Clin. Fig. IIIB1a.b

Clin. Fig. IIIB1a.b. *Subacute contact dermatitis.* Elderly woman had several-month history of pruritic scaly facial erythema and positive fragrance mix patch test.

Fig. IIIB1a.d. *Subacute allergic contact dermatitis, low power.* The stratum corneum is altered by compact orthokeratosis. The epidermis is thickened by mild spongiotic edema and by early acanthosis.

Fig. IIIB1a.e. *Subacute allergic contact dermatitis, medium power.* There is a focal scale-crust in the superficial epidermis, the site of a several-day-old vesicle. The epidermis is spongiotic. There is an inflammatory infiltrate in the edematous papillary dermis.

Fig. IIIB1a.f. *Subacute allergic contact dermatitis, medium power.* The epidermis shows spongiosis. The papillary dermis is edematous and has an infiltrate of lymphocytes and eosinophils diffusely and around dermal vessels.

Fig. IIIB1a.g. *Subacute allergic contact dermatitis, high power.* There is a parakeratotic scale overlying a spongiotic epidermis that shows exocytosis of an eosinophil.

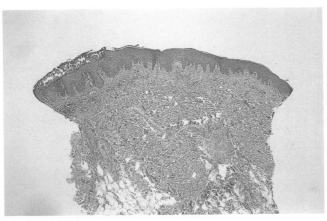

Fig. IIIB1a.d

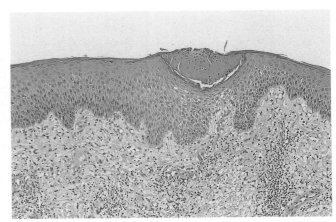

Fig. IIIB1a.e

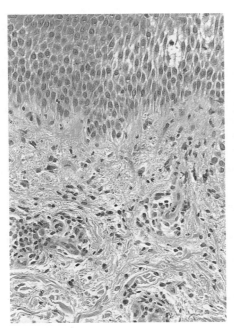

Fig. IIIB1a.f

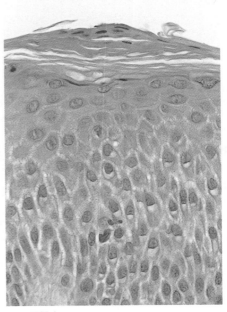

Fig. IIIB1a.g

IIIB1b. Spongiotic Dermatitis, with Plasma Cells

There is marked intercellular edema (spongiosis) within the epidermis. In the dermis, perivascular lymphocytes are predominant and plasma cells are present. Syphilis is the prototype (see Fig. IIIA1c.a).

Conditions to consider in the differential diagnosis:

syphilis, primary or secondary lesions
pinta, primary or secondary lesions
seborrheic dermatitis in HIV

IIIB1c. Spongiotic Dermatitis, with Neutrophils

There is marked intercellular edema (spongiosis) within the epidermis. Lymphocytes are present in the dermis. There is focal and shoulder parakeratosis, with a few neutrophils in the stratum corneum. *Seborrheic dermatitis* is a prototype (10).

Seborrheic Dermatitis

CLINICAL SUMMARY. Clinically, patients develop erythema and greasy scale on the scalp, paranasal areas, eyebrows, nasolabial folds, and central chest. Rarely, patients with seborrheic dermatitis develop generalized lesions. Patients with HIV infection often have severe recalcitrant disease. In infants, the scalp ("cradle cap"), face, and diaper areas are often involved.

HISTOPATHOLOGY. The histopathologic features are a combination of those observed in psoriasis and spongiotic dermatitis.

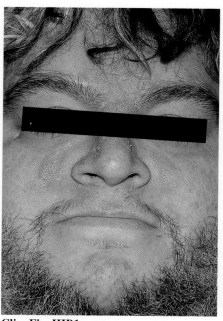

Clin. Fig. IIIB1c

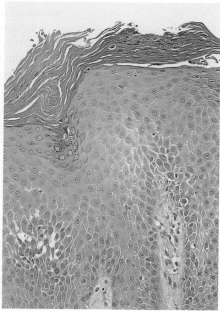

Fig. IIIB1c.a

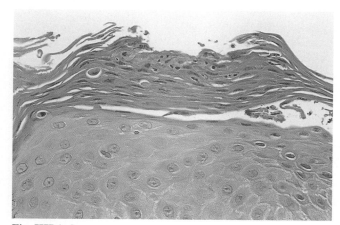

Fig. IIIB1c.b

Clin. Fig. IIIB1c. *Seborrheic dermatitis.* Greasy erythema involving the nasolabial folds, glabella, medial eyebrows, and chin characterize this persistent noninfectious condition.

Fig. IIIB1c.a. *Seborrheic dermatitis, medium power.* An ortho- and parakeratotic scale overlies an acanthotic epidermis that also has spongiosis and exocytosis.

Fig. IIIB1c.b. *Seborrheic dermatitis, high power.* Fragments of polymorphonuclear leukocytes are seen within the keratotic scale overlying an acanthotic epidermis.

Mild cases may exhibit only a slight subacute spongiotic dermatitis. The stratum corneum contains focal areas of parakeratosis, with a predilection for the follicular ostia, a finding known as "shoulder parakeratosis." Occasional pyknotic neutrophils are present within parakeratotic foci. There is moderate acanthosis with regular elongation of the rete ridges, mild spongiosis, and focal exocytosis of lymphocytes. The dermis contains a sparse mononuclear cell infiltrate. In HIV-infected patients, the epidermis may contain dyskeratotic keratinocytes and the dermal infiltrate may contain plasma cells.

Conditions to consider in the differential diagnosis:

dermatophytosis
seborrheic dermatitis
toxic shock syndrome

IIIC. SUPERFICIAL DERMATITIS WITH EPIDERMAL ATROPHY (ATROPHIC DERMATITIS)

Most inflammatory dermatoses are associated with epithelial hyperplasia. Only a few chronic conditions exhibit epidermal atrophy.

1. Atrophic Dermatitis, Scant Inflammatory Infiltrates
2. Atrophic Dermatitis, Lymphocytes Predominant
2a. Atrophic Dermatitis with Papillary Dermal Sclerosis

IIIC1. Atrophic Dermatitis, Scant Inflammatory Infiltrates

The epidermis is thinned to only a few cell layers thick. There is a scanty lymphocytic infiltrate around the superficial capillary–venular plexus.

Aged Skin

See Figs. IIIC1.a–IIIC1.b.

Radiation Dermatitis (see also section VF1)

Conditions to consider in the differential diagnosis:
aged skin
chronic actinic damage
radiation dermatitis
porokeratosis
acrodermatitis chronica atrophicans
malignant atrophic papulosis
poikiloderma atrophicans vasculare

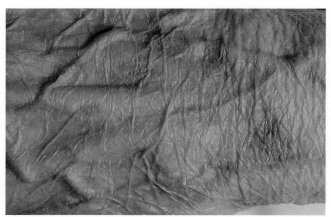

Clin. Fig. IIIC1

Clin. Fig. IIIC1. *Aged skin.* Dorsal hand has transparent wrinkled skin with prominent vessel and senile purpura.

Fig. IIIC1.a. *Aged skin, low power.* There is a thinned keratin scale overlying an effaced atrophic epidermis. The dermis shows marked solar elastosis with dilated thin-walled vessels. The inflammatory infiltrate is sparse.

Fig. IIIC1.b. *Aged skin, medium power.* The epidermis is evenly effaced. It overlies a dermis that has marked solar elastosis and a sparse inflammatory infiltrate.

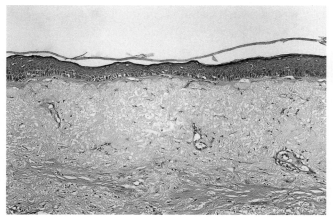

Fig. IIIC1.a

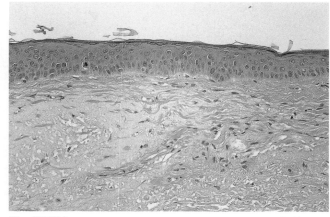

Fig. IIIC1.b

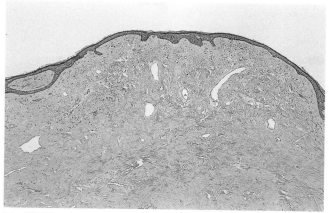

Fig. IIIC1.c

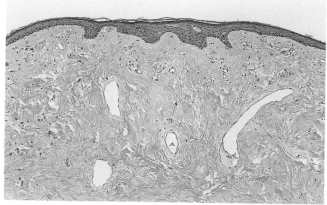

Fig. IIIC1.d

Fig. IIIC1.c. *Radiation dermatitis, low power.* The low power shows epidermal atrophy with discrete areas of acanthosis and basal layer pigmentation. The dermis is homogeneous and there is telangiectasia.

Fig. IIIC1.d. *Radiation dermatitis, medium power.* There is dermal homogenization with vascular ectasia and a sparse infiltrate around dermal vessels. The epidermis shows atrophy with basal layer pigmentation.

IIIC2. Atrophic Dermatitis, Lymphocytes Predominant

The epidermis is thinned but not as marked as in aged or irradiated skin. In the dermis there are few to many lymphocytes around the superficial capillary–venular plexus.

Poikiloderma Atrophicans Vasculare

CLINICAL SUMMARY. Clinically, the term poikiloderma atrophicans vasculare is applied to lesions that, in the early stage, show erythema with slight superficial scaling, a mottled pigmentation, and telangiectases. In the late stage the skin appears atrophic and the mottled pigmentation and the telangiectases are more pronounced. The condition may be seen in three different settings: in association with three genodermatoses, as an early stage of mycosis fungoides (11), and in association with dermatomyositis and, less commonly, lupus erythematosus.

The three genodermatoses in which the cutaneous lesions are poikilodermatous include poikiloderma congenitale of Rothmund Thomson, with the lesions present largely on the face, hands, and feet and occasionally also on the arms, legs, and buttocks (12); Bloom's syndrome, with poikiloderma-like lesions on the face, hands, and forearms (13); and dyskeratosis congenita, in which there may be extensive net-like pigmentation (14).

Poikiloderma-like lesions as features of early mycosis fungoides may be seen in one of two clinical forms: either as the large plaque (>10 cm) type of parapsoriasis en plaques, also known as poikilodermatous parapsoriasis, or as parapsoriasis variegata, which shows papules arranged in a netlike pattern. Although these two types of parapsoriasis are thought to represent an early stage of mycosis fungoides, not all cases progress clinically into fully developed mycosis fungoides.

The third group of diseases in which lesions of poikiloderma atrophicans vasculare occur is represented by dermatomyositis and systemic lupus erythematosus (SLE). Dermatomyositis is much more commonly seen as the primary disease than lupus erythematosus, and the association with dermatomyositis often is referred to as poikilodermatomyositis. In contrast to mycosis fungoides, in which poikilodermatous lesions are seen in the early stage, the lesions found in dermatomyositis and SLE generally represent a late stage.

HISTOPATHOLOGY. In early lesions of any cause, there is moderate thinning of the epidermis, with effacement of the rete ridges and hydropic degeneration of the basal cells. In the upper dermis there is a bandlike infiltrate, which in places invades the epidermis. The infiltrate consists mainly of lymphoid cells but also contains a few histiocytes. Melanophages filled with melanin as a result of pigmentary incontinence are found in varying numbers within the infiltrate. In addition, there is edema in the upper dermis and the superficial capillaries are often dilated. In the late stage the epidermis is apt to be markedly thinned and flattened, but the basal cells still show hydropic degeneration. Melanophages and edema of the upper dermis are still present, and telangiectasia may be pronounced.

The amount and type of dermal infiltrate vary with the underlying cause. In the genodermatoses and in dermatomyositis or SLE there is only slight dermal inflammation. In contrast, the inflammatory infiltrate seen in poikiloderma associated with early mycosis fungoides increases with time. Cells with large hyperchromatic nuclei, so-called mycosis cells, are likely to be present, and there is often marked epidermotropism of the infiltrate, which may result in Pautrier microabscesses. Even in developing lesions, the papillary dermis is expanded by fibrosis and collagen bundle thicken-

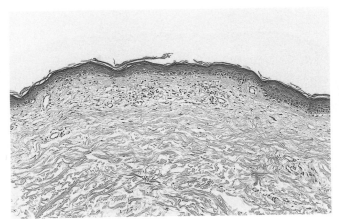

Fig. IIIC2.a

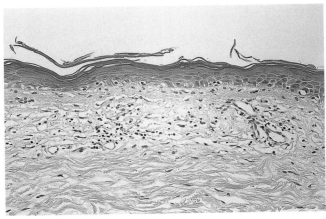

Fig. IIIC2.b

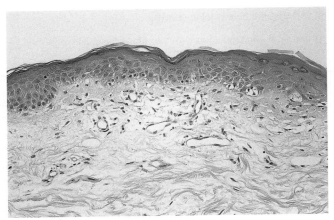

Fig. IIIC2.c

Fig. IIIC2.a. *Poikiloderma atrophicans vasculare, low power.* There is a thin keratotic scale overlying an atrophic epidermis. The papillary dermis is edematous and has a diffuse infiltrate of mononuclear cells.

Fig. IIIC2.b. *Poikiloderma atrophicans vasculare, medium power.* The thinned atrophic epidermis shows basal layer vacuolar degeneration. In the papillary dermis there is an infiltrate of lymphocytes seen diffusely and around thin-walled dermal vessels.

Fig. IIIC2.c. *Poikiloderma atrophicans vasculare, high power.* The epidermis shows focal basal layer liquefaction degeneration and a diffuse infiltrate of lymphocytes in an edematous papillary dermis, with a few lymphocytes extending among basal keratinocytes.

ing, which increases in rough proportion to lesional age. Thus, in the earliest patches, fibrosis is noticeable but subtle, whereas the papillary dermis is coarsely fibrotic late in the patch stage or in fully developed plaques. Thickened collagen bundles often lie roughly parallel to the epidermal surface, in contrast to the vertically oriented collagen bundles that develop secondary to lichenification. The overlying epidermis is nearly normal in the earliest patch lesions but typically shows slight regular psoriasiform hyperplasia and hyperkeratosis, although atrophy can be seen in poikilodermatous patches. Because the specific histologic features of mycosis fungoides are attenuated in poikilodermatous disease, multiple biopsies may be necessary for unequivocal diagnosis.

Dermatomyositis

See Figs. IIIC2.d–IIIC2.f.

Conditions to consider in the differential diagnosis:
    parapsoriasis/early mycosis fungoides
    lupus erythematous
    mixed connective tissue disease
    pinta, tertiary lesions
    dermatomyositis
    poikiloderma atrophicans vasculare

IIIC3. Atrophic Dermatitis with Papillary Dermal Sclerosis

The epidermis is thinned, and there can be hyperkeratosis. The dermis is homogenized and edematous, and inflammation is minimal. *Lichen sclerosus et atrophicus* is a prototype (15).

Lichen Sclerosus et Atrophicus

CLINICAL SUMMARY. Lichen sclerosus (LS) encompasses the disorders known as *lichen sclerosus et atrophicus, balanitis xerotica obliterans* (LS of the male glans and prepuce), and *kraurosis vulvae* (LS of the female labia majora, labia minora, perineum, and perianal region). LS is an inflammatory disorder of unknown etiology that affects patients 6 months of age to late adulthood. In both males and females, genital involvement is the most frequent, and often the only, site of

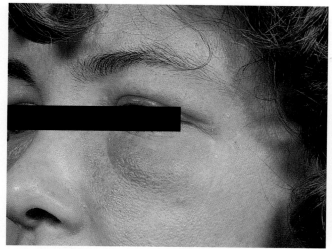

Clin. Fig. IIIC2

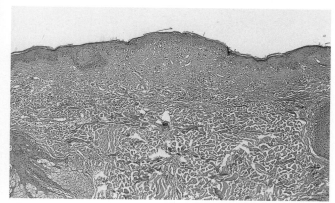

Fig. IIIC2.d

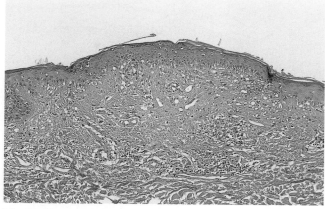

Fig. IIIC2.e

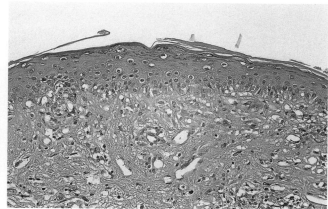

Fig. IIIC2.f

Clin. Fig. IIIC2. *Dermatomyositis.* Heliotrope lavender pruritic edematous periorbital changes in a middle-aged woman indicate a search for malignancy.

Fig. IIIC2.d. *Dermatomyositis, low power.* The epidermis is atrophic. In the dermis there is an infiltrate of mononuclear cells. The papillary dermis is expanded and edematous.

Fig. IIIC2.e. *Dermatomyositis, medium power.* The effaced thinned epidermis shows a discrete sparse lichenoid infiltrate at the dermal–epidermal junction that causes basal layer liquefaction degeneration. The papillary dermis is expanded. The infiltrate is diffuse, perivascular, and lymphocytic in type.

Fig. IIIC2.f. *Dermatomyositis, high power.* The basal layer shows distinct basal layer degeneration. The papillary dermis has telangiectatic vessels, a perivascular and diffuse infiltrate of lymphocytes.

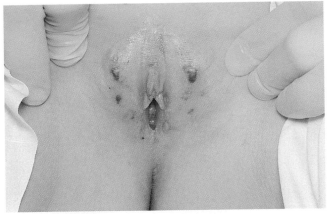

Clin. Fig. IIIC3

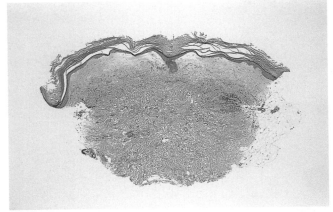

Fig. IIIC3.a

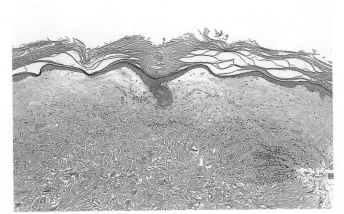

Fig. IIIC3.b

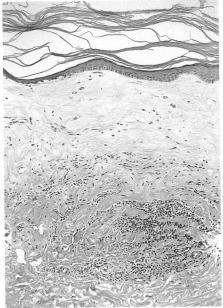

Fig. IIIC3.c

Clin. Fig. IIIC3. *Lichen sclerosus et atrophicus.* A "keyhole," ivory-colored sclerotic plaque with hemorrhage, which evolved in a child with genital pruritus.

Fig. IIIC3.a. *Lichen sclerosus et atrophicus, low power.* There is hyperkeratosis overlying an atrophic epidermis. The papillary dermis appears pale and there is an underlying perivascular infiltrate of mononuclear cells.

Fig. IIIC3.b. *Lichen sclerosus et atrophicus, medium power.* Hyperkeratosis overlies an atrophic epidermis. The papillary dermis shows homogenization and there is an underlying infiltrate of lymphocytes about dermal vessels.

Fig. IIIC3.c. *Lichen sclerosus et atrophicus, high power.* There is hyperkeratosis overlying an atrophic effaced epidermis. Underlying the area of homogenization of the papillary dermis is a perivascular and diffuse infiltrate of lymphocytes in the reticular dermis.

involvement. Extragenital lesions may occur with or without coexisting genital lesions. Lesions of LS are characterized by white polygonal papules that coalesce to form plaques. Comedolike plugs on the surface of the plaque correspond to dilated appendageal ostia. The plugs may disappear as the lesion ages, leaving a smooth porcelain-white plaque. Solitary or generalized lesions may become bullous and hemorrhagic.

HISTOPATHOLOGY.   The salient histologic findings in cutaneous lesions of lichen sclerosus et atrophicus are hyperkeratosis with follicular plugging, atrophy of the stratum malpighii with hydropic degeneration of basal cells, pronounced edema and homogenization of the collagen in the upper dermis, and an inflammatory infiltrate in the mid dermis. Beneath the hyperkeratotic and atrophic epidermis is a broad zone of pronounced lymphedema. Within this zone, the collagenous fibers are swollen and homogeneous and contain only a few nuclei. The blood and lymph vessels are dilated, and there may be areas of hemorrhage. In areas of severe lymphedema, clinically visible subepidermal bullae may form. Except in lesions of long duration, an inflammatory infiltrate is present in the dermis. In very early lesions, the infiltrate may be found in the uppermost dermis in direct apposition to the basal layer. Soon, however, a narrow zone of edema and homogenization of the collagen displaces the inflammatory infiltrate farther down so that, in well-developed lesions, the infiltrate is found in the middermis. The infiltrate can be patchy, but is often bandlike and composed of lymphoid cells admixed with plasma cells and histiocytes.

Conditions to consider in the differential diagnosis:

lichen sclerosus et atrophicus
thermal burns
parapsoriasis/early mycosis fungoides
poikiloderma atrophicans vasculare

IIID. SUPERFICIAL DERMATITIS WITH PSORIASIFORM PROLIFERATION (PSORIASIFORM DERMATITIS)

Psoriasiform proliferation is a form of epithelial hyperplasia characterized by uniform elongation of rete ridges. Although the surface may be slightly raised to form a plaque, the epidermal proliferation tends to extend downward into the dermis, in contrast to a papillomatous pattern in which the rete ridges are elongated upward above the plane of the epidermal surface and a papilloma (such as a wart) is formed. The prototype is psoriasis, in which the suprapapillary plates are thinned. In most other psoriasiform conditions, the suprapapillary plates are thickened but not as much as the elongated rete. Because of the increased epithelial turnover, there is often associated hypogranulosis and parakeratosis.

1. Psoriasiform Dermatitis, Mostly Lymphocytes
1a. Psoriasiform Dermatitis, with Plasma Cells
1b. Psoriasiform Dermatitis, with Eosinophils

2. Psoriasiform Dermatitis, Neutrophils Prominent (Neutrophilic/Pustular Psoriasiform Dermatitis)

IIID1. Psoriasiform Dermatitis, Mostly Lymphocytes

The epidermis is evenly and regularly thickened in a psoriasiform pattern, and spongiosis is variable (rare to absent in psoriasis; common in seborrheic and inflammatory dermatoses). There is an infiltrate of lymphocytes about dermal vessels. *Pityriasis rubra pilaris* is a prototypic example (16).

Pityriasis Rubra Pilaris

CLINICAL SUMMARY.   Pityriasis rubra pilaris is an erythematous squamous disorder characterized by follicular plugging and perifollicular erythema that coalesces to form orange-red scaly plaques that frequently contain islands of normal-appearing skin. As the erythema extends, the follicular component is often lost but persists longest on the dorsa of the proximal phalanges. The lesions spread caudally and may progress to a generalized erythroderma. Other clinical findings are palmoplantar keratoderma and scaling of the face and scalp. Most patients clear within 3 years, but some cases are more persistent, especially the circumscribed juvenile type, which is characterized by sharply demarcated lesions on the knees and elbows.

HISTOPATHOLOGY.   The histologic picture of a fully developed erythematous lesion shows acanthosis with broad and short rete ridges, slight spongiosis, thick suprapapillary plates, focal or confluent hypergranulosis, and alternating orthokeratosis and parakeratosis oriented in both vertical and horizontal directions. In the dermis there is a mild superficial perivascular lymphocytic infiltrate and moderately dilated blood vessels.

Areas corresponding to follicular papules show dilated infundibula filled out with an orthokeratotic plug and often display perifollicular shoulders of parakeratosis and a mild perifollicular lymphocytic. Erythrodermic lesions have a thinned or absent cornified layer, plasma exudates, and a diminished granular zone.

Mycosis Fungoides, Patch/Plaque Stage

CLINICAL SUMMARY.   Mycosis fungoides (17) is a form of T-cell lymphoma that initially involves the epidermis and papillary dermis, comprising the *patch stage* of the disease. With time, the neoplastic lymphocytes often acquire the capacity to proliferate within the reticular dermis, and plaques, nodules, and tumors (*plaque and tumor stages*) are manifest clinically. In some patients, generally after extended periods of time, the neoplasm disseminates to extracutaneous sites such as lymph nodes and viscera. The term mycosis fungoides was coined by Alibert after observing mushroomlike nodules in the tumor stage of the disease. Patches of mycosis fungoides are usually pinkish red and slightly scaly, typically distributed on the trunk and proximal extremities. The buttocks and breasts are often involved. At least some of the patches exceed 10 cm in diameter in most patients, corresponding to the morphologic pattern of "large plaque parapsoriasis." The proportion of patients with patch-stage mycosis fungoides that progresses to develop plaques is not precisely known, but it is thought to be low. Plaques of mycosis fungoides are sharply marginated and are usually red to reddish brown. The centers of plaques can involute, yielding annular or serpiginous morphology. Tumors of mycosis fungoides are morphologically indistinguishable from tumors of other cutaneous lymphomas, except that residual patch and plaques are virtually always evident.

HISTOPATHOLOGY.   The microscopic findings in the earliest patches of mycosis fungoides are subtle, consisting of a sparse intraepidermal and papillary dermal infiltrate of lymphocytes, arrayed within a fibrotic papillary dermis below an epidermis that shows slight psoriasiform hyperplasia. Because of the sparse infiltrate, multiple biopsies and close clinicopathologic correlation are often needed for diagnosis.

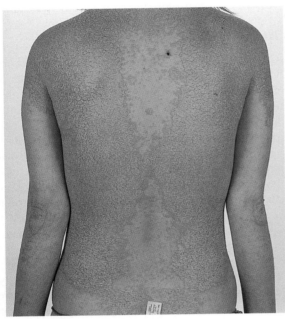

Clin. Fig. IIID1.a

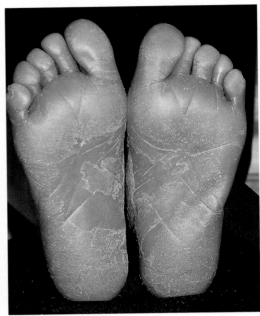

Clin. Fig. IIID1.b

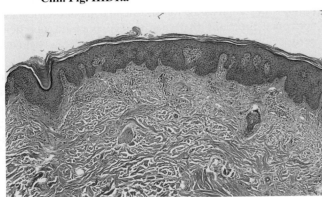

Fig. IIID1.a

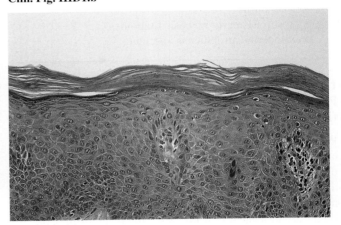

Fig. IIID1.b

Clin. Fig. IIID1.a. *Pityriasis rubra pilaris*. A 22-year-old woman developed confluent, well-demarcated, orange-red, scaling patches with prominent keratotic follicular papules on the trunk, with "skip areas" of normal skin.

Clin. Fig. IIID1.b. *Pityriasis rubra pilaris*. "Keratodermic sandals" present with thick, yellow, waxy, fissured, sometimes painful palms and soles.

Fig. IIID1.a. *Pityriasis rubra pilaris, low power*. There is follicular hyperkeratosis with an alternating scale of ortho- and parakeratin overlying an acanthotic epidermis. A perivascular infiltrate of mononuclear cells is seen in the dermis.

Fig. IIID1.b. *Pityriasis rubra pilaris, medium power*. The parakeratotic scale shows alternating vertical and linear parakeratosis. The epidermis is acanthotic with slight spongiosis. *(continues)*

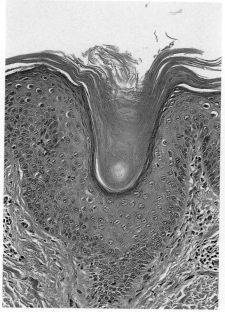

Fig. IIID1.c

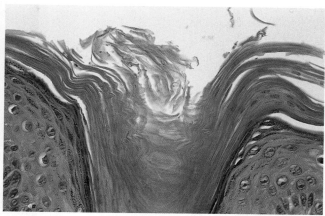

Fig. IIID1.d

Fig. IIID1.c. *Pityriasis rubra pilaris, medium power.* There is follicular hyper and parakeratosis with parakeratin at the shoulder of the follicular orifice. The papillary dermis has a sparse perivascular infiltrate of lymphocytes.

Fig. IIID1.d. *Pityriasis rubra pilaris, high power.* There is parakeratosis dipping into the follicular orifice.

Small numbers of lymphocytes, with relatively small but irregular nuclei, are arrayed within the epidermis with minimal associated spongiosis. The lymphocytes are often distributed in a linear array on the epidermal side of the basement membrane zone, an arrangement that has been likened to a string of pearls. Although clusters of intraepidermal lymphocytes, so-called "Pautrier collections," are often sought as the key to a diagnosis of mycosis fungoides, a pattern in which lymphocytes are dispersed among keratinocytes is more common in biopsies of macular lesions. Architectural alterations involve both the papillary dermis and the epidermis. The papillary dermis is expanded by fibrosis, whose degree increases in rough proportion to lesional age. Thickened collagen bundles often lie roughly parallel to the epidermal surface, in contrast to the vertically oriented collagen bundles that develop secondary to lichenification. The overlying epidermis typically shows slight regular psoriasiform hyperplasia and hyperkeratosis in the more advanced lesions. Readily discernible nuclear atypia of lymphocytes is the exception rather than the rule in conventional histologic sections of patch-stage disease, but at high magnification, some degree of nuclear convolution is usually appreciable, especially among the intraepithelial lymphocytes.

In plaque-stage mycosis fungoides, the papillary dermis is similarly expanded by coarse fibrosis and contains denser bandlike infiltrates of lymphocytes, with as a rule more prominent epidermotropism. In combination with slight regular epidermal thickening, these features account for the "lichenoid-psoriasiform" pattern that is characteristic of the late patch stage and the plaque stage. In addition to a papillary dermal infil-

trate, the reticular dermis holds superficial and deep perivascular or nearly diffuse infiltrates of lymphocytes. Cytologic atypism, particularly of intraepidermal lymphocytes, is often conspicuous in biopsies from plaques, in contrast to the subtle cytologic changes evident in macular lesions.

Parapsoriasis

See Figs. IIID1.h–IIID1.j.
Conditions to consider in the differential diagnosis:
chronic spongiotic dermatitis
atopic dermatitis
seborrheic dermatitis
nummular eczema
lichen simplex chronicus
prurigo nodularis
psoriasis
psoriasiform drug eruptions
pityriasis rosea
exfoliative dermatitis
pityriasis rubra pilaris
parapsoriasis/early mycosis fungoides
verrucous hyperkeratotic mycosis fungoides
inflammatory linear verrucous epidermal nevus
  (ILVEN)
pellagra
necrolytic migratory erythema (chronic lesions)
acrodermatitis enteropathica
kwashiorkor
reticulated hyperpigmentations (e.g., Dowling–Degos
  disease)

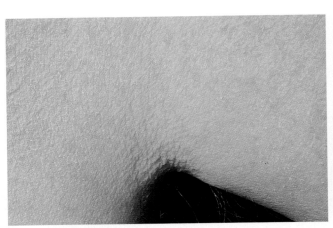

Clin. Fig. IIID1.c

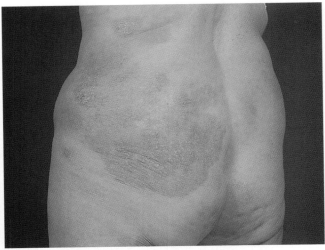

Clin. Fig. IIID1.d

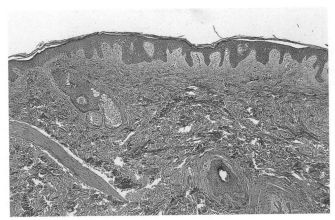

Fig. IIID1.e

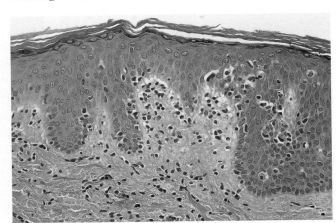

Fig. IIID1.f

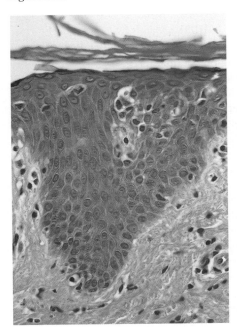

Fig. IIID1.g

Clin. Fig. IIID1.c. *Parapsoriasis/early mycosis fungoides*. Chronic pruritic maculopapular changes became increasingly indurated with erosions.

Clin. Fig. IIID1.d. *Mycosis fungoides*. A 66-year-old woman presented with a 30-year history of erythematous scaly patches and plaques with telangiectases, atrophy, and pigmentation.

Fig. IIID1.e. *Mycosis fungoides, patch stage, low power*. A thin keratin layer overlies an acanthotic epidermis. The papillary dermis is edematous. A mononuclear cell infiltrate around dermal vessels is in the upper reticular dermis.

Fig. IIID1.f. *Mycosis fungoides, patch stage, medium power*. Exocytosis of hyperchromatic lymphocytes into an acanthotic nonspongiotic epidermis is seen. The papillary dermis shows edema and a similar infiltrate that is diffuse within the papillary dermis.

Fig. IIID1.g. *Mycosis fungoides, patch stage, high power*. There is hyperkeratosis and acanthosis. Exocytosis is characterized by the presence of hyperchromatic mononuclear cells within the acanthotic epidermis. The papillary dermis is edematous.

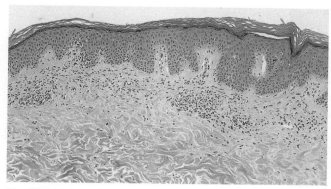

Fig. IIID1.h

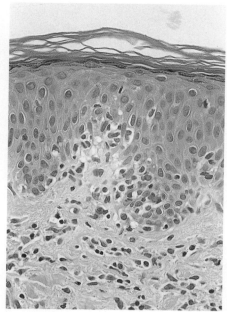

Fig. IIID1.j

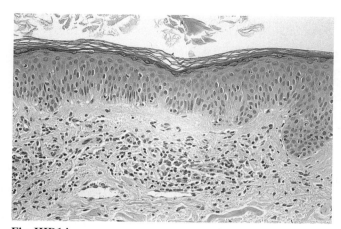

Fig. IIID1.i

Fig. IIID1.h. *Large plaque parapsoriasis/early mycosis fungoides, low power.* There is hyperkeratosis, acanthosis, and spongiosis. In the papillary dermis there is a diffuse and perivascular infiltrate of mononuclear cells.

Fig. IIID1.i. *Parapsoriasis/early mycosis fungoides, medium power.* The lymphocytic infiltrate is diffuse in the papillary dermis with associated telangiectasia, overlying epidermal acanthosis with basal layer pigmentation.

Fig. IIID1.j. *Parapsoriasis/early mycosis fungoides, high power.* An orthokeratotic basket-weave layer of keratin overlies an epidermis that is acanthotic with exocytosis of hyperchromatic mononuclear cells and little or no spongiosis. In the dermis there is fibrosis, a lymphocytic infiltrate, and melanophage pigmentation.

IIID1a. Psoriasiform Dermatitis, with Plasma Cells

The epidermis is evenly thickened and may be spongiotic. There may be exocytosis of lymphocytes. The stratum corneum is variable and often parakeratotic. Plasma cells are found around the superficial vessels in varying numbers, admixed with lymphocytes.

Lichen Simplex Chronicus

CLINICAL SUMMARY. Any patient with pruritus who chronically rubs the skin may develop lichen simplex chronicus (see also section IIIE). It often develops in the setting of atopic dermatitis or allergic contact dermatitis. The lesions are pruritic thickened plaques often with excoriation, in which the normal skin markings are accentuated, the latter finding known as lichenification.

HISTOPATHOLOGY. Lichen simplex chronicus is the prototype for chronic dermatitis. There is hyperkeratosis interspersed with areas of parakeratosis, acanthosis with irregular elongation of the rete ridges, hypergranulosis, and broadening of the dermal papillae. Slight spongiosis may be observed, but vesiculation is absent. There may be a sparse superficial perivascular infiltrate without exocytosis. In the papillary dermis, there is an increased number of fibroblasts and vertically oriented collagen bundles. As rubbing increases in intensity and chronicity, epidermal hyperplasia becomes more florid and the fibrosis more marked.

Conditions to consider in the differential diagnosis:

    arthropod bite reactions
    secondary syphilis
    cutaneous T-cell lymphoma (mycosis fungoides)
    prurigo nodularis

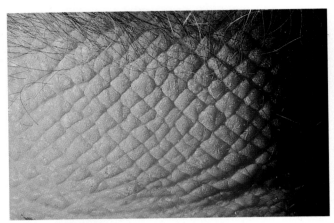

Clin. Fig. IIID1a

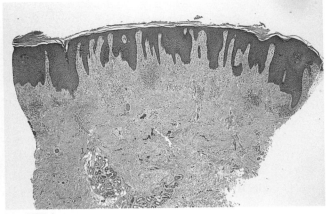

Fig. IIID1a.a

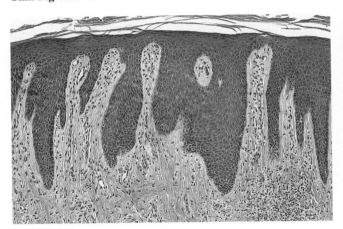

Fig. IIID1a.b

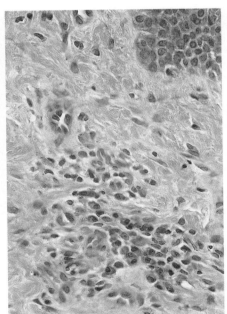

Fig. IIID1a.c

Clin. Fig. IIID1a. *Lichen simplex chronicus.* Chronic "rubbing" of posterior neck led to accentuation and thickening of skin markings.

Fig. IIID1a.a. *Lichen simplex chronicus, low power.* There is a patchy parakeratotic scale overlying an irregularly acanthotic epidermis in which there is fusion of the rete ridges. The dermis is papillomatous, with a perivascular infiltrate of mononuclear cells.

Fig. IIID1a.b. *Lichen simplex chronicus, medium power.* The epidermis shows marked acanthosis without significant exocytosis. There is papillomatosis and a diffuse and perivascular infiltrate in the fibrocellular dermis. There are vertically oriented collagen fibers in the elongated dermal papillae.

Fig. IIID1a.c. *Lichen simplex chronicus, high power.* The dermal infiltrate consists of lymphocytes and plasma cells.

IIID1b. Psoriasiform Dermatitis, with Eosinophils

The epidermis is evenly thickened and may be spongiotic, and there may be exocytosis of inflammatory cells, including eosinophils. Eosinophils are easily identified in the dermis and may be numerous in some conditions (e.g., incontinentia pigmenti). *Chronic allergic dermatitis* is the prototype (see also sections IIIB1a and IIIE).

Chronic Allergic Dermatitis

In *chronic allergic dermatitis*, there is hyperkeratosis with areas of parakeratosis, often hypergranulosis, and moderate to marked psoriasiform acanthosis. Although spongiosis may be present focally, it is minimal. The inflammatory infiltrate is sparse, often with scattered eosinophils, and papillary dermal fibrosis may be a prominent feature. With

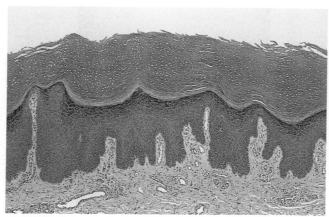

Fig. IIID1b.a

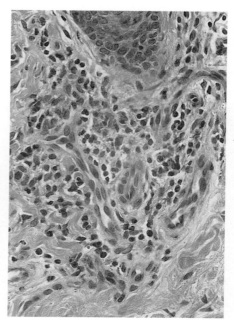

Fig. IIID1b.b

Fig. IIID1b.a. *Chronic allergic dermatitis, medium power.* There is hyperkeratosis with even acanthosis. The epidermis, covered by an orthokeratotic scale, is acanthotic and shows fusion of the rete ridges. The dermis shows vascular ectasia and a perivascular mononuclear cell infiltrate. The reaction pattern is that of lichen simplex chronicus.

Fig. IIID1b.b. *Chronic allergic dermatitis, high power.* The papillary dermis shows fibrosis. The infiltrate in the dermis consists of lymphocytes, plasma cells, and many eosinophils. The latter finding is consistent with an allergic etiology.

---

chronic rubbing and scratching, the pathology becomes that of lichen simplex chronicus (see also section IIIE).

Conditions to consider in the differential diagnosis:

    chronic spongiotic dermatitis
    chronic allergic dermatitis
    chronic atopic dermatitis
    exfoliative dermatitis
    cutaneous T-cell lymphoma
    incontinentia pigmenti, verrucous stage

IIID2. Psoriasiform Dermatitis, Neutrophils Prominent (Neutrophilic/Pustular Psoriasiform Dermatitis)

The epidermis is evenly thickened, and there is exocytosis (migration of inflammatory cells through the epidermis) of neutrophils. These may collect into abscesses in the epidermis at the level of the stratum corneum (Munro microabscess). The stratum corneum is thickened, parakeratotic, and contains neutrophils. *Psoriasis vulgaris* is the prototype (18).

Psoriasis Vulgaris

CLINICAL SUMMARY. Psoriasis vulgaris is characterized by pink to red papules and plaques that are of variable size, sharply demarcated, dry, and usually covered with layers of fine silvery scales. As the scales are removed by gentle

scraping, fine bleeding points usually are seen, the so-called Auspitz sign. The scalp, sacral region, and extensor surfaces of the extremities are commonly involved, although in some patients the flexural and intertriginous areas (inverse psoriasis) are mainly affected. An acute variant, guttate or eruptive psoriasis, is often seen in younger patients and is characterized by an abrupt eruption of small lesions associated with acute group A β-hemolytic streptococcal infections. Involvement of the nails is common; the most frequent alteration of the nail plate surface is the presence of pits. In severe cases the disease may affect the entire skin and present as generalized erythrodermic psoriasis. Pustules generally are absent in psoriasis vulgaris, although pustules on palms and soles occasionally occur, and rarely, severe psoriasis vulgaris develops into generalized pustular psoriasis. Oral lesions such as stomatitis areata migrans (geographic stomatitis) and benign migratory glossitis may be seen in psoriasis. Psoriatic arthritis characteristically involves the terminal interphalangeal joints, but frequently the large joints are also affected so that a clinical differentiation from rheumatoid arthritis often is impossible, although rheumatoid factor generally is absent.

HISTOPATHOLOGY. The histology varies considerably with the stage of the lesion, and is usually diagnostic only in early scaling papules and near the margin of advancing plaques. At

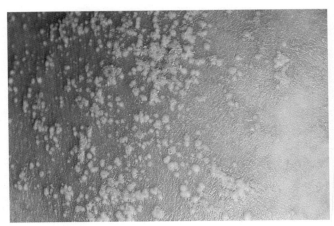

Clin. Fig. IIID2.a

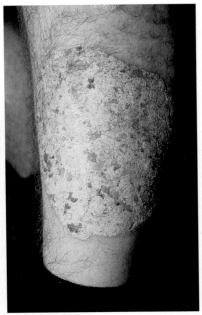

Clin. Fig. IIID2.b

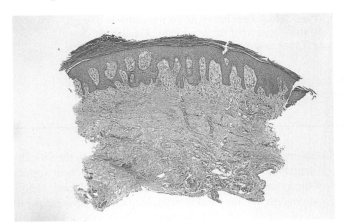

Fig. IIID2.a

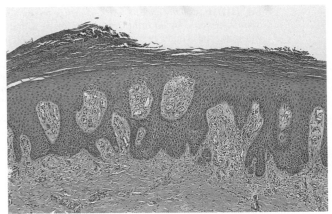

Fig. IIID2.b

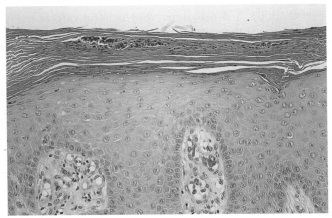

Fig. IIID2.c

Clin. Fig. IIID2.a. *Pustular psoriasis*. Rapid development of sterile pustules complicated a case of erythroderma.

Clin. Fig. IIID2.b. *Psoriasis, plaque lesion*. Well-demarcated erythematous plaque with a thick white silvery scale on extensor surfaces.

Fig. IIID2.a. *Psoriasis vulgaris, low power*. The hyperkeratotic scale is composed of ortho- and parakeratin. The epidermis is evenly acanthotic. There is papillomatosis and an infiltrate around dermal vessels and in the dermal papillae.

Fig. IIID2.b. *Psoriasis vulgaris, medium power*. The parakeratotic scale contains fragments of neutrophils. The epidermis shows even acanthosis with some rete ridge fusion. The papillary dermis is edematous and well vascularized.

Fig. IIID2.c. *Psoriasis vulgaris, high power*. The scale contains a collection of polymorphonuclear leukocytes and parakeratin. The epidermis is acanthotic. The papillary dermis is well vascularized with discrete areas of hemorrhage.

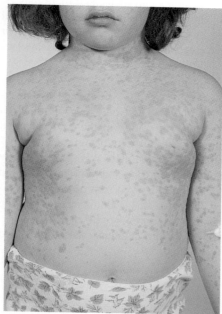

Clin. Fig. IIID2.c. *Guttate psoriasis.* Eruptive "drop-like" small plaques that cleared after therapy for β-hemolytic streptococcal infection.

Fig. IIID2.d. *Guttate psoriasis, high power.* There is a Munro microabscess located at the epidermal–stratum corneum junction with overlying parakeratosis.

Clin. Fig. IIID2.c

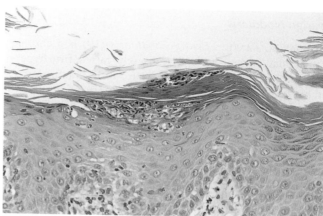

Fig. IIID2.d

first, there is capillary dilatation and edema in the papillary dermis, with a lymphocytic infiltrate surrounding the capillaries. The lymphocytes extend into the lower epidermis, where slight spongiosis develops. Then focal changes occur in the upper epidermis, where granular cells become vacuolated and disappear, and mounds of parakeratosis are formed. Neutrophils are usually seen at the summits of some of the mounds of parakeratosis and scattered through an otherwise orthokeratotic cornified layer, representing the earliest manifestation of Munro microabscesses. When there is marked exocytosis of neutrophils, they may aggregate in the uppermost portion of the spinous layer to form small spongiform pustules of Kogoj. A spongiform pustule shows aggregates of neutrophils within the interstices of a spongelike network formed by degenerated and thinned epidermal cells. Munro microabscesses are located within parakeratotic areas of the cornified layer and consist of accumulations of neutrophils and pyknotic nuclei of neutrophils that have migrated there from capillaries in the papillae through the suprapapillary epidermis. Lymphocytes remain confined to the lower epidermis, which, as more and more mitoses occur, becomes increasingly hyperplastic. The epidermal changes at first are focal but later become confluent, leading clinically to plaques.

In the fully developed lesions of psoriasis, as best seen at the margin of enlarging plaques, the histologic picture is characterized by acanthosis with regular elongation of the rete ridges with thickening in their lower portion, thinning of the suprapapillary epidermis with the occasional presence of small spongiform pustules, pallor of the upper layers of the epidermis, a diminished to absent granular layer, confluent parakeratosis, the presence of Munro microabscesses, elongation and edema of the dermal papillae, and dilated and tortuous capillaries. Of these, only the spongiform pustules of Kogoj and Munro microabscesses are most consistent with psoriasis and, in their absence, the diagnosis can rarely be made with certainty on a histologic basis. Spongiform pustules are not pathognomonic of psoriasis, as they are seen also on occasion in candidiasis, Reiter's disease, geographic tongue, and, rarely, in secondary syphilis.

Conditions to consider in the differential diagnosis:

    psoriasis vulgaris
    pustular psoriasis
    retiree's syndrome, keratoderma blenorrhagicum
    pustular drug eruption
    geographic tongue (lingua geographica)
    candidiasis
    pustular secondary syphilis (rare)
    dermatophytosis

IIIE. SUPERFICIAL DERMATITIS WITH IRREGULAR EPIDERMAL PROLIFERATION (HYPERTROPHIC DERMATITIS)

Irregular thickening and thinning of the epidermis is seen in some reactive conditions, but the possibility of squamous cell carcinoma should also be considered. As in other conditions associated with increased epithelial turnover, there may be hypogranulosis and parakeratosis.

1. Hypertrophic Dermatitis, Lymphocytes Predominant
1a. Irregular Epidermal Proliferation, Plasma Cells Present
2. Irregular Epidermal Proliferation, Neutrophils Prominent
3. Irregular Epidermal Proliferation, Above A Neoplasm

IIIE1. Hypertrophic Dermatitis, Lymphocytes Predominant

The epidermis is irregularly thickened, with areas of normal thickness, of acanthosis, and of thinning. Lymphocytes are the predominant inflammatory cell about the dermal vessels. *Prurigo nodularis* is a prototype.

Prurigo Nodularis

CLINICAL SUMMARY.   *Prurigo nodularis* (19) is a chronic skin dermatitis characterized by discrete, raised, firm hyperkeratotic papulonodules, usually from 5 to 12 mm in diameter, but occasionally larger. They occur chiefly on the extensor surfaces of the extremities and are intensely pruritic. The disease usually begins in middle age, and women are more frequently affected than men. Prurigo nodularis may coexist with lesions of lichen simplex chronicus, and there may be transitional lesions. The cause remains unknown, but local trauma, insect bites, atopic background, and metabolic or systemic diseases have been implicated as predisposing factors in some cases.

HISTOPATHOLOGY.   Sections show pronounced hyperkeratosis and irregular acanthosis. There may be papillomatosis and irregular downward proliferation of the epidermis and adnexal epithelium approaching pseudocarcinomatous hyperplasia. In the papillary dermis, there is a predominantly lymphocytic inflammatory infiltrate and vertically oriented collagen bundles. Occasionally, prominent neural hyperplasia may be observed; however, this is an uncommon finding and is not considered by some authors to be an essential feature for the diagnosis of prurigo nodularis. Eosinophils and

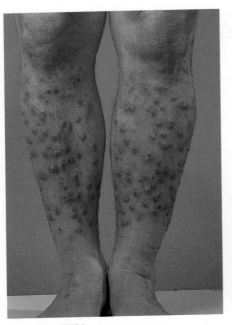

Clin. Fig. IIIE1

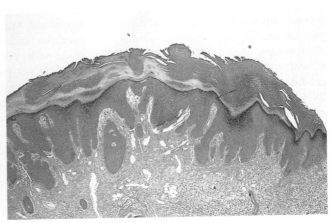

Fig. IIIE1.a

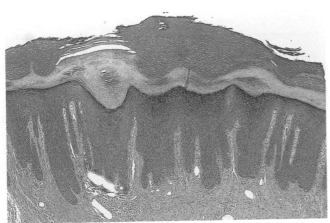

Fig. IIIE1.b

Clin. Fig. IIIE1. *Prurigo nodularis.* Hyperpigmented ill-defined papules and nodules in accessible body sites result from repeated picking and scratching.

Fig. IIIE1.a. *Prurigo nodularis/lichen simplex chronicus, low power.* There is marked irregular hyperplasia of the epidermis and hyperkeratosis. At the periphery of prurigo nodularis, the changes are those of lichen simplex chronicus.

Fig. IIIE1.b. *Prurigo nodularis/lichen simplex chronicus, medium power.* At higher magnification there may be hypergranulosis, and the hyperplastic epithelium is composed of bland-appearing keratinocytes without cytologic atypia. In a fully evolved case, there is irregular downward proliferation of the epidermis and adnexal epithelium approaching pseudocarcinomatous hyperplasia.

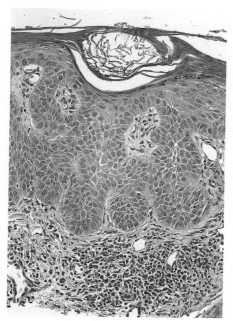

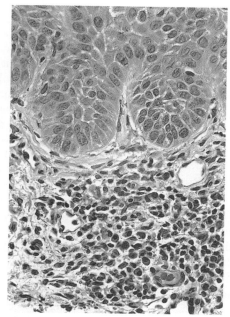

Fig. IIIE1a.a. *Actinic keratosis, medium power.* There is an ortho- and parakeratotic scale overlying an acanthotic epidermis that shows loss of natural maturation. The dermis has a dense infiltrate of mononuclear cells and discrete hemorrhage.

Fig. IIIE1a.b. *Actinic keratosis, high power* There is atypical epidermal proliferation in which there is no distinction between basal cells and epidermal keratinocytes. The dermis contains an infiltrate of plasma cells, lymphocytes, and there is vascular ectasia.

Fig. IIIE1a.a

Fig. IIIE1a.b

marked eosinophil degranulation may be seen more frequently in patients with an atopic background. Plasma cells may be present in many cases.

Conditions to consider in the differential diagnosis:

    lichen simplex chronicus
    inflammatory linear verrucous nevus (ILVEN
      psoriasiform category)
    prurigo nodularis
    lichen simplex chronicus
    incontinentia pigmenti, verrucous stage
    pellagra (niacin deficiency)
    Hartnup disease

IIIE1a. Irregular Epidermal Proliferation, Plasma Cells Present

The epidermis is irregularly acanthotic. Plasma cells are found around the dermal vessels admixed with lymphocytes.

Actinic Keratosis

See Figs. IIIE1a.a and IIIE1a.b, and section IIA1.

Conditions to consider in the differential diagnosis:

    squamous cell carcinoma *in situ* (Bowen's disease)
    erythroplasia of Queyrat
    rupial secondary syphilis, condyloma lata
    yaws, primary or secondary
    pinta, primary or secondary lesions
    actinic keratosis
    pseudoepitheliomatous hyperplasia
    pemphigus vegetans

IIIE2. Irregular Epidermal Proliferation, Neutrophils Prominent

The epidermis has focal areas of acanthosis, and neutrophils can be seen as exocytotic cells and are found in the dermis in abscesses and around dermal vessels without there being a primary vasculitis. Most examples of these epithelial reactions are associated with inflammation that involves the reticular dermis and the papillary dermis. Keratoacanthoma is a neoplastic example.

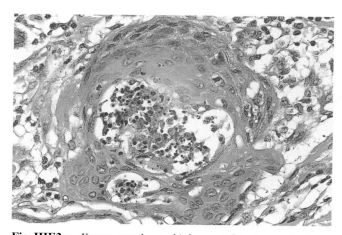

Fig. IIIE2.a. *Keratoacanthoma, high power.* Intratumor abscesses of polymorphonuclear leukocytes are seen.

Keratoacanthoma

See Fig. IIIE2.a and section VIB1.

 Conditions to consider in the differential diagnosis:

  deep fungal infections (superficial biopsy, see below)
  halogenodermas
  botryomycosis
  keratoacanthoma
  impetigo contagiosa
  granuloma inguinale

IIIE3. Irregular Epidermal Proliferation Above a Neoplasm

The epidermis is irregularly acanthotic. There is an associated neoplastic infiltrate in the epidermis or dermis, or in both. Most of these neoplasms involve the reticular dermis and the papillary dermis (see also Chapter VI).

 Conditions to consider in the differential diagnosis:

  malignant melanoma ("verrucous" pattern)
  granular cell tumor

IIIF. SUPERFICIAL DERMATITIS WITH LICHENOID INFILTRATES (LICHENOID DERMATITIS)

Lichenoid inflammation is a dense "bandlike" infiltrate of small lymphocytes clustered around the dermal–epidermal junction and obscuring the interface. The epidermis is variable in its thickness, amount of exocytotic lymphocytes, and the integrity of the basal cell zone (liquefaction degeneration). Hypergranulosis due to delayed epidermal maturation is a commonly associated feature. For the same reason, there may be orthokeratotic hyperkeratosis. Apoptotic or necrotic keratinocytes are often present. In lichen planus, these are called Civatte bodies. Pigmentary incontinence (melanin-laden macrophages in the papillary dermis) is common, as in any condition in which there is destruction of basal keratinocytes.

1. Lichenoid Dermatitis, Lymphocytes Exclusively
2. Lichenoid Dermatitis, Lymphocytes Predominant
2a Lichenoid Dermatitis, Eosinophils Present
2b. Lichenoid Dermatitis, Plasma Cells Present
2c. Lichenoid Dermatitis, with Melanophages
3. Lichenoid Dermatitis, Histiocytes Predominant
4. Lichenoid Dermatitis, Mast Cells Predominant
5. Lichenoid Dermatitis, with Dermal Fibroplasia

IIIF1. Lichenoid Dermatitis, Lymphocytes Exclusively

The bandlike infiltrate is composed almost exclusively of lymphocytes. Eosinophils and plasma cells are essentially absent. *Lichen planus* is the prototype (20).

Lichen Planus

Lichen planus is a subacute or a chronic dermatosis that may involve skin, mucous membranes, hair follicles, and nails. In glabrous skin, the eruption is characterized by small, flat-topped, shiny, polygonal, violaceous papules that may coalesce into plaques. The papules often show a network of white lines known as Wickham's striae. Itching is usually pronounced. The disease has a predilection for the flexor surfaces of the forearms, legs, and the glans penis. The eruption may be localized or extensive, and Koebner's phenomenon (exacerbation or elicitation of lesions by trauma) is commonly seen. A common variant is *hypertrophic lichen planus*, which is usually found on the shins and consists of thickened often verrucous plaques.

HISTOPATHOLOGY. Typical papules of lichen planus show compact orthokeratosis with very few, if any, parakeratotic cells, a fact that is important for the diagnosis; wedge-shaped hypergranulosis with coarse and abundant keratohyaline granules; irregular acanthosis giving rise to dome-shaped dermal papillae and to pointed or "saw-toothed" rete ridges; damage to the basal cell layer with vacuolar degeneration and apoptosis of the basal cells giving rise to the characteristic round eosinophilic apoptotic bodies (synonymously known as colloid, hyaline, cytoid, or Civatte bodies); and a bandlike dermal lymphocytic infiltrate composed almost entirely of lymphocytes intermingled with macrophages. A few eosinophils and/or plasma cells may be seen in close approximation to the epidermis, but these are rare except in some examples of hypertrophic lichen planus. Wickham's striae are believed to be caused by a focal increase in the thickness of the granular layer and of the total epidermis. Occasionally, small areas of artifactual separation between the epidermis and the dermis, known as Max–Joseph spaces, are seen. In some instances, the separation occurs *in vivo* and subepidermal blisters form (*vesicular lichen planus*). These vesicles form as a result of extensive damage to the basal cells. In old lesions the cellular infiltrate decreases in density but the number of macrophages increases. In areas in which a basal cell layer has reformed, the dermal infiltrate no longer lies in close approximation to the epidermis. Chronic lesions may show considerable acanthosis, papillomatosis, and hyperkeratosis (*hypertrophic lichen planus*).

Graft-Versus-Host Disease

 See Figs. IIIF1.d–IIIF1.f.

Mycosis Fungoides, Patch/Plaque Stage

 See Figs. IIIF1.g–IIIF1.i.
 Conditions to consider in the differential diagnosis:

  lichen planus-like keratosis (benign lichenoid keratosis)
  lichen planus
  lupus erythematous, lichenoid forms

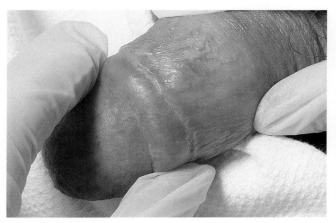

Clin. Fig. IIIF1.a

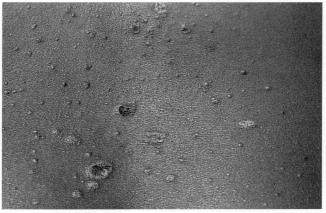

Clin. Fig. IIIF1.b

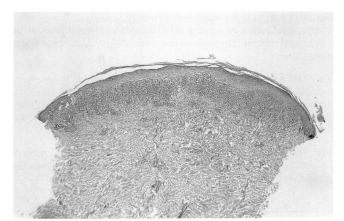

Fig. IIIF1.a

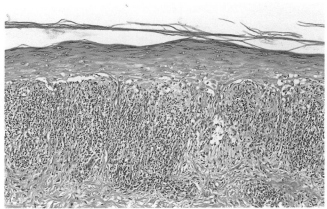

Fig. IIIF1.b

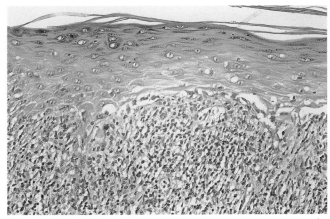

Fig. IIIF1.c

Clin. Fig. IIIF1.a. *Lichen planus*. One- to 5-mm violaceous polygonal papules on coronal sulcus with Wickham's striae followed longstanding lacy changes on buccal mucosa.

Clin. Fig. IIIF1.b. *Lichen planus*. Multiple flat-topped violaceous polygonal papules.

Fig. IIIF1.a. *Lichen planus, low power*. There is a bandlike infiltrate that occupies the papillary dermis and obscures the dermal–epidermal interface. A thin keratin scale covers the epidermis.

Fig. IIIF1.b. *Lichen planus, medium power*. The infiltrate of lymphocytes at the dermal–epidermal interface obscures and obliterates basal cells. The epidermis is thickened and there is hypergranulosis.

Fig. IIIF1.c. *Lichen planus, high power*. There is focal hypergranulosis with overlying hyperkeratosis. The infiltrate consists of lymphocytes with the presence of eosinophilic bodies (Civatte bodies) within the inflammatory infiltrate.

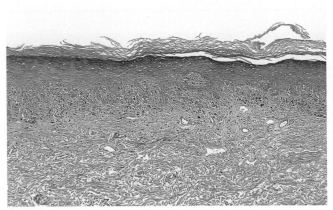

Fig. IIIF1.d

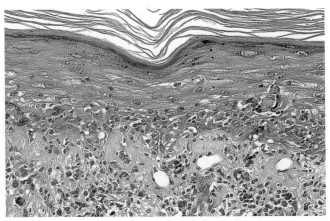

Fig. IIIF1.e

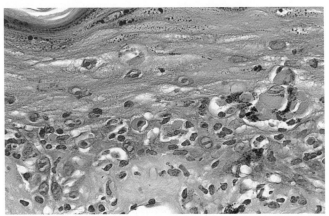

Fig. IIIF1.f

Fig. IIIF1.d. *Graft-versus-host disease, lichenoid, low power.* Lymphocytes are seen tagging at the dermal–epidermal junction in a lichenoid pattern. The stratum corneum is normal, indicative of a recent origin.

Fig. IIIF1.e. *Graft-versus-host disease, lichenoid, low power.* Lymphocytes and a few melanophages are present in the papillary dermis. There is vacuolar alteration at the dermal–epidermal junction, and there are many necrotic (apoptotic) keratinocytes near the interface.

Fig. IIIF1.f. *Graft-versus-host disease, lichenoid, low power.* Lymphocytes are adherent to some of the eosinophilic apoptotic keratinocytes, constituting so-called "satellite-cell necrosis."

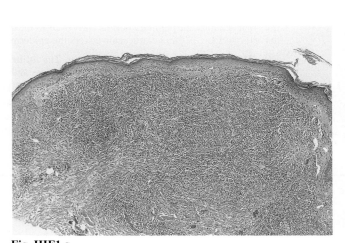

Fig. IIIF1.g

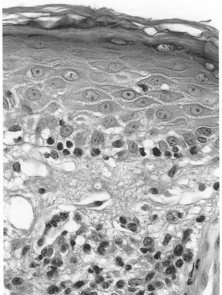

Fig. IIIF1.h

Fig. IIIF1.g. *Mycosis fungoides, patch/plaque stage, low power.* In this example, the infiltrate is more dense than most lichenoid inflammatory infiltrates.

Fig. IIIF1.h. *Mycosis fungoides, patch/plaque stage, medium power.* Lymphocytes at the dermal–epidermal junction enter the epidermis with minimal spongiosis. *(continues)*

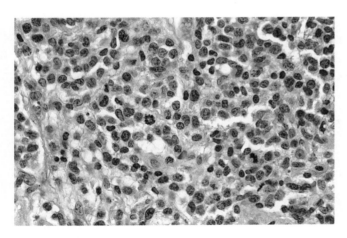

Fig. IIIF1.i. *Mycosis fungoides, patch/plaque stage, high power.* Although lymphoid atypia is not striking in this early lesion, there is some irregularity of nuclear contour.

mixed connective tissue disease
acrodermatitis chronica atrophicans
poikiloderma atrophicans vasculare
pigmented purpuric dermatitis, lichenoid type
  (Gougerot–Blum)
graft-versus-host disease, lichenoid stage
erythema multiforme
PLEVA, early lesions
parapsoriasis/mycosis fungoides, patch/plaque stage
Sezary syndrome

IIIF2. Lichenoid Dermatitis, Lymphocytes Predominant

The bandlike lichenoid infiltrate is composed almost exclusively of lymphocytes. A few plasma cells and eosinophils may also be present. *Lichen planus-like keratosis* is a prototype (21).

Lichen Planus-like Keratosis (Benign Lichenoid Keratosis)

CLINICAL SUMMARY. Lichen planus-like keratosis, also known as "benign lichenoid keratosis," is a common lesion that occurs predominantly on the trunk and upper extremities of adults between the fifth and seventh decades and consists of a nearly always solitary nonpruritic papule or slightly indurated plaque. It usually measures 5 to 20 mm in diameter, and its color varies from bright red to violaceous to brown. Its surface may be smooth or slightly verrucous. Lichen planus-like keratosis probably represents the inflammatory stage of involuting solar lentigines.

HISTOPATHOLOGY. Histologic examination shows, at least in a part of the lesion, a lichenoid pattern that may be indistinguishable from lichen planus. As in lichen planus,

there is vacuolar alteration of the basal cell layer and a bandlike lymphocytic infiltrate that obscures the dermal–epidermal junction. Necrotic keratinocytes are commonly seen and may be numerous. As in lichen planus, the epidermis often shows increased eosinophilia, hypergranulosis, and hyperkeratosis. In contrast to lichen planus, however, parakeratosis is fairly common, and eosinophils and plasma cells may be present in the infiltrate. A residual solar lentigo at the edge of the lesion supports the diagnosis of lichen planus-like keratosis. If marked keratinocytic atypia is found in association with a lichenoid inflammatory pattern, a lichenoid actinic keratosis should be considered in the differential diagnosis.

Conditions to consider in the differential diagnosis:

lichen planus-like keratosis (benign lichenoid keratosis)
parapsoriasis/mycosis fungoides, patch/plaque stage
Sezary syndrome
paraneoplastic pemphigus
secondary syphilis
halo nevus
lichenoid tattoo reaction
lichen striatus

IIIF2a. Lichenoid Dermatitis, Eosinophils Present

Eosinophils are found in the lichenoid dermal infiltrate around the dermal vessels and in some instances around the adnexal structures. *Lichenoid drug eruptions* are prototypic (22). Histiocytosis X is an important differential.

Lichenoid Drug Eruptions

CLINICAL SUMMARY. Lichenoid drug eruption is clinically similar to lichen planus. Erythematous to violaceous papules and plaques develop on the trunk and extremities in association with drug ingestion. Implicated agents include gold, antihypertensive medications (especially captopril), penicillamine, and chloroquine.

HISTOPATHOLOGY. Lichenoid drug eruption is also similar to lichen planus histologically. In comparison with erythema multiforme and toxic epidermal necrolysis, lichenoid drug eruptions are more heavily inflamed with a more prominent interstitial pattern. Differentiation from lichen planus may not be possible. Numerous eosinophils, parakeratosis, and perivascular inflammation around the mid and deep dermal plexuses are generally absent in lichen planus and should prompt consideration of a lichenoid drug eruption.

Conditions to consider in the differential diagnosis:

lichenoid drug eruptions
lichenoid actinic keratoses
lichen planus, hypertrophic
arthropod bite reactions
cutaneous T-cell lymphoma (CTCL), mycosis
  fungoides, patch/plaque stage

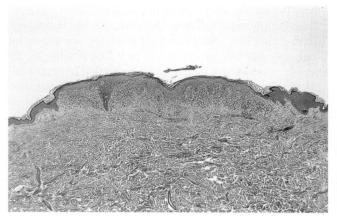

Fig. IIIF2.a

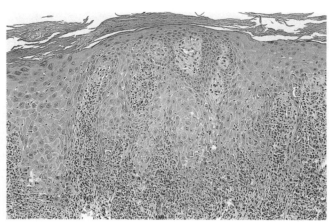

Fig. IIIF2.b

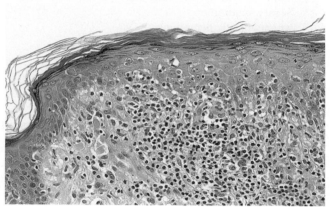

Fig. IIIF2.c

Fig. IIIF2.a. *Lichen planus-like keratosis, low power.* The features seen are those of a dense bandlike infiltrate in an expanded papillary that obscures a dermal–epidermal interface. The infiltrate is lymphocytic and fills the papillary dermis.

Fig. IIIF2.b. *Lichen planus-like keratosis, medium power.* There is patchy parakeratosis overlying acanthotic epidermis. The dermis has a dense infiltrate of lymphocytes that are exocytotic to the proliferative epidermis, destroying the basal keratinocytes.

Fig. IIIF2.c. *Lichen planus-like keratosis, high power.* There is a dense infiltrate of lymphocytes that is exocytotic to the epidermis, and there are numerous Civatte bodies in the dermis.

---

histiocytosis X (Letterer–Siwe)
mastocytosis/telangiectasia eruptiva macularis perstans

IIIF2b. Lichenoid Dermatitis, Plasma Cells Present

Plasma cells are found in the lichenoid infiltrate; their number is variable, but they do not as a rule comprise the major portion of the dermal infiltrate. *Lichenoid actinic keratosis* is a prototype (21).

Lichenoid Actinic Keratosis

This is a variant of the hypertrophic type of actinic keratosis, which demonstrates nuclear atypia, irregular acanthosis and hyperkeratosis, the presence of basal cell liquefaction, degeneration of the basal cell layer, and a bandlike "lichenoid" infiltrate in close apposition to the epidermis. Fairly numerous eosinophilic, homogeneous, apoptotic, so-called Civatte bodies are seen in the upper dermis. The presence of nuclear atypicality distinguishes these lesions from lichen planus and benign lichenoid keratosis. (See also section IIA1.)

Secondary Syphilis

See Figs. IIIF2b.d–IIIF2b.f.
   Conditions to consider in the differential diagnosis:
      lichenoid actinic keratosis
      Bowen's disease
      erythroplasia of Queyrat
      keratosis lichenoides chronica
      secondary syphilis
      pinta, primary or secondary lesions
      arthropod bite reaction
      CTCL, mycosis fungoides, patch/plaque stage
      Zoon's plasma cell balanitis

IIIF2c. Lichenoid Dermatitis, with Melanophages

Most conditions listed as lichenoid dermatoses may be associated with release of pigment from damaged basal keratinocytes into the papillary dermis "pigmentary incontinence." If a specific dermatosis cannot be identified, the appearances may be classified as postinflammatory hyperpigmentation (see section IIA1e).

   Conditions to consider in the differential diagnosis:
      postinflammatory hyperpigmentation

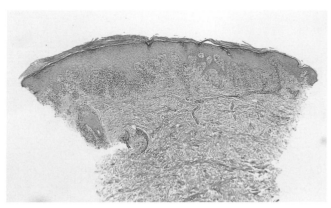

Fig. IIIF2a.a

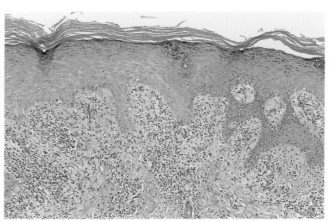

Fig. IIIF2a.b

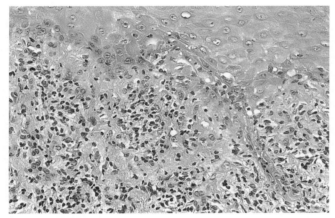

Fig. IIIF2a.c

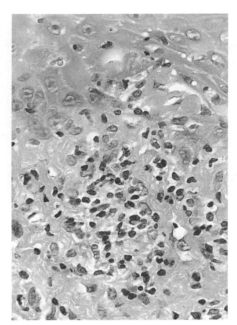

Fig. IIIF2a.d

Fig. IIIF2a.a. *Lichenoid drug eruption, low power.* There is a keratotic scale overlying a focally acanthotic epidermis. The papillary dermis is filled with an infiltrate of mononuclear cells that obscures the dermal–epidermal interface. The inflammatory infiltrate extends to the mid reticular dermis around dermal vessels.

Fig. IIIF2a.b. *Lichenoid drug eruption, medium power.* The scale is orthokeratotic overlying an acanthotic epidermis that shows irregular pointed rete (saw-toothing). The papillary dermis is edematous and filled with an infiltrate of mononuclear cells.

Fig. IIIF2a.c. *Lichenoid drug eruption, medium power.* The inflammatory infiltrate in the dermis consists of lymphocytes, histiocytes, and eosinophils. These cells are seen as exocytotic cells to the irregularly acanthotic epidermis.

Fig. IIIF2a.d. *Lichenoid drug eruption, high power.* Eosinophils are seen in the infiltrate. The epidermis shows some disorganization and exocytosis, with Civatte bodies.

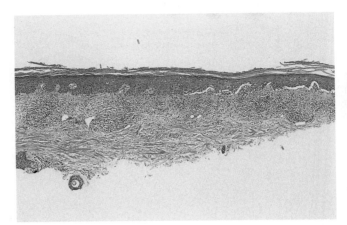

Fig. IIIF2b.a

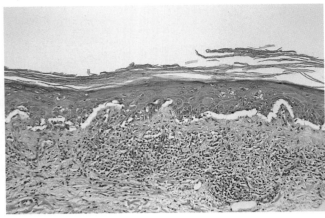

Fig. IIIF2b.b

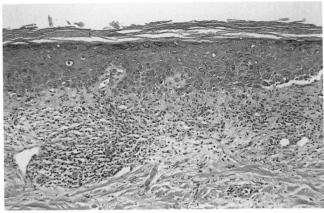

Fig. IIIF2b.c

Fig. IIIF2b.a. *Lichenoid actinic keratosis, low power.* There is an ortho- and parakeratotic scale overlying an evenly acanthotic epidermis. In the papillary dermis there is a nodular and diffuse lichenoid inflammatory infiltrate that obscures the dermal–epidermal interface.

Fig. IIIF2b.b. *Lichenoid actinic keratosis, medium power.* The basal cell zone is obliterated by the inflammatory infiltrate. The cells are lymphocytes and are exocytotic to the irregularly thickened epidermis. Necrotic keratinocytes are seen within this epidermis.

Fig. IIIF2b.c. *Lichenoid actinic keratosis, medium power.* The epidermis shows subtle keratinocyte atypia with an overlying ortho- and parakeratotic scale. Within the dermal infiltrate, there are lymphocytes and plasma cells.

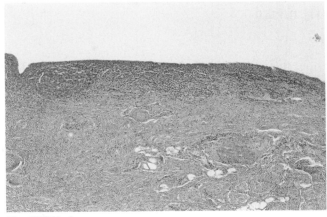

Fig. IIIF2b.d

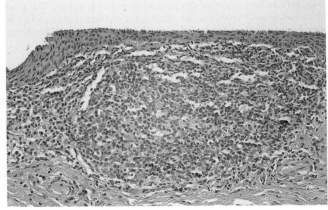

Fig. IIIF2b.e

Fig. IIIF2b.d. *Secondary syphilis, low power.* The features seen are those of conjunctival epithelium with an underlying bandlike infiltrate of mononuclear cells.

Fig. IIIF2b.e. *Secondary syphilis, medium power.* There is a mixed infiltrate of lymphocytes and plasma cells, with a germinal center.

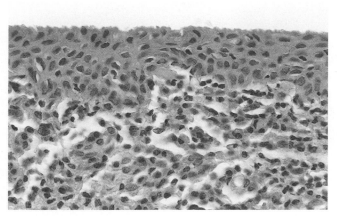

Fig. IIIF2b.f. *Secondary syphilis, high power.* The mucosal epithelium is effaced and the basal cell zone is obscured. The infiltrate consists of many plasma cells.

IIIF3. Lichenoid Dermatitis, Histiocytes Predominant

Histiocytes are the predominant cell type in the dermal infiltrate. *Lichen nitidus* is the prototype (23).

Lichen Nitidus

CLINICAL SUMMARY. This chronic, usually asymptomatic dermatitis begins commonly in childhood or early adulthood and is characterized by round, flat-topped, flesh-colored papules 2 to 3 mm in diameter that may occur in groups but do not coalesce. The lesions appear frequently as a localized eruption affecting predominantly the arms, trunk, or penis with a few cases reported to occur on palms, soles, nails, and mucous membranes. The clinical course is unpredictable; in some patients the eruption may become generalized, and in others spontaneous resolution may be seen.

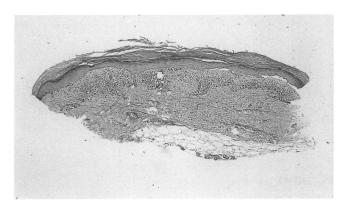

Fig. IIIF2c.a

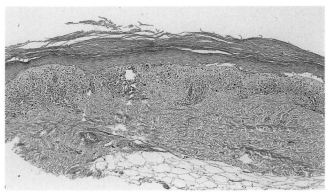

Fig. IIIF2c.b

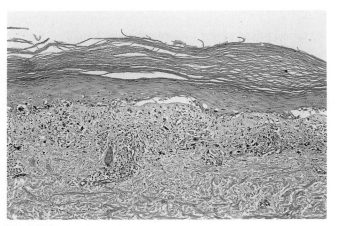

Fig. IIIF2c.c

Fig. IIIF2c.a. *Lichen planus, low power.* There is a thick orthokeratotic scale overlying an epidermis that is thinned and effaced. The papillary dermis is expanded and occupied by an infiltrate of mononuclear cells.

Fig. IIIF2c.b. *Lichen planus, medium power.* Hyperkeratosis overlies an effaced epidermis. In the dermis there is an inflammatory infiltrate of lymphocytes and melanophage pigmentation.

Fig. IIIF2c.c. *Lichen planus, high power.* The dermal–epidermal interface is obliterated by the inflammatory infiltrate that consists of lymphocytes and many melanophages.

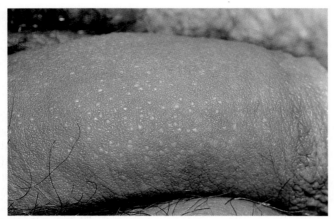

Clin. Fig. IIIF3

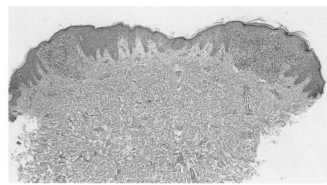

Fig. IIIF3.a

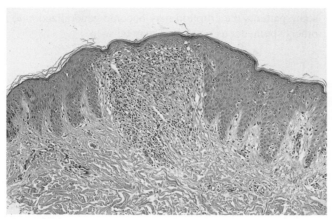

Fig. IIIF3.b

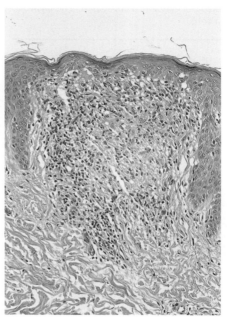

Fig. IIIF3.c

Clin. Fig. IIIF3. *Lichen nitidus.* Myriads of minute flesh-colored papules on the shaft of the penis.

Fig. IIIF3.a. *Lichen nitidus, low power.* There are two separate localized nodular infiltrates in a focally expanded papillary dermis. The epidermis surrounding the infiltrates is focally acanthotic.

Fig. IIIF3.b. *Lichen nitidus, medium power.* In an expanded dermal papilla there is a mixed inflammatory infiltrate of lymphocytes and histiocytes.

Fig. IIIF3.c. *Lichen nitidus, high power.* The nodular infiltrate within the expanded papillary dermis consists of histiocytes surrounded by a mantle of lymphocytes.

HISTOPATHOLOGY.   Each papule consists of a well-circumscribed mixed-cell granulomatous infiltrate that is closely attached to the lower surface of the epidermis and confined to a widened dermal papilla. The dermal infiltrate is composed of lymphocytes, numerous foamy or epithelioid histiocytes, and a few multinucleated giant cells. The infiltrate often extends slightly into the overlying epidermis, which is flat-tened and shows vacuolar alteration of the basal cell layer, focal subepidermal clefting, diminished granular layer, and focal parakeratosis. Transepidermal perforation of the infiltrate through the thinned epidermis may occur. At each lateral margin of the infiltrate, rete ridges tend to extend downward and seem to clutch the infiltrate in the manner of a claw clutching a ball. Follicular involvement has been described.

Conditions to consider in the differential diagnosis:

lichen nitidus
actinic reticuloid/chronic actinic dermatitis
histiocytosis X (Letterer–Siwe, Hand
   Schuller–Christian)
granulomatous slack skin

IIIF4. Lichenoid Dermatitis, Mast Cells Predominant

Mast cells are the predominant cell type in the dermis. They are frequently accompanied by eosinophils. Urticaria pigmentosa is the prototype (8).

Urticaria Pigmentosa, Lichenoid Examples

In the diffuse erythrodermic type of urticaria pigmentosa and in some papulonodular lesions, there is a dense bandlike infiltrate of mast cells in the upper dermis that may obscure the dermal–epidermal junction in a lichenoid pattern. Eosinophils may be present in small numbers (see also section IIIA2).

IIIF5. Lichenoid Dermatitis with Dermal Fibroplasia

Lymphocytes are the predominant cell type, often with an admixture of eosinophils, plasma cells, and histiocytes. In pigmented skin types and in regressed pigmented lesions,

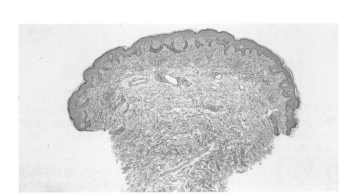

Fig. IIIF4.a

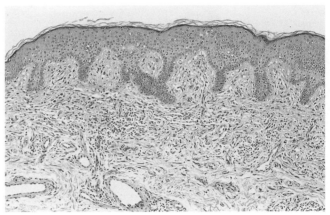

Fig. IIIF4.b

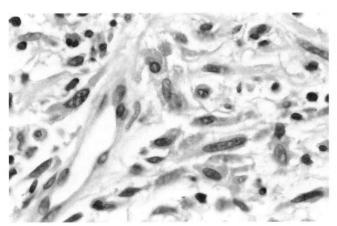

Fig. IIIF4.c

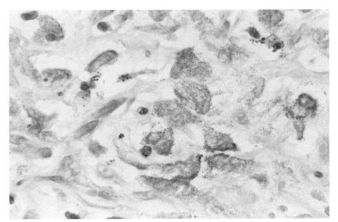

Fig. IIIF4.d

Fig. IIIF4.a. *Mastocytosis, low power.* There is a bandlike infiltrate of mast cells and lymphocytes in the papillary dermis. The overlying epidermis is acanthotic.

Fig. IIIF4.b. *Mastocytosis, medium power.* A diffuse infiltrate of mast cells and lymphocytes is seen in an edematous papillary dermis. The overlying epidermis is acanthotic with basal layer pigmentation.

Fig. IIIF4.c. *Mastocytosis, high power.* The infiltrate in the dermis consists of many mast cells and scattered eosinophils.

Fig. IIIF4.d. *Mastocytosis, high power, Giemsa stain.* Metachromatic granules are seen within dermal mast cells.

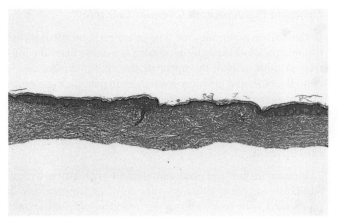

Fig. IIIF5.a

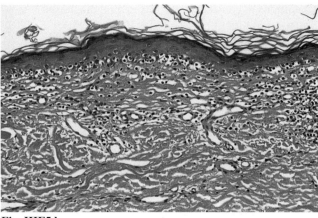

Fig. IIIF5.b

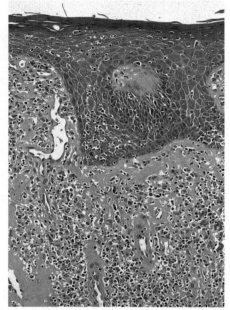

Fig. IIIF5.c

Fig. IIIF5.a. *Mycosis fungoides, atrophic patch stage, low power.* The rete ridge pattern is slightly accentuated, and there is a subtle lichenoid infiltrate in the papillary dermis. (P. LeBoit and T. Mc-Calmont)

Fig. IIIF5.b. *Mycosis fungoides, atrophic patch stage, high power.* A linear array of lymphocytes is disposed on the epidermal side of the basement membrane zone. There is delicate fibroplasia in the papillary dermis. (P. LeBoit and T. McCalmont)

Fig. IIIF5.c. *Mycosis fungoides, late plaque stage, high power.* A hyperplastic epidermis riddled with convoluted lymphocytes overlies a massively expanded fibrotic papillary dermis. (P. LeBoit and T. McCalmont)

melanophages may be prominent. Mycosis fungoides is prototypic (see section IIID).

Mycosis Fungoides, Patch Stage

See Figs. IIIF5.a–IIIF5.c.
   Conditions to consider in the differential diagnosis:
      mycosis fungoides, patch/plaque stage
      lichenoid keratosis
      actinic keratosis
      regressed pigmented lesions including regressed
         melanomas

IIIG. SUPERFICIAL VASCULITIS AND VASCULOPATHIES

Endothelial swelling, eosinophilic degeneration of the vessel wall ("fibrinoid necrosis"), and infiltration of the vessel wall by neutrophils, with nuclear fragmentation or leukocytoclasia resulting in "nuclear dust," define true vasculitis. There are extravasated red cells in the vessel walls and adjacent dermis. If the vasculitis is severe, ulceration or subepidermal separation ("bullous vasculitis") can occur. "Lymphocytic vasculitis," in which there is no vessel wall damage, is a controversial term and is discussed under lymphocytic infiltrates. A "vasculopathy" includes any abnormality of the vessel wall that does not meet the criteria above for vasculitis, such as fibrosis or hyalinization of the vessel wall without inflammation or necrosis.

1. Neutrophilic Vasculitis
2. Mixed Cell and Granulomatous Vasculitis
3. Vasculopathies with Lymphocytic Inflammation
4. Vasculopathies with Scant Inflammation
5. Thrombotic, Embolic, and Other Microangiopathies

IIIG1. Neutrophilic Vasculitis

In the dermis, vessels are necrotic, fibrinoid is present, and there are perivascular and intravascular neutrophils with leukocytoclasia and nuclear dust. *Cutaneous necrotizing (leukocytoclastic) vasculitis* is the prototype (24).

Cutaneous Necrotizing (Leukocytoclastic) Vasculitis

CLINICAL SUMMARY. A large number of different disease processes can be accompanied by small-vessel vasculitis with predominantly neutrophilic infiltrates. The clinical hallmark is palpable purpura, which may be the clinical appearance of dermal leukocytoclastic small-vessel vasculitis secondary to infection (e.g., gonococcal meningococcal or rickettsial sepsis), immune-complex–mediated vasculitis (e.g., serum sickness, cryoglobulinemia or Henoch–Schönlein purpura), antineutrophil cytoplasmic antibody (ANCA)-associated vasculitis (e.g., Wegener's granulomatosis), allergic vasculitis (e.g., reaction to a drug), vasculitis associated with connective tissue diseases, or a paraneoplastic phenomenon. It is important therefore to interpret the histologic findings in the context of clinical information to reach an appropriate diagnosis. Often, additional laboratory data, such as from microbiologic cultures, special stains for organisms, or immunofluorescence or serologic studies, are needed. Because the treatment for infectious vasculitides is so radically different from the treatment for immune-mediated diseases, the most important diagnostic step in the evaluation of a vasculitis is to rule out an infectious process. If noninfectious vasculitis is suspected, evidence for systemic vasculitis must be sought. Clinical findings—such as hematuria, arthritis, myalgia, enzymatic assays for muscle or liver enzymes, and serologic analysis for ANCAs, antinuclear antibodies, cryoglobulins, hepatitis B and C antibodies, IgA-fibronectin aggregates, and complement levels—are important to further delineate the disease process. Exposure to a potential allergen, such as a drug, that might have elicited a hypersensitivity reaction should be sought. It is also important to address the possibility that the histologic findings of vasculitis may be a secondary phenomenon as, for example, in ulceration from localized trauma.

HISTOPATHOLOGY. Neutrophilic small-vessel vasculitis is a reaction pattern of small dermal vessels, almost exclusively postcapillary venules, characterized by a combination of vascular damage and an infiltrate composed largely of neutrophils. Because there is often fragmentation of nuclei (karyorrhexis or leukocytoclasis), the term *leukocytoclastic vasculitis* is frequently used. Depending on its severity, this process may be subtle and limited to the superficial dermis or be pandermal and florid and associated with necrosis and ulceration. If edema is prominent, a subepidermal blister may form. If the neutrophilic infiltrate is dense and there is pustule formation, the term *pustular vasculitis* may be applied. In a typical case of leukocytoclastic vasculitis, the dermal vessels show swelling of the endothelial cells and deposits of strongly eosinophilic strands of fibrin within and around their walls, giving the vessel walls a "smudgy" appearance, referred to as *fibrinoid degeneration.* Actual necrosis of the perivascular collagen, however, is seen only rarely in conjunction with ulcerative lesions. If the vascular changes are severe, the vessel lumen may be occluded. The cellular infiltrate consists mainly of neutrophils and of varying numbers of eosinophils and mononuclear cells. The infiltrate also is scattered throughout the upper dermis in association with fibrin deposits between and within collagen bundles. Extravasation of erythrocytes (purpura) is commonly present (see Figs. IIIA1.a–IIIA1.d).

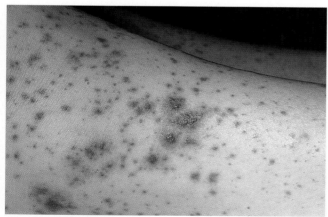

Clin. Fig. IIIG1.a

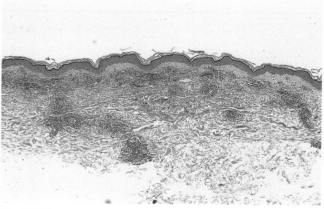

Fig. IIIG1.a

Clin. Fig. IIIG1.a. *Leukocytoclastic vasculitis.* Palpable purpuric tender papules on the legs of a 25-year-old woman resolved after therapy for streptococcal pharyngitis.

Fig. IIIG1.a. *Leukocytoclastic vasculitis, low power.* In the papillary dermis there is hemorrhage and an infiltrate around the dermal vessels. *(continues)*

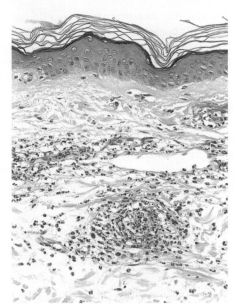

Fig. IIIG1.b

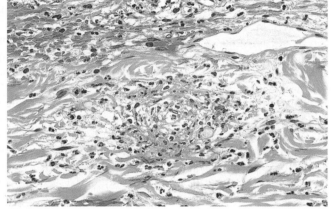

Fig. IIIG1.c

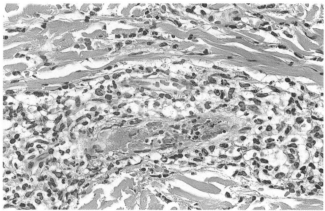

Fig. IIIG1.d

Fig. IIIG1.b. *Leukocytoclastic vasculitis, medium power.* The dermis is edematous and shows a distinct perivascular inflammatory infiltrate of lymphocytes, polymorphonuclear leukocytes, and hemorrhage.

Fig. IIIG1.c. *Leukocytoclastic vasculitis, medium power.* There is vascular destruction with an infiltrate of fragmented neutrophils and eosinophils, scattered hemorrhage, and lymphocytes.

Fig. IIIG1.d. *Leukocytoclastic vasculitis, high power.* Eosinophilic homogenous fibrinoid material is seen within a vascular structure. The inflammatory infiltrate consists of lymphocytes, polymorphonuclear leukocytes, and fragmented polymorphonuclear leukocytes.

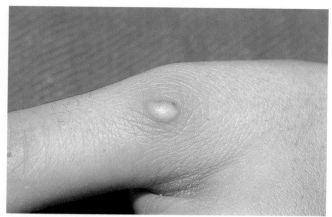

Clin. Fig. IIIG1.b

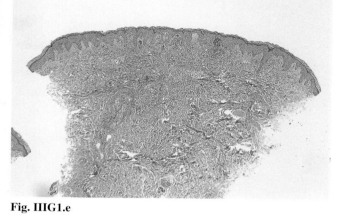

Fig. IIIG1.e

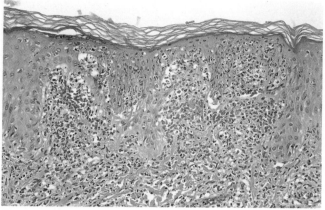

Fig. IIIG1.f

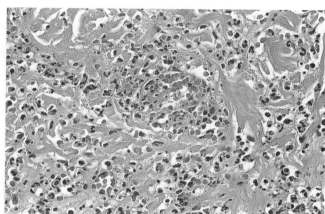

Fig. IIIG1.g

Clin. Fig. IIIG1.b. *Gonococcemia.* A 25-year-old woman developed hemorrhagic pustules of palms, knees, and elbows associated with joint tenderness and swelling. Blood and vaginal cultures were positive.

Fig. IIIG1.e. *Gonococcemia, low power.* A mixed perivascular and diffuse infiltrate of mixed cells with prominent hemorrahge in the upper and mid dermis.

Fig. IIIG1.f. *Gonococcemia, medium power.* Mixed inflammatory cells with prominent hemorrhage in the dermis and extending into the epidermis. In a slightly more advanced lesion, a necrotic hemorrhagic bulla is often produced.

Fig. IIIG1.g. *Gonococcemia, high power.* An inflammatory and thrombotic microangiopathy, with fibrin in the lumen of a small vessel and neutrophils in its wall.

Gonococcemia

See Figs. IIIG1.e–IIIG1.g.

Conditions to consider in the differential diagnosis:

cutaneous necrotizing (leukocytoclastic) vasculitis
Henoch–Schönlein purpura
cryoglobulinemia
connective tissue associated (rheumatoid, lupus)
septicemia, especially meningococcemia/
  gonococcemia
urticarial vasculitis
erythema elevatum diutinum
miscellaneous
microscopic polyarteritis nodosa
vasculitis in exanthemic pustulosis (drug-induced)

IIIG2. Mixed Cell and Granulomatous Vasculitis

There is vessel wall damage and a mixed infiltrate in the dermis that includes eosinophils, plasma cells, histiocytes, and giant cells. *Granuloma faciale* is prototypic.

Granuloma Faciale

CLINICAL SUMMARY. Granuloma faciale (25) presents clinically as one or several asymptomatic, soft, brown-red, slowly enlarging papules or plaques, almost always on the face.

HISTOPATHOLOGY. There is a dense polymorphous infiltrate, mainly in the upper half of the dermis but occasionally

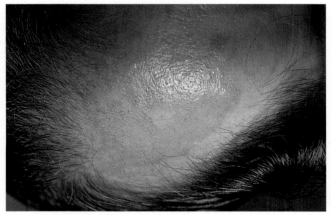

Clin. Fig. IIIG2

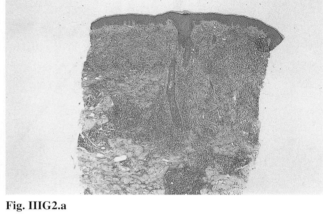

Fig. IIIG2.a

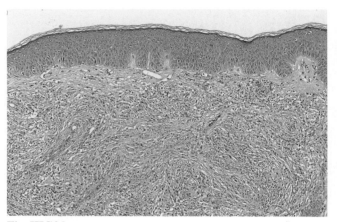

Fig. IIIG2.b

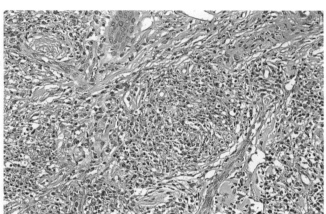

Fig. IIIG2.c

Clin. Fig. IIIG2. *Granuloma faciale.* A boggy erythematous plaque on the scalp in a middle-aged man.

Fig. IIIG2.a. *Granuloma faciale, low power.* There is a dense diffuse dermal infiltrate spanning the reticular dermis.

Fig. IIIG2.b. *Granuloma faciale, medium power.* There is a small grenz or clear zone between the epidermis and the dermal infiltrate.

Fig. IIIG2.c. *Granuloma faciale, low power.* The infiltrate is composed of mixed inflammatory cells, including neutrophils, eosinophils, lymphocytes, and histiocytes.

---

extending even into the subcutaneous tissue. The infiltrate is typically separated from the epidermis or the pilosebaceous appendages by a narrow "grenz" zone of normal collagen, and the pilosebaceous structures tend to remain intact. The infiltrate consists in large part of neutrophils and eosinophils, but mononuclear cells, plasma cells, and mast cells are also present. Frequently, there is leukocytoclasia with formation of nuclear dust, especially in the vicinity of the capillaries, and often there is some evidence of vasculitis with deposition of fibrinoid material within and around vessel walls. Occasionally, some hemorrhage is noted. Foam cells are sometimes observed and areas of fibrosis in older lesions. Direct immunofluorescence data suggest an immune-complex–mediated event with deposition of mainly IgG in and around vessels.

Conditions to consider in the differential diagnosis:

Churg–Strauss vasculitis
Wegener's granulomatosis
giant-cell arteritis
granuloma faciale
Buerger's disease

IIIG3. Vasculopathies with Lymphocytic Inflammation

A histologic diagnosis of a "lymphocytic vasculitis" may be made if there is sufficient evidence of vascular damage and the inflammatory infiltrate is predominantly lymphocytic. Often, the vascular damage is subtle, and in many cases there may be disagreement as to whether or not the term "vasculitis" is warranted. Clearcut evidence of vasculitis requires the presence of an inflammatory infiltrate together with fibrinoid necrosis of the vascular wall. These changes are not often seen in combination with a strictly lymphocytic infiltrate. The purpuric dermatoses are prototypic of a pattern of vasculopathy that usually falls short of frank vasculitis, in association with a lymphocytic infiltrate that may involve the vessel walls (26).

Pigmented Purpuric Dermatoses

CLINICAL SUMMARY. Historically, four variants of purpura pigmentosa chronica have been described: purpura annularis telangiectoides of Majocchi, progressive pigmentary dermatosis of Schamberg, pigmented purpuric dermatitis of Gougerot and Blum, and eczematoidlike purpura of Doucas and Kapentanakis. They are all closely related and often cannot be reliably distinguished on clinical and histologic grounds. Therefore, their classification as distinct entities is not necessary. It is likely that lichen aureus is a closely related variant as well, because the clinical lesion suggests a purpuric component and the histologic findings are similar to those of the other four variants of pigmented purpuric dermatitis. The general terms "pigmented purpuric dermatitis," "chronic purpuric dermatitis," and "purpura pigmentosa chronica" appear suitable for this disease spectrum.

Clinically, the primary lesion consists of discrete telangiectatic puncta as a result of capillary dilatation and pigmentation as a result of hemosiderin deposits. In some cases, telangiectasia (Majocchi's disease) predominates; in others, pigmentation (Schamberg's disease) predominates. In Majocchi's disease, the lesions are usually irregular in shape and occur predominantly on the lower legs. In some cases, the findings may mimic those of stasis. Not infrequently, clinical signs of inflammation are present, such as erythema, papules, and scaling (Gougerot–Blum disease) or papules, scaling, and lichenification (eczematoidlike purpura). The disorder is often limited to the lower extremities, but it may be extensive. Mild pruritus may be present. A localized variant of pigmented purpuric dermatitis is lichen aureus, in which one or a few closely set flat papules or macules of a rust, copper, or orange color are present, most commonly on the legs.

HISTOPATHOLOGY. The basic process is a lymphocytic perivascular infiltrate limited to the papillary dermis. Epidermal alterations may include slight acanthosis and basal layer vacuolopathy. There is variability in the pattern of the

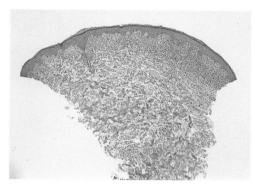

Fig. IIIG3.a

Fig. IIIG3.a. *Pigmented purpuric dermatosis, low power.* There is hyperkeratosis overlying an acanthotic epidermis. The papillary dermis is expanded with an infiltrate around the dermal vessels.

Fig. IIIG3.b. *Pigmented purpuric dermatosis, medium power.* Tufted collections of thick-walled vessels are in an edematous expanded papillary dermis. Hemorrhage is present.

Fig. IIIG3.c. *Pigmented purpuric dermatosis, high power.* The papillary dermal hemorrhage is well defined and is associated with prominent vessels.

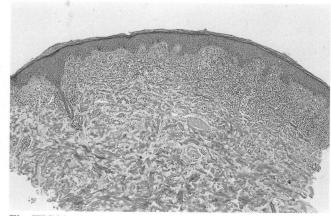

Fig. IIIG3.b

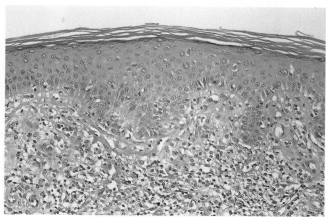

Fig. IIIG3.c

dermal infiltrate. In some instances, the infiltrate may assume a bandlike or lichenoid pattern, particularly in the lichenoid variant of Gougerot–Blum disease, and may involve the reticular dermis in a perivascular distribution. Evidence of vascular damage may be present. However, the extent of vascular injury is usually mild and often insufficient to justify the term vasculitis. Vascular damage commonly consists only of endothelial cell swelling and dermal hemorrhage. Extravasated red blood cells are usually found in the vicinity of the capillaries. Less commonly, one may observe deposition of fibrinoid material in vessel walls. In some instances, the infiltrate involves the epidermis and may be associated with mild spongiosis and patchy parakeratosis. This is observed in some cases of pigmented purpuric lichenoid dermatitis of Gougerot and Blum and eczematoidlike purpura of Doucas and Kapetanakis. The pattern of the infiltrate often is not strictly confined to the perivascular area, and may infiltrate the adjacent papillary dermis (between vessels).

In old lesions, the capillaries often show dilatation of their lumen and proliferation of their endothelium. Extravasated red blood cells may no longer be present, but one frequently finds varying amounts of hemosiderin. The inflammatory infiltrate is less pronounced than in the early stage.

In lichen aureus, a dense lymphohistiocytic infiltrate is present in the superficial dermis, typically distributed in a bandlike fashion and often associated with an increase in dermal capillaries. Exocytosis of mononuclear cells into the epidermis may be seen. Scattered within the infiltrate are hemosiderin-laden macrophages.

Conditions to consider in the differential diagnosis:

arthropod bites
hypersensitivity reactions to drugs
urticarial vasculitis
pigmented purpuric dermatoses
autoimmune and connective tissue diseases
pernio (chilblains)
polymorphous light eruption
atrophie blanche
viral processes
cutaneous T-cell infiltrates
PLEVA
pityriasis lichenoides chronica
lymphomatoid papulosis

IIIG4. Vasculopathies with Scant Inflammation

There is fibrosis or hyalinization of the vessel walls, with few inflammatory cells. *Stasis dermatitis* is a prototype.

Stasis Dermatitis

CLINICAL SUMMARY. Patients with long-standing venous insufficiency and lower extremity edema may develop pruritic, erythematous, scaly papules and plaques on the lower legs, often in association with brown pigmentation and hair loss.

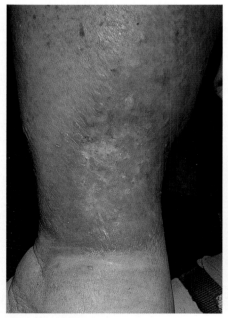

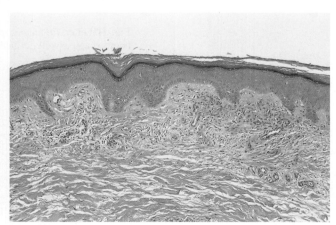

Clin. Fig. IIIG4.a   **Fig. IIIG4.a**

Clin. Fig. IIIG4.a. *Stasis dermatitis.* Lower leg brawny violaceous pigmentation, edema, and "bottle neck" deformity resulted from chronic venous insufficiency in an elderly woman.

Fig. IIIG4.a. *Stasis dermatitis, low power.* There is hyperkeratosis overlying an acanthotic epidermis. The papillary dermis is expanded with a scant infiltrate around the dermal vessels. *(continues)*

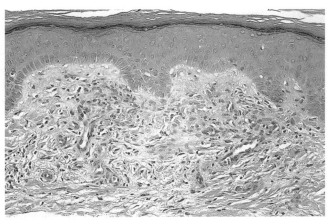

Fig. IIIG4.b

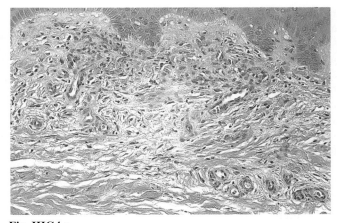

Fig. IIIG4.c

Fig. IIIG4.b. *Stasis dermatitis, medium power.* Tufted collections of thick-walled vessels are in an edematous expanded papillary dermis. Hemorrhage is present.

Fig. IIIG4.c. *Stasis dermatitis, high power.* The papillary dermal hemorrhage is well defined and is associated with vascular proliferation.

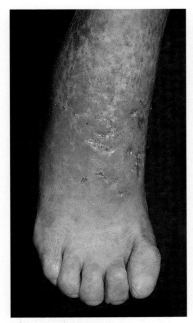

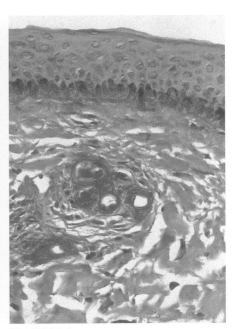

Clin. Fig. IIIG4.b

Fig. IIIG4.d

Clin. Fig. IIIG4.b. *Cryoglobulinemia.* A 73-year-old woman developed edema and reticulated erythema with extremely painful ulcerations of the lower legs and feet.

Fig. IIIG4.d. *Cryoglobulinemia, medium power [periodic acid–Schiff (PAS) stain].* PAS-positive bright-red cryoprecipitates are present in small dermal vessels. An inflammatory infiltrate is generally lacking in type I cryoglobulinemia, caused by deposition of monoclonal immunoglobulins, usually in association with an underlying lymphoproliferative disorder. (R. Barnhill and K. Busam)

HISTOPATHOLOGY.   The epidermis is hyperkeratotic with areas of parakeratosis, acanthosis, and focal spongiosis. The superficial dermal vessels may be arranged in lobular aggregates. The proliferation may be florid, mimicking Kaposi's sarcoma (acroangiodermatitis). Inflammation may be minimal or there may be a superficial, perivascular, lymphohistiocytic infiltrate around plump thickened capillaries and venules. The reticular dermis is often fibrotic. Hemosiderin is usually present superficially but may be identified about the deep vascular plexus as well.

Conditions to consider in the differential diagnosis:
   stasis dermatitis
   atrophie blanche (segmental hyalinizing vasculitis)
   malignant atrophic papulosis (Degos)
   cryoglobulinemia (type I)
   Mondor's disease
   pigmented purpuric dermatoses
      (Majocchi–Schamberg/Gougerot–Bloom)

IIIG5. Thrombotic, Embolic, and Other Microangiopathies

There are thrombi or emboli within the lumens of small vessels (27). In other microangiopathies, the vessel walls may be thickened with compromise of the lumen (amyloidosis, calciphylaxis). The *antiphospholipid syndromes* are prototypic (28).

Lupus Anticoagulant and Antiocardiolipin Syndromes

CLINICAL SUMMARY.   The *antiphospholipid syndrome* occurs in patients with SLE and other autoimmune diseases who develop immunoglobulins that can prolong phospholipid-dependent coagulation tests. These immunoglobulins occur in association with SLE and other autoimmune diseases, but are also found unassociated with these diseases. One of these is a lupus anticoagulant, which occurs in about 10% of SLE patients. Affected patients are at greater risk

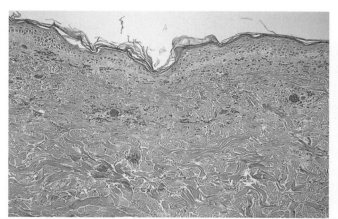

Fig. IIIG5.a

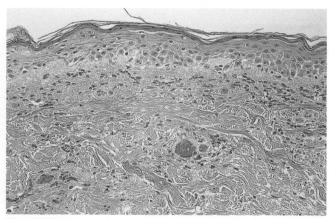

Fig. IIIG5.b

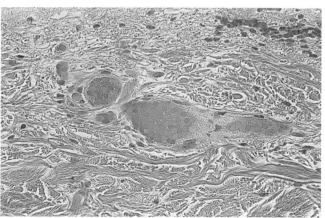

Fig. IIIG5.c

Fig. IIIG5.a. *Noninflammatory thrombi, low power.* There is an effaced epidermis with an overlying keratotic scale. The dermis shows hemorrhage with its greatest concentration in the papillary dermis but also within the reticular dermis.

Fig. IIIG5.b. *Noninflammatory thrombi, medium power.* The papillary dermis is edematous with hemorrhage. Vessels are engorged with red cell thrombi.

Fig. IIIG5.c. *Noninflammatory thrombi, high power.* Dermal vessels show red cell thrombi without an inflammatory response.

for thromboembolic disease, including deep venous thrombosis, pulmonary emboli, and other large-vessel thrombosis. Other associated findings are recurrent fetal wastage, renal vascular thrombosis, thrombosis of dermal vessels, and thrombocytopenia. Anticardiolipin antibody, a second type of antiphospholipid antibody, occurs five times more often than lupus anticoagulant antibody. It is associated with recurrent arterial and venous thrombosis, valvular abnormalities, cerebrovascular thromboses, and essential hypertension (Sneddon's syndrome). Other cutaneous findings include livedo reticularis, necrotizing purpura, disseminated intravascular coagulation, and stasis ulcers of the ankles. In severe forms of coagulopathies, large areas of ecchymosis may be present, typically located on the extremities. Large hemorrhagic bullae may overlie the ecchymoses, and some of the ecchymotic areas may undergo necrosis.

HISTOPATHOLOGY. The histologic features are nonspecific. In mild forms, the only histologic manifestation may be dermal hemorrhage—that is, extravasation of red blood cells into perivascular connective tissue. With increasing severity of the disease process, intravascular fibrin thrombi may be found. In severe cases, thrombotic vascular occlusion may lead to hemorrhagic infarcts, epidermal and dermal necrosis, or subepidermal bulla formation.

Conditions to consider in the differential diagnosis:

disseminated intravascular coagulation
thrombotic thrombocytopenic purpura
cryoglobulinemia/macroglobulinemia
antiphospholipid syndrome
lupus anticoagulant and antiocardiolipin syndromes
connective tissue disease (rheumatoid, mixed)
calciphylaxis
amyloidosis
porphyria cutanea tarda and other porphyrias
cholesterol emboli

IIIH. SUPERFICIAL DERMATITIS WITH INTERFACE VACUOLES (INTERFACE DERMATITIS)

Lymphocytes approximate the dermal–epidermal junction. Cellular degeneration and edema in the basal cell zone produce interface vacuoles. The dermis usually has perivascular lymphocytes and there may be pigment incontinence.

1. Vacuolar Dermatitis, Apoptotic/Necrotic Cells Prominent
2. Vacuolar Dermatitis, Apoptotic Cells Usually Absent
3. Vacuolar Dermatitis, Variable Apoptosis
4. Vacuolar Dermatitis, Basement Membranes Thickened

IIIH1. Vacuolar Dermatitis, Apoptotic/Necrotic Cells Prominent

Lymphocytes approximate the dermal–epidermal junction. Vacuolar degeneration is present in the basal cell zone. Apoptotic keratinocytes are found in the epidermis in variable numbers, visualized as round eosinophilic anuclear structures. The dermis usually has perivascular lymphocytes and may show pigment incontinence. *Erythema multiforme* is the prototype (29).

Erythema Multiforme

CLINICAL SUMMARY. Erythema multiforme is an acute self-limited dermatosis characterized by multiform lesions, including macules, papules, vesicles, and bullae, typically with target or iris lesions that have the form of a bull's-eye surrounded by a ring of erythema. The disease may be divided into a minor and major form, with the latter also known as Stevens–Johnson syndrome. The most frequent etiology in erythema multiforme is infection, *herpes simplex virus* being the most common agent. In Stevens–Johnson syndrome, medications, in particular sulfonamides, are the offending agents in most patients. Patients with herpes simplex virus associated erythema multiforme have recurrent lesions, affecting primarily the oral mucosa or the extremities, with typical target or iris lesions. Those with drug-induced Stevens–Johnson syndrome have truncal involvement, a more purpuric macular eruption, and atypical target lesions. Patients often present with fever. Involvement of the oral, conjunctival, nasal, and genital mucosa is common. In toxic epidermal necrolysis (Lyell's disease), which frequently overlaps with Stevens–Johnson disease and is usually regarded as a form of erythema multiforme, a widespread blotchy erythema develops. This is soon followed by the development of large flaccid bullae and detachment of the epidermis in large sheets, leaving the dermis exposed and giving a moist eroded appearance. The disease has a high mortality rate because of fluid loss and sepsis. In nearly 90% of cases it is caused by medications, most commonly sulfonamides. The "cytotoxic" or "erythema multiforme-like" drug eruptions overlap with authentic erythema multiforme and with toxic epidermal necrolysis, both of which may be drug induced. Medications associated with increased risk for these entities include sulfonamides, trimethoprim-sulfamethoxazole, phenobarbital, carbamazipine, phenytoin, oxicam nonsteroidal antiinflammatory agents, allopurinol, chlormezanone, and corticosteroids.

HISTOPATHOLOGY. Erythema multiforme is considered the prototype of the vacuolar form of interface dermatitis. Because of its acute nature, there is an orthokeratotic stratum corneum. The earliest changes include vacuolization of the basal cell layer; tagging of lymphocytes along the dermoepidermal junction; and a sparse, superficial, perivascu-

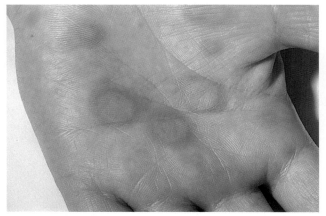

Clin. Fig. IIIH1.a

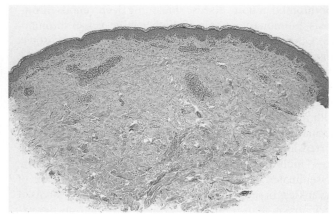

Fig. IIIH1.a

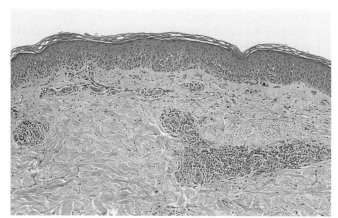

Fig. IIIH1.b

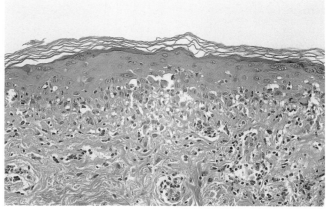

Fig. IIIH1.c

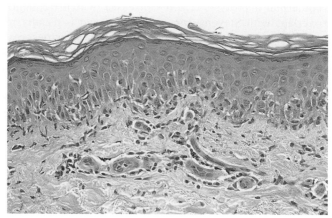

Fig. IIIH1.d

Clin. Fig. IIIH1.a. *Erythema multiforme.* Steroid responsive "target" papules characterized by central bullae with surrounding erythema appeared after antibiotic therapy.

Fig. IIIH1.a. *Erythema multiforme, low power.* The epidermis is effaced and there is a dense perivascular infiltrate of mononuclear cells.

Fig. IIIH1.b. *Erythema multiforme, medium power.* The epidermis shows spongiosis and exocytosis. The reticular and papillary dermis has a dense infiltrate of lymphocytes with scattered areas of hemorrhage.

Fig. IIIH1.c. *Erythema multiforme, medium power.* The epidermis shows necrotic keratinocytes, vacuolar degeneration at the basal cell zone, and a lichenoid inflammatory infiltrate of lymphocytic cells.

Fig. IIIH1.d. *Erythema multiforme, high power.* There is basket-weave orthokeratin overlying an epidermis that shows exocytosis basal layer liquefaction degeneration and necrotic keratinocytes. The dermal vessels are thickened and there is an infiltrate of lymphocytes.

lar lymphoid infiltrate. Mild spongiosis and exocytosis are seen. Necrosis of individual keratinocytes ("apoptosis") occurs in the stratum malpighii and is the hallmark of erythema multiforme. Satellite cell necrosis, characterized by intraepidermal lymphocytes in close association with apoptotic keratinocytes, is frequently present. In more papular edematous lesions, there is papillary dermal edema and more significant spongiosis and inflammation. Intraepider-

mal vesicles associated with exocytosis may be noted on occasion. Although some authors have noted a significant number of eosinophils in drug-induced erythema multiforme, others have not. In addition to the clinical differences, some histologic differences have been noted between drug-induced and herpes simplex-associated erythema multiforme. In the former, there is more widespread keratinocyte necrosis, microscopic blister formation, and more

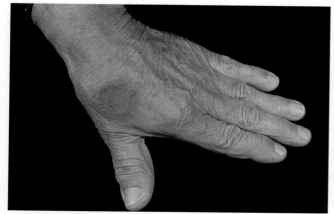

Clin. Fig. IIIH1.b

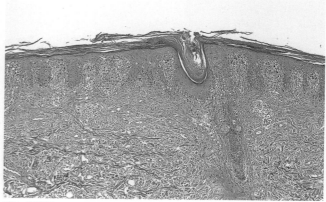

Fig. IIIH1.e

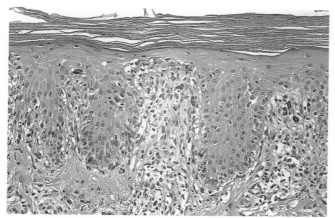

Fig. IIIH1.f

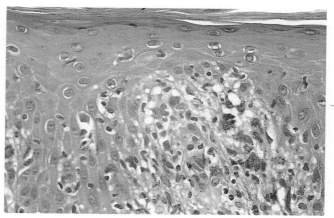

Fig. IIIH1.g

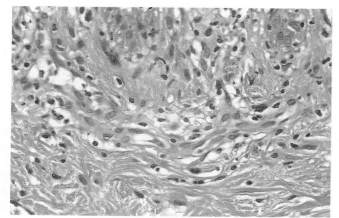

Fig. IIIH1.h

Clin. Fig. IIIH1.b. *Fixed drug eruption.* Challenge with sulfa drug resulted in recurrence of "burning" dusky vesiculated plaque on the dorsal hand. Histology (not illustrated) typically shows apoptotic dermatitis with pigmentary incontinence.

Fig. IIIH1.e. *Fixed drug eruption.* There is hyperkeratosis and a lichenoid inflammatory infiltrate in the dermis.

Fig. IIIH1.f. *Fixed drug eruption.* Vacuolar alteration is present at the dermal–epidermal junction.

Fig. IIIH1.g. *Fixed drug eruption.* Mostly in the basal epidermis, there are scattered apoptotic keratinocytes.

Fig. IIIH1.h. *Fixed drug eruption.* In the dermis, there is a lymphocytic inflammatory infiltrate with eosinophils.

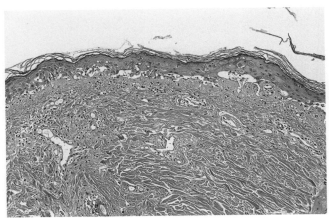

Fig. IIIH1.i

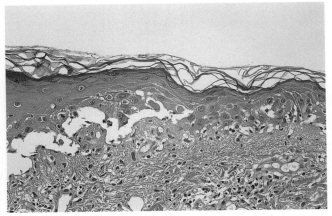

Fig. IIIH1.j

Fig. IIIH1.i. *Graft-versus-host disease, acute.* In this grade 3 graft-versus-host reaction, subepithelial separation has resulted from confluent vacuolar change.

Fig. IIIH1.j. *Graft-versus-host disease, acute.* Lymphocytes tagging at the dermal–epidermal junction and eliciting satellite-cell necrosis.

pigmentary incontinence. In cases associated with herpes simplex virus infection, there is more spongiosis, exocytosis, liquefaction degeneration of the basal layer, and papillary dermal edema. Nuclear dust may be identified in the papillary dermis in the latter.

In toxic epidermal necrolysis, in bullous lesions, and in the central portion of target lesions, there are numerous necrotic keratinocytes, even full-thickness epidermal necrosis, and a subepidermal bulla. The dermal inflammatory infiltrate is more sparse in toxic epidermal necrolysis than in erythema multiforme. Extravasated erythrocytes are commonly found within the blister cavity. Melanophages within the papillary dermis occur in late lesions.

Fixed Drug Eruption

See Figs. IIIH1.e–IIIH1.h.

Graft-Versus-Host Disease, Acute

See Figs. IIIH1.i and IIIH1.j.
Conditions to consider in the differential diagnosis:
  erythema multiforme
  toxic epidermal necrolysis (Lyell)
  Stevens–Johnson syndrome
  fixed drug eruption
  phototoxic drug eruption
  radiation dermatitis
  sunburn reaction
  thermal burn
  PLEVA
  graft-versus-host disease, acute
  eruption of lymphocyte recovery
  bullous vasculitis

IIIH2. Vacuolar Dermatitis, Apoptotic Cells Usually Absent

There is basilar keratinocyte vacuolar destruction, and apoptotic cells are rare or absent. The dermis has perivascular

lymphocytes and may show pigment incontinence. *Dermatomyositis* is a prototype (30).

Dermatomyositis

CLINICAL SUMMARY.   Dermatomyositis manifests as an inflammatory myopathy with characteristic cutaneous findings, which has peaks of incidence in children and in adults aged 45 to 65. In the absence of cutaneous findings, the diagnosis of polymyositis is applied. The cutaneous disease alone, without muscular involvement, has been termed *amyopathic dermatomyositis* or *dermatomyositis sine myositis*. In some instances the cutaneous eruption precedes the development of muscular weakness by many months or even by several years. Diagnostic criteria for dermatomyositis include proximal symmetric muscle weakness, elevated muscle enzymes, lack of neuropathy on electromyelography, consistent muscle biopsy changes, and cutaneous findings.

Two distinctive cutaneous lesions are found in dermatomyositis. One is violaceous slightly edematous periorbital patches that primarily involve the eyelids, known as the *heliotrope rash*. The other is discrete red-purple papules over the bony prominences, particularly the knuckles, knees, and elbows, known as *Gottron's papules*. These may evolve into atrophic plaques with pigmentary alterations and telangiectasia and are then known as *Gottron's sign*. Other cutaneous findings include periungual telangiectasia, hypertrophy of cuticular tissues associated with splinter hemorrhages, photosensitivity, and poikiloderma. There may be subcutaneous and periarticular calcification, usually centered in the proximal muscles of the shoulders and pelvic girdle.

Controversy exists over the association of dermatomyositis with malignancy. The pathogenesis of the disease is uncertain. Associated antibodies include PM1, Jo1 (correlates with pulmonary fibrosis), Ku (associated with sclerodermatomyositis), and M2.

HISTOPATHOLOGY.   The erythematous-edematous lesions of the skin in dermatomyositis may show only nonspecific inflammation. However, quite frequently the histologic changes are indistinguishable from those seen in SLE. There may be epidermal atrophy, basement membrane degeneration, vacuolar alteration of basilar keratinocytes, a sparse lymphocytic inflammatory infiltrate around blood vessels, and interstitial mucin deposition. With severe inflammation, there may be subepidermal fibrin deposition. Immune complexes are not detected at the dermal–epidermal junction as in lupus erythematosus. Old cutaneous lesions with the clinical appearance of poikiloderma atrophicans vasculare usu-ally show a bandlike infiltrate under an atrophic epidermis with hydropic degeneration of the basal cell layer. The Gottron's papules overlying the knuckles also show vacuolization of the basal cell layer, but acanthosis rather than epidermal atrophy. Subcutaneous tissue may show focal areas of panniculitis associated with mucoid degeneration of fat cells in early lesions. Extensive areas of calcification may be present in the subcutis at a later stage.

Three types of muscle biopsy changes may be observed in active disease: interstitial lymphohistiocytic inflammatory infiltrates; segmental muscle fiber necrosis; or vasculopathy, characterized by immune complex deposition in

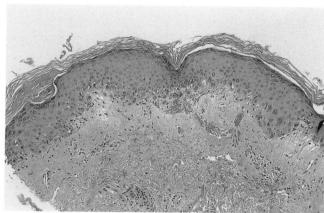

Fig. IIIH2.a

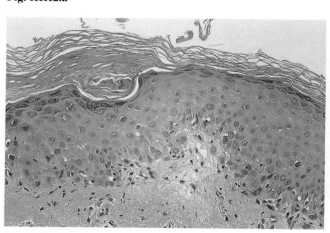

Fig. IIIH2.b

Fig. IIIH2.c

Fig. IIIH2.a. *Dermatomyositis, low power.* There is an orthokeratotic scale overlying an acanthotic epidermis. In the dermis is a patchy lichenoid inflammatory infiltrate that obscures the dermal–epidermal interface. Hemorrhage is seen within the edematous papillary dermis.

Fig. IIIH2.b. *Dermatomyositis, high power.* Focal area of parakeratosis with hemorrhage is seen overlying the acanthotic epidermis. Liquefaction degeneration is seen at the basal cell zone and there is exocytosis of lymphocytes.

Fig. IIIH2.c. *Dermatomyositis, high power.* There is a parakeratotic scale with hemorrhage overlying an epidermis that shows exocytosis and basal layer liquefaction degeneration.

vessel walls. Old lesions usually show nonspecific atrophy of the muscle fibers and diffuse interstitial fibrosis with relatively little inflammation. Changes in organs other than the skin and the striated muscles occur only rarely in dermatomyositis, in contrast to SLE and systemic scleroderma.

Conditions to consider in the differential diagnosis:

dermatomyositis
morbilliform viral exanthem
poikiloderma vasculare atrophicans
paraneoplastic pemphigus
erythema dyschromicum perstans
pinta, tertiary stage

IIIH3. Vacuolar Dermatitis, Variable Apoptosis

Vacuolar degeneration is associated with variable numbers of apoptotic cells in the epidermis. The dermis may have increased ground substance and there may be pigmentary incontinence (see section IIIH1).

Subacute Cutaneous Lupus Erythematosus

CLINICAL SUMMARY. Subacute cutaneous lupus erythematosus (SCLE) represents about 9% of all cases of lupus erythematosus. It is characterized by extensive erythematous, symmetric nonscarring, and nonatrophic lesions that arise abruptly on the upper trunk, extensor surfaces of the

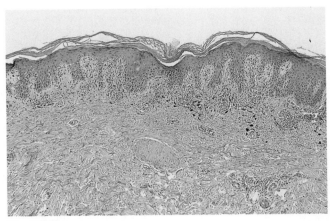

Fig. IIIH3.a

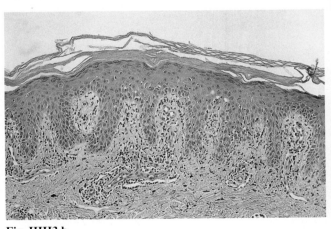

Fig. IIIH3.b

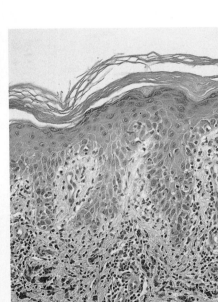

Fig. IIIH3.c

Fig. IIIH3.a. *Subacute lupus erythematosus, low power.* There is an orthokeratotic scale overlying an acanthotic epidermis. The papillary dermis is expanded, edematous, and contains a dense lichenoid inflammatory infiltrate. Melanophage pigment is seen within the upper reticular dermis.

Fig. IIIH3.b. *Subacute lupus erythematosus, medium power.* The lymphocytic infiltrate in the papillary dermis obscures the dermal–epidermal interface and is exocytotic to the acanthotic epidermis. Occasional apoptotic cells are present in the epidermis.

Fig. IIIH3.c. *Subacute lupus erythematosus, high power.* The acanthotic epidermis shows spongiosis and exocytosis. There is a dense infiltrate in the papillary dermis that is diffuse and perivascular and consists of lymphocyte and melanophage pigment.

arms, and dorsa of the hands and fingers. This eruption has two clinical variants: papulosquamous lesions and annular to polycyclic lesions. Frequently, both types of lesions are seen. In some instances, vesicular and discoid lesions with scarring may coexist. Patients with SCLE may have mild systemic involvement, particularly arthralgias.

HISTOPATHOLOGY. Histologic changes in SCLE consist of hydropic degeneration of the basilar epithelial layer, sometimes severe enough to form clefts and subepidermal vesicles, commonly with colloid (apoptotic) bodies in the lower epidermis and papillary dermis. There is often fairly prominent edema of the dermis, and there may be focal extravasation of erythrocytes and dermal fibrinoid deposits. Hyperkeratosis and inflammatory infiltrate are less prominent than in discoid lesions.

Conditions to consider in the differential diagnosis:

cytotoxic drug eruptions
SLE
drug-induced lupus

IIIH4. Vacuolar Dermatitis, Basement Membranes Thickened

Vacuolar degeneration is associated with variable numbers of apoptotic cells in the epidermis. The basement membrane zone is thickened by deposition of eosinophilic hyaline material. *Discoid lupus erythematosus* is the prototype (31).

Discoid Lupus Erythematosus

CLINICAL SUMMARY. Lupus erythematosus may affect multiple organ systems and has a broad range of clinical manifestations. It may take the form of an isolated cutaneous eruption or a fatal systemic illness. A combination of clinical and laboratory data has been set forth as Criteria for the Classification of Systemic Lupus Erythematosus by the American Rheumatism Association. These criteria, developed for classification of patients with SLE as opposed to other rheumatic diseases, are also widely used to diagnose patients with lupus erythematosus. A person is judged to have SLE if any 4 or more of the 11 following criteria are present serially or simultaneously:

- malar rash
- discoid rash
- photosensitivity
- oral ulcers
- arthritis involving two or more peripheral joints
- serositis (pleurisy or pericarditis)
- renal disorders (nephritic or nephrotic)
- neurologic disorders (seizures or psychosis)

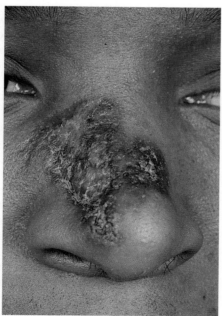

Clin. Fig. IIIH4

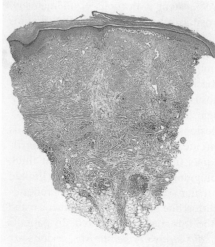

Fig. IIIH4.a

Clin. Fig. IIIH4. *Discoid lupus.* A 29-year-old man developed pigmented plaques with central depression, atrophy, and carpet tack plugging on the nose, auditory canals, and scalp.

Fig. IIIH4.a. *Discoid lupus erythematosus, low power.* The epidermis is focally atrophic and effaced, with overlying hyperkeratosis. The reticular dermis is edematous and there is an infiltrate around the dermal vessels that extends from the lower reticular dermis into the subcutaneous fat. (*continues*)

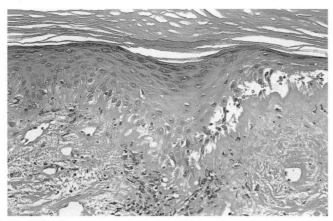

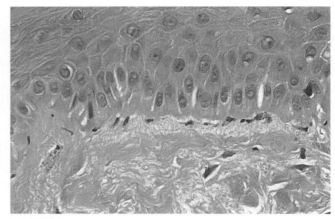

Fig. IIIH4.b   **Fig. IIIH4.c**

Fig. IIIH4.b. *Discoid lupus erythematosus, medium power.* The epidermis has basal layer vacuolar degeneration. An eosinophilic homogenized thickened basement membrane is at the dermal–epidermal interface. In the dermis is vascular ectasia, a lymphocytic infiltration, and melanophage pigmentation.

Fig. IIIH4.c. *Discoid lupus erythematosus, high power.* The eosinophilic, well-defined, thickened basement membrane is seen at the dermal–epidermal interface.

- hematologic disorders (hemolytic anemia, leukopenia, lymphopenia, thrombocytopenia)
- immunologic disorders (positive lupus erythematosus-cell test, anti-DNA abnormal titer, antibody to Sm nuclear antigen, or false-positive serologic test for syphilis)
- antinuclear antibody

Furthermore, a diagnosis of SLE is indicated in any patient who has at least three of the following four symptoms: a cutaneous eruption consistent with lupus erythematosus, renal involvement, serositis, or joint involvement. A diagnosis of SLE requires confirmation by laboratory tests.

Cutaneous changes of lupus erythematosus may be subdivided according to the morphology of the clinical lesion and/or its duration (acute, subacute, or chronic). Differentiation between lupus erythematosus subtypes is based on the constellation of clinical, histologic, and immunofluorescence findings.

Characteristically, lesions of discoid lupus erythematosus consist of well-demarcated, erythematous, slightly infiltrated, "discoid" plaques that often show adherent thick scales and follicular plugging. The lesions are often limited to the face, where the malar areas and the nose are predominantly affected. In addition, the scalp, ears, oral mucosa, and vermilion border of the lips may be involved. In patients with *disseminated discoid lupus erythematosus*, lesions are seen predominantly on the upper trunk and upper limbs, usually with lesions also on the head. Early and active lesions usually display surrounding erythema. Old lesions often appear atrophic and have hypo- or hyperpigmentation. Occasionally, lesions may show verrucous hyperkeratosis, especially at their periphery. Hypopigmentation within previously affected areas is frequent.

HISTOPATHOLOGY. In most instances of *discoid lesions*, a diagnosis of lupus erythematosus is possible on the basis of a combination of histologic findings. Changes may be apparent at all levels of the skin, but all need not be present in every case. The findings may be summarized as follows:

1. Stratum corneum: hyperkeratosis with follicular plugging. Parakeratosis is not conspicuous and may be absent. Keratotic plugs are found mainly in dilated follicular openings but may occur in the openings of eccrine ducts as well.
2. Epithelium: thinning and flattening of the stratum malpighii, hydropic degeneration of basal cells, dyskeratosis, and squamatization of basilar keratinocytes. The most significant histologic change in lupus erythematosus is hydropic degeneration of the basal layer, also referred to as liquefaction degeneration. In its absence, a histologic diagnosis of lupus erythematosus should be made with caution and only when other histologic findings greatly favor a diagnosis of lupus erythematosus. In addition to liquefaction degeneration, basilar keratinocytes may show individual cell necrosis (apoptosis) and acquire elongate contours like their superficial counterparts rather than retaining their normal columnar appearance (squamatization). Frequently, the undulating rete ridge pattern is lost and is replaced by a linear array of squamatized keratinocytes.
3. Basement membrane: thickening and tortuosity. This change, which correlates with locations of immunoreactant deposits, is more apparent with periodic acid–Schiff (PAS) stains and may be found along follicular–dermal junctions and capillary walls as well. In areas of pro-

nounced hydropic degeneration of the basal cells, the PAS-positive subepidermal basement zone may be fragmented and even absent.

4. Stroma: a predominantly lymphocytic infiltrate arranged along the dermal–epidermal junction, around hair follicles and eccrine coils, and in an interstitial pattern; interstitial mucin deposition; edema, vasodilatation, slight extravasation of erythrocytes.

5. Subcutaneous: slight extension of the inflammatory infiltrate may be present.

Conditions to consider in the differential diagnosis:

discoid lupus erythematosus
dermatomyositis

REFERENCES

1. Hulsebosch HJ, Claessen FAP, Van Ginkel CJW, et al. Human immunodeficiency virus exanthem. *J Am Acad Dermatol* 1990;23:483.

2. Soeprono FF, Schinella RA, Cockerell CJ, et al. Seborrheic-like dermatitis of acquired immunodeficiency syndrome. *J Am Acad Dermatol* 1986;14:242.

3. James WD, Redfield RR, Lupton GP, et al. A papular eruption associated with human T-cell lymphotropic virus type III disease. *J Am Acad Dermatol* 1985;13:563.

4. Kuokkanen K. Drug eruptions: a series of 464 cases in the Department of Dermatology, University of Turku, Finland, during 1966–70. *Acta Allergol* 1972;24:407.

5. Bisno AL, Stevens DL. Streptococcal infections of skin and soft tissues. *N Engl J Med* 1996;334:240.

6. Abell E, Marks R, Wilson Jones E. Secondary syphilis. A clinicopathological review. *Br J Dermatol* 1975;93:53.

7. Panizzon R, Bloch PH. Histopathology of pityriasis rosea Gibert: qualitative and quantitative light-microscopic study of 62 biopsies of 40 patients. *Dermatologica* 1982;165:551.

8. Longley J, Duffy TP, Kohn S. The mast cell and mast cell disease. *J Am Acad Dermatol* 1995;32:545.

9. Lachapelle JM. Comparative histopathology of allergic and irritant patch test reactions in man. *Arch Belg Dermatol* 1973;28:83.

10. Pinkus H, Mehregan AH. The primary histologic lesion of seborrheic dermatitis and psoriasis. *J Invest Dermatol* 1966;46:109.

11. Haeffner AC, Smoller BR, Zepter K, Wood GS. Differentiation and clonality of lesional lymphocytes in small plaque parapsoriasis. *Arch Dermatol* 1995;131:321.

12. Venos EM, Collins M, Jane WD. Rothmund-Thomson syndrome: Review of the world literature. *J Am Acad Dermatol* 1992;27:750.

13. Gretzula JL, Hevia O, Weber PJ. Bloom's syndrome. *J Am Acad Dermatol* 1987;17:479.

14. Dokal I, Luzzatto L. Dyskeratosis congenita is a chromosomal instability disorder. *Leukemia Lymphoma* 1995;15:1.

15. Meffert JJ, Davis BM, Grimwood RE. Lichen sclerosus. *J Am Acad Dermatol* 1995;32:393.

16. Soeprono FF. Histologic criteria for the diagnosis of pityriasis rubra pilaris. *Am J Dermatopathol* 1986;8:277.

17. Burg B, Dummer R, Nestle FO, et al. Cutaneous lymphomas consist of a spectrum of nosologically different entities including mycosis fungoides and small plaque parapsoriasis. *Arch Dermatol* 1996;132:567.

18. Cox AH, Watson W. Histologic variations in lesions of psoriasis. *Arch Dermatol* 1972;106:503.

19. Rowland Payne CME, Wilkinson JD, McKee PH, et al. Nodular prurigo: a clinicopathological study of 46 patients. *Br J Dermatol* 1985;113:431.

20. Boyd AS, Neldner KH. Lichen planus. *J Am Acad Dermatol* 1991;2593.

21. Prieto VG, Casal M, McNutt NS. Immunohistochemistry detects differences between lichen planus-like keratosis, lichen planus, and lichenoid actinic keratosis. *J Cutan Pathol* 1993;20:143.

22. Van den Haute V, Antoine JL, Lachapelle JM. Histopathological discriminant criteria between lichenoid drug eruption and idiopathic lichen planus: retrospective study on selected samples. *Dermatologica* 1989;179:10.

23. Lapins JA, Willoughby C, Helwig EB. Lichen nitidus: a study of forty-three cases. *Cutis* 1978;21:634.

24. Jennette JC. Vasculitis affecting the skin. *Arch Dermatol* 1994;130:899.

25. Pinkus H. Granuloma faciale. *Dermatologica* 1952;105:85.

26. Randall SJ, Kierland RR, Montgomery H. Pigmented purpuric eruptions. *Arch Dermatol Syphiligr* 1951;64:177.

27. Robboy SJ, Mihm MC, Colman RC, et al. The skin in disseminated intravascular coagulation. *Br J Dermatol* 1973;88:221.

28. Bick RL, Baker WF Jr. The antiphospholipid and thrombosis syndromes. *Med Clin North Am* 1994;78:667.

29. MacVicar DN, Graham JH, Burgoon CF Jr. Dermatitis herpetiformis, erythema multiforme and bullous pemphigoid: a comparative histopathological and histochemical study. *J Invest Dermatol* 1963;41:289.

30. Callen JP, Tuffanelli DL, Provost TT. Collagen vascular disease: an update. *J Am Acad Dermatol* 1994;28:477.

31. David-Bajar KM, Bennion SD, DeSpain JD, et al. Clinical, histologic, and immunofluorescent distinctions between subacute cutaneous lupus erythematosus and discoid lupus erythematosus. *J Invest Dermatol* 1992;99:251.

Acantholytic, Vesicular, and Pustular Disorders

Keratinocytes may separate from each other on the basis of immunologic antigen-antibody mediated damage resulting in separation and rounding up of keratinocyte cell bodies (acantholysis), on the basis of edema and inflammation (spongiosis), or perhaps on the basis of structural deficiencies of cell adhesion (Darier's disease). These processes produce intraepidermal spaces (vesicles, bullae, pustules).

IVA. SUBCORNEAL OR INTRACORNEAL SEPARATION

There is separation within or just below the stratum corneum. Inflammatory cells may be sparse or may consist predominantly of neutrophils or eosinophils, rarely.

1. Scant Inflammatory Cells
2. Neutrophils Prominent
3. Eosinophils Predominant

IVA1. Sub/Intracorneal Separation, Scant Inflammatory Cells

There is separation within or just below the stratum corneum associated with scant inflammation, usually lymphocytic. Pemphigus foliaceus is prototypic (1).

Pemphigus Foliaceus

CLINICAL SUMMARY.   Usually developing in middle-aged individuals, pemphigus foliaceus may have a chronic generalized course, or may, rarely, present as an exfoliative dermatitis. Patients present with flaccid bullae that usually arise on an erythematous base. Erythema, oozing, and crusting are present. Because of their superficial location, the blisters break easily, leaving shallow erosions rather than the denuded areas seen in pemphigus vulgaris. Oral lesions do not occur. The Nikolsky sign is positive, and Tzanck preparation reveals acantholytic granular keratinocytes. Fogo selvagem (endemic pemphigus foliaceus, which occurs in Brazil) is clinically, histologically, and immunologically indistinguishable from pemphigus foliaceus.

HISTOPATHOLOGY.   The earliest change consists of acantholysis in the upper epidermis, within or adjacent to the granular layer, leading to a subcorneal bulla in some instances. More commonly, enlargement of the cleft leads to detachment of the stratum corneum without bulla formation. The number of acantholytic keratinocytes is usually small, often requiring a careful search to identify them. Secondary clefts may develop, leading to detachment of the epidermis in its midlevel. These clefts may extend to above the basal layer, rarely giving rise to limited areas of suprabasal separation. In the setting of a subcorneal blister, dyskeratotic granular keratinocytes are diagnostic for this disorder. Eosinophilic spongiosis may be prominent with intraepidermal eosinophilic pustules. Thus, the histologic features of pemphigus foliaceus may have three patterns: eosinophilic spongiosis, a subcorneal blister, often with few acantholytic keratinocytes, and a subcorneal blister with dyskeratotic granular keratinocytes, diagnostic for this disorder. The character of the inflammatory infiltrate observed is variable.

Conditions to consider in the differential diagnosis:

staphylococcal scalded skin
bullous impetigo
miliaria crystallina
exfoliative dermatitis
pemphigus foliaceus
pemphigus erythematosus
necrolytic migratory erythema
pellagra
acrodermatitis enteropathica

IVA2. Sub/Intracorneal Separation, Neutrophils Prominent

There is separation in or just below the stratum corneum. Neutrophils are prominent in the stratum corneum and in the superficial epidermis and can often be found in the dermis. *Impetigo contagiosa* is a prototypic example (2).

Impetigo Contagiosa

CLINICAL SUMMARY.   Impetigo contagiosa is primarily an endemic disease of preschool-aged children that may occur in epidemics. Very early lesions consist of vesicopustules that rupture quickly and are followed by heavy yellow crusts. Most lesions are located in exposed areas. An occasional sequela is acute glomerulonephritis, which usually has a favorable long-term prognosis.

Impetigo contagiosa is clinically and histologically distinct from bullous impetigo and staphylococcal scalded-skin syndrome (Ritter's disease), which occur largely in the newborn and in children younger than 5 years and rarely in older individuals often in association with immunodeficiency (3,4). The disease begins abruptly with diffuse erythema and fever. Large flaccid bullae filled with clear fluid form and rupture almost immediately. Large sheets of superficial epidermis separate and exfoliate. The disease is rarely fatal in

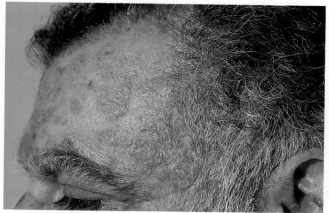

Clin. Fig. IVA1

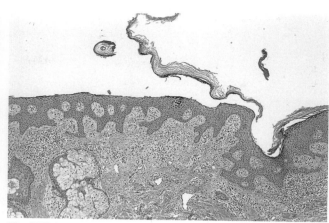

Fig. IVA1.a

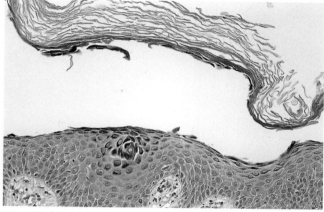

Fig. IVA1.b

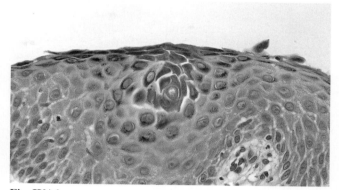

Fig. IVA1.c

Clin. Fig. IVA1. *Pemphigus foliaceus.* A middle-aged man with crusted plaques required systemic corticosteroids and immunosuppressive therapy to control his blistering disease. (W. Witmer)

Fig. IVA1.a. *Pemphigus foliaceus, low power.* A blister forms in the superficial epidermis and there is a sparse dermal infiltrate.

Fig. IVA1.b. *Pemphigus foliaceus, medium power.* The intraepidermal blister is seen within the granular cell layer; this acantholytic blister is devoid of an associated neutrophilic infiltrate. This feature is important in differentiating pemphigus foliaceus from impetigo/impetiginization.

Fig. IVA1.c. *Pemphigus foliaceus, high power.* The absence of a stratum corneum and the presence of a few acantholytic cells may be subtle clues to the diagnosis of pemphigus foliaceus.

children. In neonates with generalized lesions and in adults with severe underlying diseases, the prognosis is worse. Both bullous impetigo and staphylococcal scalded-skin syndrome are transmissible and can cause epidemics in nurseries, where they may occur together.

An important difference between the two diseases is that no staphylococci can be grown from the bullae of the staphylococcal scalded-skin syndrome, in contrast to those of bullous impetigo. In staphylococcal scalded-skin syndrome, the staphylococci are present at a distant focus, often a purulent conjunctivitis, rhinitis, or pharyngitis or rarely a cutaneous infection or a septicemia. The bullae are caused by a staphylococcal exotoxin, called exfoliatin.

HISTOPATHOLOGY. The vesicopustule arises in the upper layers of the epidermis above, within, or below the granular layer. It contains numerous neutrophils. Not infrequently, a few acantholytic cells can be observed at the floor of the vesicopustule. Occasionally, gram-positive cocci are present, both within neutrophils and extracellularly. The stratum malpighii underlying the bulla is spongiotic, and neutrophils often can be seen migrating through it. The upper dermis contains a moderately severe inflammatory infiltrate of neutrophils and lymphoid cells. At a later stage, when the bulla has ruptured, the horny layer is absent and a crust composed of serous exudate and the nuclear debris of neutrophils may be seen covering the stratum malpighii.

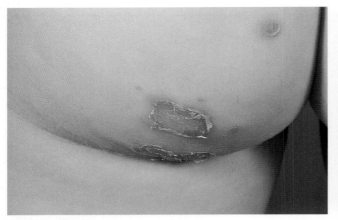

Clin. Fig. IVA2.a

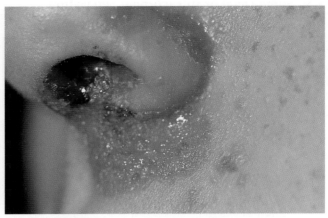

Clin. Fig. IVA2.b

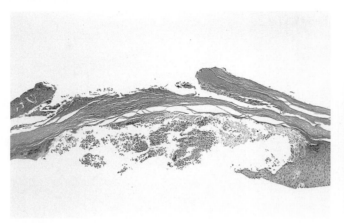

Fig. IVA2.a

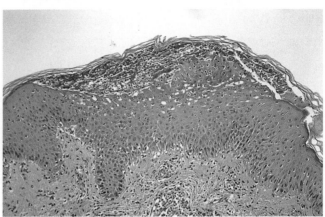

Fig. IVA2.b

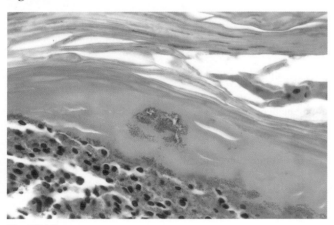

Fig. IVA2.c

Clin. Fig. IVA2.a. *Bullous impetigo.* This 4-year-old girl developed culture-positive *Staphylococcal aureus* erosions with a collarette of superficial desquamated skin on her buttock. Response to antibiotic therapy was dramatic.

Clin. Fig. IVA2.b. *Impetigo contagiosa.* Classic honey-colored crusts secondary to rupture of vesicopustules are seen in the nasal area of a child, an area commonly colonized with *Staphylococcal aureus*.

Fig. IVA2.a. *Impetigo contagiosa, medium power.* In this relatively early lesion, neutrophils are seen in the upper epidermis, forming a subcorneal pustule. There is a superficial mixed infiltrate within the dermis.

Fig. IVA2.b. *Impetigo contagiosa, low power.* In this later lesion, the subcorneal blister is filled with neutrophils. The stratum corneum is thickened and crusted.

Fig. IVA2.c. *Impetigo contagiosa, high power.* Upon closer inspection, neutrophils and bacterial colonies are seen within the stratum corneum. (J. Junkins-Hopkins)

In both bullous impetigo and staphylococcal scalded-skin syndrome, the cleavage plane of the bulla, like that in impetigo contagiosa, lies in the uppermost epidermis either below or, less commonly, within the granular layer. A few acantholytic cells are often seen adjoining the cleavage plane. In contrast to impetigo contagiosa, however, there are few or no inflammatory cells within the bulla cavity. In bullous impetigo, the upper dermis may show a polymorphous infiltrate, whereas in the staphylococcal scalded-skin syndrome, the dermis is usually free of inflammation.

Folliculitis with Subcorneal Pustule Formation

See Figs. IVA2.d and IVA2.e.

Acute Generalized Exanthematous Pustulosis

See Figs. IVA2.f and IVA2.g.

Conditions to consider in the differential diagnosis:
impetigo contagiosa
epidermis adjacent to folliculitis
impetiginized dermatitis

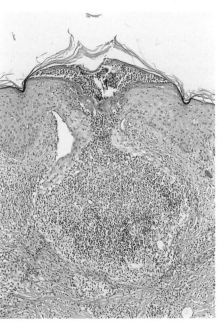

Fig. IVA2.d

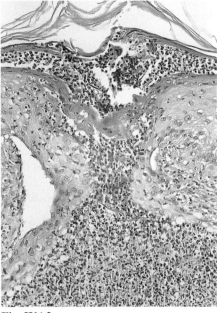

Fig. IVA2.e

Fig. IVA2.d. *Folliculitis with subcorneal pustule formation, low power*. There is an intense neutrophil-rich infiltrate that has obliterated the hair follicle.

Fig. IVA2.e. *Folliculitis with subcorneal pustule formation, medium power*. The epidermis above the follicle shows formation of a subcorneal pustule. If only a superficial shave biopsy is taken, the biopsy resembles other entities in this subgroup and the diagnosis may be missed.

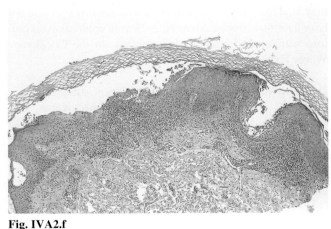

Fig. IVA2.f

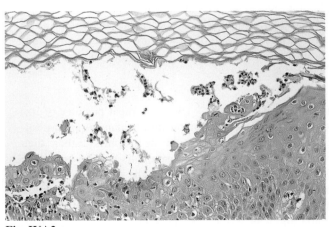

Fig. IVA2.g

Fig. IVA2.f. *Acute generalized exanthematous pustulosis, medium power*. A subcorneal separation is seen associated with a superficial dermal infiltrate in which neutrophils predominate. Most of these cases have been associated with medications and may have previously been called pustular drug eruption (see also section IVB3).

Fig. IVA2.g. *Acute generalized exanthematous pustulosis, high power*. Neutrophils are seen in the upper epidermal layers and within the blister cavity. Differentiation from an early lesion of pustular psoriasis may require clinical correlation.

candidiasis
subcorneal pustular dermatosis (Sneddon–Wilkinson)
IgA pemphigus
secondary syphilis
acropustulosis of infancy
transient neonatal pustular melanosis

IVA3. Sub/Intracorneal Separation, Eosinophils Predominant

There is separation in or just below the stratum corneum, with (pemphigus) or without acantholytic keratinocytes. Eosinophils are present in the epidermis, and occasionally there is eosinophilic spongiosis. The separation is associated with a dermal infiltrate that contains eosinophils. *Erythema toxicum neonatorum* is a prototypic example (5).

Erythema Toxicum Neonatorum

CLINICAL SUMMARY.   A benign asymptomatic eruption affecting about 40% of term infants usually within 12 to 48 hours after birth, erythema toxicum neonatorum lasts 2 to 3 days and consists of blotchy macular erythema, papules, and pustules that tend to develop at sites of pressure. The eruption is associated with blood eosinophilia.

HISTOPATHOLOGY.   The macular erythema is characterized by sparse eosinophils in the upper dermis, largely in a perivascular location, and mild papillary dermal edema. The papules show an accumulation of numerous eosinophils and some neutrophils in the area of the follicle and overlying epidermis. Papillary dermal edema is more intense and eosinophils more numerous. Mature pustules are subcorneal and are filled with eosinophils and occasional neutrophils. The pustules form as a result of the upward migration of eosinophils to the surface epidermis from within and around the hair follicles.

DIFFERENTIAL DIAGNOSIS.   The subcorneal pustules of impetigo and transient neonatal pustular melanosis are not follicular in origin and contain neutrophils rather than eosinophils. Although many eosinophils are present in the vesicles of incontinentia pigmenti, the vesicle is intraepidermal rather than subcorneal, and spongiosis is present. In addition, necrotic keratinocytes may be prominent in incontinentia pigmenti but are absent in erythema toxicum neonatorum.
Conditions to consider in the differential diagnosis:

erythema toxicum neonatorum
pemphigus foliaceus
pemphigus erythematosus
IgA pemphigus

eosinophilic pustular folliculitis
incontinentia pigmenti, vesicular
exfoliative dermatitis, drug induced

IVB. INTRASPINOUS KERATINOCYTE SEPARATION, SPONGIOTIC

There are spaces within the epidermis (vesicles, bullae). There may be dyskeratosis or acantholysis, and a few eosinophils may be present in the epidermis.

1. Intraspinous Spongiosis, Scant Inflammatory Cells
2. Intraspinous Spongiosis, Lymphocytes Predominant
2a. Intraspinous Spongiosis, Eosinophils Present
3. Intraspinous Spongiosis, Neutrophils Predominant

IVB1. Intraspinous Spongiosis, Scant Inflammatory Cells

The infiltrate in the dermis is scant, lymphocytic, or eosinophilic. Friction blister is prototypic.

Friction Blister

CLINICAL SUMMARY.   Friction blisters are caused by mechanical shearing forces, resulting in disruption to keratinocytes or cytolysis. This occurs in the normal epidermis when the structural (keratin) matrix of the keratinocyte is overwhelmed by high levels of physical agents such as friction and heat. Friction (mechanical energy applied parallel to the epidermis) leads to the shearing of keratinocytes from one another and of the keratinocytes themselves, resulting in the characteristic clear fluid-filled blisters. Minimal friction may lead to cytolysis in subjects whose keratinocytes do not have a normal structural matrix, such as in epidermolysis bullosa simplex and epidermolysis bullosa of the Cockayne–Weber type.

HISTOPATHOLOGY.   Usual friction blisters show evidence of initial spongiosis and then disruption of the keratinocytes in the spinous layer. In lesions of the palms or soles, the blisters remain intact for a time because of the thick stratum corneum in these sites. In patients with epidermolysis bullosa, the blister is likely to be subepidermal in location.
Conditions to consider in the differential diagnosis:

epidermolytic hyperkeratosis
epidermolytic acanthoma
miliaria rubra
transient acantholytic dermatosis
bullous dermatitis of diabetes and of uremia
coma bulla
friction blisters

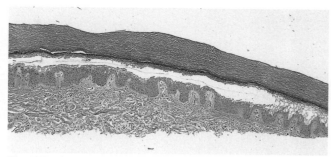

Fig. IVB1.a

Fig. IVB1.a. *Friction blister, low power.* There is a blister in the midepidermis.

Fig. IVB1.b. *Friction blister, medium power.* The blister is formed by cytolysis of keratinocytes with spongiotic edema, but there is scant associated inflammation.

Fig. IVB1.c. *Friction blister, medium power.* There may be evidence of damage to the surface epithelium or it may be relatively intact, especially on the palms or soles, as in this example.

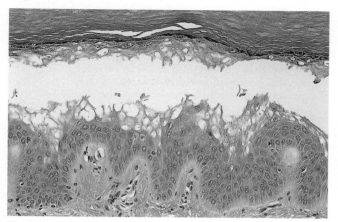

Fig. IVB1.b

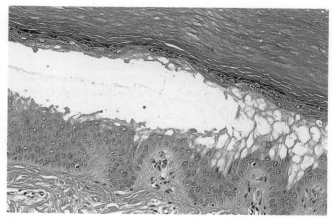

Fig. IVB1.c

IVB2. Intraspinous Spongiosis, Lymphocytes Predominant

In the dermis, lymphocytes predominate. Eosinophils can be found in most examples of atopy and in allergic contact dermatitis.

Dyshidrotic Dermatitis (Eczema)

CLINICAL SUMMARY. This entity is characterized by recurrent, severely pruritic, deep-seated vesicles that classically involve the lateral aspects of the fingers and, in some cases, the toes. Emotional stress may exacerbate the eruption. In chronic cases, there may be more extensive involvement of the palms and soles. Although the eruption develops acutely, it may become chronic with erythema, lichenification, and fissuring. Secondary impetiginization is common.

HISTOPATHOLOGY. Spongiosis and intraepidermal vesiculation occur in acute lesions. There is a superficial perivascular lymphohistiocytic infiltrate with exocytosis of lymphocytes into spongiotic zones. The infiltration is usually mild. In acute lesions, the compact thickened stratum corneum of acral skin remains intact and the epidermal thickness is normal. With chronicity, spongiosis diminishes, acanthosis and parakeratosis predominate, and serum may be identified within the stratum corneum. Difficulty in diagnosis may occur because of the formation of vesiculopustules in older lesions.

Conditions to consider in the differential diagnosis:

spongiotic (eczematous) dermatitis (see section IIIB1)
atopic dermatitis
allergic contact dermatitis
photoallergic drug eruption
irritant contact dermatitis
nummular eczema
dyshidrotic dermatitis
"id" reaction
seborrheic dermatitis
stasis dermatitis
erythroderma
miliaria rubra
pityriasis rosea

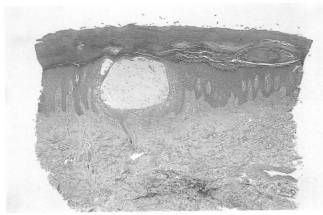

Fig. IVB2.a

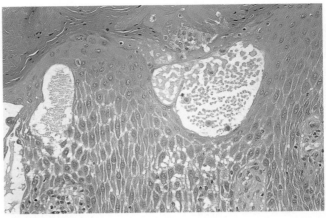

Fig. IVB2.b

Fig. IVB2.a. *Spongiotic dermatitis, dyshidrotic eczema, low power.* This biopsy of acral skin shows an intraepidermal vesicle and an associated superficial inflammatory infiltrate. A collection of serous fluid in the stratum corneum seen in the right upper corner of this photomicrograph is a common finding in spongiotic processes.

Fig. IVB2.b. *Dyshidrotic eczema, high power.* There is diffuse spongiosis within the epidermis manifested by white spaces separating the keratinocytes. Several intraepidermal vesicles also form. The lymphocytic infiltrate can be seen at the lower margin of the epidermis in this photomicrograph.

IVB2a. Intraspinous Spongiosis, Eosinophils Present

The number of eosinophils seen is variable from many in incontinentia pigmenti and pemphigus vegetans to few in atopic dermatitis.

Acute Contact Dermatitis

See Figs. IVB2.a.a and IVB2.a.b. See also section IIIB1A.

Bullous Pemphigoid, Urticarial Phase

See Figs. IVB2.a.c and IVB2.a.d. See also section IVE3.

Incontinentia Pigmenti

See Figs. IVB2.a.e and IVB2.a.f.
Conditions to consider in the differential diagnosis:
spongiotic (eczematous) dermatitis
atopic dermatitis

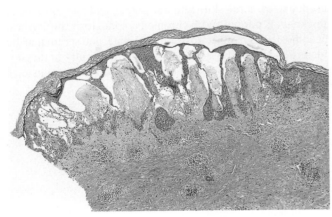

Fig. IVB2a.a

Fig. IVB2a.a. *Spongiotic dermatitis (acute contact dermatitis), low power.* In this acute lesion, the stratum corneum shows a basket-weave pattern. Intraepidermal vesicles are seen associated with a perivascular inflammatory infiltrate.

Fig. IVB2a.b. *Spongiotic dermatitis (acute contact dermatitis), high power.* There is diffuse spongiosis with intraepidermal vesicles. The infiltrate is mixed but contains many eosinophils in the dermis.

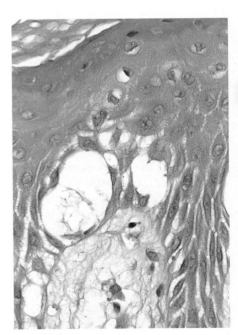

Fig. IVB2a.b

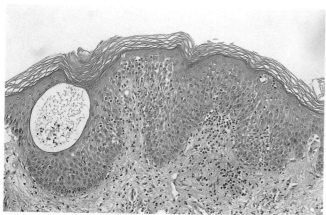

Fig. IVB2a.c

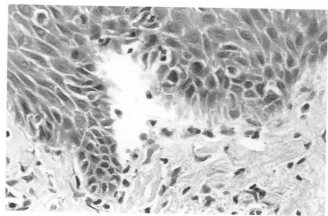

Fig. IVB2a.d

Fig. IVB2a.c. *Bullous pemphigoid, urticarial phase, medium power.* In this example of bullous pemphigoid, it mimics an acute contact dermatitis with intraepidermal spongiosis and eosinophilic spongiosis.

Fig. IVB2a.d. *Bullous pemphigoid, urticarial phase, high power.* Eosinophils are seen accumulating at the dermal–epidermal junction and within the dermal papillae, a feature that may be a clue to the diagnosis of pemphigoid. In many instances, if blister formation has not occurred, direct immunofluorescence may be necessary to distinguish early pemphigoid from acute contact dermatitis.

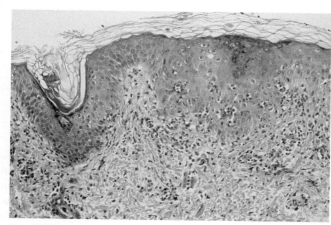

Clin. Fig. IVB2a

Clin. Fig. IVB2a. *Incontinentia pigmenti, verrucous stage.* A 5-month-old developed blisters followed by hyperpigmented and verrucous changes in a swirled pattern. Mother and maternal grandmother had skin and dental abnormalities.

Fig. IVB2a.e. *Incontinentia pigmenti, medium power.* The transition stage between vesicular and acanthotic. Many eosinophils are seen in the dermis and in the focally acanthotic and spongiotic epidermis.

Fig. IVB2a.f. *Incontinentia pigmenti, high power.* Eosinophilic spongiosis and early acanthosis, with numerous dyskeratotic keratinocytes.

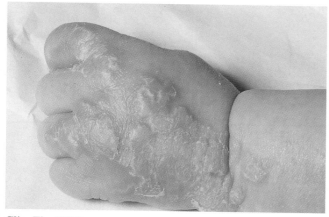

Fig. IVB2a.e

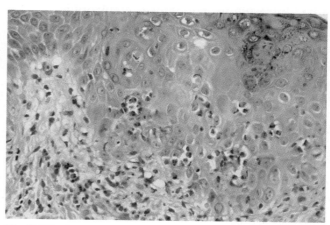

Fig. IVB2a.f

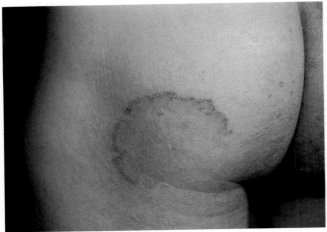

Clin. Fig. IVB3

Clin. Fig. IVB3. *Dermatophytosis.* A large erythematous patch showing central clearing and a polycyclic scaling border, which is quite narrow and threadlike.

Fig. IVB3.a. *Dermatophytosis, low power.* There is both papillary dermal edema and spongiosis of the epidermis. The stratum corneum is thickened and focally parakeratotic with neutrophils.

Fig. IVB3.b. *Dermatophytosis, high power.* Periodic acid–Schiff stain reveals septate hyphae within the stratum corneum.

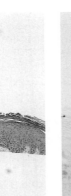

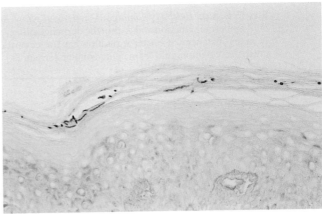

Fig. IVB3.a

Fig. IVB3.b

allergic contact dermatitis
photoallergic drug eruption
bullous pemphigoid, urticarial phase
incontinentia pigmenti, vesicular stage

IVB3. Intraspinous Spongiosis, Neutrophils Predominant

Neutrophils are seen in the epidermis, stratum corneum, and in the dermis. Aggregations of neutrophils in the superficial spinous layer constitute the spongiform pustules of Kogoj characteristic of psoriasis.

Dermatophytosis

See Figs. IVB3.a and IVB3.b.
   Conditions to consider in the differential diagnosis:
      pustular psoriasis
      Reiter's syndrome
      IgA pemphigus
      subcorneal pustular dermatosis (Sneddon–Wilkinson)
      exanthemic pustular drug eruptions

impetiginized dermatosis
dermatophytosis
rupial secondary syphilis
seborrheic dermatitis (see section IIIB1.c)
epidermis adjacent to folliculitis
impetigo contagiosa
hydroa vacciniforme
mucocutaneous lymph node syndrome (Kawasaki
   disease, pustular variant)

IVC. INTRASPINOUS KERATINOCYTE SEPARATION, ACANTHOLYTIC

There are spaces within the epidermis (vesicles, bullae). The process of separation is acantholysis. Keratinocytes within the spinous layer detach or separate from each other or from basal keratinocytes. There may be dyskeratosis, and a few eosinophils may be present in the epidermis. The infiltrate in the dermis is variable and composed of lymphocytes with or without eosinophils.

1. Intraspinous Acantholysis, Scant Inflammatory Cells
2. Intraspinous Acantholysis, Predominant Lymphocytes
2a. Intraspinous Acantholysis, Eosinophils Present
3. Intraspinous Separation, Neutrophils or Mixed Cell Types

IVC1. Intraspinous Acantholysis, Scant Inflammatory Cells

The infiltrate in the dermis is scant, lymphocytic, or eosinophilic. Hailey–Hailey disease and Grover's disease are prototypic.

Familial Benign Pemphigus (Hailey–Hailey Disease)

CLINICAL SUMMARY. Familial benign pemphigus is inherited as an autosomal dominant trait, with a family history obtainable in about two-thirds of the patients. It is characterized by a localized recurrent eruption of small vesicles on an erythematous base (6). By peripheral extension, the lesions may assume a circinate configuration. The sites of predilection are the intertriginous areas, especially the axillae and the groin. Only very few instances of mucosal lesions have been reported.

HISTOPATHOLOGY. Although early lesions may show small suprabasal separations, so-called lacunae, in fully developed lesions, there are large separations, that is, vesicles and even bullae. Villi, which are elongated papillae lined by a single layer of basal cells, protrude upward into the bullae, and, in some cases, narrow strands of epidermal cells proliferate downward into the dermis. Many cells of the detached stratum malpighii show loss of their intercellular bridges, so that acantholysis affects large portions of the epidermis. Individual cells and groups of cells usually are seen in large numbers in the bulla cavity. Some acantholytic cells may exhibit premature keratinization, resembling the grains of Darier's disease. Despite the extensive loss of intercellular bridges, in many places the cells of the detached epidermis are only slightly separated from one another because a few intact intercellular bridges still hold them together loosely. This quite typical feature gives the detached epidermis the appearance of a dilapidated brick wall.

Transient Acantholytic Dermatosis (Grover's Disease)

CLINICAL SUMMARY. Transient acantholytic dermatosis is characterized by pruritic discrete papules and papulovesicles on the chest, back, and thighs (7,8). In rare instances, vesicles and even bullae are seen. Most patients are middle-aged or elderly men. Although the disorder is transient in most patients, lasting from 2 weeks to 3 months, it can persist for several years.

HISTOPATHOLOGY. Focal acantholysis and dyskeratosis ("focal acantholytic dyskeratosis") are present. Because

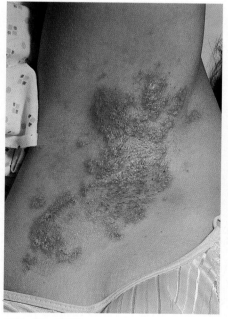

Clin. Fig. IVC1.a

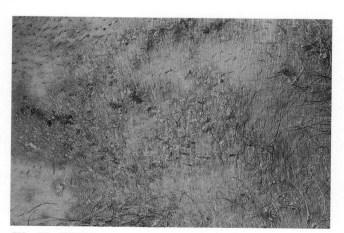

Clin. Fig. IVC1.b

Clin. Fig. IVC1.a. *Hailey–Hailey disease.* A 39-year-old woman presented with malodorous, vegetating, erythematous crusted erosions, peripheral flaccid bullae, and scattered pustules in the axillae and groin.

Clin. Fig. IVC1.b. *Hailey–Hailey disease.* The patient's 43-year-old brother has similar macerated plaques with pustules in the intertriginous areas, characteristic of this autosomal dominant disorder. (*continues*)

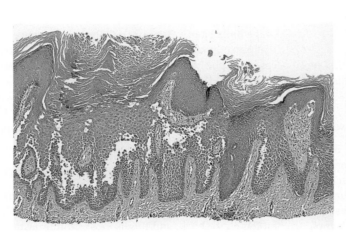

Fig. IVC1.a

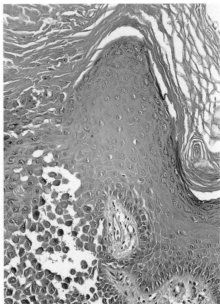

Fig. IVC1.b

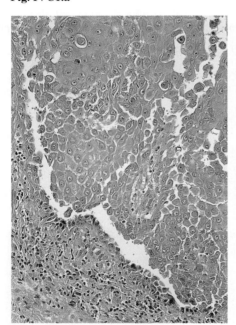

Fig. IVC1.c

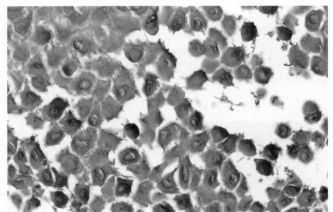

Fig. IVC1.d

Fig. IVC1.a. *Hailey–Hailey disease, low power.* The epidermis is hyperplastic and focally hyperkeratotic. There is diffuse intraepidermal separation of keratinocytes at all levels of the epidermis.

Fig. IVC1.b. *Hailey–Hailey disease, medium power.* The acantholysis involves the full thickness of the epidermis, forming the dilapidated brick wall.

Fig. IVC1.c. *Hailey–Hailey disease, medium power.* Hailey–Hailey disease may also show suprabasal separation and dyskeratosis. The dyskeratosis is generally less prominent than what is seen in Darier's disease.

Fig. IVC1.d. *Hailey–Hailey disease, high power.* High magnification of the acantholysis demonstrating separation of keratinocytes from one another and rounding up within the blister cavity.

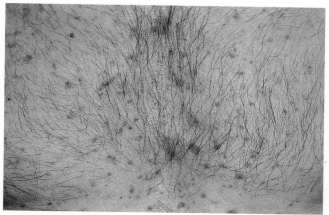

Clin. Fig. IVC1.c

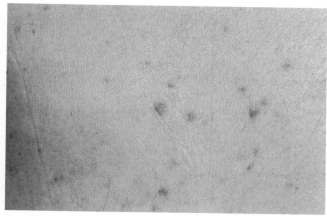

Clin. Fig. IVC1.d

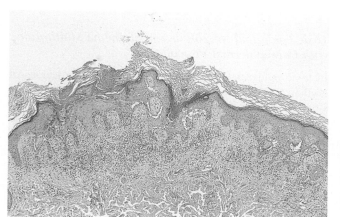

Fig. IVC1.e

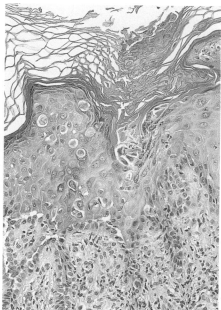

Fig. IVC1.f

Clin. Fig. IVC1.c. *Grover's disease.* An elderly man presented with pruritic lesions on the chest and back.

Clin. Fig. IVC1.d. *Grover's disease.* The lesions are discrete pruritic brown keratotic papules.

Fig. IVC1.e. *Transient acantholytic dermatosis (Grover's disease), low power.* At scanning magnification, multiple foci of intraepidermal separation are seen. There is a mild superficial dermal inflammatory infiltrate. Multiple histologic changes can be seen in these areas of intraepidermal separation, including the most common pattern seen here that mimics Darier's disease but also patterns of Hailey–Hailey disease, pemphigus vulgaris, pemphigus foliaceus, and spongiotic dermatitis.

Fig. IVC1.f. *Grover's disease, Darier's pattern, medium power.* There is suprabasal acantholysis with parakeratosis and corps ronds in the upper epidermal layer.

these foci are small, they are sometimes found only when step sections are obtained. The acantholysis may occur in five histologic patterns, resembling Darier's disease, Hailey–Hailey disease, pemphigus vulgaris, superficial pemphigus, or spongiotic dermatitis. Two or more of these patterns may be found in the same specimen.

Conditions to consider in the differential diagnosis:

    epidermolytic hyperkeratosis
    epidermolytic acanthoma
    Darier's disease
    isolated keratosis follicularis (warty dyskeratoma)
    Hailey–Hailey disease
    transient acantholytic dermatosis
    focal acantholytic dyskeratosis
    acantholytic solar keratosis
    pemphigus erythematosus
    pemphigus foliaceus
    friction blister (cytolytic blister)

IVC2. Intraspinous Acantholysis, Predominant Lymphocytes

In the dermis, lymphocytes are predominant. In erythema multiforme and related lesions there is necrosis of individual cells (apoptosis) that may become confluent. Herpes simplex and varicella-zoster are prototypic examples (9).

Herpes Simplex

Two immunologically distinct viruses can cause herpes simplex: herpes simplex virus type 1 (HSV-1; orofacial type) and herpes simplex virus type 2 (HSV-2; genital type). Primary infection with HSV-1 is usually subclinical in childhood. In about 10% of the cases, acute gingivostomatitis occurs, usually in childhood and only rarely in early adult life. HSV-2 generally is acquired venereally. Occasionally, an infant contracts HSV-2 in utero or by direct contact in the birth canal. Recurrent infections of the oral cavity, the skin, or the genitals can result either from reactivation of a latent infection or from a new infection.

Both primary and recurrent herpes simplex, in their earliest stages, show one or several groups of vesicles on an inflamed base. If located on a mucous surface, the vesicles erode quickly, whereas if located on the skin, they may become pustular before crusting.

HISTOPATHOLOGY. Herpes simplex of the skin produces profound degeneration of keratinocytes, resulting in acantholysis. Degeneration of epidermal cells occurs in two forms, ballooning degeneration and reticular degeneration, both of which are changes typical of viral vesicles. The earliest changes include nuclear swelling of keratinocytes. With hematoxylin and eosin stains, these nuclei appear slate gray and homogeneous. Ballooning degeneration (swelling of epidermal cells) then follows. Eosinophilic inclusion bodies are frequently observed in the centers of enlarged round nuclei of balloon cells. Reticular degeneration is a process in which epidermal cells are distended by intracellular edema so that cell walls rupture. Through coalescence, a multilocular vesicle results, the septa of which are formed by resistant cellular walls. In older vesicles, the cellular walls disappear and the vesicle becomes unilocular. Reticular degeneration is not specific for viral vesicles, because it also occurs in the vesicles of dermatitis. The upper dermis beneath viral vesicles contains an inflammatory infiltrate of variable density. In some cases of herpes simplex, vascular damage is present, showing necrosis of vessel walls, microthrombi, and hemorrhage. In addition, eosinophilic inclusions may be found in endothelial cells and fibroblasts.

Varicella-Zoster Infection

See Figs. IVC2.c and IVC2.d.

Toxic Epidermal Necrolysis and Erythema Multiforme with Intraepidermal Vesiculation

In toxic epidermal necrolysis (TEN), in bullous lesions of erythema multiforme, and in the central portion of target lesions of erythema multiforme, there are numerous necrotic keratinocytes, with full-thickness epidermal necrosis in TEN, and a subepidermal separation to form a bulla or to result in extensive desquamation of the necrotic epithelium in TEN. The dermal inflammatory infiltrate is more sparse in TEN than in erythema multiforme. Extravasated erythrocytes are commonly found within the blister cavity. Melanophages within the papillary dermis occur in late lesions (see also section IIIH1).

Conditions to consider in the differential diagnosis:

    erythema multiforme (with vacuolar and apoptotic
       changes)
    Stevens–Johnson
    toxic epidermal necrolysis (TEN)
    herpes simplex, varicella-zoster
    hydroa vacciniforme (epidermal necrosis)
    cowpox
    hand-foot and mouth disease (Coxsackie virus)
    orf
    paraneoplastic pemphigus

IVC2a. Intraspinous Acantholysis, Eosinophils Present

The number of eosinophils seen is variable from many in incontinentia pigmenti and pemphigus vegetans to few in atopic dermatitis. *Pemphigus vegetans* is a prototypic example (10).

Pemphigus Vegetans

CLINICAL SUMMARY. This is an uncommon variant of pemphigus vulgaris, which historically has been divided into the Neumann type and Hallopeau type. In the Neumann type, the disease begins and ends as pemphigus vulgaris, but many of

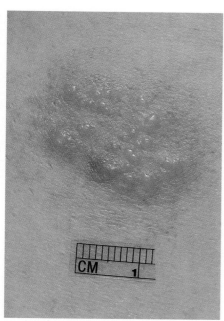

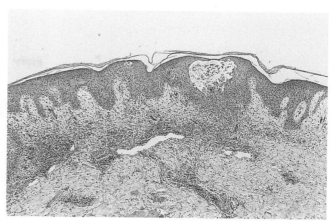

Clin. Fig. IVC2.a. *Herpes simplex.* A 28-year-old woman gave a history of burning and pruritus and recurrent clusters of vesicles on an edematous erythematous base on her thigh.

Fig. IVC2.a. *Herpes simplex infection, low power.* There is diffuse epidermal spongiosis and intraepidermal vesicle formation. There is an associated mixed dermal inflammatory infiltrate.

Fig. IVC2.b. *Herpes simplex infection, high power.* Multiple keratinocytes of the epithelium show typical nuclear changes of herpes viral infection. There is peripheral rimming of nuclear chromatin; also, several multinucleated keratinocytes are present.

Clin. Fig. IVC2.a

Fig. IVC2.a

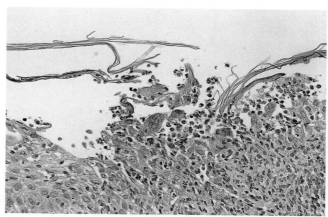

Fig. IVC2.b

the denuded areas heal with verrucous vegetations that may contain small pustules in early stages. The Hallopeau type is relatively benign, having pustules as the primary lesions instead of bullae. Their development is followed by the formation of gradually enlarging verrucous vegetations, especially in intertriginous areas.

HISTOPATHOLOGY. In the Neumann type, the early lesions consist of bullae and denuded areas that have the same histologic picture as that of pemphigus vulgaris (see section IVD3). As the lesions age, however, there is formation of villi and verrucous epidermal hyperplasia. Numerous eosinophils are present within the epidermis and dermis, producing both eosinophilic spongiosis and eosinophilic pustules. Acantholysis may not be present in older lesions.

In the Hallopeau type, the early lesions consist of pustules arising on normal skin with acantholysis and formation of small clefts, many in a suprabasal position. The clefts are filled with numerous eosinophils and degenerated acantholytic epidermal cells. Early lesions may reveal more eosinophilic abscesses than in the Neumann type. The subsequent verrucous lesions are histologically identical to the Neumann type. Direct immunofluorescence (DIF) examination reveals squamous intercellular IgG.

Conditions to consider in the differential diagnosis:

pemphigus vegetans
pemphigus vulgaris
incontinentia pigmenti
drug-induced pemphigus
paraneoplastic pemphigus

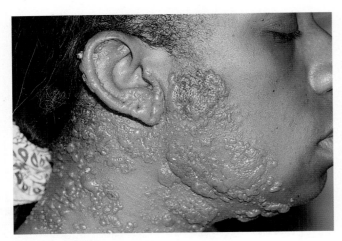

Clin. Fig. IVC2.b

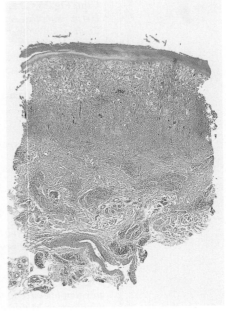

Fig. IVC2.c

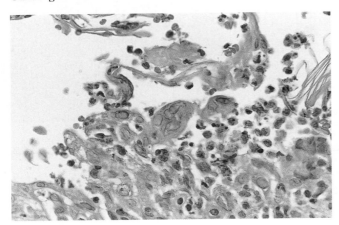

Fig. IVC2.d

Clin. Fig. IVC2.b. *Herpes zoster.* Lakes of umbilicated vesicles in a dermatomal distribution appeared in this human immunodeficiency virus-positive middle-aged woman.

Fig. IVC2.c. *Varicella-zoster infection, low power.* The epidermis shows diffuse spongiosis and necrosis. There is a moderately intense superficial and deep inflammatory infiltrate that may extend into the subcutaneous fat. Although varicella-zoster cannot always be distinguished from herpes simplex using histology, the infiltrate in varicella-zoster is generally more intense and extends more deeply into the dermis.

Fig. IVC2.d. *Varicella-zoster infection, high power.* Similar to what is seen in herpes simplex infection, keratinocytes show multinucleation and the nuclei show peripheral rimming of the chromatin.

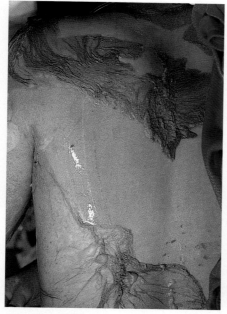

Clin. Fig. IVC2.c

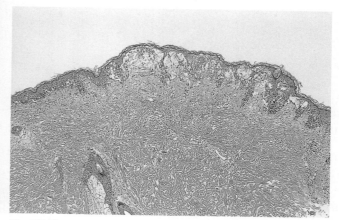

Fig. IVC2.e

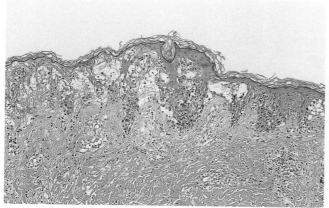

Fig. IVC2.f

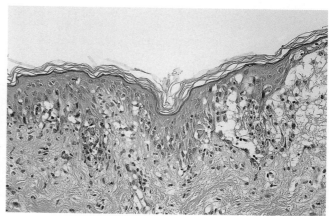

Fig. IVC2.g

Clin. Fig. IVC2.c. *Toxic epidermal necrolysis.* The patient initially presented with a painful widespread erythematous rash that soon developed into sheets of peeling skin with erosions. This is a serious skin condition with a mortality of 25% to 50% and requires intensive medical care in a burn unit.

Fig. IVC2.e. *Erythema multiforme/toxic epidermal necrolysis, low power.* There is a focus of prominent epidermal spongiosis and necrosis. There is a sparse dermal infiltrate of lymphocytes.

Fig. IVC2.f. *Erythema multiforme/toxic epidermal necrolysis, medium power.* The intact basket-weave stratum corneum portrays the acute nature of this lesion. The epidermis shows multiple zones of intraspinous separation and blister formation.

Fig. IVC2.g. *Erythema multiforme/toxic epidermal necrolysis, medium power.* At the periphery of the lesion, a few lymphocytes are seen tagging the dermal–epidermal interface and are associated with vacuolar alteration, the earliest change in this process.

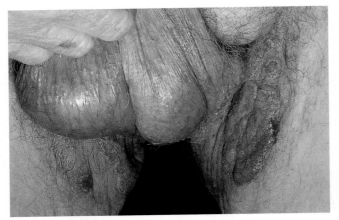

Clin. Fig. IVC2a.a

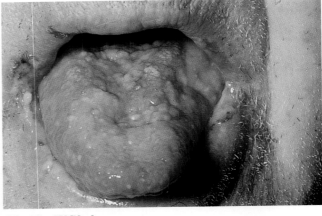

Clin. Fig. IVC2a.b

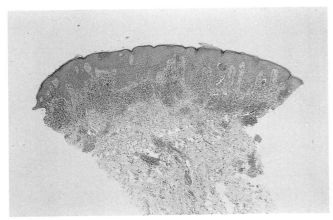

Fig. IVC2a.a

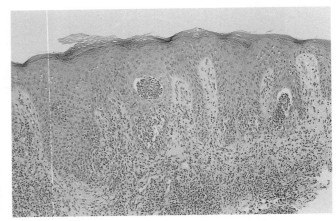

Fig. IVC2a.b

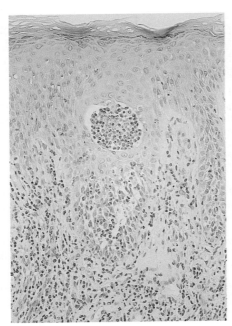

Fig. IVC2a.c

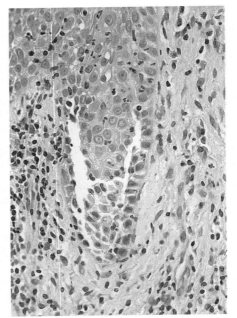

Fig. IVC2a.d

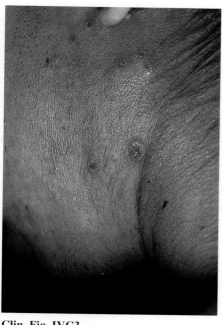

Clin. Fig. IVC3

Clin. Fig. IVC3. *IgA pemphigus.* A Vietnamese man suffered from recurrent pustular and crusted lesions for years.

Fig. IVC3.a. *IgA pemphigus, medium power.* A subcorneal and intraepidermal blister is filled with fluid and numerous neutrophils. A few small clusters of acantholytic cells may be evident. (L. Cohen)

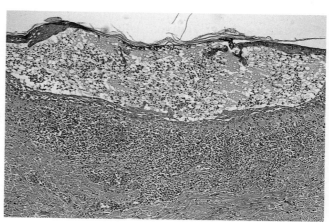

Fig. IVC3.a

IVC3. Intraspinous Separation, Neutrophils or Mixed Cell Types

Inflammatory cells in the dermis include lymphocytes and plasma cells with or without eosinophils, neutrophils, mast cells, and histiocytes. *IgA pemphigus* is a prototypic example (11).

IgA Pemphigus

CLINICAL SUMMARY. This is a pruritic vesiculopustular eruption characterized by squamous intercellular IgA deposits and intraepidermal neutrophils. It occurs primarily, but not exclusively, in middle-aged and elderly individuals.

The clinical findings are similar to those in pemphigus foliaceus or subcorneal pustular dermatosis. There are flaccid vesicles, pustules, or bullae that arise on an erythematous base and may be annular. There may be mild leukocytosis, eosinophilia, and IgA kappa paraproteinemia. Two types have been distinguished: a subcorneal pustular dermatosis-like disorder or an intraepidermal pustular eruption.

HISTOPATHOLOGY. Two patterns are observed that parallel the two clinical presentations. In the first, there are subcorneal neutrophilic vesicopustules or pustules with minimal acantholysis. In the second, intraepidermal vesicopustules or pustules contain small to moderate numbers of neutrophils. One case without neutrophil infiltration has been described.

Clin. Fig. IVC2a.a. *Pemphigus vegetans.* Hallopeau type. An 80-year-old man had a 20-year history of verrucous plaques in the groin, intergluteal cleft, and parietal scalp controlled with avlosulfone.

Clin. Fig. IVC2a.b. *Pemphigus vegetans.* The oral mucous membranes, including the lips and tongue, presented with painful erosive and crusting plaques.

Fig. IVC2a.a. *Pemphigus vegetans, low power.* The epidermis reveals irregular acanthosis, and there is a superficial and mid dermal inflammatory infiltrate. In most cases of pemphigus vegetans, the acantholytic areas require careful inspection and may require multiple deeper levels.

Fig. IVC2a.b. *Pemphigus vegetans, medium power.* At this magnification one can identify the characteristic intraepidermal abscesses.

Fig. IVC2a.c. *Pemphigus vegetans, medium power.* The intraepidermal abscesses are composed almost entirely of eosinophils. Small foci of suprabasal acantholysis, similar to those seen in pemphigus vulgaris, are also seen.

Fig. IVC2a.d. *Pemphigus vegetans, high power.* The acantholysis is suprabasal and may be present in only minute foci.

IMMUNOFLUORESCENCE TESTING. DIF testing typically reveals IgA deposition in the squamous intercellular substance throughout the epidermis with increased intensity in the upper layers in some cases of the subcorneal pustular type. Complement and other immunoglobulins are usually absent. The antibodies are directed against neither the pemphigus vulgaris nor the foliaceus antigen but bind with proteins in desmosomes (desmocollins).

Conditions to consider in the differential diagnosis:

    acantholytic solar keratosis
    acantholytic squamous cell carcinoma
    hydroa vacciniforme (epidermal necrosis)
    IgA pemphigus

IVD. SUPRABASAL KERATINOCYTE SEPARATION

There is separation between the keratinocytes of the basal layer and those of the spinous layer.

1. Suprabasal Vesicles, Scant Inflammatory Cells
2. Suprabasal Separation, Lymphocytes and Plasma Cells
3. Suprabasal Vesicles, Lymphocytes and Eosinophils

IVD1. Suprabasal Vesicles, Scant Inflammatory Cells

The suprabasal separation may be associated with scant inflammation and frequently with dyskeratotic or atypical keratinocytes. *Darier's disease (keratosis follicularis)* and *warty dyskeratoma (isolated keratosis follicularis)* are prototypic (12).

Keratosis Follicularis (Darier's Disease)

CLINICAL SUMMARY. In this disease, which is usually transmitted in an autosomal dominant pattern, there is a more or less extensive, persistent, slowly progressive eruption consisting of hyperkeratotic or crusted papules or verrucous lesions often showing a follicular distribution. The so-called seborrheic areas are the sites of predilection. The oral mucosa is involved occasionally. Special clinical variants are a hypertrophic type, a vesiculobullous type, and a linear or zosteriform type. In the hypertrophic type, widespread, markedly thickened, hyperkeratotic lesions are seen, especially in the intertriginous areas. In the vesiculobullous type, vesicles and small bullae are seen in addition to papules. In the linear or zosteriform type, usually limited to one side, there are either localized or widespread lesions that may occasionally be present at birth or may arise in infancy, childhood, or adult life. This type of lesion may represent a linear epidermal nevus with acantholytic dyskeratosis rather than Darier's disease, and the designation *acantholytic dyskeratotic epidermal nevus* has been suggested.

HISTOPATHOLOGY. The characteristic changes in Darier's disease are a peculiar form of dyskeratosis, resulting in the formation of corps ronds and grains; suprabasal acantholysis, leading to the formation of suprabasal clefts or lacunae; and irregular upward proliferation into the lacunae of papillae lined with a single layer of basal cells, so-called villi. There are also papillomatosis, acanthosis, and hyperkeratosis. The dermis shows a chronic inflammatory infiltrate. In some cases, there is downward proliferation of epidermal cells into the dermis.

The corps ronds occur in the upper stratum malpighii, particularly in the granular and horny layers; grains are found in the horny layer and as acantholytic cells within the lacunae. Corps ronds possess a central homogeneous, basophilic, pyknotic nucleus that is surrounded by a clear halo, peripheral to which there is a shell of basophilic dyskeratotic material. The grains resemble parakeratotic cells but are somewhat larger. Their nuclei are elongated and often grain shaped and are surrounded by homogeneous dyskeratotic basophilic or eosinophilic material. The lacunae represent small, slitlike intraepidermal vesicles most commonly located directly above the basal layer and containing acantholytic partial keratinized cells. The changes seen in particular lesions of Grover's disease may be indistinguishable from Darier's disease, but usually the lesions are smaller, and if multiple lesions are available from the same patient, the pattern typically varies from lesion to lesion.

Warty Dyskeratoma

CLINICAL SUMMARY. Warty dyskeratoma usually occurs as a solitary lesion, most commonly on the scalp, face, or neck (13). It often occurs as a slightly elevated papule or nodule with a keratotic umbilicated center, which after having reached a certain size, persists indefinitely.

HISTOPATHOLOGY. The center of the lesion is occupied by a large cup-shaped invagination connected with the surface by a channel filled with keratinous material. The large invagination contains numerous acantholytic dyskeratotic cells in its upper portion. The lower portion of the invagination is occupied by numerous villi, markedly elongated dermal papillae that are often lined with only a single layer of basal cells and project upward from the base of the cup-shaped invagination. Typical corps ronds can usually be seen in the thickened granular layer lining the channel at the entrance to the invagination.

Conditions to consider in the differential diagnosis:

    transient acantholytic dermatosis (Grover)
    benign familial pemphigus (Hailey–Hailey)
    Darier's disease (keratosis follicularis)
    acantholytic solar keratosis
    acantholytic squamous cell carcinoma

Clin. Fig. IVD1.a

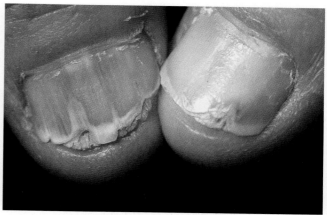

Clin. Fig. IVD1.b

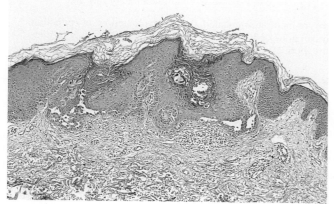

Fig. IVD1.a

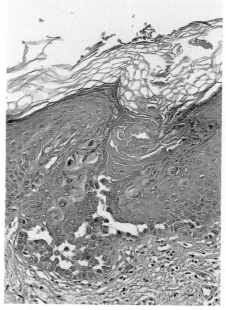

Fig. IVD1.b

Clin. Fig. IVD1.a. *Darier's disease.* A 54-year-old woman with this lifelong autosomal dominant disease presented with dirty brown papules on the neck and trunk.

Clin. Fig. IVD1.b. *Darier's disease.* The nails show characteristic changes of V-shaped nicking, linear striations, onycholysis, and subungual keratotic reaction.

Fig. IVD1.a. *Darier's disease, medium power.* There is mild verrucous acanthosis of the epidermis, and several foci of acantholysis are seen in the lower epidermal layers.

Fig. IVD1.b. *Darier's disease, high power.* The acantholysis is suprabasal, and several corps ronds are seen in the upper epidermal layers associated with a focus of parakeratosis.

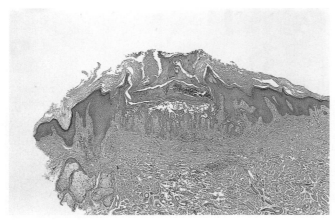

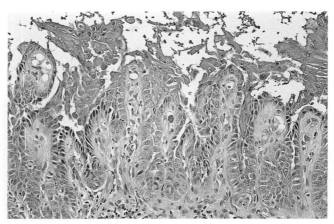

Fig. IVD1.c   Fig. IVD1.d

Fig. IVD1.c. *Warty dyskeratoma, low power.* A solitary focus of verrucous epidermal hyperplasia with an invaginated architecture is seen in the center of this biopsy. There is a sparse dermal inflammatory infiltrate.

Fig. IVD1.d. *Warty dyskeratoma, high power.* There are multiple, elongated, fingerlike projections of epithelium that show suprabasal acantholysis. There are also dyskeratotic cells and corps ronds. The pathology may be identical to Darier's disease. However, the solitary nature, both clinically and histologically, allows easy differentiation between these two entities.

IVD2. Suprabasal Separation, Lymphocytes and Plasma Cells

Suprabasal separation, associated with keratinocyte atypia, may be seen with a lymphoplasmacytic infiltrate in the dermis in an acantholytic solar keratosis (14).

Acantholytic Actinic Keratosis

Five types of actinic keratosis can be recognized histologically: hypertrophic, atrophic, bowenoid, acantholytic, and pigmented. In all types, there is random atypia of basal keratinocytes, with hyperkeratosis intermingled with areas of parakeratosis. Keratinocytes in the stratum malpighii show a loss of polarity and thus a disorderly arrangement. Some of these cells show crowding, pleomorphism, and atypicality of their nuclei, which appear large, irregular, and hyperchromatic, and some of the cells are dyskeratotic or apoptotic; acantholytic keratoses show dyshesion of lesional cells that may simulate a glandular pattern. The acantholysis is usually suprabasal but may involve the full thickness of the epidermis (see also section IIA1).

Conditions to consider in the differential diagnosis:
    acantholytic solar keratosis
    acantholytic squamous cell carcinoma

IVD3. Suprabasal Vesicles, Lymphocytes and Eosinophils

There is suprabasal separation with eosinophils in the epidermis (eosinophilic spongiosis) and in the dermis. *Pemphigus vulgaris* is the prototype (1).

Pemphigus Vulgaris

CLINICAL SUMMARY. This condition develops primarily in older individuals, presenting with large and flaccid bullae. These break easily and leave denuded areas that tend to increase in size by progressive peripheral detachment of the epidermis (positive Nikolsky sign), leading in some cases to widespread cutaneous involvement. The lesions characteristically involve the oral mucosa, scalp, midface, sternum, and groin. Oral lesions are almost invariably present and are often the first manifestation of the disease. Before corticosteroids became available, the mortality of this disease was high because of fluid loss and superinfection.

HISTOPATHOLOGY. The earliest recognized change may be either eosinophilic spongiosis or, more commonly, spongiosis in the lower epidermis. Acantholysis leads first to the formation of clefts and then to blisters in a predominantly suprabasal location, although intraepithelial separation may occasionally be higher in the stratum spinosum. The basal keratinocytes, although separated from one another through the loss of attachment to each other, remain firmly attached to the dermis like a "row of tombstones" lining the blister base. The blister roof consists of the remaining intact squamous epithelium. Within the blister cavity, there are acantholytic keratinocytes that have rounded condensed cytoplasm around an enlarged nucleus with peripherally palisaded chromatin and enlarged nucleoli. These may reside singularly or in clusters. They may be recognized cytologically in a Tzanck preparation, which is a smear taken from the underside of the roof and from the base of an early freshly opened bulla. Acantholysis may extend into adnexal structures. There is little inflammation in the early phase of blister formation. If present,

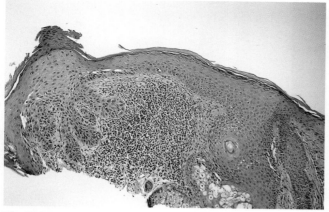

Fig. IVD2.a

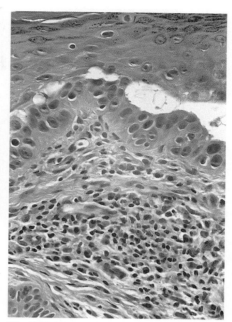

Fig. IVD2.b

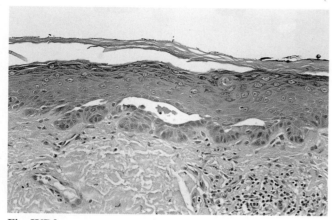

Fig. IVD2.c

Fig. IVD2.a. *Acantholytic actinic keratosis, low power.* The epidermis shows acanthosis with fingerlike projections of atypical epithelium associated with a parakeratotic scale. There is a moderately intense infiltrate in the superficial dermis.

Fig. IVD2.b. *Acantholytic actinic keratosis, high power.* Within this solar (actinic) keratosis there are foci of suprabasal acantholysis, a pattern that may mimic pemphigus vulgaris. In this keratosis, the infiltrate is composed of lymphocytes and plasma cells. The character of the infiltrate (eosinophils predominate in pemphigus vulgaris) and the presence of keratinocyte atypia aid in differentiating these two entities.

Fig. IVD2.c. *Acantholytic actinic keratosis, medium power.* In this example, the keratosis also shows suprabasal acantholysis. There is prominent solar elastosis within the dermis associated with a mononuclear cell infiltrate, which is scant in this example.

---

it is usually a sparse lymphocytic perivascular infiltrate accompanied by dermal edema. If, however, eosinophilic spongiosis is apparent, numerous eosinophils may infiltrate the dermis, and as the lesions age, a mixed inflammatory cell reaction consisting of neutrophils, lymphocytes, macrophages, and eosinophils may develop. Because of the instability of the blister roof, erosion and ulceration may occur. Older blisters may also have several layers of keratinocytes at the blister base because of keratinocyte migration and proliferation, and there may be considerable downward growth of epidermal strands, giving rise to so-called villi.

IMMUNOFLUORESCENCE TESTING. DIF testing is a very reliable and sensitive diagnostic test for pemphigus vulgaris in that it demonstrates IgG in the squamous intercellular substance in 80% to 95% of cases, including early cases and those with very few lesions, and in up to 100% of cases with active disease. It remains positive, often for many years after the disease has subsided. Indirect testing is less specific than the direct test.

Conditions to consider in the differential diagnosis:
    pemphigus vulgaris
    pemphigus vegetans

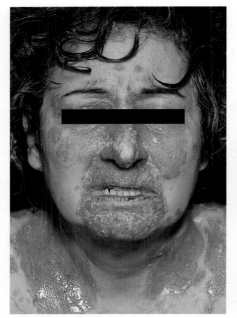

Clin. Fig. IVD3.a

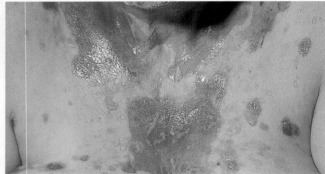

Clin. Fig. IVD3.b

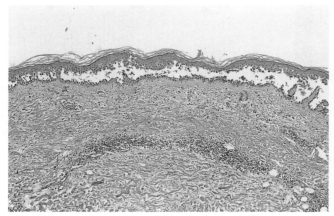

Fig. IVD3.a

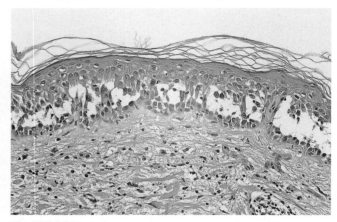

Fig. IVD3.b

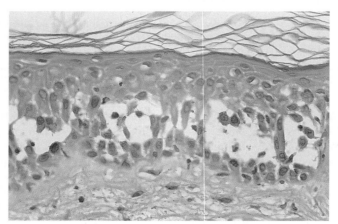

Fig. IVD3.c

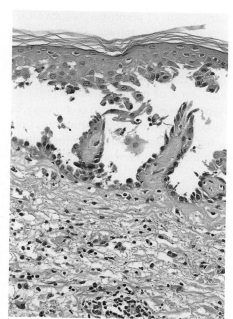

Fig. IVD3.d

Fig. IVD3.d. *Pemphigus vulgaris, medium power.* Another example shows a characteristic single-cell tombstone layer of basal keratinocytes at the floor of the blister.

Fig. IVD3.e. *Pemphigus vulgaris, direct immunofluorescence, medium power.* There is cell surface (intercellular) IgG deposition. C3 deposition is also frequently seen in pemphigus vulgaris.

Fig. IVD3.f. *Pemphigus vulgaris, indirect immunofluorescence, high power.* Using monkey esophagus as a substrate there is prominent cell surface (intercellular) staining with IgG.

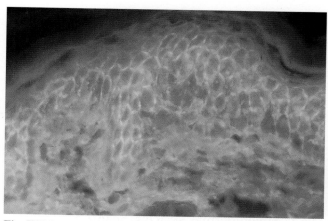

Fig. IVD3.e

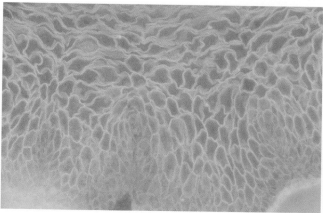

Fig. IVD3.f

Clin. Fig. IVD3.a. *Pemphigus vulgaris.* A 52-year-old woman developed mouth erosions and fragile flaccid bullae with expanding erosions and skin denudation.

Clin. Fig. IVD3.b. *Pemphigus vulgaris.* The lesions progressed over the entire body, requiring burn unit therapy. Indirect immunofluorescence was 1:5,120 on guinea pig esophagus and 1:2,560 on monkey esophagus.

Fig. IVD3.a. *Pemphigus vulgaris, low power.* At scanning magnification there is formation of an intraepidermal vesicle and an associated perivascular inflammatory infiltrate.

Fig. IVD3.b. *Pemphigus vulgaris, medium power.* There is intraspinous separation that is predominantly in the suprabasal region. The stratum corneum is intact and shows a basket-weave pattern.

Fig. IVD3.c. *Pemphigus vulgaris, medium power.* A solitary row of basal layer keratinocytes remain attached to the floor of the blister. The roof of the blister is composed of relatively intact superficial epidermal layers. The dermal infiltrate is composed of lymphocytes and eosinophils. Eosinophilic spongiosis may also be seen.

IVE. SUBEPIDERMAL VESICULAR DERMATITIS

A subepidermal blister refers to separation of the epidermis from the dermis. The roof of the blister is composed of an intact or (partially) necrotic epithelium.

1. Subepidermal Vesicles, Scant /No Inflammation
2. Subepidermal Vesicles, Lymphocytes Predominant
3. Subepidermal Vesicles, Eosinophils Prominent
4. Subepidermal Vesicles, Neutrophils Prominent
5. Subepidermal Vesicles, Mast Cells Prominent

IVE1. Subepidermal Vesicles, Scant/ No Inflammation

The infiltrate in the dermis in most of these conditions is scant (few lymphocytes, eosinophils, neutrophils). *Porphyria cutanea tarda and other porphyrias* are prototypic (15).

Porphyria Cutanea Tarda and Other Porphyrias

CLINICAL SUMMARY.   Three forms of the dominantly inherited disorder porphyria cutanea tarda can be distinguished: sporadic, familial, and hepatoerythropoietic. In the *sporadic form*, only the hepatic activity of uroporphyrinogen decarboxylase is decreased. Almost all patients are adults, and no clinical evidence of porphyria cutanea tarda is found in other members of the patient's family. In most instances, in addition to the inherited enzymatic defect, an acquired damaging factor to liver function such as ethanol or estrogens is needed. In the *familial form*, in addition to the hepatic activity, the extrahepatic activity of uroporphyrinogen decarboxylase is decreased to about 50% of normal, and often, but not always, there is a family history of overt porphyria cutanea tarda. In the very rare *hepatoerythropoietic form*, the skin lesions appear in childhood, the activity of uroporphyrinogen decarboxylase in all organs is decreased to less than 10% of normal, and family studies suggest that these patients are homozygous for the causative gene.

Clinically, the sporadic form of porphyria cutanea tarda, by far the most common type of porphyria, shows blisters that arise through a combination of sun exposure and minor trauma, mainly on the dorsa of the hands but sometimes also on the face. Scarring and milia formation may result. The skin of the face and the dorsa of the hands often are thickened and sclerotic. Hypertrichosis of the face is common. In the familial and in the hepatoerythropoietic forms, the clinical picture is similar, but the changes are more pronounced. Evidence of hepatic cirrhosis with siderosis is regularly present in the sporadic form.

In *erythropoietic porphyria*, a very rare disease that typically develops during infancy or childhood, recurrent vesiculobullous eruptions in sun-exposed areas of the skin gradually result in mutilating ulcerations and scarring. In *erythropoietic protoporphyria*, the usual reaction to light is erythema and edema followed by thickening and superficial scarring of the skin. In rare instances, vesicles are present that may resemble those seen in hydroa vacciniforme. The protoporphyrin is formed in reticulocytes in the bone marrow and is carried in circulating erythrocytes and in the plasma. In porphyria variegata, different members of the same family may have either cutaneous manifestations identical to those of porphyria cutanea tarda or systemic involvement analogous to acute intermittent porphyria, or both, or the condition may remain latent.

HISTOPATHOLOGY.   The histologic changes in the skin lesions are the same in all six types of porphyria with cutaneous lesions. Differences are based on the severity rather than on the type of porphyria. Homogeneous eosinophilic material is regularly observed, and bullae are present in some instances. In addition, sclerosis of the collagen is present in old lesions. In mild cases, homogeneous, pale, eosinophilic deposits are limited to the immediate vicinity of the blood vessels in the papillary dermis. These deposits are periodic acid–Schiff (PAS) positive and diastase resistant. In severely involved areas, which are most common in erythropoietic protoporphyria, the perivascular mantles of homogeneous material are wide enough in the papillary dermis to coalesce

Clin. Fig. IVE1. *Porphyria cutanea tarda.* A 33-year-old man presented with intact vesicles and bullae and crusted erosions without milia on dorsal hands. His history of excessive alcohol intake and hepatitis C positivity is typical for the sporadic form of the disease.

Fig. IVE1.a. *Porphyria cutanea tarda, low power.* This biopsy of acral skin shows a subepidermal blister. There is little or no inflammation within the dermis.

Fig. IVE1.b. *Porphyria cutanea tarda, medium power.* At the edge of the blister, one can see that the roof of the blister is composed of full-thickness epidermis and the floor of the blister is composed of underlying dermis. Again, almost no inflammation is seen at the periphery of the blister.

Fig. IVE1.c. *Porphyria cutanea tarda, medium power.* At the floor of the blister, one can identify a dermal papilla that has retained its architecture (festooning). A periodic acid–Schiff stain may reveal basement membrane thickening of the blood vessels within this dermal papilla.

Fig. IVE1.d. *Porphyria cutanea tarda, direct immunofluorescence, high power.* There is smudgy positive staining with IgG of the blood vessels in the papillary dermis.

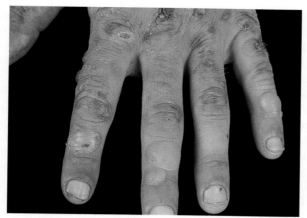

Clin. Fig. IVE1

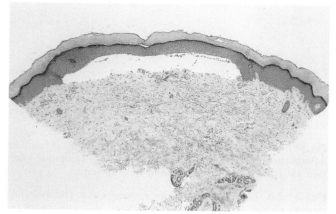

Fig. IVE1.a

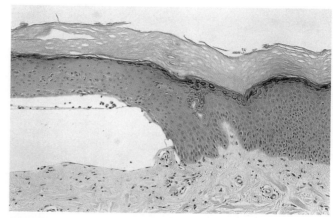

Fig. IVE1.b

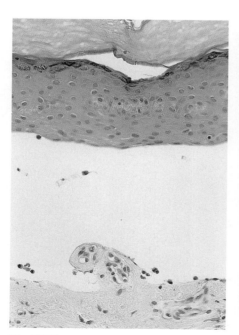

Fig. IVE1.c

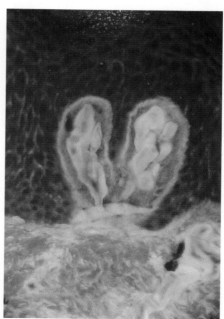

Fig. IVE1.d

with those of adjoining capillaries. In addition, deeper blood vessels may show homogeneous material around them, and similar homogeneous material may be found occasionally around eccrine glands. In addition, the PAS-positive epidermal–dermal basement membrane zone may be thickened. In areas of sclerosis, which occur especially in porphyria cutanea tarda, the collagen bundles are thickened.

The bullae, which are most common in porphyria cutanea tarda, arise subepidermally. Some blisters are dermolytic and arise beneath the PAS-positive basement membrane zone; others form in the lamina lucida and are situated above the PAS-positive basement membrane zone. It is quite characteristic of the bullae of porphyria cutanea tarda that the dermal papillae often extend irregularly from the floor of the bulla into the bulla cavity. This phenomenon, referred to as festooning, is explained by the rigidity of the upper dermis induced by the presence of eosinophilic material within and around the capillary walls in the papillae and the papillary dermis. The epidermis forming the roof of the blister often contains eosinophilic bodies that are elongate and sometimes segmented. These caterpillar bodies are PAS positive and diastase resistant. There are only a few inflammatory cells in the dermis.

Conditions to consider in the differential diagnosis:

porphyria cutanea tarda and other porphyrias
drug-induced pseudoporphyria
bullous pemphigoid, cell poor
epidermolysis bullosa simplex
epidermolysis bullosa letalis
epidermolysis bullosa acquisita (classic)
graft-versus-host disease (GVHD), acute
acute radiation dermatitis
bullous dermatosis of diabetes

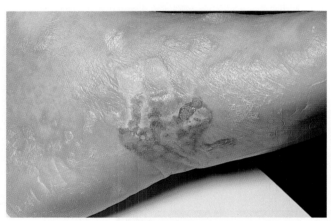

Clin. Fig. IVE2.a

Clin. Fig. IVE2.a. *Bullous lichen planus.* A 93-year-old woman with a history of hypertrophic lichen planus presented with a sudden eruption of hemorrhagic ruptured bullae on a background of violaceous plaques on the soles of her feet. The eruption was treated successfully with a short course of systemic steroids.

Fig. IVE2.a. *Bullous lichen planus, low power.* There is a bandlike inflammatory infiltrate that obscures the dermal–epidermal interface. Inflammation is not seen within the deep dermis.

Fig. IVE2.b. *Bullous lichen planus, medium power.* The epidermis shows irregular acanthosis, hypergranulosis, and a thickened orthokeratotic scale. The epidermis has separated from the underlying dermis, forming a subepidermal cleft. There is an intense bandlike infiltrate composed predominantly of lymphocytes.

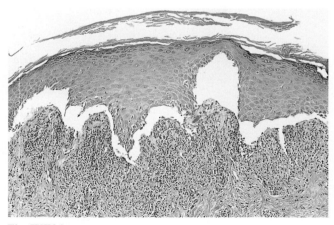

Fig. IVE2.b

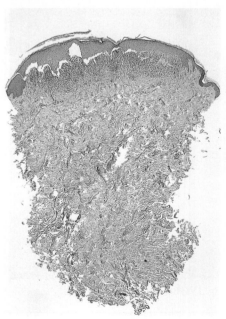

Fig. IVE2.a

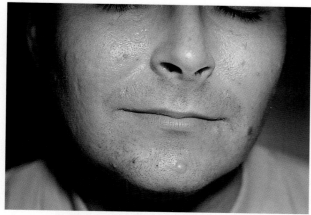

Clin. Fig. IVE2.b

Clin. Fig. IVE2.b. *Polymorphous light eruption.* Pruritic papules and vesicles developed on an intermittent basis several hours after sun exposure.

Fig. IVE2.c. *Polymorphous light eruption, low power.* There is both intraepidermal spongiosis and edema of the papillary dermis. There is an associated superficial and deep inflammatory infiltrate. The papillary dermal edema is frequently more intense, a helpful feature in making a diagnosis at low power.

Fig. IVE2.d. *Polymorphous light eruption, medium power.* The papillary dermal edema shows early subepidermal separation. The infiltrate may be mixed but is largely composed of lymphocytes.

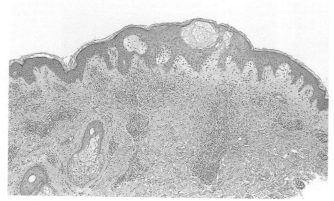

Fig. IVE2.c

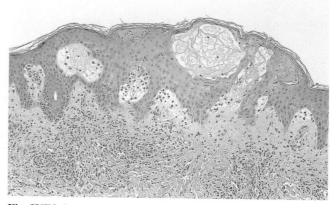

Fig. IVE2.d

bullous dermatosis of uremia
electrical burn (polarized epidermis)
thermal burn (epidermal necrosis)
suction blister
vibrio vulnificus septicemia (necrotic bullae)

IVE2. Subepidermal Vesicles, Lymphocytes Predominant

The epidermis is separated from the dermis, predominantly due to liquefaction of the basal cell layer. In polymorphous light eruption (PMLE), massive papillary dermal edema is the cause. The infiltrate in the dermis is primarily lymphocytic. *Bullous lichen planus* is an example (16).

Bullous Lichen Planus

In lichen planus, a dense dermal infiltrate obscures the dermal–epidermal junction with vacuolar degeneration and necrosis of the basal cells. Necrotic keratinocytes, also referred to as apoptotic, colloid, hyaline, cytoid, or Civatte bodies, are present in most cases in the lower epidermis and especially in the papillary dermis. Because of this disruption of the dermal–epidermal junction, small areas of artifactual

separation between the epidermis and the dermis, known as Max–Joseph spaces, are occasionally seen. In some instances, the separation occurs *in vivo* and subepidermal blisters form (vesicular or bullous lichen planus). These vesicles form as a result of extensive damage to the basal cells (see also section IIIF1).

Polymorphous (Polymorphic) Light Eruption

CLINICAL SUMMARY. This is a commonly occurring, transient, intermittent, ultraviolet radiation-induced eruption of nonscarring, erythematous, itchy papules, plaques, or vesicles of exposed skin, most severe in spring and summer and most common in young women (17). Attacks develop during sunny vacations and summer weather, often persisting or recurring, sometimes with gradual reduction in severity, from spring until fall. They typically follow around 15 minutes to a few hours of sun exposure and last for hours, days, or, rarely, weeks.

HISTOPATHOLOGY. This may vary, but usually there is variable epidermal spongiosis and dermal, perivascular, predominantly mononuclear cell infiltration with edema, which in older

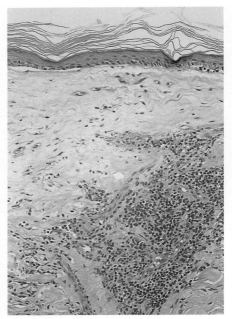

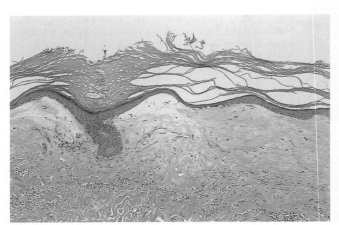

Fig. IVE2.e   **Fig. IVE2.f**

Fig. IVE2.e. *Lichen sclerosus et atrophicus, low power.* The epidermis shows atrophy and has lost the rete ridge architecture. The stratum corneum is thickened and orthokeratotic. There is pallor and homogenization of the expanded papillary dermis.

Fig. IVE2.f. *Lichen sclerosus et atrophicus, medium power.* Early subepidermal blister formation is seen. Beneath the homogenized papillary dermis, there is a predominantly lymphocytic infiltrate that extends into the superficial reticular dermis.

---

lesions may extend into the deeper dermis and may be so severe as to occasionally result in an apparent subepidermal blister. The cells of the infiltrate are usually T lymphocytes, but occasionally eosinophils and neutrophils are present as well.

Lichen Sclerosus et Atrophicus

See Figs. IVE2.e and IVE2.f. See also section IIIC3.
    Conditions to consider in the differential diagnosis:

bullous lichen planus (more often histologic than
    clinical)
erythema multiforme
fixed drug eruption
lichen sclerosus et atrophicus
bullous erythematosus, mononuclear type
GVHD
PMLE
epidermolysis bullosa acquisita (usually neutrophils)

Clin. Fig. IVE3. *Bullous pemphigoid.* An elderly man presented with multiple tense bullae on an erythematous base and erosions, distributed primarily on the medial thighs and trunk.

Fig. IVE3.a. *Bullous pemphigoid, low power.* At scanning magnification there is a subepidermal blister with an associated superficial inflammatory infiltrate.

Fig. IVE3.b. *Bullous pemphigoid, medium power.* The blister contains inflammatory cells, and there is an associated superficial dermal inflammatory infiltrate.

Fig. IVE3.c. *Bullous pemphigoid, high power.* At the edge of the blister, eosinophils are seen within the blister and in the papillary dermis.

Fig. IVE3.d. *Bullous pemphigoid, medium power.* At the edge of an early lesion, eosinophils are seen within the papillary dermis and focally extending into the overlying epidermis.

Fig. IVE3.e. *Bullous pemphigoid, medium power.* Eosinophilic spongiosis is a common finding in pemphigoid where numerous eosinophils extend into the overlying spongiotic epidermis. (*continues*)

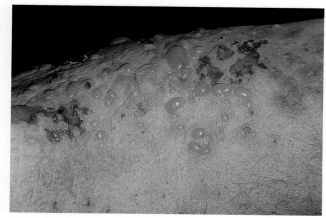

Clin. Fig. IVE3

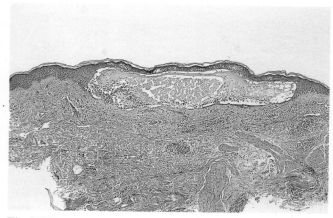

Fig. IVE3.a

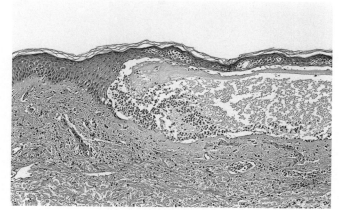

Fig. IVE3.b

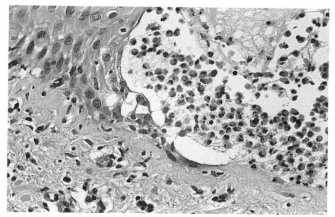

Fig. IVE3.c

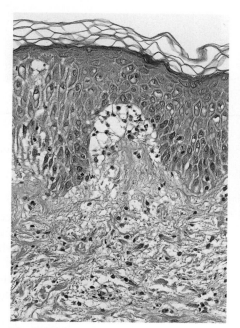

Fig. IVE3.d

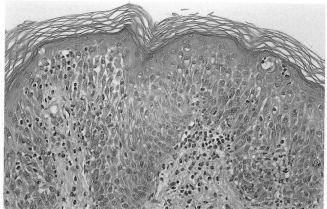

Fig. IVE3.e

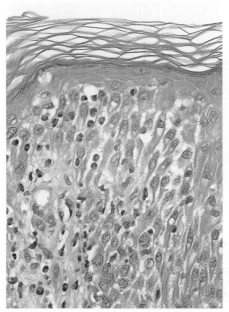

Fig. IVE3.f

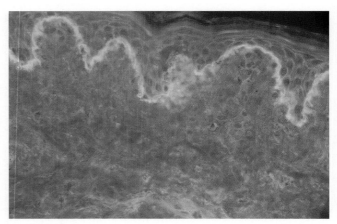

Fig. IVE3.g

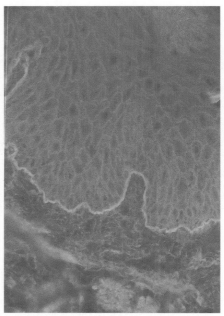

Fig. IVE3.h

Fig. IVE3.f. *Bullous pemphigoid, high power.* High magnification reveals that most inflammatory cells in the epidermis are eosinophils (eosinophilic spongiosis).

Fig. IVE3.g. *Bullous pemphigoid, medium power.* Direct immunofluorescence reveals linear staining of C3 at the basement membrane zone. Other immune reactants, including IgG, IgA, and IgM, may also be detected. C3 is the most common reactant, followed by IgG.

Fig. IVE3.h. *Bullous pemphigoid, high power.* Indirect immunofluorescence using monkey esophagus as the substrate and patient's serum as the test sample. Linear staining of IgG is seen at the basement membrane zone.

IVE3. Subepidermal Vesicles, Eosinophils Prominent

The subepidermal blister is associated with a dermal infiltrate rich in eosinophils. Eosinophils may extend into the overlying epidermis. *Bullous pemphigoid* is a prototypic example (18).

Bullous Pemphigoid

CLINICAL SUMMARY. First described by Lever in 1953 (19), bullous pemphigoid affects primarily elderly patients with large tense bullae arising on an urticarial erythematous base or on nonerythematous skin. The course is chronic and benign. In contrast to pemphigus, the Nikolsky sign is negative. The lesions involve the trunk, the extremities, and the intertriginous areas, with the oral mucosa involved in about one-third of the cases. Bullous pemphigoid may start as a non-specific eruption suggestive of urticaria or dermatitis and can persist for weeks or months.

HISTOPATHOLOGY. In early lesions, papillary dermal edema in combination with a variably cell-poor or cell-rich perivascular lymphocytic and eosinophilic infiltrate is present. The cell-poor pattern is observed when blisters develop on relatively normal skin and the cell-rich pattern when the blisters arise on erythematous skin. In the cell-poor pattern, there is usually scant perivascular lymphocytic inflammation with few eosinophils, some scattered throughout the dermis and others near the epidermis. In the cell-rich pattern, eosinophilic dermal abscesses may develop with numerous perivascular and interstitial eosinophils intermingled with lymphocytes and neutrophils in the papillary and deeper dermis. Eosinophilic spongiosis may occur. The blister arises at the dermoepidermal junction, although epithelial migration and regeneration may result in an intraepidermal location in older blisters. Similar to pemphigus vegetans, a pseudoepitheliomatous hyperplasia of the epidermis, subepidermal bullae, and accumulations of eosinophils and lymphocytes may be seen.

IMMUNOFLUORESCENCE TESTING. DIF testing of perilesional skin has shown linear C3 deposition at the dermoepidermal junction in virtually all cases and IgG in most. IIF studies reveal circulating antibasement membrane zone IgG antibodies in most cases, with IgA and IgM in some. No correlation exists between the antibody titer and the clinical severity of the disease. The IgG is located within the lamina lucida, where it appears bound specifically to the hemidesmosomes. Specimens submitted for DIF examination may also be salt-split (direct salt-split skin technique). When this technique is used in pemphigoid, IgG is present on the roof or on the roof and the floor of the blister.

Bullous Drug Eruption

See Figs. IVE3.i and IVE3.j.

Herpes Gestationis

See Figs. IVE3.k and IVE3.l.
  Conditions to consider in the differential diagnosis:
    bullous pemphigoid
    cicatricial pemphigoid
    bullous drug eruption
    herpes gestationis
    bullous insect bite reaction
    dermatitis herpetiformis (certain old bullae)

IVE4. Subepidermal Vesicles, Neutrophils Prominent

A neutrophilic infiltrate is seen often in dermal papillae at the dermal–epidermal junction adjacent to the subepidermal blister or in the blister. *Dermatitis herpetiformis* is a prototypic example (20).

Dermatitis Herpetiformis

CLINICAL SUMMARY. This is an intensely pruritic chronic recurrent dermatitis that has a slight male predilection. The lesions usually develop in young to middle-aged adults as symmetric grouped papulovesicles, vesicles, or crusts on erythematous bases. Oral lesions are absent. The elbows, knees, buttocks, scapula, and scalp are commonly involved. Most patients have asymptomatic gluten-sensitive enteropathy. There is a small increased risk of lymphoma.

HISTOPATHOLOGY. The typical histologic features are best observed in erythematous skin adjacent to early blisters. In these zones, neutrophils accumulate at the tips of dermal papillae. With an increase in size to microabscesses, a significant admixture of eosinophils may be noted. As the neutrophilic or mixed microabscesses form, a separation develops between the tips of the dermal papillae and the overlying epidermis, so that early blisters are multiloculated. The presence of fibrin in the papillae may give them a bluish appearance. Within 1 to 2 days, the rete ridges lose their attachment to the dermis, and the blisters then become unilocular and clinically apparent. At this time, the characteristic papillary microabscesses may be observed at the blister periphery. The dermis beneath the papillae may have a relatively intense inflammatory infiltrate of lymphocytes, neutrophils, and some eosinophils. Apoptotic keratinocytes may be noted above the papillary microabscesses.

IMMUNOFLUORESCENCE TESTING. Granular deposits of IgA are found alone or in combination with other immune reactants within the dermal papillae in both lesional and nonlesional skin in most cases. Early in the course of the disease, IgA deposits may be absent, and repeat DIF is necessary. False-negative results may occur when blistered or inflamed skin is evaluated. Circulating IgA antibodies that react against reticulin, smooth muscle endomysium, the dietary antigen gluten, bovine serum albumin, and β-lactoglobin may be present. Using monkey or pig gut as substrate, IIF has been used to detect antiendomysial antibodies.

Linear IgA Dermatosis

CLINICAL SUMMARY. Two relatively definitive clinical phenotypes are based on patient age and clinical features (21). These are adult linear IgA dermatosis and childhood linear IgA dermatosis (chronic benign bullous dermatosis of childhood) (22). Other cases may be associated with drug therapy at any age. In the adult type, vesicles and bullae are present, which are less symmetric and less pruritic than those in dermatitis herpetiformis but are distributed in similar locations. Ocular and oral lesions may be present in up to 50% of cases. It is not infrequent for adult-type linear IgA dermatosis to be associated with drug therapy. Vancomycin, lithium, diclofenac, captopril, cifinmandol, and somatostatin have been associated with such presentations. Histologically, the changes are identical to idiopathic linear IgA dermatosis in most cases. In some cases, there is an associated lymphoeosinophilic infiltrate in combination with an interface neutrophilic infiltration.

  The childhood type of linear IgA dermatosis, originally known as chronic bullous dermatosis of childhood, is a unique disorder that presents in prepubertal, often preschool, children and rarely in infancy. Vesicles or bullae develop on an erythematous or normal base, occasionally giving rise to a so-called string of pearls, a characteristic lesion in which peripheral vesicles develop on a polycyclic plaque. They involve the buttocks, lower abdomen, and genitalia and characteristically have a perioral distribution on the face. Oral lesions may occur. The disorder usually remits by age 6 to 8.

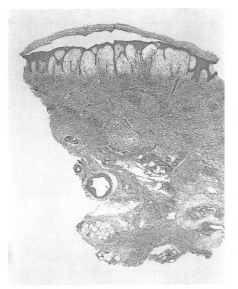

Fig. IVE3.i

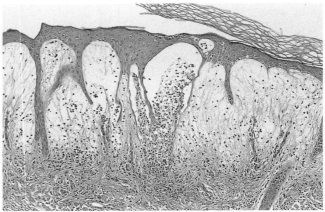

Fig. IVE3.j

Fig. IVE3.i. *Bullous drug eruption, low power.* There is marked edema of the papillary dermis forming a subepidermal blister. This is associated with a superficial and deep inflammatory infiltrate.

Fig. IVE3.j. *Bullous drug eruption, medium power.* The subepidermal separation is associated with a mixed inflammatory infiltrate that contains eosinophils. Eosinophilic spongiosis, however, is less common than in pemphigoid. However, immunofluorescence may still be necessary for definitive diagnosis.

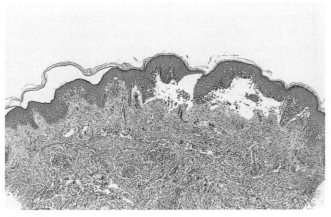

Fig. IVE3.k

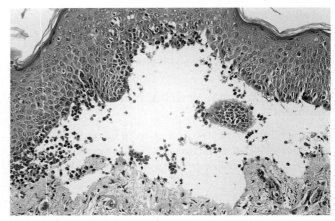

Fig. IVE3.l

Fig. IVE3.k. *Herpes gestationis, low power.* There is subepidermal blister formation and a superficial predominantly perivascular infiltrate.

Fig. IVE3.l. *Herpes gestationis, medium power.* The subepidermal blister shows eosinophils within the blister cavity at the dermal–epidermal interface and within the epidermal layer. Scattered dyskeratotic cells may also be present. The histology is generally indistinguishable from that of bullous pemphigoid.

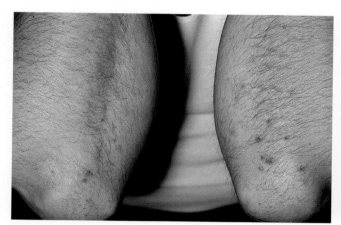

Clin. Fig. IVE4.a

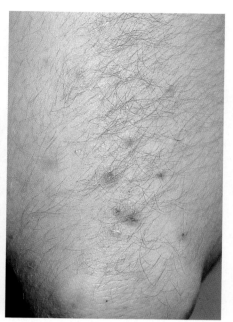

Clin. Fig. IVE4.b

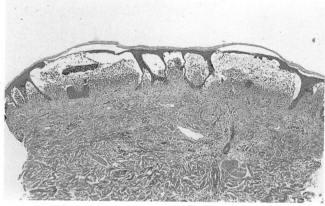

Fig. IVE4.a

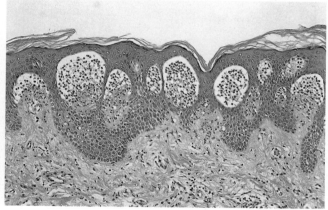

Fig. IVE4.b

Clin. Fig. IVE4.a. *Dermatitis herpetiformis.* A 27-year-old man developed pruritic symmetric grouped vesicles on an erythematous base on the elbows and knees. (W. Witmer)

Clin. Fig. IVE4.b. *Dermatitis herpetiformis.* Single and grouped discrete vesicles that later responded to avlosulfone and a gluten free diet. (W. Witmer)

Fig. IVE4.a. *Dermatitis herpetiformis, low power.* At scanning magnification there is subepidermal blister formation associated with a superficial inflammatory infiltrate.

Fig. IVE4.b. *Dermatitis herpetiformis, medium power.* The stratum corneum shows a normal basket-weave pattern. Within the dermis there is a mild mixed inflammatory infiltrate. (*continues*)

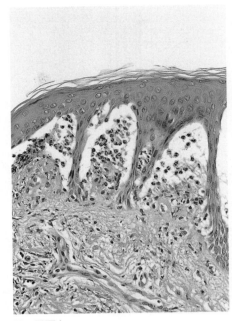

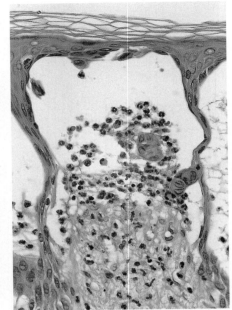

Fig. IVE4.c   **Fig. IVE4.d**

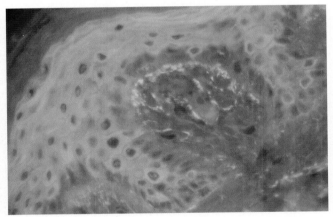

Fig. IVE4.c. *Dermatitis herpetiformis, medium power.* There are numerous papillary dermal microabscesses that are seen adjacent to the subepidermal blisters.

Fig. IVE4.d. *Dermatitis herpetiformis, high power.* The papillary dermal abscesses are composed almost entirely of neutrophils.

Fig. IVE4.e. *Dermatitis herpetiformis, high power, direct immunofluorescence.* Granular deposition of IgA is seen in dermal papillae, concentrated at the dermal–epidermal junction.

Fig. IVE4.e

HISTOPATHOLOGY.   The features are similar, if not identical, to dermatitis herpetiformis. According to some, there is less tendency for papillary microabscess formation and greater tendency for uniform neutrophil infiltration along the entire dermoepidermal junction and rete in inflamed skin. DIF reveals linear IgA along the basement membrane zone in perilesional skin in 100% of cases. If IgG and IgA are present, the differential diagnosis with bullous pemphigoid may be difficult or impossible (linear IgA/IgG dermatosis). The antibodies are deposited principally within the lamina lucida and less commonly beneath the lamina densa. The histologic and immunofluorescent features of childhood linear IgA disease are similar to those of the adult-type disease.

Bullous Lupus Erythematosus

CLINICAL SUMMARY.   Vesicles and bullae may develop in patients with systemic lupus erythematosus (23). In contrast to dermatitis herpetiformis, they are nonpruritic and neither symmetric nor do they have a predilection for extensor surfaces of arms, elbows, or scalp. The lesions may be photodistributed. These patients rarely have classic lesions of discoid, systemic, or subacute cutaneous lupus erythematosus when they develop blisters.

HISTOPATHOLOGY.   Three histologic patterns have been identified in such lesions. The first is striking basal layer vac-

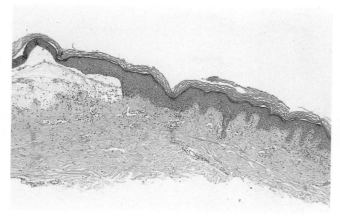

Fig. IVE4.f

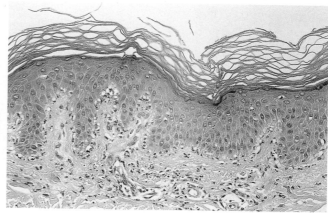

Fig. IVE4.g

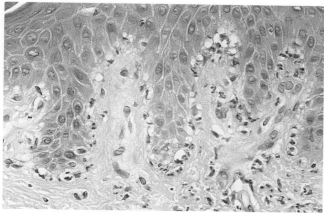

Fig. IVE4.h

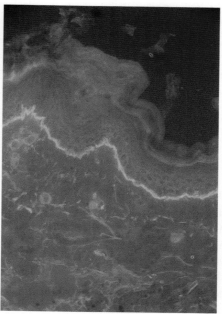

Fig. IVE4.i

Fig. IVE4.f. *Linear IgA disease, low power.* There is a subepidermal blister associated with a superficial inflammatory infiltrate.

Fig. IVE4.g. *Linear IgA disease, medium power.* At the edge of the blister, where the dermal–epidermal junction is intact, inflammatory cells are seen tagging along the basal cell layer.

Fig. IVE4.h. *Linear IgA disease, high power.* At high magnification, one can see that the inflammatory cells are neutrophils and they are seen not only at the tips of papillae (as is seen in dermatitis herpetiformis) but are also quite prominent along the tips of the rete ridges, a feature that may help distinguish linear IgA disease from dermatitis herpetiformis.

Fig. IVE4.i. *Linear IgA disease, direct immunofluorescence, high power.* IgA is deposited in a linear fashion at the dermal–epidermal junction. Other immune reactants may be seen less commonly and intensely than IgA.

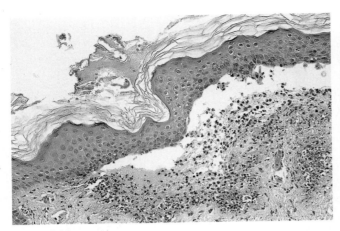

Fig. IVE4.j

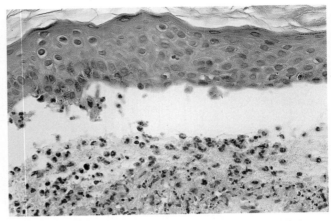

Fig. IVE4.k

Fig. IVE4.j. *Bullous lupus erythematosus, medium power.* There is a large subepidermal bulla containing inflammatory cells.

Fig. IVE4.k. *Bullous lupus erythematosus, high power.* The inflammatory cells in the bulla are mostly neutrophils.

uolization with subsequent blister formation. The second is vasculitis with subepidermal blister and pustule formation. The third and most common is a dermatitis herpetiformis-like histologic pattern. Approximately 25% of cases are said to have a small-vessel neutrophil-rich leukocytoclastic vasculitis beneath the blister. Histologic features more routinely identified with lupus erythematosus are not present, other than the presence of dermal mucin and hyaluronic acid in the dermis. By immunofluorescence, IgG and C3 deposits are demonstrated at the epidermal basement membrane zone. The pattern may be linear or "granular bandlike." A salt-split skin preparation using patient serum reveals localization to the split floor as in epidermolysis bullosa acquisita (EBA). Antibodies to type VII collagen may be present. Immunoelectron microscopic examination reveals electron-dense deposits of IgG at the lower edge of the basal lamina and immediately subjacent dermis in an identical location to the antibody in EBA.

Conditions to consider in the differential diagnosis:

dermatitis herpetiformis
bullous lupus erythematosus, neutrophilic type
bullous vasculitis
linear IgA dermatosis (adult, childhood, drug associated)
epidermolysis bullosa acquisita (inflammatory)
vesiculopustular eruption of hepatobiliary disease
toxic shock syndrome

IVE5. Subepidermal Vesicles, Mast Cells Prominent

The epidermis is separated from the dermis. There is an infiltrate in the superficial dermis composed almost entirely of mast cells, with or without a few eosinophils. This may be associated with separation of the epidermis from the dermis. *Bullous mastocytosis* is the only example (24).

Bullous Mastocytosis

CLINICAL SUMMARY. Vesicles or bullae may be seen in all types of cutaneous mastocytosis (urticaria pigmentosa) except telangiectasia macularis eruptiva perstans. The maculopapular type, which is the most common type, may be seen in children or adults and consists usually of dozens or even hundreds of brown lesions that urticate on stroking; the multinodular type exhibits multiple brown nodules or plaques and, on stroking, shows urtication and occasionally blister formation. The nodular type seen almost exclusively in infants is characterized by a usually solitary large cutaneous nodule, which on stroking often shows not only urtication but also large bullae. The diffuse erythrodermic type always starts in early infancy and shows generalized brownish-red soft infiltration of the skin, with urtication on stroking. Multiple blisters may form during the first 2 years of life on stroking and also spontaneously. If bullae are a predominant clinical feature, the term *bullous mastocytosis* has been applied.

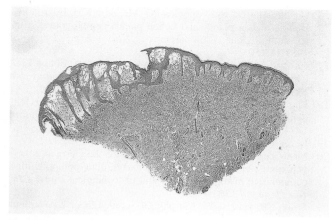

Fig. IVE5.a

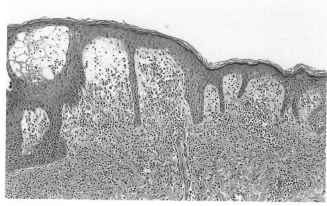

Fig. IVE5.b

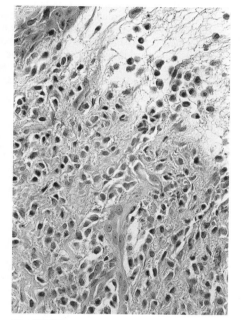

Fig. IVE5.c

Fig. IVE5.d

Fig. IVE5.a. *Bullous mastocytosis, low power.* There is subepidermal blister formation, with a moderately intense infiltrate involving the superficial and middermis.

Fig. IVE5.b. *Bullous mastocytosis, medium power.* The subepidermal blister is associated with a diffuse interstitial mononuclear cell infiltrate.

Fig. IVE5.c. *Bullous mastocytosis, high power.* The infiltrate is composed almost entirely of mast cells with small uniform oval nuclei. There are scattered eosinophils.

Fig. IVE5.d. *Bullous mastocytosis, high power.* Giemsa stain metachromatically stains the granules of mast cells purple.

HISTOPATHOLOGY. The bullae that may occur in infants with multiple or solitary nodules or with the diffuse erythrodermic type arise subepidermally. Because of regeneration of the epidermis at the base of the bulla, older bullae may be located intraepidermally. The bullous cavity often contains mast cells and eosinophils.

REFERENCES

1. Thivolet J. Pemphigus: past, present, and future. *Dermatology* 1994;189(suppl):26.
2. Dagan R. Impetigo in childhood: changing epidemiology and new treatments. *Pediatr Ann* 1993;22:235.
3. Elias PM, Fritsch P, Epstein EH Jr. Staphylococcal scalded skin syndrome [Review]. *Arch Dermatol* 1977;113:207

4. Coskey RJ, Coskey LA. Diagnosis and treatment of impetigo. *J Am Acad Dermatol* 1987;17:62.

5. Freeman RG, Spiller R, Knox JM. Histopathology of erythema toxicum neonatorum. *Arch Dermatol* 1960;82:586.

6. Peluso AM, Bonifast J, Ikeda S, et al. Hailey-Hailey disease sublocalization of the gene on chromosome 3Q and identification of a kindred with an apparent deletion. *J Invest Dermatol* 1995;104:598.

7. Grover RW. Transient acantholytic dermatosis. *Arch Dermatol* 1970;101:426.

8. Chalet M, Grover R, Ackerman AB. Transient acantholytic dermatosis. *Arch Dermatol* 1977;113:431.

9. Blank H, Haines H. Viral diseases of the skin, 1975: a 25-year perspective. *J Invest Dermatol* 1976;67:169–176.

10. Ahmed AR, Blose DA. Pemphigus vegetans, Neumann type and Hallopeau type. *Int J Dermatol* 1984;23:135.

11. Beutner EH, Chorzelski TP, Wilson RM, et al. IgA pemphigus foliaceus. *J Am Acad Dermatol* 1989;20:89.

12. Gottlieb SK, Lutzner MA. Darier's disease. *Arch Dermatol* 1973;107:225.

13. Tanay A, Mehregan AH. Warty dyskeratoma [Review]. *Dermatologica* 1969;138:155

14. Carapeto FJ, García-Pérez A. Acantholytic keratosis. *Dermatologica* 1974;148:233.

15. Meola T, Lim HW. The porphyrias. *Dermatol Clin* 1993;11:583.

16. Gawkrodger DJ, Stavropoulos PG, McLaren KM, Buxton PK. Bullous lichen planus and lichen planus pemphigoides: clinico-pathological comparisons. *Clin Exp Dermatol* 1989;14:150.

17. Hawk JLM. Cutaneous photobiology. In: Rook A, Ebling FJG, Champion RH, Burton JL, eds. *Textbook of dermatology.* 5th ed. Oxford: Blackwell Scientific Publications, 1991;849.

18. Eng AM, Moncada B. Bullous pemphigoid and dermatitis herpetiformis: histologic differentiation. *Arch Dermatol* 1974;110:51.

19. Lever WF. Pemphigus. *Medicine (Baltimore)* 1953;32:1.

20. MacVicar DN, Graham JH, Burgoon CF Jr. Dermatitis herpetiformis, erythema multiforme and bullous pemphigoid: a comparative histopathological and histochemical study. *J Invest Dermatol* 1963;41:289.

21. Smith SB, Harrist TJ, Murphy GF, et al. Linear IgA bullous dermatosis v. dermatitis herpetiformis. *Arch Dermatol* 1984;120:324.

22. Wojnarowska F, Whitehead P, Leigh IM, et al. Identification of the target antigen in chronic bullous disease of childhood and linear IgA disease of adults. *Br J Dermatol* 1991;124:157.

23. Tsuchida T, Furue M, Kashiwado T, Ishibashi Y. Bullous systemic lupus erythematosus with cutaneous mucinosis and leukocytoclastic vasculitis. *J Am Acad Dermatol* 1994;31:387.

24. Orkin M, Good RA, Clawson CC, et al. Bullous mastocytosis. *Arch Dermatol* 1970;101:547.

Perivascular, Diffuse, and Granulomatous Infiltrates of the Reticular Dermis

The dermis serves as a reaction site for a variety of inflammatory, infiltrative, and desmoplastic processes. These include infiltrations of a variety of cells (lymphocytes, histiocytes, eosinophils, plasma cells, melanocytes), perivascular and vascular reactions, infiltration with organisms and foreign bodies, proliferations of dermal fibers, and precursors of dermal fibers as reactions to a variety of stimuli.

VA. SUPERFICIAL AND DEEP PERIVASCULAR INFILTRATES WITHOUT VASCULAR DAMAGE OR VASCULITIS

In some of the diseases considered here, the infiltrates are predominantly in the upper reticular dermis (urticarial eruptions), whereas others are both superficial and deep (gyrate erythemas). Most of these also involve the superficial plexus. A few diseases are mainly deep (some examples of lupus erythematosus, scleroderma).

1. Perivascular Infiltrates, Lymphocytes Predominant
2. Perivascular Infiltrates, Neutrophils Predominant
3. Perivascular Infiltrates, Lymphocytes and Eosinophils
4. Perivascular Infiltrates, With Plasma Cells
5. Perivascular Infiltrates, Mixed Cell Types

VA1. Perivascular Infiltrates, Lymphocytes Predominant

There is no vasculitis in the dermis, only a perivascular surround of lymphocytes as the predominant cell. Erythema annulare centrifigum is prototypic (1).

Erythema Annulare Centrifugum

CLINICAL SUMMARY. Also known as gyrate erythema, this disorder represents a hypersensitivity reaction manifesting as arcuate and polycyclic areas of erythema. The condition has been categorized into superficial and deep variants. The deep form is characterized clinically by annular areas of palpable erythema with central clearing and absence of surface changes. The superficial variant differs only by the presence of a characteristic trailing scale, a delicate annular rim of scale that trails behind the advancing edge of erythema. Small vesi-cles may occur. The lesions may attain considerable size (up to 10 cm across) over a period of several weeks, may be mildly pruritic, and have a predilection for the trunk and proximal extremities. Most cases resolve spontaneously within 6 weeks; however, the condition may persist for years.

HISTOPATHOLOGY. In the classic deep or indurated type, a perivascular lymphocytic infiltrate characterized by a tightly cuffed "coat-sleeve–like" pattern is present in the middle and lower portions of the dermis. In the superficial variant, there is a superficial perivascular tightly cuffed lymphohistiocytic infiltrate with endothelial cell swelling and focal extravasation of erythrocytes in the papillary dermis, and focal epidermal spongiosis and parakeratosis can be seen. Erythema chronicum migrans is an important differential, but usually presents with plasma cells and lymphocytes, and is also discussed in section VA5.

Erythema Chronicum Migrans

See Figs. VA1.d–VA1.f and section VA5.

Tumid Lupus Erythematosus

See Figs. VA1.g–VA1.i.
  Conditions to consider in the differential diagnosis:
    pityriasis lichenoides et varioliformis acuta
    stasis dermatitis
    acne rosacea
    discoid lupus erythematosus
    polymorphous light eruption
    deep gyrate erythemas
    erythema annulare centrifigum
    erythema chronicum migrans
    Jessner's lymphocytic infiltrate
    reticulated erythematous mucinosis

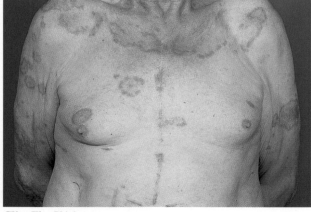

Clin. Fig. VA1.a

Clin. Fig. VA1.b

Clin. Fig. VA1.a. *Erythema annulare centrifugum.* Multiple annular lesions developed on the trunk of a middle-aged man.

Clin. Fig. VA1.b. *Erythema annulare centrifugum.* An annular area of palpable erythema with central clearing and a delicate annular rim of scale trailing behind the advancing edge of the erythema.

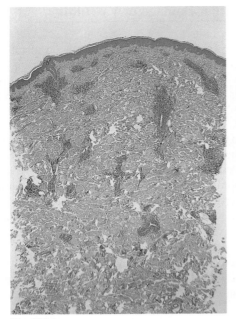

Fig. VA1.a

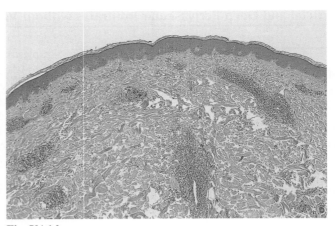

Fig. VA1.b

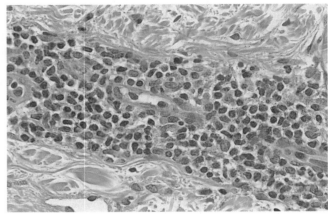

Fig. VA1.c

Fig. VA1.a. *Erythema annulare centrifugum, low power.* A tight cuff of small round cells surrounds the vessels of the superficial and middermal plexuses.

Fig. VA1.b. *Erythema annulare centrifugum, medium power.* The vessels at the center of the infiltrates show no evidence of damage other than slight endothelial cell swelling.

Fig. VA1.c. *Erythema annulare centrifugum, high power.* The infiltrate is composed almost entirely of mature small lymphocytes.

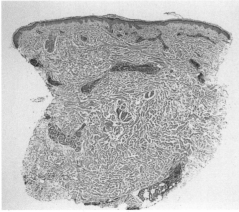

Fig. VA1.d

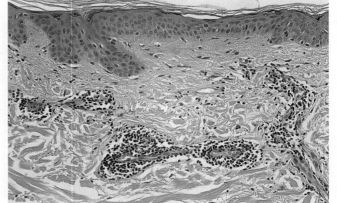

Fig. VA1.e

Fig. VA1.d. *Erythema chronicum migrans, low power.* Similar to erythema annulare centrifugum, there is a tight cuff of small cells around the vessels of the superficial and deep-dermal plexuses.

Fig. VA1.e. *Erythema chronicum migrans, medium power.* The infiltrate surrounds vessels quite tightly, without a significant interstitial infiltrate.

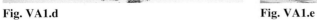

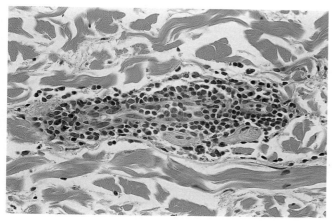

Fig. VA1.f. *Erythema chronicum migrans, high power.* Although plasma cells are usually present, in some instances, as here, the infiltrate is composed almost entirely of mature small lymphocytes.

perioral dermatitis
papular acrodermatitis (Gianotti–Crosti)
leprosy, indeterminant
"tumid" lupus erythematosus
perniosis (chilblains)

VA2. Perivascular Infiltrates, Neutrophils Predominant

In this pattern, neutrophils are seen in perivascular or perivascular and diffuse patterns in the dermis. Edema is prominent in some instances. Sweet's syndrome can present as a perivascular infiltrate but is more often nodular, and is discussed in section VC2. Neutrophil-rich urticaria may present as a predominantly neutrophilic infiltrate, but eosinophils are usually also present (see section VA3). The other conditions listed are mostly infections. Biopsies from the periphery of a lesion may appear perivascular, but the fully developed center of these lesions will consist of diffuse infiltrates (see section VA3).

Cellulitis

See Figs. VA2.a–VA2.b.
Conditions to consider in the differential diagnosis:
acute febrile neutrophilic dermatosis (Sweet's)
erysipelas
necrotizing fasciitis
pyoderma gangrenosum (early)
ecthyma gangrenosum
neutrophil-rich urticaria
solar urticaria
rheumatoid arthritis

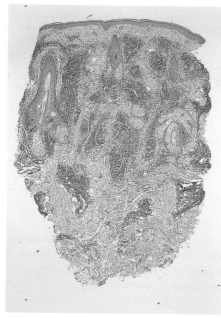

Fig. VA1.g

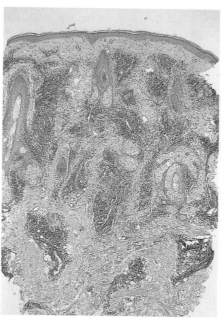

Fig. VA1.h

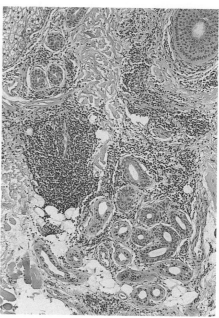

Fig. VA1.i

Fig. VA1.g. *"Tumid" lupus erythematosus, low power.* A dense lymphocytic infiltrate is present around the vessels of the superficial, mid- and deep-dermal plexuses, and around adnexal structures.

Fig. VA1.h. *"Tumid" lupus erythematosus, medium power.* In contrast to erythema annulare centrifugum and erythema chronicum migrans, the cuff of small lymphocytes appears less tight around the vessels of the superficial, mid- and deep-dermal plexuses, because there is also an interstitial component to the infiltrate.

Fig. VA1.i. *"Tumid" lupus erythematosus, high power.* Although plasma cells are usually present, the infiltrate is often as here composed almost entirely of mature small lymphocytes. Involvement of skin appendages (sweat glands) is a clue to the diagnosis of lupus.

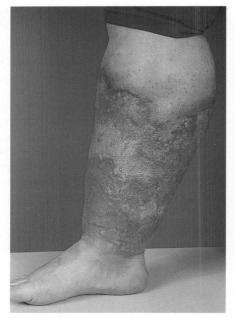

Clin. Fig. VA2

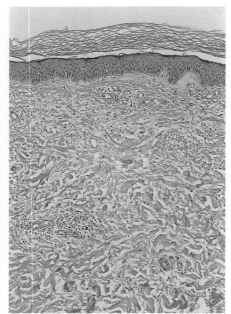

Fig. VA2.a

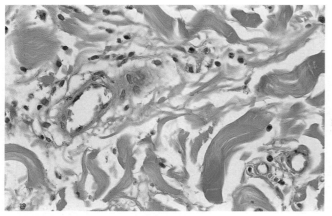

Fig. VA2.b

Clin. Fig. VA2. *Cellulitis.* This middle-aged woman was admitted with septic shock secondary to her cellulitis. She had marked erythema and bullous changes and rapidly improved on intravenous antibiotics.

Fig. VA2.a. *Cellulitis, low power.* There is edema and a patchy infiltrate in the reticular dermis, appearing at this magnification to be mainly perivascular.

Fig. VA2.b. *Cellulitis, high power.* The neutrophils are mainly perivascular. In other areas, the infiltrate appears more diffuse (see section VC2).

VA3. Perivascular Infiltrates, Lymphocytes and Eosinophils

Lymphocytes and eosinophils are mixed in the infiltrate. Lymphocytes are always seen, and eosinophil numbers may vary, being greatest in bite reactions and often (although variable and sometimes very few) in eosinophilic fasciitis. Papular urticaria is a prototypic example (2).

Papular Urticaria

CLINICAL SUMMARY.   Also known as lichen urticatus, this condition is the result of hypersensitivity to bites from certain insects, especially mosquitoes, fleas, and bedbugs. One observes edematous papules and papulovesicles, which, because of severe itching, usually are excoriated. The eruption

is more common in children than adults and, if caused by mosquitoes, is limited to the summer months. The lesions of papular urticaria are clinically and often also histologically indistinguishable from those of prurigo simplex.

HISTOPATHOLOGY.   The stratum malpighii shows intercellular and intracellular edema and occasionally a spongiotic vesicle. A chronic inflammatory infiltrate is present around the vessels of the dermis, often extending into the lower dermis and containing a significant admixture of eosinophils.

Pruritic Urticarial Papules and Plaques of Pregnancy

CLINICAL SUMMARY.   Pruritic urticarial papules and plaques of pregnancy is a fairly common entity that has a predilection

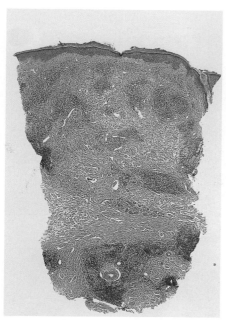

Fig. VA3.a

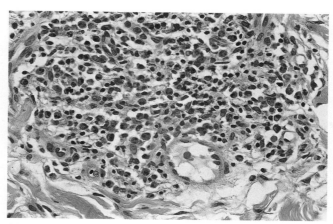

Fig. VA3.b

Fig. VA3.a. *Papular urticaria/arthropod bite, low power*. A dense perivascular infiltrate of lymphocytes and eosinophils, more conspicuous than in many instances of typical papular urticaria.

Fig. VA3.b. *Papular urticaria/arthropod bite, high power*. The infiltrate is composed primarily of lymphocytes, with a striking component of eosinophils. Plasma cells may also be present in some cases.

for primigravidas in the third trimester of pregnancy (3). The rash usually starts on the abdomen and is composed of intensely pruritic erythematous urticarial papules, which may be surmounted by vesicles. The proximal parts of the extremities are also affected. There is no increased incidence of the rash in subsequent pregnancies. The rash usually involutes spontaneously after delivery. Fetal outcome appears to be unaffected.

HISTOPATHOLOGY. Microscopic findings most commonly show a superficial and middermal perivascular lymphohistiocytic infiltrate with variable numbers of eosinophils and neutrophils together with edema of the superficial dermis. Epidermal involvement is variable and consists of focal spongiosis with exocytosis, parakeratosis, and mild acanthosis.

Conditions to consider in the differential diagnosis:

  urticaria/angioedema
  pruritic and urticarial papules and plaques of
    pregnancy
  prurigo simplex
  papular urticaria
  morbilliform drug eruption
  photoallergic reaction
  eosinophilic fasciitis/scleroderma
  angiolymphoid hyperplasia with eosinophilia (AHLE)
  insect bite reaction

VA4. Perivascular Infiltrates, with Plasma Cells

In addition to lymphocytes, plasma cells are found in the dermal infiltrate. Secondary syphilis is a prototypic example (4).

Secondary Syphilis

CLINICAL SUMMARY. Secondary syphilis results from the hematogenous dissemination of *Treponema pallidum*, resulting in widespread clinical signs accompanied by constitutional symptoms such as fever, malaise, and generalized lymphadenopathy. A generalized eruption occurs, comprising brown-red macules and papules and, rarely, pustules. Lesions may be follicular, annular, or serpiginous. Other skin findings include alopecia and condylomata lata, the latter comprising broad, raised, gray, confluent papular lesions arising in anogenital areas and mucous patches composed of multiple, shallow, painless ulcers.

HISTOPATHOLOGY. The two fundamental pathologic changes in syphilis are swelling and proliferation of endothelial cells and a predominantly perivascular infiltrate composed of lymphoid cells, and often plasma cells. However, plasma cells and endothelial swelling are not invariably present. Frank necrotizing vasculitis is distinctly unusual. In late secondary and tertiary syphilis, there are also granulomatous infiltrates of epithelioid histiocytes and giant cells.

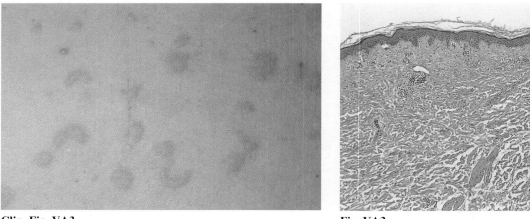

Clin. Fig. VA3

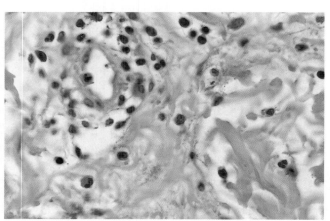

Fig. VA3.c

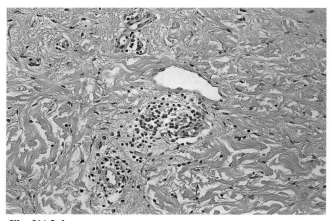

Fig. VA3.d

Fig. VA3.e

Clin. Fig. VA3. *Urticaria*. Edematous plaques with central clearing and geographic configuration are typical of urticaria.

Fig. VA3.c. *Urticaria, low power*. A patchy perivascular infiltrate of lymphocytes and eosinophils, which could be seen in papular urticaria or in idiopathic urticaria.

Fig. VA3.d. *Urticaria, medium power*. There is dermal edema separating collagen fibers. Lymphatic channels are dilated (a clue to the presence of edema).

Fig. VA3.e. *Urticaria, high power*. The perivascular infiltrate includes a few lymphocytes and eosinophils and neutrophils.

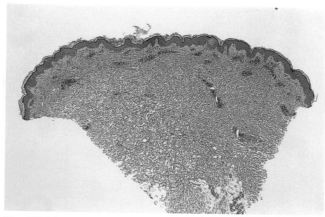

Fig. VA3.f

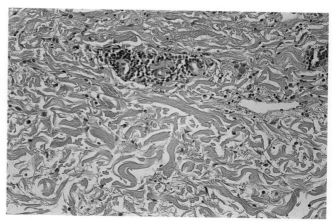

Fig. VA3.g

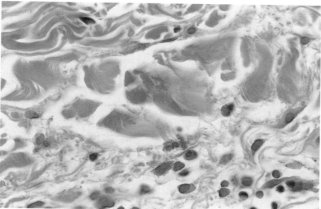

Fig. VA3.h

Fig. VA3.f. *Pruritic and urticarial papules and plaques of pregnancy (PUPPP), low power.* There is a tight perivascular infiltrate of lymphocytes and eosinophils about the superficial and mid plexuses.

Fig. VA3.g. *PUPPP, medium power.* As in usual urticaria, there is dermal edema separating collagen fibers, and lymphatic channels are dilated.

Fig. VA3.h. *PUPPP, high power.* The perivascular and interstitial infiltrate includes lymphocytes and eosinophils, which may not be numerous as in this case.

Biopsies generally reveal psoriasiform hyperplasia of the epidermis with spongiosis and basilar vacuolar alteration, exocytosis of lymphocytes, spongiform pustulation, and parakeratosis. The parakeratosis may be patchy or broad, with or without intracorneal neutrophilic abscesses. Scattered necrotic keratinocytes may be observed. Ulceration is not usual except in *lues maligna*. The dermal changes include marked papillary dermal edema and a perivascular and/or periadnexal and often lichenoid infiltrate that may be lymphocyte predominant, lymphohistiocytic, histiocytic predominant, or frankly granulomatous. This infiltrate is of greatest intensity in the papillary dermis, and extends as loose perivascular aggregates into the reticular dermis. In a few cases, atypical-appearing nuclei may be present and may suggest the possibility of lymphoma. Neutrophils are not infrequent and may permeate the eccrine coil to produce a neutrophilic eccrine hidradenitis. Granulomatous inflammation develops after a few months. A silver stain is positive for spirochetes in about a third of the cases. The organisms are

seen in the epidermis, follicular epithelium, and blood vessels. Lesions of condylomata lata show all of the aforementioned changes, with more florid epithelial hyperplasia and intraepithelial microabscess formation.

Tertiary Syphilis

See Clin. Fig. VA4.c.

Morphea

See Figs. VA4.e–VA4.g and section VF.
    Conditions to consider in the differential diagnosis:
        primary syphilitic chancre
        erythema chronicum migrans
        acne rosacea
        perioral dermatitis
        scleroderma/morphea
        secondary syphilis
        Kaposi's sarcoma, early lesions

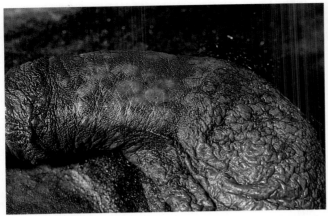

Clin. Fig. VA4.a

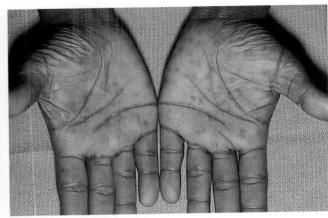

Clin. Fig. VA4.b

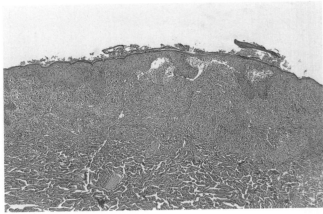

Fig. VA4.a

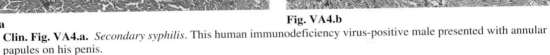

Fig. VA4.b

Clin. Fig. VA4.a. *Secondary syphilis.* This human immunodeficiency virus-positive male presented with annular papules on his penis.

Clin. Fig. VA4.b. *Secondary syphilis.* Brown-red macules were present on the palms of the same patient. RPR was positive.

Fig. VA4.a. *Secondary syphilis, low power.* There is hyperplasia of the epidermis. Within the dermis, there is a perivascular to diffuse infiltrate of mixed cell types.

Fig. VA4.b. *Secondary syphilis, medium power.* Epidermal changes include spongiosis and basilar vacuolar alteration, exocytosis of lymphocytes, and parakeratosis. A perivascular to mixed infiltrate is present in the dermis.

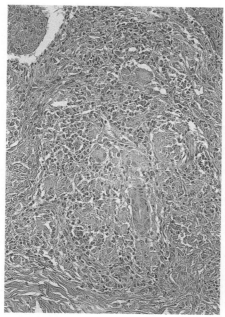

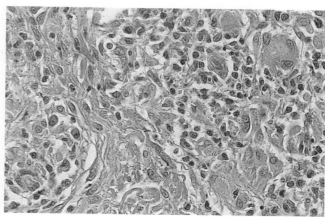

Fig. VA4.c   **Fig. VA4.d**

Fig. VA4.c. *Secondary syphilis, medium power.* The cells in the dermis include lymphocytes and prominent plasma cells, as a well as a few histiocytes and giant cells in this example, forming ill-defined noncaseating granulomas.

Fig. VA4.d. *Secondary syphilis, high power.* A mixed infiltrate of lymphocytes, histiocytes, and plasma cells, often also including neutrophils and eosinophils, is present.

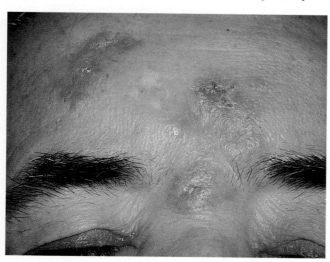

Clin. Fig. VA4.c. *Tertiary syphilis.* This man with positive syphilis serology presented with gummatous lesions characterized by subcutaneous swellings and ulceration.

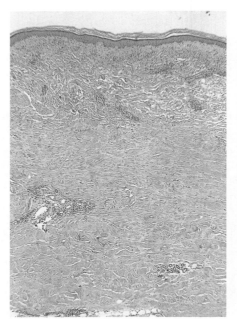

Fig. VA4.e

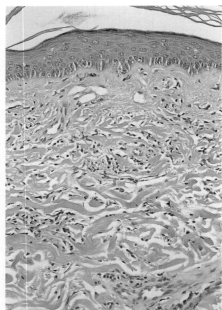

Fig. VA4.f

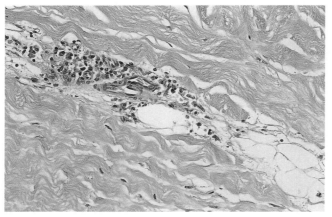

Fig. VA4.g

Fig. VA4.e. *Morphea, low power.* Scanning magnification reveals a perieccrine infiltrate associated with sclerosis of the lower portion of the reticular dermis. The eccrine glands appear "trapped" within the sclerotic collagen. In the inflammatory stage of morphea, sclerosis, although usually detectable as here, may not be as prominent as it is in later stages of the disease.

Fig. VA4.f. *Morphea, medium power.* Inflammatory stage morphea may present as a perivascular dermatitis.

Fig. VA4.g. *Morphea, high power.* The infiltrate usually includes plasma cells and lymphocytes and is frequently present at the dermal–subcutaneous junction.

VA5. Perivascular Infiltrates, Mixed Cell Types

In addition to lymphocytes, plasma cells and eosinophils are found in the dermal infiltrate. Erythema chronicum migrans is a prototypic example (5).

Erythema Chronicum Migrans

CLINICAL SUMMARY. Erythema chronicum migrans is the distinctive cutaneous manifestation of stage I Lyme disease and represents the site of primary tick inoculation. The lesion starts as an area of scaly erythema or a distinct red papule within 3 to 30 days after the tick bite, before spreading centrifugally with central clearing after a few weeks, occasionally reaching a diameter of 25 cm. Average lesional duration is a few weeks, but in some cases, lesions may persist for as long as 12 months. The lesions may be solitary or multiple, the latter reflecting hematogenous dissemination of the spirochete, which may be accompanied by fever, fatigue, headaches, cough, and arthralgias.

HISTOPATHOLOGY. An intense superficial and deep angiocentric, neurotropic, and eccrinotropic infiltrate predominated by lymphocytes with a variable admixture of plasma cells and eosinophils is the principal histopathology. Plasma cells have been identified most frequently in the peripheries of lesions of erythema chronicum migrans, whereas eosinophils are identified in the centers of the lesions. Not infrequently, these florid dermal alterations are accompanied by eczematous epithelial alterations and interstitial infiltration of the reticular dermis with a concomitant incipient sclerosing reaction. A Warthin–Starry stain may be positive, especially if taken from the advancing border of the lesion.

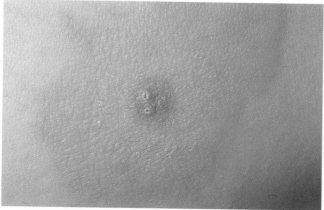

Clin. Fig. VA5

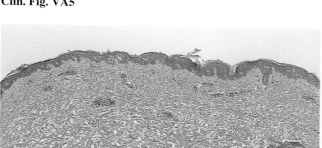

Fig. VA5.a

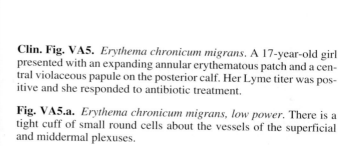

Clin. Fig. VA5. *Erythema chronicum migrans.* A 17-year-old girl presented with an expanding annular erythematous patch and a central violaceous papule on the posterior calf. Her Lyme titer was positive and she responded to antibiotic treatment.

Fig. VA5.a. *Erythema chronicum migrans, low power.* There is a tight cuff of small round cells about the vessels of the superficial and middermal plexuses.

Fig. VA5.b. *Erythema chronicum migrans, high power.* Plasma cells and eosinophils are present in the perivascular infiltrate.

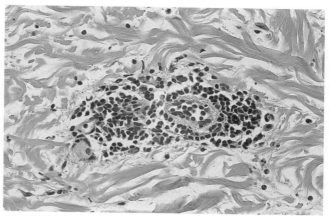

Fig.VA5.b

Conditions to consider in the differential diagnosis:

    secondary syphilis
    erythema chronicum migrans
    arthropod bite reaction

VB. VASCULITIS AND VASCULOPATHIES

True vasculitis is defined by eosinophilic degeneration of the vessel wall ("fibrinoid necrosis"), infiltration of the vessel wall by neutrophils, with neutrophils, nuclear dust, and extravasated red cells in the vessel walls and adjacent dermis. Some conditions mentioned here lack these prototypic findings and may be termed "vasculopathies" (e.g., Degos' disease).

1. Vascular Damage, Scant Inflammatory Cells
2. Vasculitis, Lymphocytes Predominant
3. Vasculitis, Neutrophils Prominent
4. Vasculitis, Mixed Cell Types and/or Granulomas
5. Thrombotic and Other Microangiopathies

VB1. Vascular Damage, Scant Inflammatory Cells

Although there is significant vascular damage, there is little early inflammatory response. Degos' syndrome is an example (6).

Degos' Syndrome

CLINICAL SUMMARY. The clinical manifestations include crops of asymptomatic, slightly raised, yellowish-red papules that gradually develop an atrophic porcelain-white center. These papules tend to affect the trunk and proximal extremities. Degos initially described a cutaneointestinal syndrome, in which distinct skin findings ("drops of porcelain") were associated with recurrent attacks of abdominal pain that often ended in death from intestinal perforations. He chose the name *malignant atrophic papulosis* to emphasize the serious clinical course of the disease. Today, it is believed that malignant atrophic papulosis is a clinicopathologic reaction pattern associated with a number of conditions that are not always lethal. Lesions similar, if not identical, to

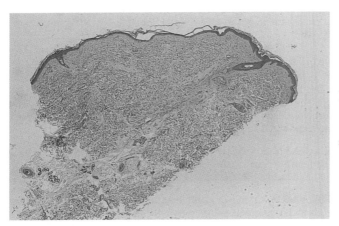

Fig. VB1.a

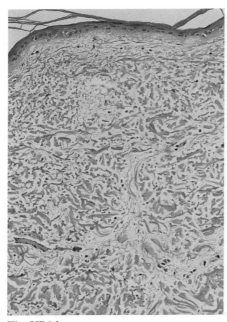

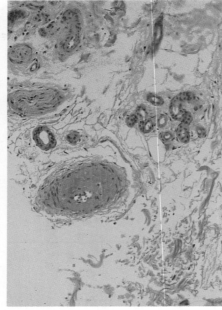

Fig. VB1.a. *Degos' lesion, low power.* Atrophic epidermis overlies a wedge-shaped area of altered dermis. (R. Barnhill and K. Busam)

Fig. VB1.b. *Degos' lesion, medium power.* Within the wedge, there is interstitial mucin deposition. (R. Barnhill and K. Busam)

Fig. VB1.c. *Degos' lesion, high power.* At the base of the lesion, there is a thrombosed vessel with a thickened wall. This lesion occurred in a patient with dermatomyositis. (R. Barnhill and K. Busam)

Fig. VB1.b   **Fig. VB1.c**

malignant atrophic papulosis have been noted, in particular, in connective tissue diseases such as lupus erythematosus, dermatomyositis, and progressive systemic sclerosis, in atrophie blanche, and in Creutzfeldt–Jakob disease.

HISTOPATHOLOGY. Although the pathogenesis of Degos' syndrome is poorly understood, a thrombotic vasculopathy is a characteristic associated finding. A typical lesion shows a wedge-shaped area of altered dermis covered by atrophic epidermis with slight hyperkeratosis. Dermal alterations may include frank necrosis but more common are edema, extensive mucin deposition, and slight sclerosis. There may be a sparse perivascular lymphocytic infiltrate, but the vessel walls are not inflamed. Typically, vascular damage is noted in the vessels at the base of the "cone of necrobiosis." This

damage may be limited to endothelial swelling, but more characteristically, intravascular fibrin thrombi may be noted, suggesting that the dermal and epidermal changes result from ischemia.

Conditions to consider in the differential diagnosis:

Degos' syndrome (malignant atrophic papulosis)
atrophie blanche

VB2. Vasculitis, Lymphocytes Predominant

The term "lymphocytic vasculitis" is controversial, but there are some conditions in which perivascular and intramural lymphocytes may be associated with some degree of vessel wall damage, not usually including frank fibrinoid necrosis.

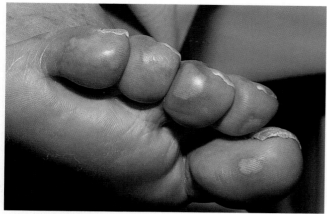

Clin. Fig. VB2

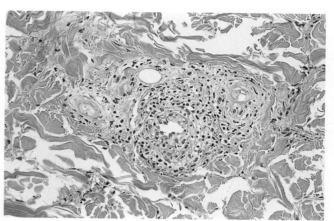

Fig. VB2.a

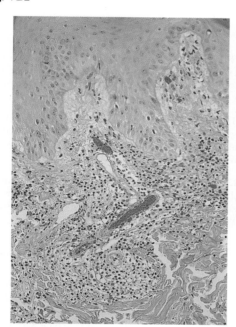

Fig. VB2.b

Fig. VB2.c

Clin. Fig. VB2. *Perniosis.* A 62-year-old man presented with tender, edematous, erythematous macules and plaques with a hint of bullous change after spending a considerable time out in the cold. Lesions improved with avoidance of and protection from the cold.

Fig. VB2.a. *Pernio, low power.* There is edema of the papillary dermis, with a superficial and deep perivascular and interstitial infiltrate.

Fig. VB2.b. *Pernio, medium power.* The infiltrate tends to be localized about and within the walls of vessels of the superficial plexus.

Fig. VB2.c. *Pernio, high power.* The vessel walls are edematous and are infiltrated by lymphocytes.

Most of these conditions are discussed elsewhere (see sections IIIA and VA) as "perivascular lymphocytic infiltrates." In angiocentric lymphomas, the cells infiltrating the vessel walls are neoplastic, but the process may be mistaken for an inflammatory reaction. *Pernio* is a prototypic inflammatory example (7).

Pernio

CLINICAL SUMMARY. Pernio or chilblain usually consists of tender or painful, raised, violaceous plaques on the fingers or toes referred to as superficial pernio. Occasionally, it is found at a more proximal portion of an extremity in a deeper location in the skin or subcutis. Pernio is caused in suscepti-

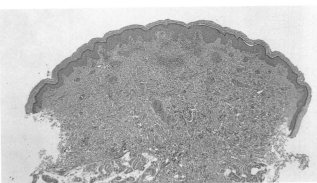

Fig. VB2.d

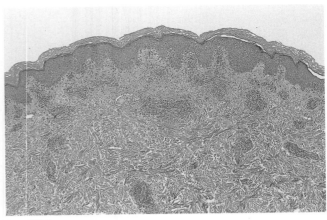

Fig. VB2.e

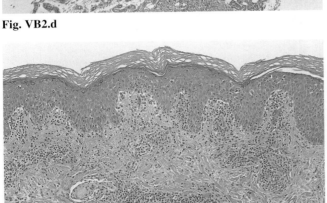

Fig. VB2.f

Fig. VB2.d. *Pityriasis lichenoides et varioliformis acuta (PLEVA), low power.* There is a dense perivascular, predominantly lymphocytic infiltrate in the papillary dermis and extending into the reticular dermis in a wedge-shaped pattern.

Fig. VB2.e. *PLEVA, medium power.* The infiltrate obscures the dermal–epidermal junction with pronounced vacuolar alteration of the basal layer, marked exocytosis of lymphocytes and erythrocytes, with intercellular and intracellular edema.

Fig. VB2.f. *PLEVA, medium power.* Vessel walls are obscured by a dense lymphocytic infiltrate, often with endothelial swelling, and extravasated erythrocytes are seen in most cases. However, there is no true vessel wall necrosis.

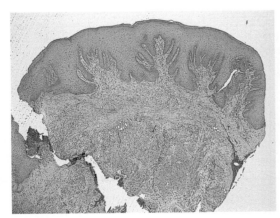

Fig. VB2.g

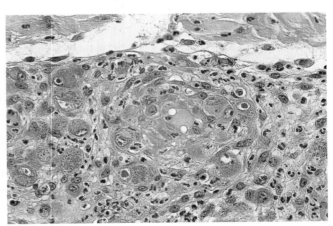

Fig. VB2.h

Fig. VB2.g. *Cytomegalovirus infection of endothelial cells, low power.* A biopsy of an oral lesion in a patient with acquired immune deficiency syndrome shows a perivascular and diffuse infiltrate composed mainly of lymphocytes with a few plasma cells.

Fig. VB2.h. *Cytomegalovirus, medium power.* Endothelial cells are markedly swollen, and some contain inclusions (intranuclear and/or cytoplasmic). (*continues*)

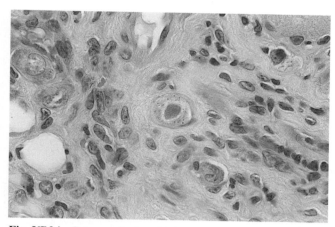

Fig. VB2.i. *Cytomegalovirus, high power.* A cell contains a characteristic large eosinophilic intranuclear inclusion body.

ble individuals by prolonged exposure to cold above the freezing point, especially in damp climates.

HISTOPATHOLOGY. In superficial pernio, intense edema of the papillary dermis is observed. A marked perivascular mononuclear cell infiltrate is seen in the upper dermis, sparing the edematous papillary dermis. The blood vessels are said to show a diffuse, "fluffy" edema of their walls. The mononuclear infiltrate of the vascular walls is consistent with a lymphocytic vasculitis. In deep pernio, an intense mononuclear cell perivascular infiltrate extends throughout the dermis into the subcutaneous fat. The blood vessels show a similar edema as the superficial form of pernio.

Pityriasis Lichenoides et Varioliformis Acuta

See Figs. VB2.d–VB2.f.

Cytomegalovirus Infection

See Figs. VB2.g–VB2.i.

Erythema Chronicum Migrans`

See Figs. VB2.j–VB2.k.
   Conditions to consider in the differential diagnosis:
      "lymphocytic vasculitis"
      lupus erythematosus
      lymphomatoid papulosis
      pityriasis lichenoides et varioliformis acuta
      pityriasis lichenoides chronica
      purpura pigmentosa chronica
      morbilliform viral infections
      Lyme disease
      perniosis (chilblains)
      angiocentric mycosis fungoides
      angiocentric T-cell lymphoma/lymphomatoid
         granulomatosis
      cytomegalovirus inclusion disease
      Behçet's syndrome

VB3. Vasculitis, Neutrophils Prominent

Neutrophils are prominent in the infiltrate, with fibrinoid necrosis and nuclear dust; eosinophils and lymphocytes are also found. Polyarteritis nodosa is prototypic (8).

Polyarteritis Nodosa and Microscopic Polyangiitis

CLINICAL SUMMARY. *Classic polyarteritis nodosa* (PAN) is a systemic vasculitic disorder in which large arteries are involved and in which ischemic glomerular lesions are common, but glomerulonephritis is rare. *Microscopic PAN,* also termed *microscopic polyangiitis* (MPA), refers to a systemic small-vessel vasculitis primarily affecting arterioles and capillaries, typically associated with focal necrotizing

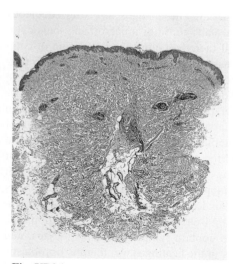

Fig. VB2.j

Fig. VB2.j. *Erythema chronicum migrans, low power.* A tight perivascular cuff of lymphocytes about the superficial and middermal vessels.

Fig. VB2.k. *Erythema chronicum migrans, high power.* In this example, the lymphocytes diffusely infiltrate the vessel wall. However, there is no vessel wall necrosis (see section VA5).

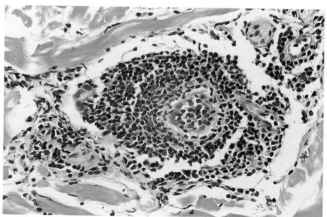

Fig. VB2.k

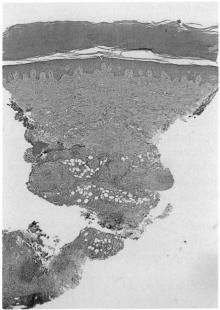

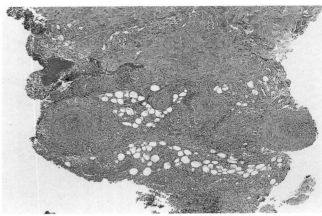

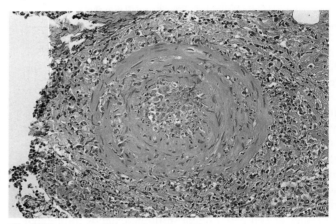

Fig. VB3.a. *Polyarteritis nodosa, low power.* Vessels in the deep dermis and subcutis are thick-walled, and there is a diffuse subcutaneous infiltrate.

Fig. VB3.b. *Polyarteritis nodosa, medium power.* The infiltrate is predominantly in the panniculus but also extends into the deep dermis.

Fig. VB3.c. *Polyarteritis nodosa, high power.* There are areas of eosinophilic change ("fibrinoid necrosis"), with neutrophilic infiltration, in the walls of large vessels (small muscular arteries).

Fig. VB3.a

Fig. VB3.b

Fig. VB3.c

glomerulonephritis with crescents. Most patients with MPA have antineutrophil, cytoplasmic antibodies (ANCA) to myeloperoxidase (MPO). Some cases of vasculitis present with an *overlapping syndrome* affecting both small- and medium-sized arteries.

Most patients with MPA are male and over 50 years of age. Prodromal symptoms include fever, myalgias, arthralgias, and sore throat. The most common clinical feature is renal disease manifesting as microhematuria, proteinuria, or acute oliguric renal failure. Although cutaneous involvement is rare in classic PAN, 30% to 40% of patients with MPA exhibit skin changes. These changes include palpable purpura, splinter hemorrhages, and ulcerations.

HISTOPATHOLOGY. The characteristic lesion of classic PAN is a panarteritis involving medium-sized and small arteries. Even though in classic PAN the arteries show the characteristic changes in many visceral sites, affected skin often shows only small-vessel disease, and arterial involve-

ment is typically focal. The changes affecting cutaneous small vessels are usually those of a necrotizing leukocytoclastic vasculitis. If there is a clinical presentation of cutaneous nodules, panarteritis similar to visceral lesions is usually detected. In classic PAN, the lesions typically are in different stages of development (i.e., fresh and old). Early lesions show degeneration of the arterial wall with deposition of fibrinoid material and partial to complete destruction of the external and internal elastic laminae. An infiltrate present within and around the arterial wall is composed largely of neutrophils showing evidence of leukocytoclasis, although it often contains eosinophils. At a later stage, intimal proliferation and thrombosis lead to complete occlusion of the lumen with subsequent ischemia, and possibly ulceration. The infiltrate may also contain lymphocytes, histiocytes, and some plasma cells. In the healing stage, there is fibroblastic proliferation extending into the perivascular area. The small vessels of the middle and upper dermis often exhibit a nonspecific lymphocytic perivascular infiltrate.

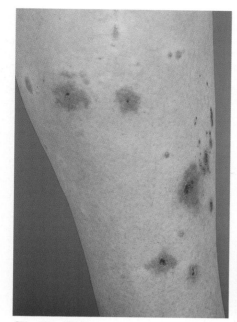

Clin. Fig. VB3.a

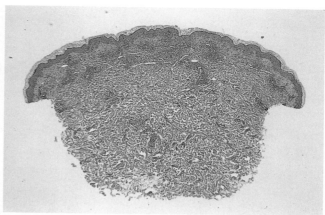

Fig. VB3.d

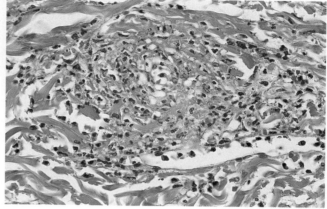

Fig. VB3.e

Clin. Fig. VB3.a. *Leukocytoclastic vasculitis (LCV).* Hemorrhagic purpuric papules and plaques on the lower leg in a middle-aged woman were believed to be secondary to a nonsteroidal antiinflammatory drug.

Fig. VB3.d. *LCV, low power.* Although LCV is often confined to the superficial plexus, deeper small vessels including frequently those in the middermis, are often involved, as in this example.

Fig. VB3.e. *LCV, high power.* There is fibrinoid necrosis of vessel walls, with neutrophilic infiltration and leukocytoclasia around the involved vessels.

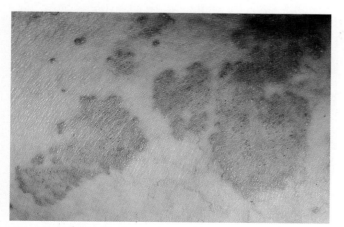

Clin. Fig. VB3.b. *Erythema elevatum diutinum.* Brownish-yellow annular plaques with an infiltrated border developed on the extensor surface of the lower extremity. No monoclonal or polyclonal gammopathy was detected. (S. Binnick)

Leukocytoclastic Vasculitis

See Figs. VB3.d and VB3.e.

Erythema Elevatum Diutinum

See Clin. Fig. VB3.b.

Conditions to consider in the differential diagnosis:
   small vessel leukocytoclastic vasculitis
   neutrophilic dermatoses
   Sweet's syndrome
   granuloma faciale
   bowel-associated dermatosis-arthrosis syndrome
   septic/embolic lesions of gonococcemia/meningococcemia
   Rocky Mountain spotted fever ("Rickettsia rickettsii")
   polyarteritis nodosa
   erythema elevatum diutinum
   Behçet's syndrome
   papulonecrotic tuberculid

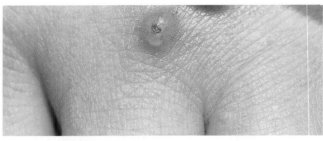

Clin. Fig. VB4

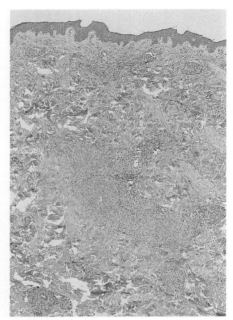

Fig. VB4.a

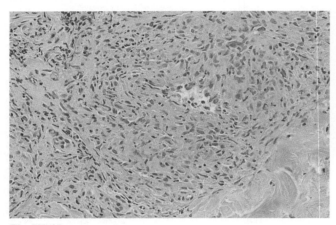

Fig. VB4.b

Clin. Fig. VB4. *Granulomatous vasculitis.* This inflammatory nodule histologically showed evidence of a granulomatous vasculitis.

Fig. VB4.a. *Granulomatous vasculitis, low power.* There is a perivascular granulomatous infiltrate of histiocytes and lymphocytes in the reticular dermis. (R. Barnhill and K. Busam)

Fig. VB4.b. *Granulomatous vasculitis, medium power.* The wall of a middermal vessel is damaged. The differential diagnosis for this lesion could include several of the conditions listed below in the differential diagnosis of this condition. Most cases of Churg–Strauss syndrome would likely have a more prominent component of eosinophils in the inflammatory infiltrate. (R. Barnhill and K. Busam)

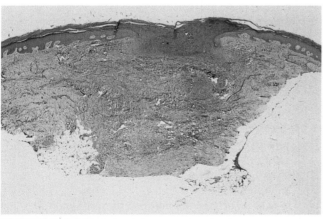

Fig. VB4.c

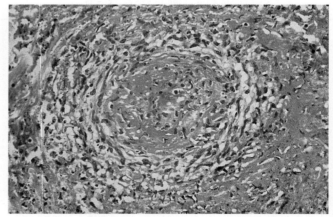

Fig. VB4.d

Fig. VB4.c. *Papulonecrotic tuberculid, low power.* Wedge-shaped infarction of the dermis and epidermis, caused by vasculitis. (S. Lucas)

Fig. VB4.d. *Papulonecrotic tuberculid, high power.* Necrotizing vasculitis of a dermal artery, with surrounding granulomatous inflammation. (S. Lucas)

VB4. Vasculitis, Mixed Cell Types and/or Granulomas

Histiocytes and giant cells are a part of the infiltrate. Lymphocytes and eosinophils can also be found depending on the diagnosis. Giant cell arteritis is a true inflammation of the artery wall (true arteritis), although there is no fibrinoid necrosis. Most cases of giant cell arteritis involve vessels of the subcutis. Allergic granulomatosis (Churg–Strauss) is prototypic (9).

Churg–Strauss Syndrome (Allergic Granulomatosis)

CLINICAL SUMMARY.   Churg–Strauss syndrome is a systemic disease which occurs in asthmatic patients, and is characterized by vasculitis, eosinophilic infiltration of multiple organs, and peripheral eosinophilia. There is considerable overlap of this disease process with other systemic vasculitides and with other inflammatory disorders exhibiting eosinophils, such as eosinophilic pneumonitis. The internal organs most commonly involved are the lungs, the gastrointestinal tract, and, less commonly, the peripheral nerves and the heart. In contrast to PAN, renal failure is rare. A slightly broader definition of Churg–Strauss syndrome has been proposed requiring asthma, blood hypereosinophilia, and systemic vasculitis involving two or more extrapulmonary organs.

Two types of cutaneous lesions may occur: hemorrhagic lesions similar to Henoch–Schönlein purpura, varying from petechiae to extensive ecchymoses, often with areas of erythema and sometimes with necrotic ulcers, and cutaneous-subcutaneous nodules. The extremities are the most common sites of skin lesions, but the trunk may also be involved, and some cases are generalized. ANCA tests obtained during an active phase of the disease contain p-ANCA in most cases. There is also a limited form, in which the lesions are confined to the conjunctiva, the skin, and subcutaneous tissue.

HISTOPATHOLOGY.   The areas of cutaneous hemorrhage typically show changes of leukocytoclastic vasculitis. Eosinophils may be conspicuous. In some instances, the dermis shows a granulomatous reaction composed predominantly of radially arranged histiocytes and, frequently, multinucleated giant cells centered around degenerated collagen fibers. The central portions of the granulomas contain not only degenerated collagen fibers but also dense aggregates of disintegrated cells, particularly eosinophils. These granulomas have been referred to as Churg–Strauss granulomas. However, they are not always present, and similar findings can also be observed in other disease processes, such as connective tissue diseases (rheumatoid arthritis and lupus erythematosus), Wegener's granulomatosis, PAN, lymphoproliferative disorders, subacute bacterial endocarditis, chronic active hepatitis, and inflammatory bowel disease. The granulomas in the subcutaneous tissue may attain considerable size through expansion and confluence, thus giving rise to the clinically apparent cutaneous-subcutaneous nodules. They are embedded in a diffuse inflammatory exudate rich in eosinophils. Similar changes have also been observed in other diseases, such as PAN.

Papulonecrotic Tuberculid

See Figs. VB4.c and VB4.d.

Conditions to consider in the differential diagnosis:
allergic granulomatosis (Churg–Strauss)
Wegener's granulomatosis
giant cell arteritis (temporal arteritis)
erythema chronicum migrans
erythema nodosum leprosum
some insect bite reactions
"secondary vasculitis" at the base of ulcers of diverse etiology
Behçet's syndrome

VB5. Thrombotic and Other Microangiopathies

The dermal vessels contain fibrin, red cells and platelet thrombi, and/or eosinophilic protein precipitates. Coagulopathies of diverse etiologies may have similar histologic features (see section IIIG). Calciphylaxis is a microangiopathy that appears to be caused by calcification of the media of small arteries, followed by fibroplasia affecting the intima and occluding the lumen (10).

Calciphylaxis

CLINICAL SUMMARY.   Calciphylaxis is a life-threatening condition in which there is progressive calcification of small and medium-sized vessels of the subcutis, with thickening of the intima by fibrosis and subsequent vascular compromise resulting in ischemia and necrosis. It most frequently arises in the setting of hyperparathyroidism associated with chronic renal failure, and is often, but not always, associated with an elevated serum calcium/phosphate product. Clinically, the lesions present as a panniculitis or vasculitis. Bullae, ulcerations, or a livedo reticularis-like eruption can be present.

HISTOPATHOLOGY.   The histologic changes in calciphylaxis include calcium deposits in the subcutis, chiefly within the walls of small and medium-sized arteries. These deposits can be associated with endovascular fibrosis, thrombosis, or global calcific obliteration. Calcification can also be identified within the soft tissues. The vascular lesions result in ischemic and/or gangrenous necrosis of the subcutaneous fat and overlying skin.

Livedo Reticularis

See Clin.Fig. VB5.b.

Conditions to consider in the differential diagnosis:
septicemia
disseminated intravascular coagulation
thrombotic thrombocytopenic purpura
purpura fulminans

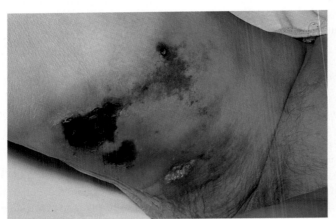

Clin. Fig. VB5.a

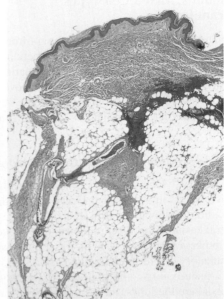

Fig. VB5.a

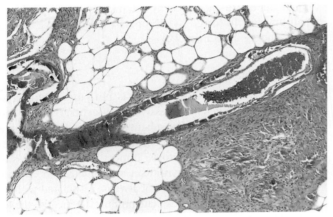

Fig. VB5.b

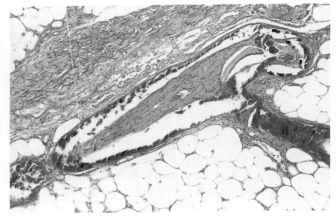

Fig. VB5.c

Clin. Fig. VB5.a. *Calciphylaxis.* This elderly woman with end-stage renal disease and elevated parathyroid hormone level developed widespread induration of the lower extremities that led to purpuric and necrotic ulcerations.

Fig. VB5.a. *Calciphylaxis, low power.* There is a vessel in the subcutis with a calcified and thickened wall, associated with fat necrosis and hemorrhage.

Fig. VB5.b. *Calciphylaxis, medium power.* There is necrosis of fat adjacent to the abnormal vessel. Necrosis is often much more extensive than in this example and often involves the dermis.

Fig. VB5.c. *Calciphylaxis, high power.* The calcification affects the media of this small artery. In the same vessel, the intima is thickened by delicate fibroplasia, greatly compromising the lumen. The intimal fibrosis has retracted from the stiffened calcified wall due to fixation artifact.

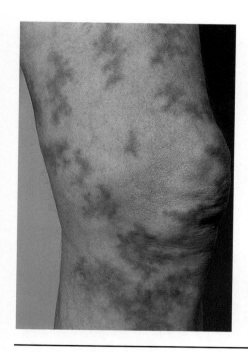

Clin. Fig. VB5.b. *Livedo reticularis.* Persistent red-blue mottling of the skin in a netlike pattern is a nonspecific sign of sluggish blood flow that may occur in association with a vasculitis or a vasculopathy in several different contexts, such as infection, atrophie blanche, cholesterol emboli, and connective tissue disease. A biopsy from an affected area may show a thick-walled vessel with the lumen occluded by a thrombus.

coumarin necrosis
lupus anticoagulant
amyloidosis
porphyria cutanea tarda and other porphyrias
calciphylaxis
thrombophlebitis and superficial migratory
  thrombophlebitis
Lucio reaction

VC. DIFFUSE INFILTRATES OF THE RETICULAR DERMIS

Diffuse infiltrates of the reticular dermis may show some relation to vessels or to skin appendages or may be randomly distributed in the reticular dermis.

1. Lymphocytes Predominant
2. Neutrophils Predominant
3. "Histiocytoid" Cells Predominant
4. Plasma Cells Prominent
5. Mast Cells Predominant
6. Eosinophils Predominant
7. Mixed Cell Types
8. Pigment Cells
9. Extensive Necrosis

VC1. Diffuse Infiltrates, Lymphocytes Predominant

Lymphocytes are seen almost to the exclusion of other cell types. Jessner's lymphocytic infiltration is prototypic (11).

Jessner's Lymphocytic Infiltration of the Skin

CLINICAL SUMMARY. This poorly understood entity is characterized by asymptomatic papules or well-demarcated, slightly infiltrated red plaques, which may develop central clearing. In contrast to lesions of chronic lupus erythematosus, the surface shows no follicular plugging or atrophy. The eruption may be precipitated or aggravated by sunlight. Lesions arise most often on the face but may also involve the neck and upper trunk. Affected patients are usually middle-aged men and women. Variable numbers of lesions (one to many) often persist for several months or several years. They may disappear without sequelae, or recur at previously involved sites or elsewhere.

HISTOPATHOLOGY. The epidermis may be normal, but often appears slightly flattened. In the dermis, there are moderately dense perivascular and diffuse infiltrates composed of small mature lymphocytes admixed with occasional histiocytes and plasma cells. The infiltrate may extend around folliculosebaceous units and into subcutaneous adipose tissue.

Leukemia Cutis

See Figs. VC1.d–VC1.g

Conditions to consider in the differential diagnosis:
cutaneous lymphoid hyperplasia/lymphocytoma cutis
Jessner's lymphocytic infiltrate
leukemia cutis [chronic lymphocytic lymphoma (CLL)]

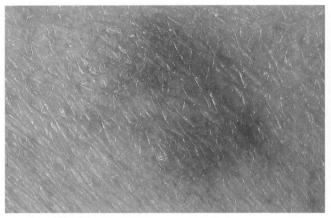

Clin. Fig. VC1.a

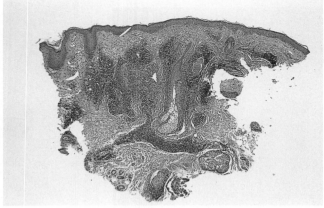

Fig. VC1.a

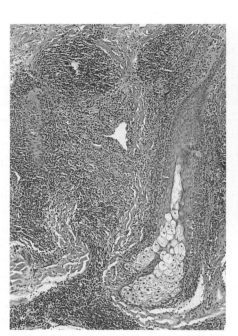

Fig. VC1.b

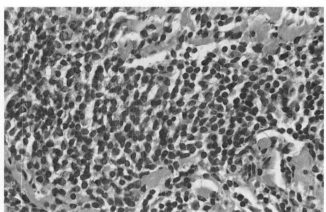

Fig. VC1.c

Clin. Fig. VC1.a. *Jessner's lymphocytic infiltrate.* Typical infiltrated red plaques with central clearing are seen on the forehead.

Fig. VC1.a. *Jessner's lymphocytic infiltration, low power.* A dense perivascular and interstitial infiltrate extends through the full thickness of the dermis.

Fig. VC1.b. *Jessner's lymphocytic infiltration, medium power.* The infiltrate is partly perivascular but mainly diffuse.

Fig. VC1.c. *Jessner's lymphocytic infiltration, high power.* The lesional cells are mature small lymphocytes.

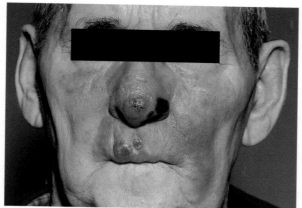

Clin. Fig. VC1.b

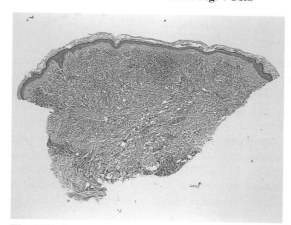

Fig. VC1.d

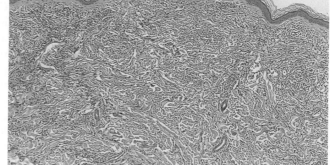

Fig. VC1.e

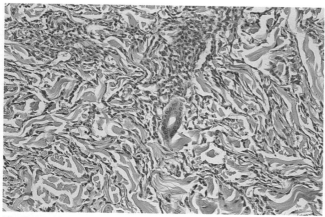

Fig. VC1.f

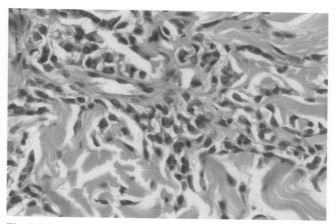

Fig. VC1.g

Clin. Fig. VC1.b. *Leukemia cutis*. An elderly man with chronic lymphocytic leukemia developed recurrent ulcerated nodules on an infiltrated violaceous plaque. Local radiation therapy was successful.

Fig. VC1.d. *Leukemia cutis, low power*. In this example of acute myelogenous leukemia, there is a dense diffuse infiltrate in the reticular dermis. The cells could easily be mistaken for lymphocytes.

Fig. VC1.e. *Leukemia cutis, medium power*. The infiltrate shows little tendency to perivascular or periadnexal orientation.

Fig. VC1.f. *Leukemia cutis, medium power*. The lesional cells tend to dissect between collagen bundles.

Fig. VC1.g. *Leukemia cutis, high power*. The lesional cells have ovoid or indented nuclei and an appreciable amount of eosinophilic cytoplasm, consistent with acute myelogenous leukemia. Phenotyping should be done on blood or bone marrow if possible.

VC2. Diffuse Infiltrates, Neutrophils Predominant

Neutrophils are the main infiltrating cell, although lymphocytes can be found. Sweet's syndrome is prototypic (12). Erysipelas is another good example (13).

Acute Febrile Neutrophilic Dermatosis (Sweet's Syndrome)

CLINICAL SUMMARY. Classic Sweet's syndrome is characterized by acute onset of fever, leukocytosis, and erythematous plaques, vesicles, or pustules infiltrated by neutrophils. This condition typically occurs in middle-aged women after nonspecific infections of the respiratory or gastrointestinal tract. In addition to classic Sweet's syndrome, sterile lesions with neutrophilic infiltrates that improve on steroid treatment can be found in a variety of other clinical conditions. Such infiltrates can be associated with inflammatory diseases, such as autoimmune disorders or with recovery from infection. They may also develop in patients with hemoproliferative disorders or solid tumors, and in pregnant women.

HISTOPATHOLOGY. There is a dense perivascular infiltrate composed largely of neutrophils, often with leukocytoclasia. In addition, there are mononuclear cells, such as lymphocytes and histiocytes, and occasional eosinophils. The in-flammatory cells typically assume a bandlike distribution throughout the papillary dermis. The density of the infiltrate varies, and may be limited in a small proportion of cases. There is usually vasodilation and swelling of endothelium with moderate erythrocyte extravasation. The prominent edema of the upper dermis in some instances may result in subepidermal blister formation. Extensive vascular damage is not a feature of Sweet's syndrome. The histologic appearance varies depending on the stage of the process. In later stages, lymphocytes and histiocytes may predominate. It is important to realize that the composition and distribution of the infiltrate are not specific enough to histologically rule out an infectious process.

Erysipelas/Cellulitis

CLINICAL SUMMARY. Erysipelas is an acute superficial cellulitis of the skin caused by group *A streptococci*. It is characterized by a well-demarcated, slightly indurated, dusky-red area with an advancing palpable border. In some patients, erysipelas has a tendency to recur periodically in the same areas. In the early antibiotic era, the incidence of erysipelas appeared to be on the decline and most cases occurred on the face. More recently, however, there appears to have been an increase in the incidence, and facial sites are now less common, whereas erysipelas of the legs is predominant.

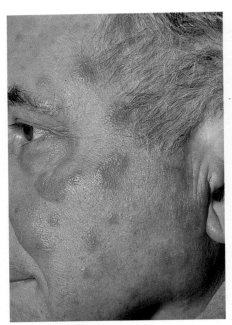 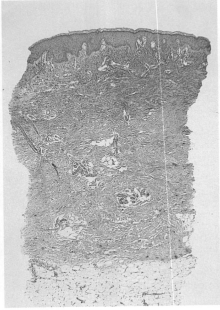 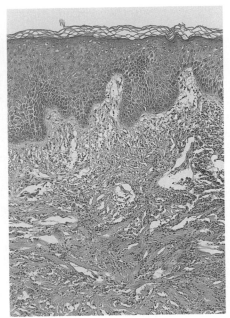

Clin. Fig. VC2   **Fig. VC2.a**   **Fig. VC2.b**

Clin. Fig. VC2. *Sweet's syndrome.* A middle-aged man experienced the acute onset of fever and erythematous plaques on the face. (W. Witmer)

Fig. VC2.a. *Sweet's syndrome, low power.* There is edema of the upper dermis and a diffuse cellular infiltrate in the reticular dermis.

Fig. VC2.b. *Sweet's syndrome, medium power.* The infiltrate is composed almost entirely of neutrophils. Diagnostic changes of leukocytoclastic vasculitis are not observed. (*continues*)

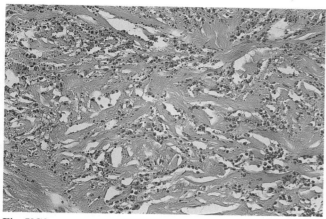

Fig. VC2.c

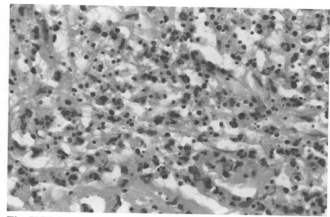

Fig. VC2.d

Fig. VC2.c. *Sweet's syndrome, high power.* The infiltrate is variable but often very dense, as in this example.

Fig. VC2.d. *Sweet's syndrome, high power.* The dense neutrophilic infiltrate shows extensive leukocytoclasia.

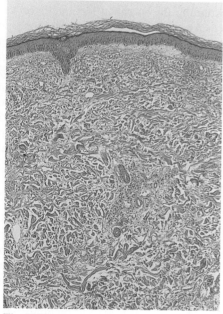

Fig. VC2.e

Fig. VC2.e. *Erysipelas/cellulitis, low power.* The dermis is edematous and there is a patchy infiltrate in the reticular dermis.

Fig. VC2.f. *Erysipelas/cellulitis, medium power.* The infiltrate is partly perivascular but also diffuse.

Fig. VC2.g. *Erysipelas/cellulitis, high power.* Most of the cells in the infiltrate are neutrophils. There is no necrosis, and bacteria are frequently not demonstrable in the dermis.

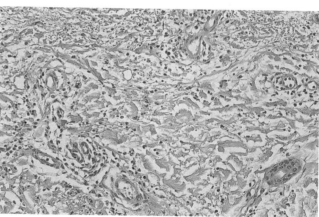

Fig. VC2.f

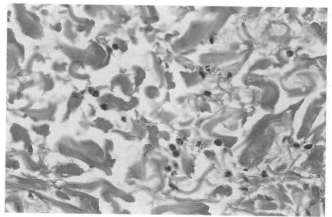

Fig. VC2.g

HISTOPATHOLOGY.   The dermis shows marked edema and dilatation of the lymphatics and capillaries. There is a diffuse infiltrate, composed chiefly of neutrophils, that extends throughout the dermis and occasionally into the subcutaneous fat. It is loosely arranged around dilated blood and lymph vessels. If sections are stained with the Giemsa or Gram stain, streptococci may be found in the tissue and within lymphatics. In cases of recurring erysipelas, the lymph vessels of the dermis and subcutaneous tissue show fibrotic thickening of their walls with partial or complete occlusion of the lumen. Erysipelas and cellulitis must be distinguished from Sweet's-like eruptions and vice versa. This distinction cannot always be made on histologic grounds alone.

Conditions to consider in the differential diagnosis:

acute neutrophilic dermatosis (Sweet's syndrome)
erythema elevatum diutinum
rheumatoid neutrophilic dermatosis
granuloma faciale
cutaneous reaction to cytokines, especially granulocyte
    colony-stimulating factor
bowel arthrosis dermatosis syndrome
erysipelas
cellulitis
pyoderma gangrenosum
dermis adjacent to folliculitis
abscess
Behçet's syndrome

VC3. Diffuse Infiltrates, "Histiocytoid" Cells Predominant

Histiocytes, or histiocytoid cells, are found in great numbers in the dermal infiltrate. Some may be foamy, whereas others may contain organisms. The leukemic cells of myeloid leukemia may be easily mistaken for histiocytes, and may have histiocytic differentiation (myelomonocytic leukemia). Lepromatous leprosy is a good example (14).

Lepromatous Leprosy

CLINICAL SUMMARY.   Lepromatous leprosy initially has cutaneous and mucosal lesions, with neural changes occurring later. The lesions usually are numerous and are symmetrically arranged. There are three clinical types: macular, infiltrative-nodular, and diffuse. In the macular type, numerous ill-defined, confluent, either hypopigmented or erythematous macules are observed. They are frequently slightly infiltrated. The infiltrative-nodular type, the classic and most common variety, may develop from the macular type or arise as such. It is characterized by papules, nodules, and diffuse infiltrates that are often dull red in color. Involvement of the eyebrows and forehead often results in a leonine facies, with a loss of lateral eyebrows and eyelashes. The lesions themselves are not notably hypoesthetic, although, through involvement of the large peripheral nerves, disturbances of sensation and nerve paralyses develop. The nerves that are most commonly involved are the ulnar, radial, and common peroneal nerves. The diffuse type of leprosy, called Lucio leprosy, most common in Mexico and Central America, shows diffuse infiltration of the skin without nodules. This infiltration may be quite inconspicuous except for the alopecia of the eyebrows and eyelashes it produces. Acral symmetric anesthesia is generally present. Rarely, lepromatous leprosy can present as a single lesion rather than as multiple lesions.

HISTOPATHOLOGY.   In the usual macular or infiltrative-nodular lesions, there is an extensive cellular infiltrate that is almost invariably separated from the flattened epidermis by a narrow grenz zone of normal collagen. The infiltrate causes destruction of the cutaneous appendages and extends into the subcutaneous fat. In florid early lesions, the macrophages have abundant eosinophilic cytoplasm and contain a mixed population of solid and fragmented bacilli. There is no macrophage activation to form epithelioid cell granulomas. Lymphocyte infiltration is not prominent, but there may be many plasma cells. In time, and with antimycobacterial chemotherapy, degenerate bacilli accumulate in the macrophages constituting the so-called lepra cells or Virchow cells, which then have foamy or vacuolated cytoplasm. The Wade–Fite stain reveals that the bacilli are fragmented or granular and, especially in very chronic lesions, disposed in large basophilic clumps called globi. In lepromatous leprosy, in contrast to tuberculoid leprosy, the nerves in the skin may contain considerable numbers of leprosy bacilli but remain well preserved for a long time and slowly become fibrotic. The histopathology of Lucio (diffuse) leprosy is similar but with a characteristic heavy bacillation of the small blood vessels in the skin.

Langerhans Cell Histiocytosis (Histiocytosis X)

CLINICAL SUMMARY.   Langerhans cell histiocytosis (LCH), or histiocytosis X, is characterized by a proliferation of dendritic or Langerhans histiocytes (15). If LCH occurs during the first year of life, it is usually characterized by significant, potentially fatal visceral involvement and classified as acute disseminated LCH (Letterer–Siwe disease). If LCH develops during early childhood, the disease is predominantly manifested by osseous lesions with less extensive visceral involvement, and known as chronic multifocal LCH or Hand–Schüller–Christian disease. In older children and adults, LCH is usually of the chronic focal type, often presenting one or few bone lesions known as eosinophilic granuloma. Cutaneous lesions are very commonly encountered in Letterer–Siwe disease and occur occasionally in the two other forms. The cutaneous lesions usually consist of petechiae and papules. In some cases, there are numerous,

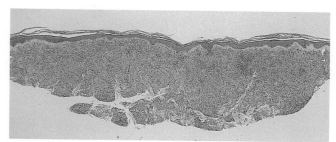

Fig. VC3.a

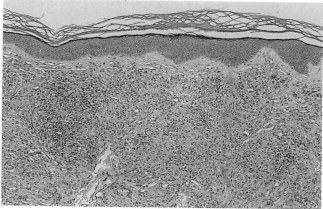

Fig. VC3.b

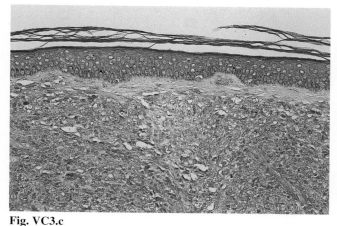

Fig. VC3.c

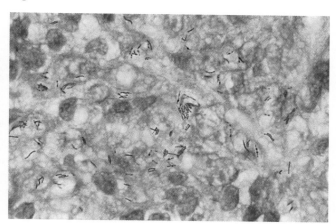

Fig. VC3.d

Fig. VC3.a. *Lepromatous leprosy, low power.* There is a diffuse to nodular infiltrate, nearly obliterating the architecture of the dermis.

Fig. VC3.b. *Lepromatous leprosy, medium power.* The infiltrate is composed of large histiocytes and small lymphocytes.

Fig. VC3.c. *Lepromatous leprosy, medium power, Fite stain.* Even at this magnification, the presence of acid-fast organisms can be appreciated.

Fig. VC3.d. *Lepromatous leprosy, high power, Fite stain.* The organisms are arranged in clumps within the cytoplasm of the histiocytes.

---

closely set brownish papules covered with scales or crusts, particularly involving the scalp, face, and trunk. The clinical course and the prognosis of LCH are difficult to predict.

HISTOPATHOLOGY. The key to diagnosis is identifying the typical LCH or histiocytosis X cell in the appropriate surroundings. The cell has a distinct folded or lobulated, often kidney-shaped, nucleus. Nucleoli are not prominent, and the slightly eosinophilic cytoplasm is unremarkable. A typical clinical and light microscopic picture leads to a presumptive diagnosis; confirmation by typical S-100 or peanut agglutinin staining produces a diagnosis. A definite diagnosis requires either a positive CD1a stain or electron microscopic demonstration of Birbeck granules. Although three kinds of

histologic reactions have been described in LCH histiocytosis—proliferative, granulomatous, and xanthomatous—only the first two are commonly seen. In general, the proliferative reaction with its almost purely histiocytic infiltrate is typical of acute disseminated LCH and the granulomatous reaction of chronic focal or multifocal LCH, as the name *eosinophilic granuloma* suggests. Xanthomatous lesions in the skin are rare. The proliferative reaction is characterized by the presence of an extensive infiltrate of histiocytes. The infiltrate usually lies close to or involves the epidermis, resulting in ulceration and crusting. Inflammatory cells are also present, most often lymphocytes, but also eosinophils. The granulomatous reaction shows extensive aggregates of histiocytes often extending deep into the dermis, with variable

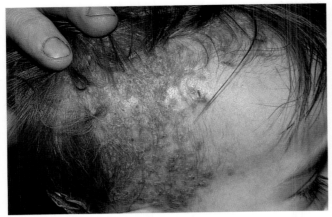

Clin. Fig. VC3.a

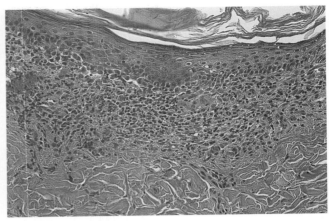

Fig. VC3.e

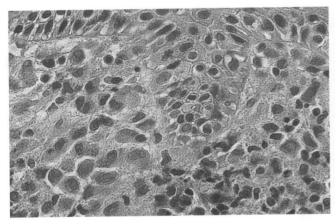

Fig. VC3.f

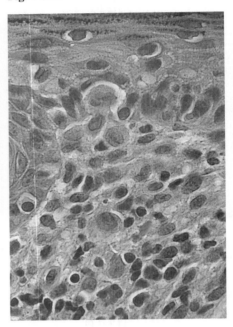

Fig. VC3.g

Clin. Fig. VC3.a. *Histiocytosis X.* An 18-month-old boy with a persistent scalp eruption characterized by closely set brownish papules covered with scales and crust required hospital admission for chemotherapy. A similar eruption was present in the diaper area.

Fig. VC3.e. *Histiocytosis X, low power.* There is a diffuse infiltrate in the dermis, close to the epidermis.

Fig. VC3.f. *Histiocytosis X, high power.* The lesional cells are large with abundant pink cytoplasm and reniform nuclei. There is an admixture of inflammatory cells including occasional eosinophils.

Fig. VC3.g. *Histiocytosis X, high power.* The infiltrate is focally epidermotropic.

eosinophils, multinucleated giant cells, neutrophils, lymphoid cells, and plasma cells present.

Xanthelasma

See Figs. VC3.h and Vc3.i.
 Conditions to consider in the differential diagnosis:
  xanthelasma, xanthomas (usually nodular)
  atypical mycobacteria
  Mycobacterium avium-intracellulare

deep fungus infection
cryptococcosis
histoplasmosis
paraffinoma
silicone granuloma
talc and starch granuloma
annular elastolytic giant cell granuloma (actinic granuloma)
lepromatous leprosy

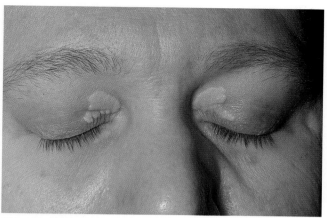

Clin. Fig. VC3.b

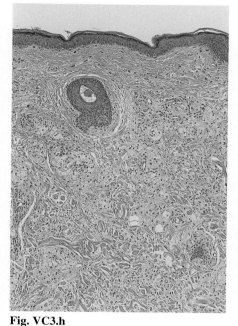

Fig. VC3.h

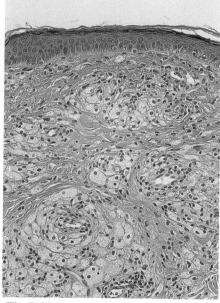

Fig. VC3.i

Clin. Fig. VC3.b. *Xanthelasma.* Most often, no underlying lipid abnormalities are present when patients present with these typical yellowish plaques on the eyelids.

Fig. VC3.h. *Xanthelasma, low power.* There is a diffuse infiltrate of pale-staining cells in the dermis.

Fig. VC3.i. *Xanthelasma, high power.* The lesional cells are large with abundant foamy cytoplasm. There is no admixture of inflammatory cells.

---

histoid leprosy
cutaneous leishmaniasis
rhinoscleroma (Klebsiella rhinoscleromatis)
histiocytosis X
leukemia cutis (myeloid, myelomonocytic)
anaplastic large cell lymphoma (Ki-1)
reticulohistiocytic granuloma
malakoplakia

VC4. Diffuse Infiltrates, Plasma Cells Prominent

Plasma cells are found in the diffuse dermal infiltrate, although they may not be the predominant cell. Secondary syphilis may be predominantly perivascular and has been discussed as such in section VA4. Other examples present as a diffuse infiltrate.

Secondary Syphilis

See Figs. VC4.a and VC4.b.
   Conditions to consider in the differential diagnosis:
     insect bite reaction
     plasmacytoma, myeloma
     circumorificial plasmacytosis
     Zoon's balanitis circumscripta plasmacellularis
     syphilis, secondary or tertiary
     yaws, primary or secondary
     acne keloidalis nuchae

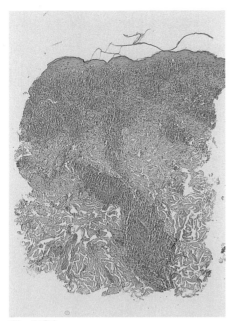

Fig. VC4.a. *Secondary syphilis, low power.* There is a dense diffuse and perivascular infiltrate in the superficial and deep dermis.

Fig. VC4.b. *Secondary syphilis, medium power.* In this example, the infiltrate is band-like in architecture and is composed mostly of plasma cells and lymphocytes.

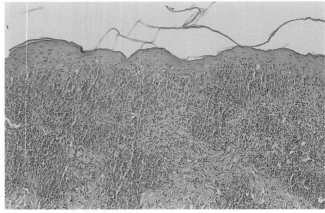

Fig. VC4.b

Fig. VC4.a

VC5. Diffuse Infiltrates, Mast Cells Predominant

Mast cells compose almost the entire dermal infiltrate. There may be an admixture of eosinophils (see sections IIIA2, IVE4, and VIB10).

    Conditions to consider in the differential diagnosis:

        urticaria pigmentosa (nodular or diffuse)

VC6. Diffuse Infiltrates, Eosinophils Predominant

Eosinophils are prominent, although not the only infiltrating cell. Lymphocytes are also found, and plasma cells may also be present. Eosinophilic cellulitis is a good example (16).

Eosinophilic Cellulitis (Wells' Syndrome)

CLINICAL SUMMARY. This rare dermatosis presents as a sudden eruption of a variable number of bright erythematous patches, which over a period of a few days expand into indurated erythematous plaques that may be painful. The overlying epidermis may produce vesicles or small blisters. The disease, if untreated, may persist for a few weeks or months, and may be recurrent. Associated or provoking stimuli may include insect bites and cutaneous parasitosis, cutaneous viral infections and drug reactions, leukemic and myeloproliferative disorders, and atopic dermatitis and fungal infections. Patients are usually adults. Peripheral blood eosinophilia is usually present.

HISTOPATHOLOGY. Early lesions demonstrate diffuse but dense dermal infiltrates of eosinophils; eosinophil degranula-

tion is prominent. Infiltrates generally extend throughout the dermis and may involve the subcutaneous tissue, or, occasionally, the underlying muscle. When the epidermis is substantially involved, multilocular spongiotic intraepidermal vesicles develop, but blistering is usually of subepidermal type. Eosinophils are found in the epidermis. Older lesions show more extensive eosinophil degranulation; the granular material aggregates focally around collagen fibers, forming the characteristic "flame figures." These foci may develop a palisade of macrophages and sometimes giant cells. In florid lesions, necrobiosis may develop within the palisading histiocytic reaction.

Tick Bite

See Figs. VC6.e–VC6.g.
    Conditions to consider in the differential diagnosis:
        eosinophilic cellulitis (Well's syndrome)
        insect bite reaction
        granuloma faciale

VC7. Diffuse Infiltrates, Mixed Cell Types

The diffuse infiltrate contains plasma cells, lymphocytes, histiocytes, and a variety of acute inflammatory cells. Leishmaniasis is a good example (17).

Cutaneous Leishmaniasis

CLINICAL SUMMARY. Leishmaniasis is transmitted by a number of different strains of the protozoan parasite *Leish-*

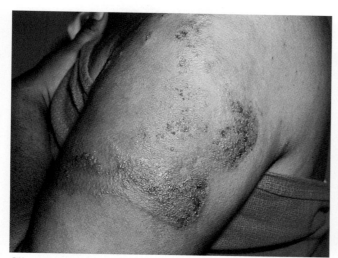

Clin. Fig. VC6.a

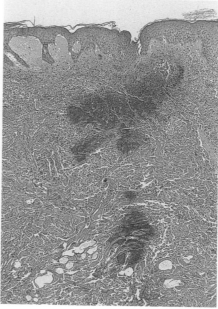

Fig. VC6.a

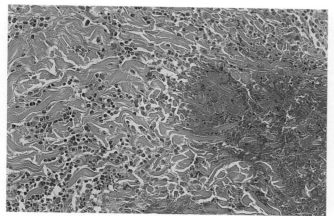

Fig. VC6.b

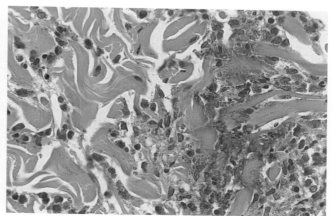

Fig. VC6.c

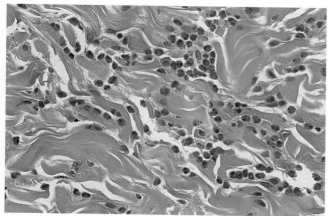

Fig. VC6.d

Clin. Fig. VC6.a. *Well's syndrome.* A middle-aged woman presented with an erythematous indurated plaque with vesiculation at the borders. Peripheral blood eosinophilia was present.

Fig. VC6.a. *Eosinophilic cellulitis (Well's), low power.* Striking flame figures are present in the reticular dermis. There is intense subepidermal edema.

Fig. VC6.b. *Eosinophilic cellulitis (Well's), medium power.* The flame figure is composed of eosinophil granules.

Fig. VC6.c. *Eosinophilic cellulitis (Well's), high power.* Numerous eosinophils are present in the dermis at the edge of the flame figure.

Fig. VC6.d. *Eosinophilic cellulitis (Well's), high power.* There is a diffuse infiltrate of eosinophils in the dermis away from the flame figure.

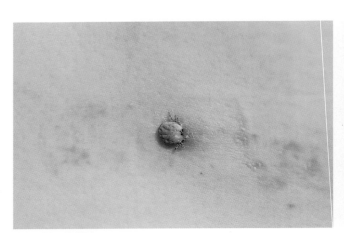

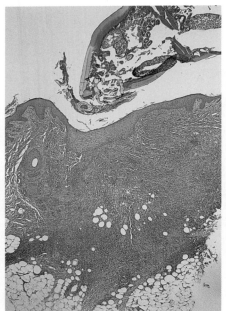

Clin. Fig. VC6.b   **Fig. VC6.e**

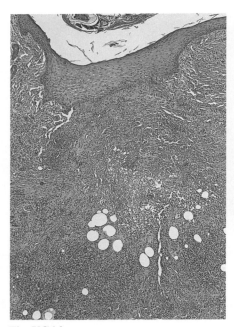

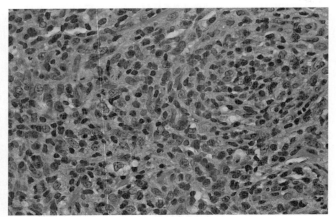

Fig. VC6.g

Fig. VC6.f

Clin. Fig. VC6.b. *Insect bite*. A punch biopsy was required to remove the engorged tick embedded in an edematous erythematous papule on the lower back.

Fig. VC6.e. *Tick bite, low power*. A tick is seen above a reepithelializing wound.

Fig. VC6.f. *Tick bite, medium power*. There is a diffuse mixed cellular infiltrate with eosinophils in the dermis.

Fig. VC6.g. *Tick bite, high power*. The infiltrate includes many eosinophils and lymphocytes and plasma cells.

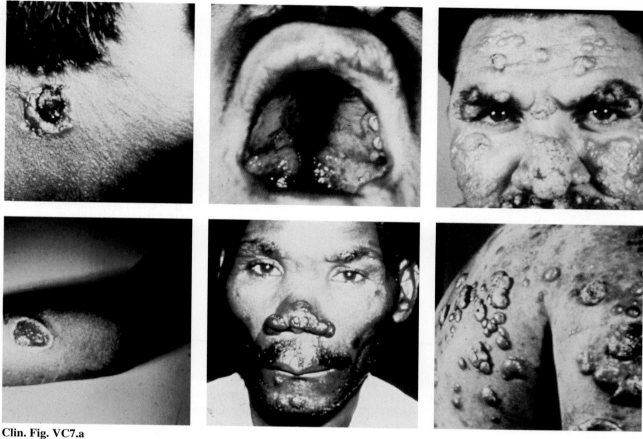

Clin. Fig. VC7.a

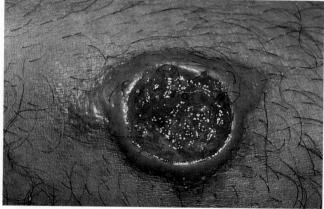

Clin. Fig. VC7.b

Clin. Fig. VC7.a. *Spectrum of American cutaneous leishmaniasis.* **Left:** localized cutaneous leishmaniasis. Middle panels: Mucocutaneous leishmaniasis (espundia). **Right:** Diffuse cutaneous leishmaniasis. (J. Convit)

Clin. Fig. VC7.b. *American cutaneous leishmaniasis.* Lesion of localized cutaneous leishmaniasis presenting as an indurated nodule with an ulcerated crateriform center. (J. Convit)

mania. Cutaneous leishmaniasis occurs initially as single or multiple erythematous papules on exposed areas of the body weeks to months after the bite of an infected sandfly. The papules may enlarge to form indurated nodules, which frequently ulcerate to form a central crater. Cutaneous leishmaniasis can be placed both along a clinical and immunopathologic spectrum in which the clinical features depend on the response of the host to the parasite. At one pole of the spectrum is the localized form, characterized by the occurrence of one or a few lesions with very few parasites and a well-developed immunologic response. These cases generally respond very well to treatment. At the other pole is the diffuse form, characterized by multiple lesions, large numbers of parasites, absence of immunologic response, and a poor response to treatment. More than 90% of cutaneous leishmaniasis cases can be placed in the localized end of the spectrum. There are intermediate forms called mucocutaneous, verrucous, or relapse cutaneous leishmaniasis, that taken together

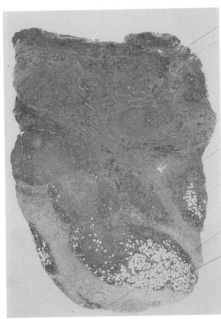

Fig. VC7.a

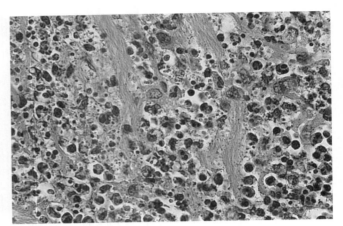

Fig. VC7.a. *Localized cutaneous leishmaniasis, low power.* A diffuse infiltrate extends into the subcutis. The epidermis is ulcerated.

Fig. VC7.b. *Localized cutaneous leishmaniasis, high power.* The infiltrate is mixed, with many plasma cells and neutrophils but with histiocytes predominating. In this stage, many organisms are seen within the histiocytes.

Fig. VC7.b

account for about 8% of cutaneous leishmaniasis in the Americas. Diffuse cases are extremely rare. They are characterized by plaquelike or nodular lesions that can be localized in a single area of the body in the early stages and then extend until they cover most of the skin and start to slowly compromise nasal, buccal, and laryngeal mucous tissue. Clinically, these lesions can be confused with lepromatous leprosy or with cutaneous lymphomas.

HISTOPATHOLOGY.　Early lesions of localized cutaneous leishmaniasis are characterized by a macrophagic infiltrate with a slight tendency to epithelioid differentiation (related to time of evolution), with associated infiltration by lymphoid cells. In this stage there are variably abundant parasites inside macrophages, facilitating diagnosis both through direct lesional touch smears and in biopsy sections. In the intermediate or late stages, most lesions are ulcerated. In the few lesions that are not ulcerated, the morphology is characterized by a tuberculoid-type granuloma with prominent lymphoid infiltration. When the lesions are ulcerated, they show a subacute or chronic mixed-cell reaction provoked by secondary infection. The latter may present with macrophagic infiltrates, formation of small abscesses, necrotic areas, plasma-cell infiltrates, and proliferation of small vessels. In this stage, parasites in lesions become increasingly difficult to find. The histopathology of acute lesions is usually characterized by epithelial loss, but in chronic lesions there can be a variable degree of epithelial hypertrophy. The microscopic morphology of diffuse cutaneous leishmaniasis is a macrophagic infiltrate with sparse lymphocytes and with enormous numbers of parasites inside macrophages.

Conditions to consider in the differential diagnosis:

B-cell cutaneous lymphoid hyperplasia
pseudolymphoma
lymphocytoma cutis
syphilis, primary, secondary, or tertiary
acrodermatitis chronica atrophicans
cutaneous reactions to cytokines
chronic actinic dermatitis (actinic reticuloid)
rhinosporidiosis
rhinoscleroma
histoplasmosis
dermal hematopoiesis (extramedullary hematopoiesis)
cutaneous leishmaniasis
granuloma inguinale
granuloma gluteale infantum

VC8. Diffuse Infiltrates, Pigment Cells

The diffuse infiltrate contains bipolar, cuboidal, or dendritic cells with brown cytoplasmic pigment. Nevus of Ota is a well-known example (18).

Nevi of Ota and Ito and Dermal Melanocyte Hamartoma

CLINICAL SUMMARY.　The *nevus of Ota* presents as a usually unilateral discoloration of the face composed of blue and brown, partially confluent macular lesions. The periorbital region, temple, forehead, malar area, and nose are usually involved, giving rise to the term "nevus fuscocaeruleus ophthalmomaxillaris." There is frequently a patchy blue discoloration of the sclera of the ipsilateral eye, and occasionally of the conjunctiva, cornea, and retina. In some instances, the

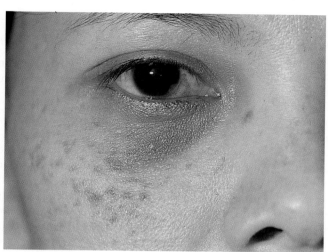

Clin. Fig. VC8

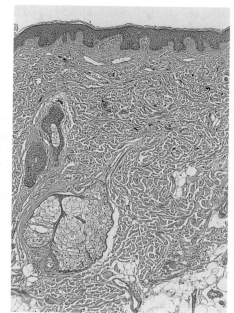

Fig. VC8.a

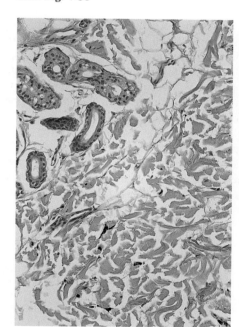

Fig. VC8.b

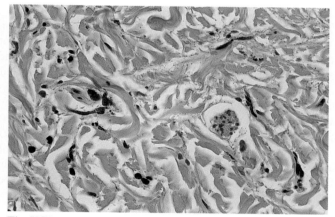

Fig. VC8.c

Clin. Fig. VC8. *Nevus of Ota.* Mottled and even colored slate-blue discoloration with scleral involvement in the typical location of the periorbital area.

Fig. VC8.a. *Nevus of Ota, low power.* The melanocytic infiltrate is easily missed at scanning magnification. There is no melanocytic proliferation in the epidermis. Small areas of brown pigment are seen within the upper dermis.

Fig. VC8.b. *Nevus of Ota, medium power.* Pigmented cells are present between otherwise normal reticular dermis collagen bundles.

Fig. VC8.c. *Nevus of Ota, high power.* The lesional cells are elongated dendritic-spindle shaped heavily pigmented melanocytes.

oral and nasal mucosae are similarly affected. In a few cases, the lesions of the nevus of Ota are bilateral rather than unilateral. The involved areas of the skin show a brown to slate-blue even or mottled discoloration, usually without any infiltration. Occasionally, some areas are slightly raised, and sometimes discrete nodules of highly variable size (up to a few centimeters) and with the appearance of blue nevi are found within the lesion. The *nevus of Ito* has a similar clinical appearance but differs by its location in the supraclavicular, scapular, and deltoid regions. It may occur alone or in association with an ipsilateral or bilateral nevus of Ota. In the *dermal melanocyte hamartoma*, a single, very extensive area of gray-blue pigmentation may be present from the time of birth. The involvement may be nearly generalized, or there may be several coalescing blue macules that gradually extend within a circumscribed area from childhood.

HISTOPATHOLOGY.   The noninfiltrated areas of the nevus of Ota and the nevus of Ito and the dermal melanocyte hamartoma contain elongated dendritic melanocytes scattered among the collagen bundles. Although most of the fusiform melanocytes lie in the upper third of the reticular dermis, they may also occur in the papillary layer and may extend as far down as the subcutaneous tissue. Melanophages are uncommon. Slightly raised and infiltrated areas show a larger number of elongated dendritic melanocytes than do noninfiltrated areas, thus approaching the histologic picture of a blue nevus, and nodular areas are indistinguishable histologically from a blue nevus. Malignant changes in lesions of nevus of Ota have been reported in a handful of cases. The histologic appearance of the tumors is typically that of a malignant or cellular blue nevus. Rarely, a primary melanoma of the choroid, iris, orbit, or brain has developed in patients with a nevus of Ota involving an eye.

Conditions to consider in the differential diagnosis:
>   Mongolian spot
>   nevus of Ota, nevus of Ito
>   dermal melanocytic hamartoma

VC9. Diffuse Infiltrates, Extensive Necrosis

Vascular and dermal necrosis are found secondary to vascular occlusion or to destruction by organisms. Gangrenous ischemic necrosis is a good example (19).

Gangrenous Ischemic Necrosis

CLINICAL SUMMARY.   Gangrenous necrosis is usually seen in the distal extremity as a consequence of peripheral vascular disease, most often related to atherosclerosis. The onset is usually in old age. Diabetics are at special risk and tend to present at a younger age with severe disease, which is more likely to be complicated by infection. In chronic ischemia, there may be evidence of atrophy, with thin shiny skin and loss of skin appendages, or there may be hypertrophic changes with hyperkeratosis and thickening of the nails. The latter changes are especially likely when there is associated venous stasis. When an extremity or a digit becomes necrotic, there may be initial pallor or duskiness, depending on the degree of occlusion and/or stasis. Ultimately, the affected portion will become black. If an ulcer develops, it is likely to be come infected, often with the development of osteomyelitis of the underlying digit.

HISTOPATHOLOGY.   There may be evidence of chronic ischemia in the form of atrophy of skin, appendages, and muscle fibers. The early changes of acute ischemia, which may be seen at the edges of areas of infarction, include basal vac-

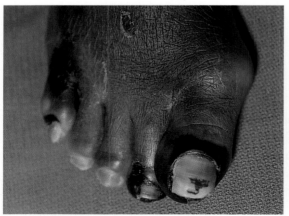

Clin. Fig. VC9

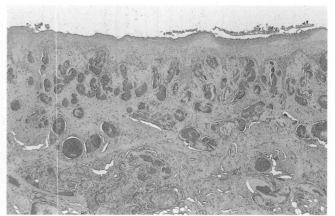

Fig. VC9.a

Clin. Fig. VC9. *Gangrene.* Severe peripheral vascular disease in a patient with a longstanding history of insulin-dependent diabetes mellitus led to cold feet with dusky and black patches of necrosis.

Fig. VC9.a. *Gangrene, low power.* Full-thickness coagulation necrosis of skin with loss of nuclear and fine cytologic detail is evident even at scanning magnification. The dermal vessels are acutely congested.

uolar change, coagulation necrosis of surface keratinocytes beginning superficially, and necrosis of appendages, especially the metabolically active sweat glands. In established infarcts, the architecture may be evident as a ghostly outline, with loss of cell nuclei but with some preservation of cell shape and connective tissue matrix. At the edge of the infarct, there is an inflammatory zone of neutrophils, with leukocytoclasia in the ischemic area itself. There may be occlusive thrombi in small and sometimes large vessels. In general, changes of severe atherosclerosis are confined to proximal vessels, which are not present in amputation specimens from the distal extremity.

Conditions to consider in the differential diagnosis:

tertiary syphilis
sporotrichosis
deep fungus
atypical mycobacteria
infarcts
vasculitis and deep vasculitis
thrombi and deep thrombi
calciphylaxis (cutaneous necrosis/calcification syndrome)
gangrenous ischemic necrosis

VD. DIFFUSE OR NODULAR INFILTRATES OF THE RETICULAR DERMIS WITH EPIDERMAL PROLIFERATION

Ill-defined nodules or diffuse infiltrates of inflammatory cells, usually including lymphocytes, plasma cells, and neutrophils, are present in the dermis, and the epidermis is irregularly thickened.

1. Epidermal Proliferation with Mixed Cellular Infiltrates

VD1. Epidermal Proliferation with Mixed Cellular Infiltrates

There is a dermal inflammatory infiltrate composed of a variable mixture of lymphocytes, plasma cells, eosinophils, neutrophils, and histiocytes. There may be central necrosis forming an abscess, and there may be ill-defined or well-defined granulomas. The overlying epidermis is irregularly hyperplastic, with tongues of epithelium penetrating into the dermis. The epithelium in general shows evidence of good maturation from a well-defined basal layer to a thickened stratum corneum. Eruptions that may be associated with ingestion of halogens are a good example (20).

North American Blastomycosis

CLINICAL SUMMARY. North American blastomycosis, caused by *blastomyces dermatitidis*, occurs in three forms: primary cutaneous inoculation blastomycosis, pulmonary blastomycosis, and systemic blastomycosis. Primary cutaneous inoculation blastomycosis is very rare and occurs almost exclusively as a laboratory or autopsy room infection.

It starts at the site of injury on a hand or wrist as an indurated, ulcerated, chancriform solitary lesion. Lymphangitis and lymphadenitis may develop in the affected arm. Small nodules may be present along the involved lymph vessel. Spontaneous healing takes place within a few weeks or months.

Pulmonary blastomycosis, the usual route of acquisition of the infection, may be asymptomatic or may produce mild to moderately severe acute pulmonary signs, such as fever, chest pain, cough, and hemoptysis. The pulmonary lesions either resolve or progress to chronic pulmonary blastomycosis with cavity formation.

In systemic blastomycosis, the lungs are the primary site of infection. Granulomatous and suppurative lesions may occur in many different organs, but, aside from the lungs, they are most commonly found in the skin, followed by the bones, the male genital system, the oral and nasal mucosa, and the central nervous system. Cutaneous lesions are very common in systemic blastomycosis, occurring in about 70% of the patients. They may be solitary or numerous. They occur in two types, either as verrucous lesions, the more common type, or as ulcerative lesions. Verrucous lesions show central healing with scarring and a slowly advancing, raised, verrucous border that is beset by a large number of pustules or small crusted abscesses. Ulcerative lesions begin as pustules and rapidly develop into ulcers with a granulating base. In addition, subcutaneous abscesses may occur; they usually develop as an extension of bone lesions.

HISTOPATHOLOGY. In primary cutaneous inoculation blastomycosis, the primary lesion shows at first a nonspecific inflammatory infiltrate without epithelioid or giant cells. Numerous organisms, many in a budding state, are present. After a few weeks, occasional giant cells may be seen, and later on the primary lesion may show the verrucous histologic pattern usually seen in skin lesions of systemic blastomycosis. In the verrucous lesions of systemic blastomycosis, in a biopsy taken from the active border, there is considerable downward proliferation of the epidermis, often amounting to pseudocarcinomatous hyperplasia. Intraepidermal abscesses often are present. Occasionally, multinucleated giant cells are completely enclosed by the proliferating epidermis. There is a polymorphous dermal infiltrate dominated by neutrophils that often form small abscesses. Multinucleated giant cells are scattered throughout the dermis, with only occasional ill-formed granulomas. The spores of *B dermatitidis* are found in histologic sections often only after a diligent search, usually in clusters of neutrophils or within giant cells. The spores have a thick wall, which gives them a double-contoured appearance. They measure 8 to 15 μm in diameter (average 10 μm).

Deep Fungal Infections (General)

HISTOPATHOLOGY. Histologic reactions in deep cutaneous fungal infections, including primary cutaneous aspergillosis, chromomycoses, phaeohyphomycosis, phaeomycetoma, rhinosporidiosis, and lobomycosis, typically consist of a mixed

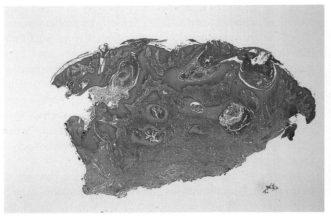

Fig. VD1.a

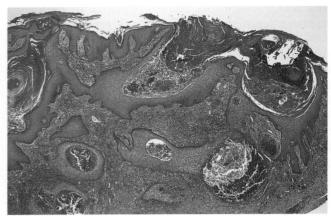

Fig. VD1.b

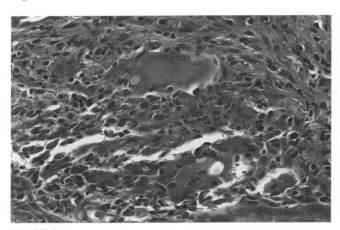

Fig. VD1.c

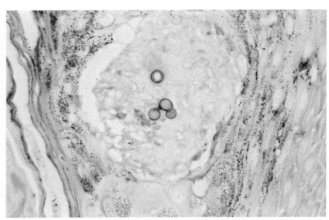

Fig. VD1.d

Fig. VD1.a. *North American blastomycosis, low power.* There is pseudoepitheliomatous hyperplasia of squamous epithelium, extending down into the reticular dermis in relation to a dense, diffuse infiltrate.

Fig. VD1.b. *North American blastomycosis, medium power.* Microabscesses are present within the epithelial tongues.

Fig. VD1.c. *North American blastomycosis, high power.* The inflammatory infiltrate is mixed, with neutrophils predominating, but with an admixture of lymphocytes, plasma cells, and giant cells. One of the latter contains an organism, which can be visualized as a circular defect in its cytoplasm.

Fig. VD1.d. *North American blastomycosis, high power, silver stain for fungi.* The silver stain or a periodic acid–Schiff stain highlight the organisms, which are thick-walled spores 8 to 15 mm in diameter. One of the organisms demonstrates broad-based budding.

dermal infiltrate that is often associated with pseudoepitheliomatous hyperplasia and occasionally with dermal fibrosis. Incidental cutaneous infections by fungi that usually primarily involve other organs, such as blastomycosis or coccidioidomycosis, typically show a pattern similar to that seen with the deep primary cutaneous fungi: a mixed dermal infiltrate with multinucleated giant cells associated with pseudoepitheliomatous hyperplasia (21). A few organisms, such as *Histoplasma* and *Loboa loboi*, are more likely to be associated with epidermal thinning than with hyperplasia, and other systemic fungal infections, such as disseminated can-

didiasis with its microabscess formation, cryptococcosis with its gelatinous and granulomatous reaction patterns, or zygomycosis and aspergillosis with their tendency for vascular invasion and infarction, show special tissue reaction patterns. A similar reaction pattern is seen in eruptions associated with halogen ingestion—bromoderma, fluoroderma, iododerma.

Conditions to consider in the differential diagnosis:

squamous cell carcinoma
pseudoepitheliomatous hyperplasia
halogenodermas

deep fungal infections
North American blastomycosis
paracoccidioidomycosis
chromoblastomycosis
coccidioidomycosis
rhinosporidiosis
protothecosis
verrucous cutaneous leishmaniasis
verrucous lupus vulgaris
tuberculosis verrucosa cutis
Mycobacterium marinum
granuloma inguinale (*Calymmatobacterium granulomatis*)
pyoderma vegetans
verruciform xanthoma
verrucose sarcoidosis
granuloma gluteale infantum
verrucous lupus erythematosus

VE. NODULAR INFLAMMATORY INFILTRATES OF THE RETICULAR DERMIS: GRANULOMAS, ABSCESSES, AND ULCERS

A granuloma may be defined as a localized collection of histiocytes, which may have abundant cytoplasm and confluent borders ("epithelioid histiocytes"), often with Langhans-type giant cells. Granulomas may be associated with necrosis or may palisade around areas of necrobiosis, may be mixed with other inflammatory cells, may include foreign-body giant cells, and may contain ingested foreign material or pathogens (acid-fast bacilli, fungi). An abscess is a localized area of suppurative necrosis, containing abundant neutrophils mixed with necrotic debris and usually surrounded by a reaction of granulation tissue and fibrosis.

1. Epithelioid Cell Granulomas without Necrosis
2. Epithelioid Cell Granulomas with Necrosis
3. Palisading Granulomas
4. Mixed Cell Granulomas
5. Inflammatory Nodules with Prominent Eosinophils
6. Inflammatory Nodules with Mixed Cell Types
7. Inflammatory Nodules with Necrosis and Neutrophils (Abscesses)
8. Inflammatory Nodules with Prominent Necrosis
9. Chronic Ulcers and Sinuses Involving the Reticular Dermis

VE1. Epithelioid Cell Granulomas without Necrosis

Large epithelioid histiocytes are common in the infiltrate, as well as giant cells. The infiltrate may also contain a few plasma cells and lymphocytes. Sarcoidosis is prototypic (22).

Sarcoidosis

CLINICAL SUMMARY. Sarcoidosis is a systemic granulomatous disease of undetermined etiology. A distinction is made between the rare, subacute transient type of sarcoidosis and the usual chronic persistent type. In subacute transient sarcoidosis, which subsides in almost all patients within a few months without sequelae, cutaneous manifestations other than erythema nodosum do not occur.

In chronic persistent sarcoidosis, cutaneous lesions are quite common and may be the only manifestation. The most common type of cutaneous lesion consists of brown-red or purple papules and plaques. Through central clearing, annual or circinate lesions may result. When the papules or plaques are situated on the nose, cheeks, and ears, the term *lupus pernio* is applied. Rare manifestations of sarcoidosis include the lichenoid form, in which small papular lesions are found, and the very rare erythrodermic, ichthyosiform, atrophic, ulcerating, verrucous, angiolupoid, hypopigmented, and alopecic forms. Subcutaneous nodules of sarcoidosis are infrequent.

HISTOPATHOLOGY. Like lesions in other organs, the cutaneous lesions of chronic persistent sarcoidosis are characterized by the presence of circumscribed granulomas of epithelioid cells, so-called epithelioid cell tubercles showing little or no necrosis. Occasionally, a slight degree of necrosis showing eosinophilic staining is found in the center of some of the granulomas. Classically, sarcoid has been associated with only a sparse lymphocytic infiltrate, particularly at the margins of the epithelioid cell granulomas. Because of this sparse infiltrate of lymphocytes, the granulomas have been referred to as "naked" tubercles. However, lymphocytic infiltrates in sarcoid may occasionally be dense, as in tuberculosis.

In typical lesions of sarcoidosis of the skin, the well-demarcated islands of epithelioid cells contain only few, if any, giant cells, usually of the Langhans type (with their nuclei arranged at the periphery of the cytoplasm). A moderate number of giant cells can be found in old lesions. These may contain asteroid bodies or Schauman bodies, which are star-shaped eosinophilic structures or round/oval, laminated, partly calcified blue structures, respectively. Neither of the two bodies is specific for sarcoidosis.

The papules, plaques, and lupus pernio-type lesions show variously sized aggregates of epithelioid cells scattered irregularly through the dermis with occasional extension into the subcutaneous tissue. In the erythrodermic form, the infiltrate shows rather small granulomas of epithelioid cells in the upper dermis intermingled with numerous lymphocytes and rare giant cells. Typical epithelioid cell tubercles are found in the ichthyosiform lesions. Verrucous sarcoid shows prominent acanthosis and hyperkeratosis. In the common form of tuberculosis of the skin, lupus vulgaris, epidermal involvement is often a feature, and there is often a more prominent lymphocytic infiltrate between the granulomas.

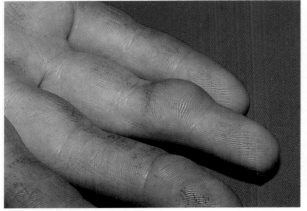

Clin. Fig. VE1.a

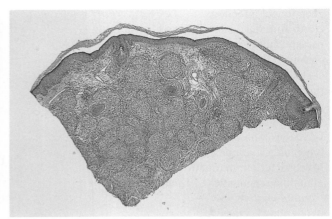

Fig. VE1.a

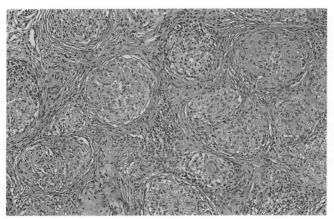

Fig. VE1.b

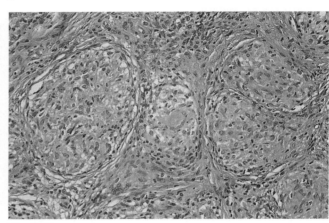

Fig. VE1.c

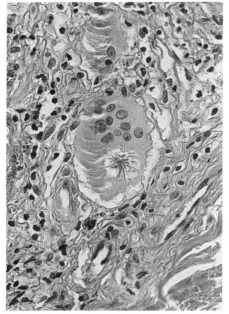

Fig. VE1.d

Clin. Fig. VE1.a. *Sarcoidosis.* A 39-year-old man with pulmonary sarcoidosis developed several fleshy subcutaneous nodules on his palmar digits. The lesions resolved with intralesional steroids.

Fig. VE1.a. *Sarcoidosis, low power.* A nodular infiltrate diffusely replaces the architecture of the reticular dermis.

Fig. VE1.b. *Sarcoidosis, medium power.* The nodules are granulomas composed of epithelioid histiocytes, with relatively sparse surrounding lymphocytes.

Fig. VE1.c. *Sarcoidosis, medium power.* The granulomas contain occasional giant cells and are noncaseating.

Fig. VE1.d. *Sarcoidosis, high power.* A giant cell contains a prominent asteroid body. Although characteristic, these are not diagnostic of sarcoidosis.

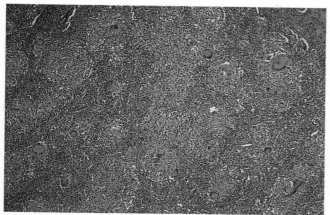

Fig. VE1.e

Fig. VE1.f

Fig. VE1.e. *Lupus vulgaris, low power.* Near-confluent nonnecrotizing granulomas in the dermis. The lymphocytic infiltrate is more intense than in sarcoidosis. (S. Lucas)

Fig. VE1.f. *Lupus vulgaris, high power.* Same lesion as Fig. VE1.e, showing an epithelioid cell granuloma, and interstitial lymphocytes. (S. Lucas)

Lupus Vulgaris

See Figs. VE1.e and VE1.f.

Conditions to consider in the differential diagnosis:

sarcoidosis (lupus pernio and other types)
granulomatous granuloma annulare
foreign body granulomas
secondary or tertiary syphilis
granulomatous rosacea
cheilitis granulomatosa
 (Miescher–Melkersson–Rosenthal)
tuberculoid leprosy
tuberculosis
lupus vulgaris
lichen scrofulosorum
Crohn's disease
allergic granulomatous reactions to chemical agents
silica, zirconium, aluminum, beryllium (may have
 necrosis)
collagen implant granuloma
granulomatous mycosis fungoides
chronic cutaneous leishmaniasis

VE2. Epithelioid Cell Granulomas with Necrosis

The presence of necrosis in an epithelioid cell granuloma of the skin strongly suggests cutaneous tuberculosis except in lesions of the face. Further, some cutaneous tuberculous eruptions do not contain prominent necrosis. However, tuberculosis is prototypic of necrotizing granulomas (23).

Tuberculosis

CLINICAL SUMMARY. Infection of the skin and subcutis by *Mycobacterium tuberculosis* occurs by three routes: by direct inoculation into the skin (causing a primary chancre, or tuberculosis verrucosa cutis, or tuberculosis cutis orificialis lesions), by hematogenous spread from an internal lesion (causing lupus vulgaris, miliary tuberculosis, and tuberculous gumma lesions), and from an underlying tuberculous lymph node by direct extension (causing scrofuloderma). In clinical practice, many cases do not readily fit into these clinical and histologic categories. The necrotic granuloma is typical of tuberculosis and other mycobacterial infections, but is not specific.

HISTOPATHOLOGY. In *lupus vulgaris,* tuberculoid granulomas composed of epithelioid cells and giant cells are present. Caseation necrosis within the tubercles is slight or may be absent. The giant cells usually are of the Langhans type, with peripheral arrangement of the nuclei, but some can be of the foreign-body type. There is an associated infiltrate of lymphocytes, which are sometimes more prominent than the granulomatous component. There is destruction of the cutaneous appendages. In areas of healing, extensive fibrosis may be present. Tubercle bacilli may be difficult to demonstrate. In *miliary tuberculosis,* the center of the papular lesions is necrotic, constituting a microabscess containing neutrophils, cellular debris, and numerous tubercle bacilli, surrounded by a zone of macrophages with occasional giant cells. In *scrofuloderma,* the center of the lesion usually exhibits nonspecific acute inflammatory changes, but in the deeper portions and at the periphery of the lesion, there are tuberculoid granulomas with considerable necrosis and inflammation. *Tuberculosis verrucosa cutis* represents inoculation infection in an individual with prior immunity. There is epithelial hyperkeratosis and acanthosis, and in the dermis there are epithelioid cell granulomas with necrosis. The lesions of *tuberculosis cutis orificialis* are shallow ulcers with a granulating base occurring near mucosal orifices due to spread by direct contamination from an internal lesion that is excreting bacilli. In most instances, tuberculoid granulomas with pronounced necrosis are found deep in the dermis. Tubercle bacilli are usually readily demonstrated in the sections, even when the histologic appearance is nonspecific. In a *tuberculous gumma*, most of the lesion is caseation necrosis with a rim of epithelioid cells and giant cells. Acid-fast bacilli are scant.

Secondary changes in the epidermis are common, and are most pronounced in tuberculosis verrucosa cutis. The epidermis may undergo atrophy and subsequent destruction, causing ulceration, or it may become hyperplastic, showing acanthosis, hyperkeratosis, and papillomatosis. At the margins of ulcers, pseudoepitheliomatous hyperplasia often exists. In rare instances, squamous cell carcinoma supervenes.

Tuberculoid Leprosy

See Figs. VE2.e–VE2.g

Lupus Miliaris Disseminatus Facei (Granulomatous Rosacea)

CLINICAL SUMMARY. Although now considered a variant of rosacea, lupus miliaris disseminatus facei has its own distinct clinical presentation. Characteristic lesions are discrete papules—single papules or small groups of flesh-colored or mildly erythematous papules—involving the face but specifically involving the eyelids and upper lip, areas where rosacea lesions are uncommon and lack the erythema and telangiectasia of rosacea.

HISTOPATHOLOGY. Biopsy specimens sectioned through the central portion of a papular lesion demonstrate one of the most highly characteristic patterns of cutaneous histopathology. Surrounding a usually large area of caseous necrosis, aggregates of epithelioid histiocytes and occasional multinucleate giant cells form a substantial "tubercle." There are sparse lymphoid infiltrates peripheral to the granulomas.

Conditions to consider in the differential diagnosis:

tuberculosis
tuberculosis verrucosa cutis
miliary tuberculosis
lupus vulgaris (necrosis usually slight or absent)
nontuberculosis mycobacteria (e.g., *M. ulcerans*)
type 1 reaction in tuberculoid leprosy
lupus miliaris disseminatus facei (granulomatous rosacea)
tertiary syphilis
epithelioid sarcoma
cryptococcosis
histoplasmosis

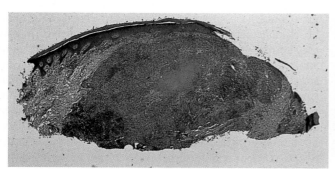

Fig. VE2.a

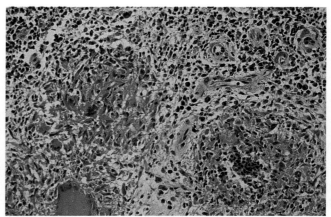

Fig. VE2.b

Fig. VE2.a. *Inoculation tuberculosis, low power.* A prosector's wart from inoculation of a finger from an infected cadaver. There is central caseation necrosis with dense surrounding macrophages and lymphocytes. (S. Lucas)

Fig. VE2.b. *Inoculation tuberculosis, medium power.* An epithelioid cell granuloma at left, a Langhans giant cell at left lower, and a granuloma with central necrosis and acute inflammation. Occasional acid-fast bacilli were observed in this case. (S. Lucas)

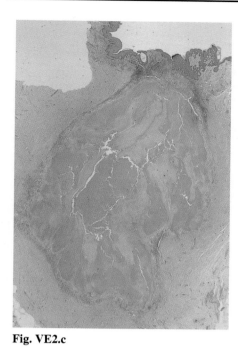

Fig. VE2.c. *Tuberculous gumma, low power.* A tuberculoma-like appearance with extensive caseation necrosis in the dermis, with a surrounding cellular infiltrate. (S. Lucas)

Fig. VE2.d. *Tuberculous gumma, high power.* The edge of the necrosis (*right*) with histiocytes, lymphocytes, and a Langhans giant cell at left of the image.

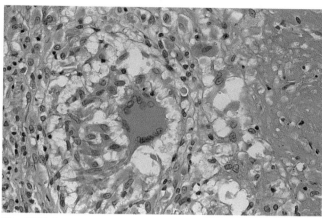

Fig. VE2.d

Fig. VE2.c

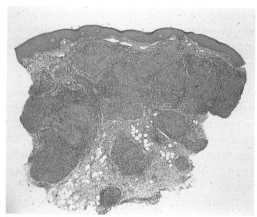

Fig. VE2.e

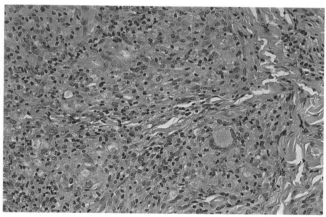

Fig. VE2.f

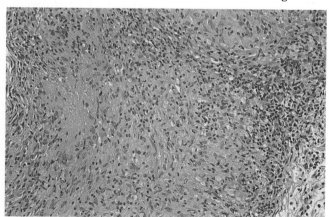

Fig. VE2.g

Fig. VE2.e. *Tuberculoid leprosy, low power.* The reticular dermis is replaced by epithelioid cell granulomas. The epidermis is not much involved.

Fig. VE2.f. *Tuberculoid leprosy, medium power.* The granulomas are admixed with lymphocytes.

Fig. VE2.g. *Tuberculoid leprosy, high power.* There is focal fibrinoid necrosis, as may be seen in an upgrading delayed-type hypersensitivity (type 1) reaction.

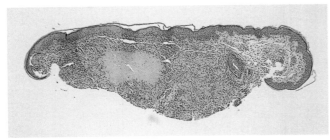

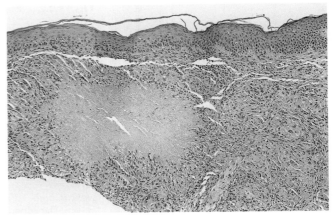

Fig. VE2.h   **Fig. VE2.i**

Fig. VE2.h. *Lupus miliaris disseminatus facei, low power.* A papular lesion characterized by a dense lymphohistiocytic infiltrate with a conspicuous area of caseous necrosis.

Fig. VE2.i. *Lupus miliaris disseminatus facei, medium power.* The caseous necrosis characteristic of this condition is not indicative of mycobacterial or other infection.

VE3. Palisading Granulomas

There are foci of altered collagen ("necrobiosis") surrounded by histiocytes and lymphocytes. Histiocytic giant cells are also seen in the infiltrate. The lesions of epithelioid sarcoma are associated with true tumor necrosis but may superficially resemble rheumatoid nodules. Granuloma annulare is the prototype (24).

Granuloma Annulare

CLINICAL SUMMARY. The lesions of granuloma annulare consist of small, firm, asymptomatic papules that are flesh-colored or pale red and are often grouped in a ringlike or circinate fashion, found most commonly on the hands and feet. Although chronic, they subside after a number of years. Unusual variants of granuloma annulare include a generalized form, consisting of hundreds of papules that are either discrete or confluent but only rarely show an annular arrangement; perforating granuloma annulare, with umbilicated lesions that may be local or generalized; erythematous granuloma annulare, showing large slightly infiltrated erythematous patches, with a palpable border, on which scattered papules may subsequently arise; and subcutaneous granuloma annulare, in which subcutaneous nodules similar to rheumatoid nodules occur, especially in children, either alone or in association with intradermal lesions.

HISTOPATHOLOGY. Histologically, granuloma annulare is characterized by an infiltrate of histiocytes and lymphocytes, which may be present in an interstitial pattern without organization or in a well-developed palisade completely surrounding areas with prominent mucin. Patterns between these two extremes occur. Although degenerated collagen and small quantities of fibrin may be present, it is the increased mucin (hyaluronic acid) that is the hallmark of granuloma annulare (although it may be absent from some lesions, especially those that lack good palisading). The

Clin. Fig. VE3.a. *Granuloma annulare.* A middle-aged woman with generalized granuloma annulare presents a typical annular plaque on her dorsal right hand.

Clin. Fig. VE3.b. *Granuloma annulare.* Multiple orangish papules of granuloma annulare on the left dorsal hand in the same patient.

Fig. VE3.a. *Granuloma annulare, low power.* There are ill-defined areas of pallor in the reticular dermis, surrounded by a somewhat palisaded infiltrate.

Fig. VE3.b. *Granuloma annulare, medium power.* Histiocytes and lymphocytes are arranged around the areas of mucin deposition and collagen alteration.

Fig. VE3.c. *Granuloma annulare, low power.* Another example showing the hypocellular areas alternating with an interstitial inflammatory infiltrate.

Fig. VE3.d. *Granuloma annulare, medium power.* In this example, giant cells are more prominent in the histiocytic infiltrate.

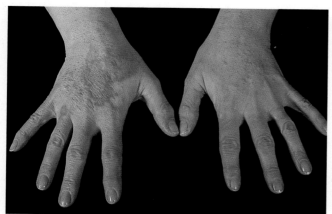

Clin. Fig. VE3.a

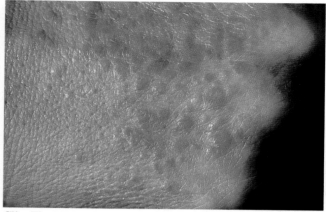

Clin. Fig. VE3.b

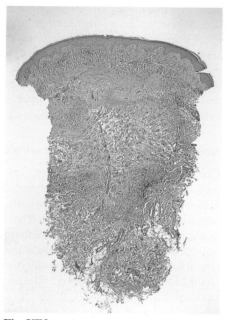

Fig. VE3.a

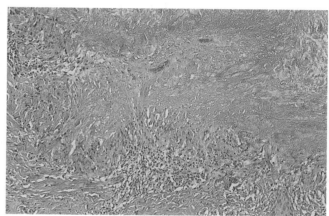

Fig. VE3.b

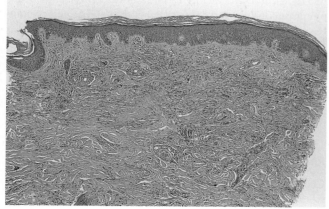

Fig. VE3.c

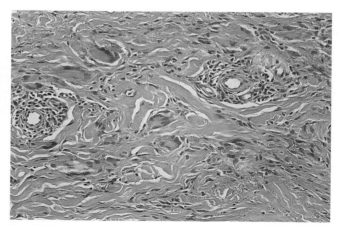

Fig. VE3.d

increased mucin is usually apparent on routinely stained sections as faint blue material with a stringy, finely granular appearance. Stains such as colloidal iron and Alcian blue can be used to highlight it. Plasma cells are present rarely, and a sparse to moderately dense infiltrate of eosinophils can occur. Multinucleated histiocytes are present more often than not, but they are usually few and often subtle. They can occasionally be seen to have engulfed short, thick, blue-gray elastic fibers. On rare occasions, there are granulomas resembling those of sarcoidosis ("granulomatous granuloma annulare"). In perforating granuloma annulare, at least part of the palisading granulomatous process is located very superficially and is associated with disruption of the epidermis. The nodules of subcutaneous granuloma annulare usually show large foci of palisaded histiocytes surrounding areas of degenerated collagen and prominent mucin with a pale appearance.

Necrobiosis Lipoidica Diabeticorum

CLINICAL SUMMARY. Most patients with necrobiosis lipoidica have or will have diabetes, abnormal glucose tolerance, or a family history of diabetes, although of all patients with diabetes, less than 1% develop necrobiosis lipoidica. The lesions present as one or several sharply but irregularly demarcated patches or plaques often with central telangiectases, usually on the shins, elsewhere on the lower extremities, or occasionally elsewhere (25).

HISTOPATHOLOGY. The epidermis may be normal, atrophic, hyperkeratotic, or ulcerated. Usually the entire thickness of the dermis or its lower two thirds is affected by variable degrees of granulomatous inflammation, degeneration of collagen, and sclerosis. Giant cells are usually of the Langhans or foreign-body type, occasionally with Touton cells or asteroid bodies. There may or may not be histiocytes arranged in a palisade, which may tend to be somewhat horizontally oriented and vaguely tiered. Histiocytes may encircle altered connective tissue, particularly degenerated collagen, referred to as "necrobiosis," and differing from normal collagen tinctorially by having a paler grayer hue and structurally by appearing more fragmented and more haphazardly arranged or more compact. Increased mucin is usually inapparent or just subtle, in contrast to granuloma annulare. Other findings include a sparse to moderately dense primarily perivascular lymphocytic infiltrate, plasma cells in the deep dermis in some biopsies, involvement of the upper subcutis with thickened fibrous septa, and lipids in foamy histiocytes or in cholesterol clefts. Older lesions show telangiectases superficially. Blood vessels, particularly in the middle and lower dermis, often exhibit thickening of their walls with periodic acid–Schiff- (PAS) positive diastase-resistant material and proliferation of their endothelial cells. The process may lead to partial, and, rarely, complete occlusion of the lumen.

DIFFERENTIAL DIAGNOSIS. Although histologic distinction between necrobiosis and granuloma annulare may be difficult or impossible, it can usually be accomplished by using the following criteria. Necrobiosis lipoidica rarely involves just one focus of the dermis or predominantly the upper half of the dermis, whereas granuloma annulare commonly does. Histiocytes in palisades that completely encircle altered connective tissue are more common in granuloma annulare, whereas histiocytes in linear array that are horizontally oriented in a somewhat tiered fashion are more typical of necrobiosis lipoidica. Abundant mucin is typical of granuloma annulare and distinctly uncommon in necrobiosis lipoidica. Necrobiosis lipoidica often shows dermal sclerosis and thickened subcutaneous septa, whereas granuloma annulare does not (the sclerosis often produces a straight edge to the sides of a punch biopsy, in contrast to the inward retraction and/or more irregular edge seen in biopsies without sclerosis). Other features that are more characteristic of necrobiosis lipoidica include more numerous giant cells, more pronounced vascular changes such as thickened blood vessel walls, and prominent plasma cells in the deep dermis and occasionally extensive deposits of lipids or nodular lymphocytic infiltrates in the deep dermis or subcutis.

Necrobiotic Xanthogranuloma with Paraproteinemia

CLINICAL SUMMARY. Necrobiotic xanthogranuloma with paraproteinemia, a rare disorder, presents with large, often yellow, indurated plaques with atrophy, telangiectasia, and occasionally also ulceration (26). The most common location is periorbital, and the thorax is also commonly involved. In most patients, serum protein electrophoresis shows an IgG monoclonal gammopathy that usually consists of kappa light chains. In several patients, bone marrow examination has revealed multiple myeloma.

HISTOPATHOLOGY. Granulomatous masses are present either as focal aggregates or as large intersecting bands occupying the dermis and subcutaneous tissue. The intervening tissue separating the granulomas shows extensive necrobiosis. The granulomas contain histiocytes, foam cells, and often also an admixture of inflammatory cells, often arranged as lymphoid follicles. A distinctive feature is the presence of numerous large giant cells, both of the Touton type with a peripheral rim of foamy cytoplasm and of the foreign-body type. Aggregates of cholesterol clefts are also common.

Rheumatoid Nodules

CLINICAL SUMMARY. Rheumatoid nodules vary in size from a few millimeters to 5 cm, and may be solitary or numerous. They occur in patients with rheumatoid arthritis, particularly over extensor surfaces (27) and rarely in extracutaneous sites. *Pseudorheumatoid nodule* refers to nodules in the subcutis that mimic rheumatoid nodules histologi-

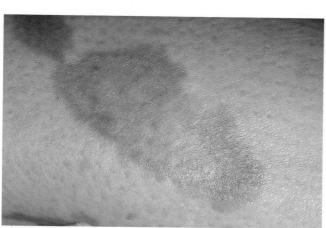

Clin. Fig. VE3.c

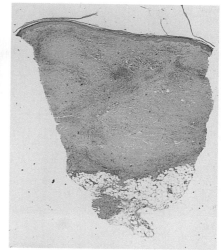

Fig. VE3.e

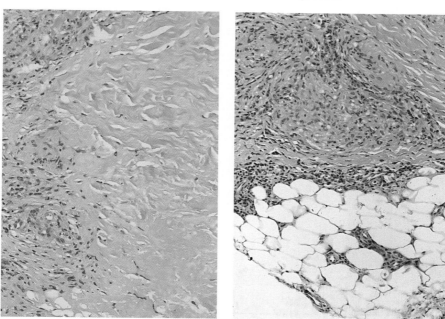

Fig. VE3.f   **Fig. VE3.g**

Clin. Fig. VE3.c. *Necrobiosis lipoidica (NLD).* A solitary plaque of the anterior tibial region shows a pink-brown color, atrophy, and telangiectasia. (W. Witmer)

Fig. VE3.e. *Necrobiosis lipoidica, low power.* The presence of fibrosis can be identified because of the straight edges of the biopsy. The infiltrate involves the full thickness of the dermis and is arranged in a tierlike fashion. (P. Shapiro)

Fig. VE3.f. *Necrobiosis lipoidica, medium power.* Histiocytes and lymphocytes on the left surrounding degenerated collagen in the lower right corner. Compared with the normal collagen above it, the degenerated collagen has a more compact appearance and appears more gray-blue than pink. (P. Shapiro)

Fig. VE3.g. *Necrobiosis lipoidica, high power.* Epithelioid granulomas in the deep dermis and lymphocytes and plasma cells at the dermal–subcutaneous junction are features that favor NLD over granuloma annulare. (P. Shapiro)

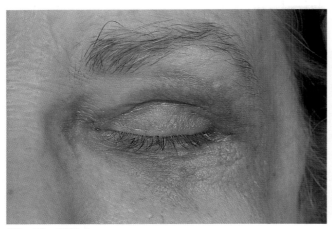

Clin. Fig. VE3.d

Clin. Fig. VE3.d. *Necrobiotic xanthogranuloma.* A 65-year-old woman developed asymmetric periorbital induration with violaceous color change.

Fig. VE3.h. *Necrobiotic xanthogranuloma, low power.* A diffuse infiltrate spans the dermis and subcutaneous tissue.

Fig. VE3.i. *Necrobiotic xanthogranuloma, low power.* The infiltrate is vaguely granulomatous, with intersecting bands of acellular necrosis and cellular infiltrates that are present either as focal aggregates or as large intersecting bands occupying the dermis and subcutaneous tissue.

Fig. VE3.j. *Necrobiotic xanthogranuloma, high power.* The granulomatous infiltrate contains histiocytes, foam cells, and an admixture of lymphocytes and plasma cells, with numerous large giant cells of the Touton type with a peripheral rim of foamy cytoplasm, or of foreign-body type.

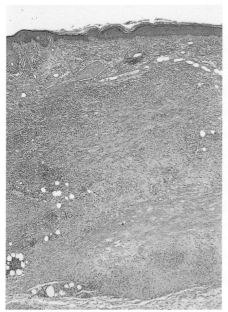

Fig. VE3.h

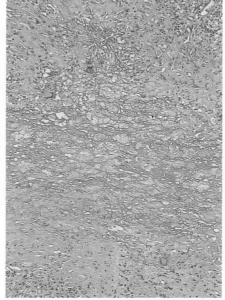

Fig. VE3.i

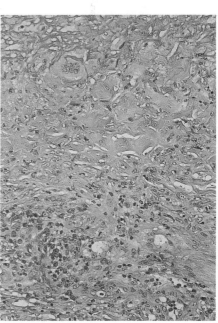

Fig. VE3.j

cally but that develop in the absence of rheumatoid arthritis (or systemic lupus erythematosus). The subsequent development of rheumatoid arthritis occurs infrequently in adults and rarely, if ever, in children. These nodules have been considered to represent a subcutaneous variant of granuloma annulare.

HISTOPATHOLOGY. Rheumatoid nodules occur in the subcutis and lower dermis and show one or several areas of fibrinoid degeneration of collagen that stain homogeneously red. Nuclear fragments and basophilic material may be present, but mucin is almost always minimal or absent. These areas are surrounded by histiocytes in a palisaded arrangement, often with scattered foreign-body giant cells. In the surrounding stroma, there is a proliferation of blood vessels, with fibrosis and a fairly sparse infiltrate of other inflammatory cells, including predominantly lymphocytes and a few neutrophils but also mast cells, plasma cells, and eosinophils occasionally.

Conditions to consider in the differential diagnosis:

granuloma annulare
necrobiosis lipoidica
subcutaneous granuloma annulare
necrobiotic xanthogranuloma with paraproteinemia
annular elastolytic giant cell granuloma (actinic granuloma)
rheumatic nodule
epithelioid sarcoma
occasional examples of deep fungus infections

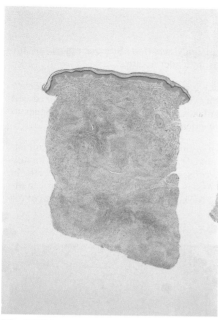

Fig. VE3.k.
Rheumatoid nodule, low power. There are patches of hypocellular collagen surrounded by a cellular infiltrate in the reticular dermis.

Fig. VE3.l.
Rheumatoid nodule, medium power. The patches are areas of degenerate acellular collagen.

Fig. VE3.m.
Rheumatoid nodule, high power. The necrobiotic areas are surrounded by histiocytes in a vaguely palisaded arrangement.

Fig. VE3.k

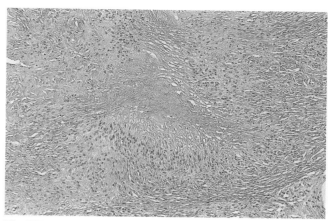

Fig. VE3.l

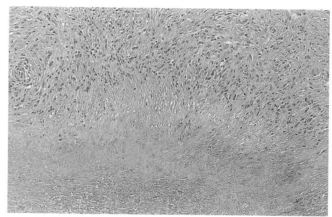

Fig. VE3.m

VE4. Mixed Cell Granulomas

Lymphocytes and plasma cells are present in addition to epithelioid histiocytes, which may form loose clusters, and giant cells, which may be quite inconspicuous. In many of these granulomatous infiltrates, organisms are found. Keratin granuloma is the most common mixed granuloma. Flakes of keratin may be appreciated as fibers, often gray rather than pink, in the cytoplasm of giant cells. Foreign-body reactions may present as mixed-cell granulomas (28).

Foreign Body Reactions

CLINICAL SUMMARY. Foreign substances, when injected or implanted accidentally into the skin, can produce a focal nonallergic foreign-body reaction or, in persons specifically sensitized to them, a focal allergic response. In addition, certain substances formed within the body may produce a nonallergic foreign-body reaction when deposited in the dermis or the subcutaneous tissue. Such endogenous foreign-body reactions are produced, for instance, by urates in gout and by keratinous material in pilomatricoma and in ruptured epidermoid and trichilemmal cysts.

HISTOPATHOLOGY. A *nonallergic* foreign-body reaction typically shows a granulomatous response with histiocytes and giant cells around the foreign material. Often, some of the giant cells are of the foreign-body type, in which the nuclei are in haphazard array. In addition, lymphocytes are usually present, such as plasma cells and neutrophils, constituting a mixed-cell granuloma. Frequently, some of the foreign material is seen within macrophages and giant cells, a finding that is of great diagnostic value. The most common cause of a foreign-body granuloma is rupture of a hair follicle or follicular cyst, and sometimes only the cyst content, rather than residual cyst wall, is identifiable. Exogenous substances producing nonallergic foreign-body reactions are, for instance, silk and nylon sutures, wood, paraffin and other oily substances, silicone gel, talc, surgical glove starch powder, and cactus spines. Some of these substances—nylon sutures, wood, talc, surgical glove starch powder, and sea-urchin spines—are doubly refractile on polarizing examination. Double refraction often is very helpful in localizing foreign substances.

An *allergic* granulomatous reaction to a foreign body typically shows a sarcoidal or tuberculoid pattern consisting of epithelioid cells with or without giant cells. Phagocytosis of the foreign substance is slight or absent. Substances that may produce allergic granulomatous reactions in sensitized per-

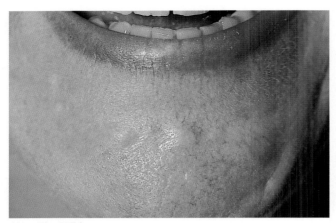

Clin. Fig. VE4

Clin. Fig. VE4. *Foreign body reaction.* Silicone injections for wrinkles led to whitish, firm, tender nodules.

Fig. VE4.a. *Foreign body granuloma in ruptured epidermal cyst, low power.* Remnants of a cyst are present adjacent to a mixed-cell inflammatory infiltrate. Flakes of keratin from the cyst appear to elicit the inflammatory response.

Fig. VE4.b. *Ruptured epidermal cyst, high power.* The inflammatory reaction contains a mixed cell-granulomatous infiltrate including lymphocytes, plasma cells, some neutrophils, and giant cells. In lesions where a remnant cyst is not identified, the diagnosis can often be made by searching for keratin flakes in the cytoplasm of giant cells.

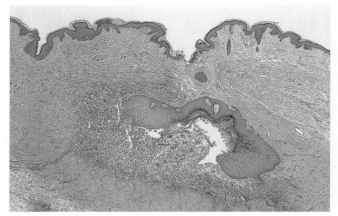

Fig. VE4.a

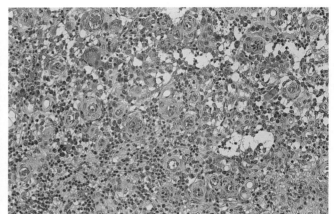

Fig. VE4.b

sons include zirconium, beryllium, and certain dyes used in tattoos. Some substances that act as foreign material at first may act as allergens later on, after sensitization has occurred, as in the case of sea-urchin spines and silica.

Conditions to consider in the differential diagnosis:

> keratin granuloma
> ruptured cyst
> folliculitis
> foreign-body granulomas
> sporotrichosis
> persistent arthropod bite
> syphilis, secondary and tertiary
> cryptococcosis
> candidal granuloma
> nontuberculosis mycobacteria
> cat-scratch disease
> North American blastomycosis
> South American blastomycosis
> chromomycosis
> phaeohyphomycosis
> coccidioidomycosis

VE5. Inflammatory Nodules with Prominent Eosinophils

The nodular dermal infiltrates contain many eosinophils often admixed with lymphocytes. Angiolymphoid hyperplasia is the best example (29).

Angiolymphoid Hyperplasia with Eosinophilia and Kimura's Disease

CLINICAL SUMMARY. Lesions of angiolymphoid hyperplasia with eosinophilia may arise superficially in the dermis or in the subcutaneous or deeper tissues. Superficial lesions, which have been referred to as pseudopyogenic granuloma, present often in young to middle-aged women with pruritic papules and plaques often at or around the external ear or elsewhere on the head and neck. Lesions of subcutaneous and deeper tissues typically present as a solitary, slowly growing, firm, subcutaneous swelling up to 10 cm in size, usually in the head and neck region with some predilection for the pre- or postauricular sites. Blood eosinophilia and modest enlargement of neighboring lymph nodes and salivary tissue may occur. The conditions are chronic, but serious complications do not occur.

When angiolymphoid hyperplasia with eosinophilia was first described in western Europe, similarities to *Kimura's disease* as reported in the Far East were noted. However, more recently, most authorities emphasize differences between the two entities. Angiolymphoid hyperplasia and Kimura's disease occur most commonly in the head and neck region in adults and both share the histologic features of extensive lymphoid proliferation, tissue eosinophilia, and evidence of vascular hyperplasia. Kimura's disease, however, demonstrates a wider age span with male predominance and a tendency for more extensive lesions to occur, often with involvement of salivary tissue and lymph nodes and at sites distant from the head and neck region.

HISTOPATHOLOGY.   The main components of the pathology are proliferation of small to medium-sized blood vessels of-ten showing a lobular architecture and lined by greatly enlarged (epithelioid) endothelial cells, a perivascular inflammatory cell infiltrate composed mainly of lymphocytes and eosinophils, nodular areas of lymphocytic infiltrate occurring with or without follicle formation, and inflammatory vascular occlusive changes in medium-sized arteries associated with endothelial cell proliferation.

In superficial lesions, there is variable vascular hyperplasia that can include areas in which the proliferation is almost angiomatous. A distinctive feature is the "cobblestone" appearance of enlarged endothelial cells that project into the lumina of some vessels. These cells lack atypia or mitotic activity. Affected vessels often contain endothelial cells with intracytoplasmic vacuoles, the so-called "histiocytoid hemangioma" pattern. In subcutaneous lesions, the inflammatory cell infiltrate is usually more massive, with a

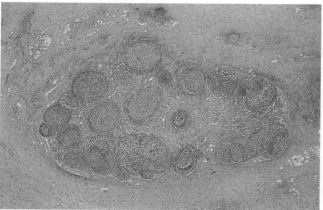

Fig. VE5.a

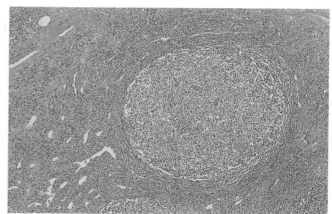

Fig. VE5.b

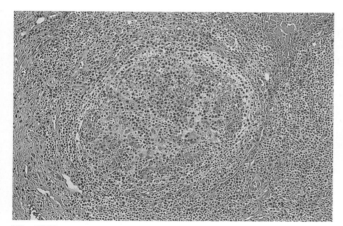

Fig. VE5.c

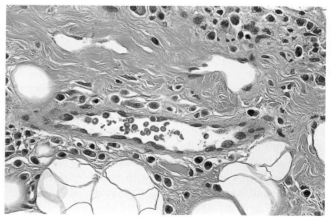

Fig. VE5.d

Fig. VE5.a. *Kimura's disease, low power.* A nodular cluster of lymphoid follicles in the deep dermis and subcutaneous tissue.

Fig. VE5.b. *Kimura's disease, medium power.* The follicles are surrounded by fibrosis and separated by a meshwork of prominent small vessels.

Fig. VE5.c. *Kimura's disease, medium power.* A cluster of lymphocytes admixed with eosinophils.

Fig. VE5.d. *Kimura's disease, high power.* The endothelial cells lining the small vessels are swollen and some of them protrude into the lumen, imparting a cobblestone appearance.

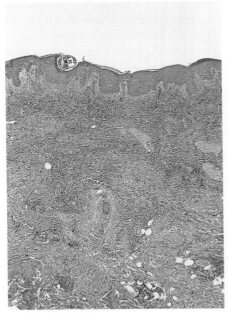

Fig. VE5.e

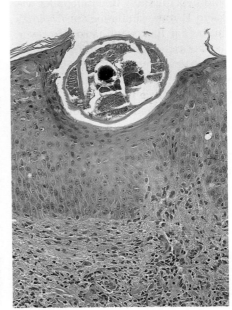

Fig. VE5.f

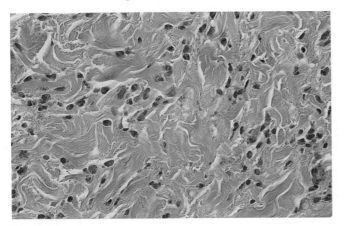

Fig. VE5.g

Fig. VE5.e. *Scabetic nodule, low power.* A patchy to diffuse infiltrate in the reticular dermis. If mites are not appreciated in the epidermis, the diagnosis of scabies may be missed.

Fig. VE5.f. *Scabetic nodule, medium power.* A scabies mite is present in the stratum corneum.

Fig. VE5.g. *Scabetic nodule, high power.* In the dermis, eosinophils are a conspicuous component of the inflammatory infiltrate.

central, poorly circumscribed nodule that replaces the fat. The nodule is composed of confluent sheets of small lymphocytes and eosinophils in which a network of poorly canalized thick-walled capillaries is embedded. Satellite smaller islands of lymphoid cells with lymphoid follicles usually surround the central nodule. Commonly, there is involvement of medium- to large-sized arteries, with infiltration of the vessel wall by inflammatory cells and occlusion of the lumen.

Histologic differences between angiolymphoid hyperplasia with eosinophilia and Kimura's disease include the lesser degree of exuberant vascular hyperplasia lacking prominent eosinophilic endothelial cells and the absence of uncanalized blood vessels in Kimura's disease. Other points of difference are eosinophilic abscesses and marked fibrosis around the lesions in Kimura's disease and the absence of lesions centered around damaged arteries. There is an important association between Kimura's disease and nephrotic syndrome.

Scabetic Nodule

See Figs. VE5.e–VE5.g.

Conditions to consider in the differential diagnosis:

angiolymphoid hyperplasia with eosinophils
Kimura's disease
scabetic nodule

VE6. Inflammatory Nodules with Mixed Cell Types

A variety of cells occurs in the infiltrate, including neutrophils, histiocytes, plasma cells, giant cells, and lymphocytes. Sporotrichosis is a good example (30).

Sporotrichosis

CLINICAL SUMMARY. Clinical sporotrichosis usually occurs as one of two primary cutaneous forms, either the fixed cutaneous or the lymphocutaneous form. Both result from direct inoculation at a site of minor trauma. Systemic sporotri-

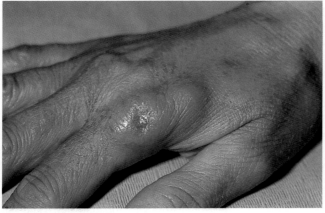

Clin. Fig. VE6.a

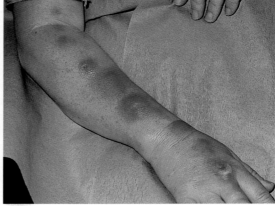

Clin. Fig. VE6.b

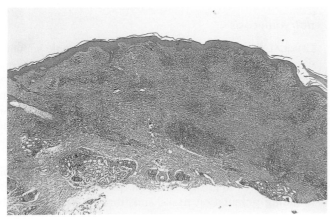

Fig. VE6.a

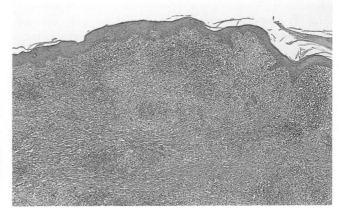

Fig. VE6.b

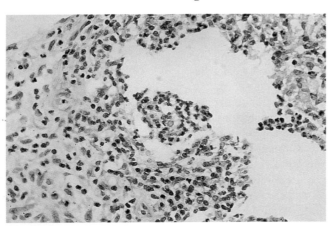

Fig. VE6.c

Clin. Fig. VE6.a. *Sporotrichosis.* An ulcerated nodule developed after the area was pricked by a rose bush.

Clin. Fig. VE6.b. *Sporotrichosis.* Subsequently nodules along the draining lymph vessels appeared (a sporotrichoid pattern of spread).

Fig. VE6.a. *Sporotrichosis, low power.* A patchy to diffuse infiltrate spanning the dermis.

Fig. VE6.b. *Sporotrichosis, medium power.* Focal areas of necrosis can be appreciated within the infiltrate, which in some areas is granulomatous.

Fig. VE6.c. *Sporotrichosis, high power.* The cells in the infiltrate include neutrophils, admixed with histiocytes and lymphocytes and some plasma cells. A single organism is present, visualized as a round pink-walled body about the size of a lymphocyte near the center of the image. (S. Lucas)

chosis is rare, and more commonly follows pulmonary infection in association with immunosuppression. The lymphocutaneous form of sporotrichosis starts with a painless papule that grows into an ulcer, usually on a finger or hand. Subsequently, a chain of asymptomatic nodules appears along the lymph vessel, draining the area. These lymphatic nodules may undergo suppuration with subsequent ulceration. In the fixed cutaneous form, a solitary plaque or occasionally a group of lesions is seen, most commonly on an arm or the face. It may show superficial crusting or a verrucous surface. There is no tendency toward lymphatic spread.

HISTOPATHOLOGY. Early lesions of primary cutaneous sporotrichosis usually show a nonspecific inflammatory infiltrate composed of neutrophils, lymphoid cells, plasma cells, and histiocytes. In an older lesion with an elevated border or a verrucous appearance, small abscesses are often found in the hyperplastic epidermis, and the dermis contains small abscesses and granulomas often associated with asteroid bodies and scattered through a lymphoplasmacytic infiltrate with eosinophils and giant cells. Later, through coalescence, a characteristic arrangement of the infiltrate in three zones may develop. These include a central "suppurative" zone composed of neutrophils; a "tuberculoid" zone with epithelioid cells and multinucleated histiocytes; and, peripherally, a "round cell" zone of lymphoid cells and plasma cells.

The lymphatic nodules of lymphocutaneous sporotrichosis, as well as the cutaneous nodules of multifocal systemic sporotrichosis, at first show scattered granulomas within an inflammatory infiltrate, predominantly in the deep dermis and subcutaneous fat. These enlarge and run together to form irregularly shaped suppurative granulomata and eventually a large abscess surrounded by zones of histiocytes and lymphocytes as described for primary lesions.

In many instances, it is not possible to recognize the causative organisms of *S. schenckii* in tissue sections. Immunohistochemical staining may increase the yield. If present, the spores of *S. schenckii* appear as round to oval bodies 4 to 6 mm in diameter that stain more strongly at the periphery than in the center. Single or occasionally multiple buds are present. In some instances, small cigar-shaped bodies up to 8 mm long are also present. Asteroid bodies in sporotrichosis consist a central spore 5 to 10 mm in diameter surrounded by radiating elongations of a homogeneous eosinophilic material, known as the Splendore–Hoeppli phenomenon and thought to represent deposition of antigen–antibody complexes and host debris.

Conditions to consider in the differential diagnosis:

chronic bacterial infections
keratin granuloma
ruptured cyst
folliculitis
sporotrichosis
rhinoscleroma (Klebsiella rhinoscleromatis)
atypical mycobacteria
Mycobacterium avium-intracellulare
Mycobacterium marinum
nocardiosis
lobomycosis
protothecosis

VE7. Inflammatory Nodules with Necrosis and Neutrophils (Abscesses)

Inflammatory nodules are characterized by central suppurative necrosis, with neutrophils adjacent to the necrosis and often with granulation tissue, mixed inflammatory cells including epithelioid histiocytes and giant cells, and fibrosis at the periphery. Botryomycosis is prototypic (31).

Botryomycosis

CLINICAL SUMMARY. Botryomycosis is a chronic suppurative infection of skin (and other organs such as lungs and meninges) in which pyogenic bacteria form granules similar to those seen in mycetoma. Most patients have no known immune defect. The skin lesions are local nodules, ulcers, or sinuses communicating with deep abscesses. They occur mainly on the extremities.

HISTOPATHOLOGY. The dermal inflammation is predominantly that of neutrophil polymorph abscesses with surrounding granulation tissue and fibrosis. Within the abscesses are granules (grains) shaped like a bunch of grapes, hence the name of the disease. The grains, which may range up to 2 mm in diameter, are composed of closely aggregated nonfilamentous bacteria with a peripheral radial deposition

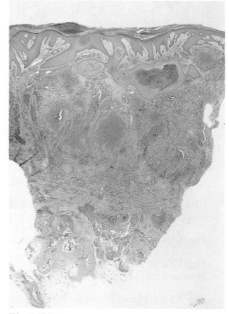

Fig. VE7.a

Fig. VE7.a. *Botryomycosis, low power.* There is pseudoepitheliomatous hyperplasia of the epidermis, and there are small abscesses in the dermis. (S. Lucas) *(continues)*

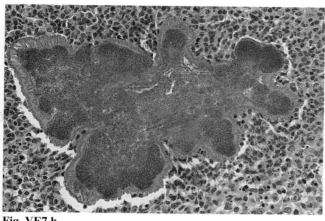

Fig. VE7.b

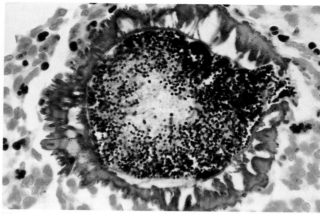

Fig. VE7.c

Fig. VE7.b. *Botryomycosis, medium power.* An abscess within that is a basophilic bacterial colony with a surrounding eosinophilic Hoeppli–Splendore phenomenon. (S. Lucas)

Fig. VE7.c. *Botryomycosis, high power.* A staphylococcal lesion showing gram-positive cocci (centrally they are degenerate and nonstaining). (S. Lucas)

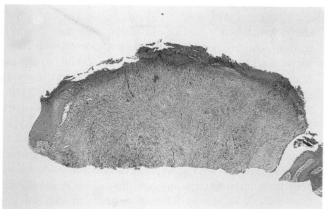

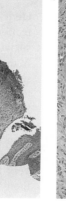

Fig. VE7.d

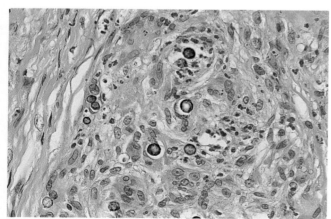

Fig. VE7.e

Fig. VE7.d. *Chromoblastomycosis, low power.* An ulcerated epidermis overlies a mixed-cell inflammatory infiltrate in the dermis.

Fig. VE7.e. *Chromoblastomycosis, medium power.* The infiltrate includes lymphocytes and epithelioid cells with giant cells but without well-formed epithelioid cell granulomas.

Fig. VE7.f. *Chromoblastomycosis, high power.* The organisms appear as dark brown, thick-walled, ovoid, or spherical spores lying within giant cells and free in the tissue.

Fig. VE7.f

of intensely eosinophilic material a Hoeppli–Splendore reaction. The bacteria are usually *Staphylococcus aureus*, but streptococci and certain gram-negative bacilli such as *Proteus*, *Pseudomonas*, and *Escherichia coli* are sometimes found. The overlying epithelium often exhibits pseudoepitheliomatous hyperplasia. Transepithelial elimination of grains may be observed.

Chromoblastomycosis

CLINICAL SUMMARY. Chromoblastomycosis is a slowly progressive cutaneous mycosis caused by pigmented (dematiaceous) fungi that occur as round nonbudding forms in tissue sections. Inasmuch as budding is absent, the designation chromoblastomycosis is somewhat inappropriate. The causative fungi are saprophytes that can be found growing in soil, decaying vegetation, or rotten wood in subtropical and tropical countries. The primary lesion is thought to develop as a result of traumatic implantation of the fungus into the skin. The lesions are most common on the lower extremities and consist of verrucous papules, nodules, and plaques that may itch.

HISTOPATHOLOGY. The cutaneous type of chromoblastomycosis resembles North American blastomycosis in histologic appearance with a lichenoid-granulomatous inflammatory pattern, with pseudoepitheliomatous epidermal hyperplasia and an extensive dermal infiltrate composed of many epithelioid histiocytes, and multinucleated giant cells, small abscesses with clusters of neutrophils, and variable numbers of lymphocytes, plasma cells, and eosinophils. Tuberculoid formations may be present, but caseation necrosis is absent. The causative organisms are found within giant cells and free in the tissue, especially in the abscesses. They appear as conspicuous, dark brown, thick-walled, ovoid or spherical spores varying in size from 6 to 12 mm and lying either singly or in chains or clusters.

  Conditions to consider in the differential diagnosis:

    acute or chronic bacterial abscesses
    deep fungal infections
    phaeohyphomycotic cyst
    North American blastomycosis
    chromoblastomycosis
    cutaneous alternariosis
    paracoccidioidomycosis
    coccidioidomycosis
    sporotrichosis
    botryomycosis
    actinomycosis
    nocardiosis
    cat-scratch disease
    erythema nodosum leprosum (type 2 leprosy reaction)
    scrofuloderma
    tuberculous gumma
    protothecosis

VE8. Inflammatory Nodules with Prominent Necrosis

Necrosis is a striking feature along with variable but sometimes sparse infiltrates of inflammatory cells that may include plasma cells, epithelioid histiocytes, neutrophils, lymphocytes, and hemorrhage. Organisms may be demonstrable. Aspergillosis is prototypic (32).

Aspergillosis

CLINICAL SUMMARY. Cutaneous aspergillosis may occur as a primary infection or may be secondary to disseminated aspergillosis. The lesions of primary cutaneous aspergillosis are usually found at an intravenous infusion site. One observes either one or several macules, papules, plaques, or hemorrhagic bullae, which may rapidly progress into necrotic ulcers that are covered by a heavy black eschar. Death often results from secondary systemic dissemination of the aspergillosis. Primary cutaneous infection has been seen in patients with acquired immunodeficiency syndrome (AIDS). In addition, *Aspergillus* may colonize burn or surgical wounds and subsequently invade viable tissue; in these cases, the prognosis is generally good. Secondary cutaneous aspergillosis, usually associated with invasive lung disease, shows multiple scattered lesions as a result of embolic hematogenous spread and has a poor prognosis.

HISTOPATHOLOGY. Unlike most deep cutaneous fungal infections, cutaneous aspergillosis is not characteristically associated with pseudoepitheliomatous epidermal hyperplasia. In the more serious primary forms and in the secondary disseminated form, numerous *Aspergillus* hyphae are seen in the dermis with hematoxylin-eosin stained sections or with PAS or silver methenamine staining. The 2- to 4-mm hyphae are often arranged in a radiate fashion, are septate, and branch at an acute angle. Hyphae characteristically invade blood vessels, giving rise to areas of ischemic necrosis with very little inflammation in some instances. In other cases, there may be an acute inflammatory reaction with polymorphonuclear leukocytes in addition to lymphocytes and histiocytes. In patients with primary cutaneous or subcutaneous aspergillosis who are otherwise in good health, the number of hyphae present is relatively small, and there may be a well-developed granulomatous reaction.

  Conditions to consider in the differential diagnosis:

    tertiary syphilis
    tertiary yaws
    aspergillosis
    zygomycosis (mucormycosis)
    tuberculosis
    atypical mycobacteria
    infarcts
    deep vasculitis
    deep thrombi
    calciphylaxis
    frostbite
    necrobiotic xanthogranuloma with paraproteinemia

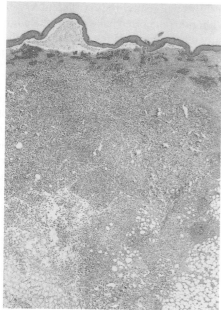

Fig. VE8.a

Fig. VE8.a. *Cutaneous aspergillosis, low power.* There is an extensive dermal inflammatory infiltrate throughout most of the field, with a less cellular area of necrosis at the lower left of the image. The epidermis has separated due to ischemic changes of basal keratinocytes.

Fig. VE8.b. *Cutaneous aspergillosis, medium power.* At the periphery of the necrotic area (*lower left*), there is an inflammatory infiltrate in the viable dermis. Both areas are extensively infiltrated by fungal hyphae.

Fig. VE8.c. *Cutaneous aspergillosis, high power.* A thrombosed vessel surrounded by acute inflammatory cells, with fungal hyphae of *Aspergillus* organisms in typical pose spanning the vessel wall.

Fig. VE8.d. *Cutaneous aspergillosis, medium power, silver stain for fungi.* Black-stained fungal hyphae in the vessel lumen and wall.

Fig. VE8.e. *Cutaneous aspergillosis, high power, silver stain for fungi.* The hyphae are narrow, fairly uniform, septate, and tend to branch at acute angles.

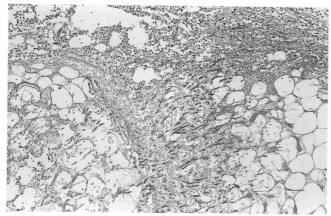

Fig. VE8.b

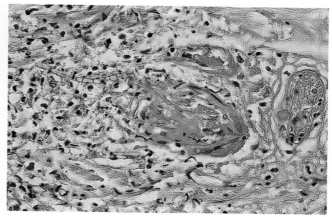

Fig. VE8.c

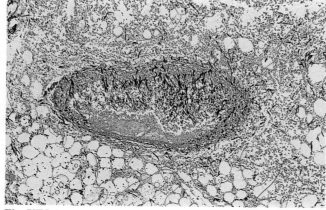

Fig. VE8.d

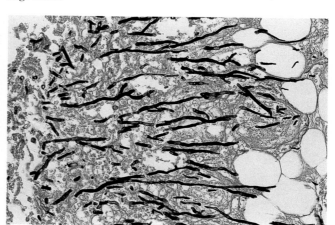

Fig. VE8.e

gangrenous ischemic necrosis
epithelioid sarcoma

VE9. Chronic Ulcers and Sinuses Involving the Reticular Dermis

A chronic ulcer is characterized by central suppurative necrosis, with neutrophils adjacent to the necrosis and often with granulation tissue, fibrosis, and reactive epithelium at the periphery. A sinus extends deeper into the dermis than most ulcers in a serpentine fashion. A fistula is an abnormal communication between two epithelial-lined surfaces. The histologic architecture of fistulas and sinuses is similar to that of chronic ulcers. Chancroid is a good example of a chronic ulcer (33).

Chancroid

CLINICAL SUMMARY.   Chancroid, caused by *Haemophilus ducreyi*, is a sexually transmitted disease leading to one or several ulcers, chiefly in the genital region. The ulcers exhibit little if any induration, and often have undermined borders. They are usually tender. Inguinal lymphadenitis, either unilateral or bilateral, is common and, unless treated, often results in an inguinal abscess.

HISTOPATHOLOGY.   The histologic changes beneath the ulcer are sufficiently distinct to permit a presumptive diagnosis of chancroid in many instances. The lesion consists of three zones overlying each other and shows characteristic vascular changes. The surface zone at the floor of the ulcer is rather narrow and consists of neutrophils, fibrin, erythrocytes, and necrotic tissue. The next zone is fairly wide and contains many newly formed blood vessels showing marked proliferation of their endothelial cells. As a result of the endothelial proliferation, the lumina of the vessels are often occluded, leading to thrombosis. In addition, there are degenerative changes in the walls of the vessels. The deep zone is composed of a dense in-

Fig. VE9.a

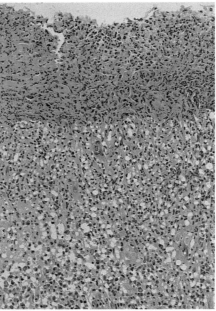

Fig. VE9.b

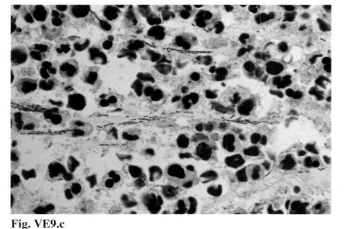

Fig. VE9.c

Fig. VE9.a. *Chancroid, low power.* Cutaneous ulcer with the characteristic three-zone pattern of inflammation-superficial acute inflammatory exudate, a midzone of granulation tissue, and a deep zone of plasma cells and lymphocytes. (S. Lucas)

Fig. VE9.b. *Chancroid, medium power.* A superficial necrotic zone, and underlying granulation tissue. (S. Lucas)

Fig. VE9.c. *Chancroid, high power.* A Giemsa-stained image from the superficial necrotic zone, containing bacilli lying in parallel chains. (S. Lucas, courtesy of A. Freinkel)

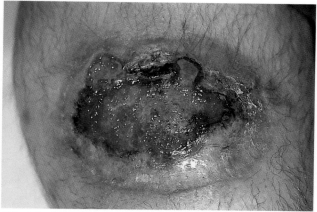

Clin. Fig. VE9

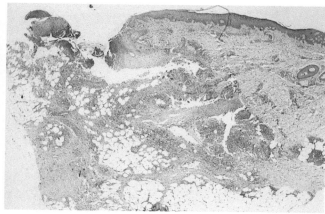

Fig. VE9.d

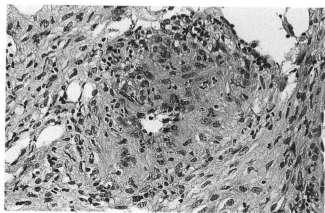

Fig. VE9.e

Fig. VE9.f

Clin. Fig. VE9. *Pyoderma gangrenosum.* A 25-year-old man with ulcerative colitis developed a fluctuant calf nodule that broke down into a painful enlarging ulcer with purple-red undermined borders.

Fig. VE9.d. *Pyoderma gangrenosum, low power.* A punched-out ulcer with an undermined edge extending deeply into the dermis.

Fig. VE9.e. *Pyoderma gangrenosum, medium power.* The ulcer base is lined by an intense infiltrate of neutrophils.

Fig. VE9.f. *Pyoderma gangrenosum, high power.* Neutrophils are present in a vessel wall without true vasculitis, which requires fibrinoid necrosis. Necrotizing vasculitis that may be seen at the surface of acute ulcers may be secondary to the ulcer and should not necessarily be considered pathogenic.

---

filtrate of plasma cells and lymphoid cells. Demonstration of bacilli in tissue sections stained with Giemsa stain or Gram stain is occasionally possible. The bacilli are most apt to be found between the cells of the surface zone. *H. ducreyi* is a fine, short, gram-negative coccobacillus, measuring about 1.5 by 0.2 mm, often arranged in parallel chains.

Pyoderma Gangrenosum

CLINICAL SUMMARY. The lesions begin as tender papulopustules or as folliculitis that eventually may ulcerate. In the fully developed stage, the lesions have a raised undermined border, which has a dusky-purple hue. Pyoderma gangrenosum may occur as an isolated cutaneous phenomenon or may be a cutaneous manifestation associated with various systemic dis-

ease processes, such as inflammatory bowel disease, connective tissue diseases, and lymphoproliferative lesions (34).

HISTOPATHOLOGY. The histologic findings are nonspecific and the diagnosis is primarily clinical. Most authors studying early lesions have reported a primarily neutrophilic infiltrate, which frequently involves follicular structures but is often also diffuse. Others, however, have stated that the lesions begin with a lymphocytic reaction. Degrees of vessel involvement range from none to fibrinoid necrosis. In most lesions, a neutrophilic infiltrate is present with some, but limited, vascular damage. Outright vasculitis has been reported and has led to speculations about its possible role in the etiology of pyoderma gangrenosum. Focal vasculitis is often observed in fully developed lesions but appears secondary to

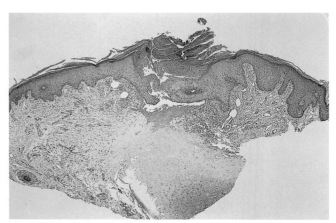

Fig. VE9.g

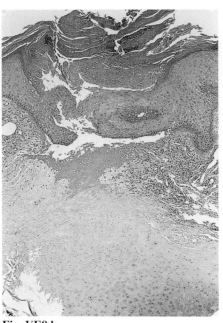

Fig. VE9.h

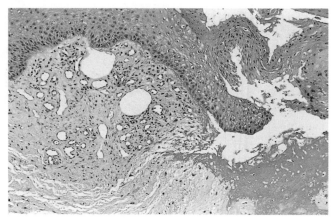

Fig. VE9.i

Fig. VE9.g. *Chondrodermatitis nodularis helicis.* Hyperkeratosis and a hyperplastic epithelium are associated with a focal ulcer and an inflammatory reaction that extends to the cartilage of the ear.

Fig. VE9.h. *Chondrodermatitis nodularis helicis.* Beneath the focal ulcer there is a zone of eosinophilic degeneration of collagen extending to the cartilage.

Fig. VE9.i. *Chondrodermatitis nodularis helicis.* Around the zone of eosinophilic degeneration, there is a lymphocytic infiltrate with fibrosis.

the inflammatory process. The infiltrate tends to be deeper and more extensive than that in classic Sweet's syndrome. Fully developed lesions exhibit ulceration, necrosis, and a mixed inflammatory cell infiltrate. Involvement of the deep reticular dermis and subcutis may exhibit primarily mononuclear cell and granulomatous inflammatory reactions.

Chondrodermatitis Nodularis Helicis

See Figs. VE9.g–VE9.i.

Conditions to consider in the differential diagnosis:

pyoderma gangrenosum
ecthyma gangrenosum
deep fungal infection
North American blastomycosis
eumycetoma
tuberculosis cutis orificialis
enterocutaneous fistula

chondrodermatitis nodularis helicis
ecthyma
papulonecrotic tuberculid
Buruli ulcer (*M. ulcerans*)
chancroid (*Haemophilus ducreyi*)
granuloma inguinale (*Calymmatobacterium granulomatis*)
lymphogranuloma venereum (*Chlamydia trachomatis*)
follicular occlusion disorder
pilonidal sinus
hidradenitis suppurativa
acne conglobata
perifolliculitis capitis abscedens et suffodens (dissecting cellulitis of the scalp)
anthrax (*Bacillus anthracis*)
tularemia (*Francisella tularensis*)
cutaneous leishmaniasis

necrotizing sialometaplasia of hard palate
eosinophilic ulcer of the tongue

VF. DERMAL MATRIX FIBER DISORDERS

The dermis serves as a reaction site for a variety of inflammatory, infiltrative, and desmoplastic processes. These may include accumulations or deficiencies of dermal fibrous and nonfibrous matrix constituents as reactions to a variety of stimuli.

1. Fiber Disorders, Collagen Increased
2. Fiber Disorders, Collagen Reduced
3. Fiber Disorders, Elastin Increased or Prominent
4. Fiber Disorders, Elastin Reduced
5. Fiber Disorders, Perforating

VF1. Fiber Disorders, Collagen Increased

Dermal collagen is increased with production at the dermal subcutaneous interface. Inflammation is seen at this site. The inflammatory cells are lymphocytes, plasma cells, and eosinophils. Fibroblasts are increased in some instances. Scleroderma is the prototype (35).

Scleroderma

CLINICAL SUMMARY. Scleroderma is a connective tissue disorder characterized by thickening and fibrosis of the skin. Two types of scleroderma exist: circumscribed scleroderma (*morphea*) and systemic scleroderma (*progressive systemic sclerosis*). In morphea, the lesions usually are limited to the skin and to the subcutaneous tissue beneath the cutaneous lesions. Morphea may be divided according to morphology and distribution of lesions into six types: guttate, plaque, linear, segmental, subcutaneous, and generalized.

Lesions of the plaque type, the most common, are indurated, with a smooth surface and an ivory color with a violaceous border in growing lesions, the so-called lilac ring. Guttate lesions are small and superficial. Linear lesions may have the configuration of a saber-cut (*coup de sabre*). Segmental morphea occurs on one side of the face, resulting in hemiatrophy. In subcutaneous morphea (morphea profunda) the involved skin is thickened and bound to the underlying fascia and muscle. Generalized morphea comprises very extensive cases showing a combination of several of the five types just described.

In systemic scleroderma, visceral lesions are present in addition to involvement of the skin and the subcutaneous tissue, leading to death in some patients. The indurated lesions of the skin are not sharply demarcated or circumscribed, as in morphea. Facial changes include a masklike, expressionless face and tightening of the skin around the mouth associated with radial folds. There may be diffuse hyperpigmentation, mainly in diffuse systemic sclerosis. The hands show nonpitting edema involving the dorsa of the fingers, hands, and forearms. Gradually the fingers become tapered, the skin be-

comes hard, and flexion contractures form. These changes, referred to as *acrosclerosis*, are associated with Raynaud's phenomenon. Macular telangiectasias on the face and hands, calcinosis cutis on the extremities, and ulcerations, especially on the tips of the fingers, over the knuckles, and on the lower extremities, occur predominantly in acrosclerosis.

Systemic sclerosis with limited scleroderma, known as CREST syndrome, is a variant of acrosclerosis that consists of several or all of the following manifestations: *C*alcinosis cutis, *R*aynaud's phenomenon, involvement of the *E*sophagus with dysphagia, *S*clerodactyly and *T*elangiectases. Death from visceral lesions is infrequent in CREST syndrome.

HISTOPATHOLOGY. The different types of morphea cannot be differentiated histologically. Early inflammatory and late sclerotic stages can be distinguished. In the early inflammatory stage, particularly at the active violaceous border, the reticular dermis collagen bundles are thickened and there is a moderately intense interstitial and perivascular inflammatory infiltrate, which is predominantly lymphocytic admixed with plasma cells. A much more pronounced inflammatory infiltrate often involves the subcutaneous fat and extends upward toward the eccrine glands. Trabeculae subdividing the subcutaneous fat are thickened by an inflammatory infiltrate and deposition of new collagen. Large areas of subcutaneous fat are replaced by newly formed collagen composed of fine wavy fibers. Vascular changes in the early inflammatory stage may consist of endothelial swelling and edema of the walls of the vessels.

In the late sclerotic stage, as seen in the center of old lesions, the inflammatory infiltrate has disappeared almost completely, except in some areas of the subcutis. The epidermis is normal. The collagen bundles in the reticular dermis often appear thickened, closely packed, hypocellular, and hypereosinophilic. In the papillary dermis, homogeneous collagen may replace the normal loosely arranged fibers. The eccrine glands are atrophic, have few or no adipocytes surrounding them, and are surrounded by newly formed collagen. Few blood vessels are seen within the sclerotic collagen; they often have a fibrotic wall and a narrowed lumen. Hair follicles and sebaceous glands are absent. The fascia and striated muscles underlying lesions of morphea may be affected in the linear, segmental, subcutaneous, and generalized types, showing fibrosis and sclerosis similar to that seen in subcutaneous tissue. The muscle fibers appear vacuolated and separated from one another by edema and focal collections of inflammatory cells.

The histologic appearance of the skin lesions in systemic scleroderma is similar to that of morphea so that their histologic differentiation is not possible. However, in early lesions of systemic scleroderma, the inflammatory reaction is less pronounced than in morphea. The vascular changes in early lesions are slight, as in morphea. In contrast, in the late stage, systemic scleroderma shows more pronounced vascular changes than morphea, particularly in the subcutis. These changes include a paucity of blood vessels, thickening and hyalinization of their walls, and narrowing of the lumen.

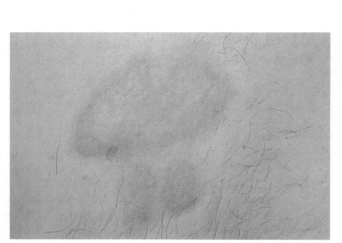

Clin. Fig. VF1.a

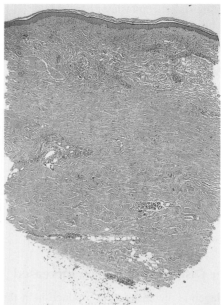

Fig. VF1.a

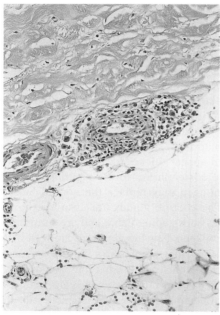

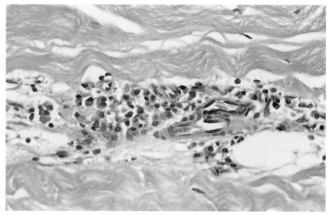

Fig. VF1.c

Fig. VF1.b

Clin. Fig. VF1.a. *Morphea.* Asymptomatic, indurated depressed plaques with white-appearing sclerotic centers are seen on the back of an otherwise healthy elderly man.

Fig. VF1.a. *Morphea, low power.* A late inflammatory lesion, with a patchy interstitial and perivascular inflammatory infiltrate, and partial sclerosis of dermal collagen.

Fig. VF1.b. *Morphea, medium power.* The infiltrate tends to be especially pronounced at the dermal–subcutaneous junction.

Fig. VF1.c. *Morphea, high power.* Lymphocytes and plasma cells are admixed in the infiltrate.

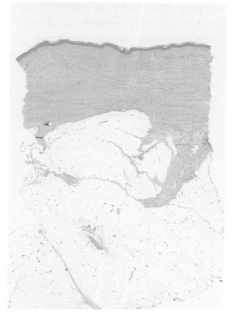

Fig. VF1.d

Fig. VF1.e

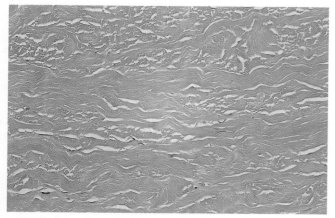

Fig. VF1.f

Fig. VF1.d. *Morphea, low power.* A late sclerotic lesion. The presence of dermal sclerosis is indicated by the straight sides of the punch biopsy.

Fig. VF1.e. *Morphea, medium power.* Skin appendages are lost within the sclerotic reticular dermis.

Fig. VF1.f. *Morphea, high power.* The collagen bundles in the reticular dermis appear thickened, closely packed, hypocellular, and hypereosinophilic. Blood vessels are few within the sclerotic collagen.

Even in late lesions, the epidermis usually appears normal. Aggregates of calcium may also be seen in the late stage within areas of sclerotic, homogeneous collagen of the subcutaneous tissue.

Radiation Dermatitis

CLINICAL SUMMARY. Early or acute radiation dermatitis develops after large doses of x-rays or radium. Erythema develops within about a week and may heal with desquamation and pigmentation. If the dose was high enough, painful blisters may develop at the site of erythema. In that case, healing usually takes place with atrophy, telangiectasia, and irregular hyperpigmentation. Subsequent to very large doses ulceration occurs, generally within 2 two months. Such an ulcer may heal ultimately with severe atrophic scarring, or it may not heal.

Late (chronic) radiation dermatitis occurs from a few months to many years after the administration of fractional doses of x-rays or radium. The skin shows atrophy, telangiectasia, and irregular hyper- and hypopigmentation. Ulceration, as well as foci of hyperkeratosis, may be seen within the areas of atrophy. Squamous cell carcinomas or basal cell epitheliomas may develop.

HISTOPATHOLOGY. In early radiation dermatitis, there is intracellular edema of the epidermis with pyknosis of the nuclei of epidermal and adnexal cells. An inflammatory infiltrate is present throughout the dermis and may permeate the epidermis. Some of the blood vessels are dilated, whereas others, especially large ones in the deep dermis, show edema of their walls, endothelial proliferation, and even thrombosis. The collagen bundles are edematous. In cases with blisters, the degenerated epidermis is detached from the dermis, and there may be ulceration, with necrosis and neutrophilic infiltration.

In late radiation dermatitis, the epidermis is irregular, with variable atrophy and hyperplasia, often with hyperkeratosis. The cells of the stratum malpighii may be disorderly, with individual cell keratinization, and some of the nuclei may be atypical. The epidermis may also show irregular downward growth and may even grow around telangiectatic vessels, nearly enclosing them. In the dermis, the collagen bundles are swollen and often hyalinized. Large, bizarre, stellate radiation fibroblasts may be found, with nuclei that are enlarged, irregular, and hyperchromatic. This radiation atypia differs from that seen in neoplasms because the cellularity is low and the atypical nuclei are scattered among other less atypical cells. Thus, the atypia is random rather than uniform. Blood vessels in the deep dermis often show fibrous thickening of

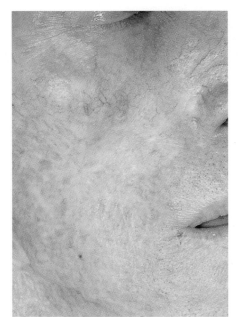

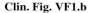

Clin. Fig. VF1.b

Clin. Fig. VF1.b. *Radiation dermatitis.* Chronic radiation changes of atrophy, hypopigmentation, hyperpigmentation, and telangiectases developed many years after radiation therapy for acne.

Fig. VF1.g. *Late radiation dermatitis, low power.* The dermal collagen is homogenized, telangiectatic vessels are apparent, and there are irregular downgrowths of the epidermis. Adnexal structures are markedly diminished.

Fig. VF1.h. *Late radiation dermatitis, medium power.* Stellate fibroblasts are prominent in the sclerotic collagen.

Fig. VF1.i. *Late radiation dermatitis, high power.* Randomly scattered fibroblasts exhibit nuclear enlarged and hyperchromatic nuclei. There are no mitoses, and there is no contiguous proliferation of the atypical cells.

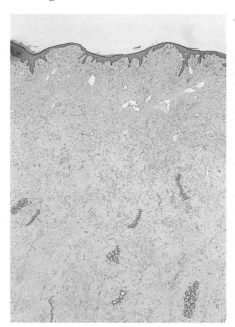

Fig. VF1.g

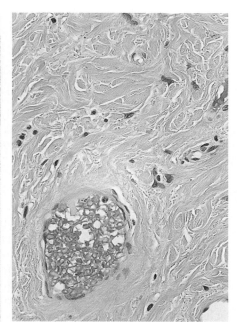

Fig. VF1.h   **Fig. VF1.i**

their walls, nearly or entirely occluding the lumen. Some vessels show thrombosis and recanalization. In contrast, the vessels of the upper dermis may be telangiectatic, and there may be lymphedema in the subepidermal region. Hair structures and sebaceous glands are absent, but the sweat glands usually are preserved at least in part, except in areas of severe injury.

Conditions to consider in the differential diagnosis:

scar, keloid
scleroderma/morphea
sclerodermoid graft-versus-host disease
phytonadione-induced pseudoscleroderma
necrobiosis lipoidica
eosinophilic fasciitis
radiation fibrosis
acrodermatitis chronica atrophicans
facial hemiatrophy
chronic lymphedema
necrobiosis lipoidica
acroosteolysis

VF2. Fiber Disorders, Collagen Reduced

Collagen may be reduced focally or diffusely as part of an inborn error of collagen fiber metabolism or as an acquired phenomenon. Focal dermal hypoplasia is a prototypic example (36).

Focal Dermal Hypoplasia Syndrome (Goltz)

CLINICAL SUMMARY. The focal dermal hypoplasia syndrome, or Goltz's syndrome, is probably due to an X-linked dominant gene lethal in homozygous males. Therefore, the syndrome occurs largely in females. The cutaneous manifestations include widely distributed linear areas of hypoplasia of the skin resembling striae distensae, soft yellow

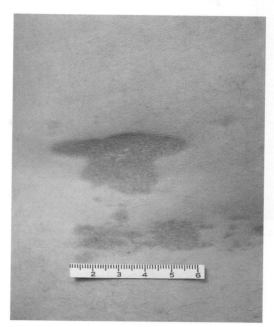

Clin. Fig. VF2. *Atrophoderma.* Sharply demarcated brown plaques with cliff-drop borders on the trunk are typical.

nodules, often in linear arrangement, and large ulcers due to congenital absence of skin that gradually heal with atrophy. The presence of fine, parallel, vertical striations in the metaphysis of long bones on radiography, referred to as osteopathia striata, is a reliable diagnostic marker of Goltz's syndrome.

HISTOPATHOLOGY. The linear areas of hypoplasia of the skin show a marked diminution in the thickness of the dermis, the collagen being present as thin fibers not united into

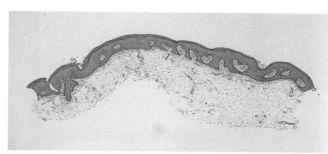

Fig. VF2.a

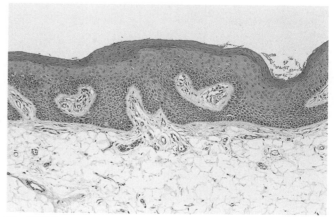

Fig. VF2.b

Fig. VF2.a. *Focal dermal hypoplasia syndrome (Goltz), low power.* The dermis is essentially absent. The epidermis in this example shows reactive changes.

Fig. VF2.b. *Focal dermal hypoplasia syndrome (Goltz), medium power.* Lobules of the subcutaneous fat extend up to the basal layer of the epidermis, partially separated only by a few wisps of collagen.

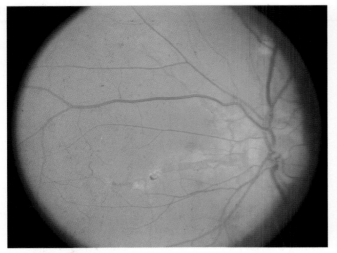

Clin. Fig. VF3.a

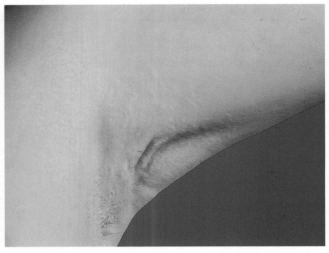

Clin. Fig. VF3.b

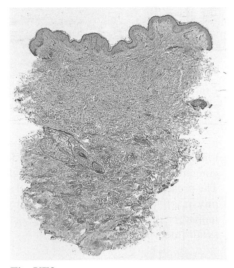

Fig. VF3.a

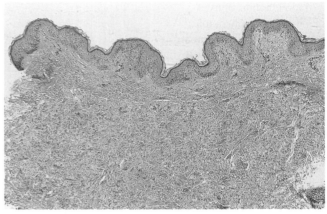

Fig. VF3.b

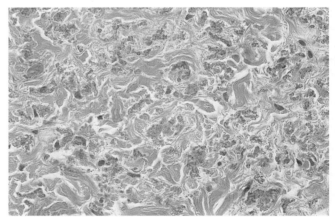

Fig. VF3.c

Clin. Fig. VF3.a. *Pseudoxanthoma elasticum (PXE).* An ophthalmologist detected angioid streaks in the retina of a middle-aged woman.

Clin. Fig. VF3.b. *Pseudoxanthoma elasticum.* Referral to dermatology confirmed the diagnosis of PXE with multiple yellowish waxy papules present in her axillae as shown here and in her antecubital fossae and neck region.

Fig. VF3.a. *Pseudoxanthoma elasticum, low power.* In this example, there is little calcification. The architecture of the reticular dermis appears subtly altered at scanning magnification.

Fig. VF3.b. *Pseudoxanthoma elasticum, medium power.* The collagen fibers are not arranged in their normal interlacing pattern.

Fig. VF3.c. *Pseudoxanthoma elasticum, high power.* At this power, the abnormal fibers, here staining a bright pink color, can be appreciated. (*continues*)

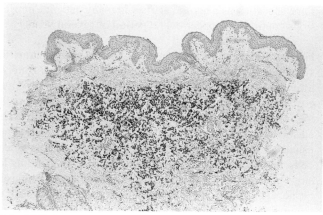

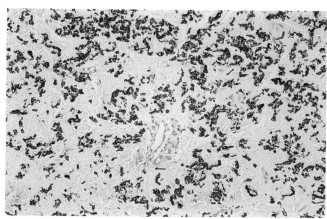

Fig. VF3.d

Fig. VF3.e

Fig. VF3.d. *Pseudoxanthoma elasticum, low power.* An elastic stain reveals the tangle of abnormal elastic fibers in the dermis.

Fig. VF3.e. *Pseudoxanthoma elasticum, medium power.* The fibers are abnormally short, swollen, and irregularly clumped.

bundles. The soft yellow nodules represent accumulations of fat that largely replace the dermis, so that the subcutaneous fat extends upward to the epidermis in some areas. Thin fibers of collagen and even some bundles of collagen resembling those of normal dermis may be located between the subepidermal adipose tissue and the subcutaneous fat.

Conditions to consider in the differential diagnosis:

Ehlers–Danlos syndrome
Marfan's syndrome
penicillamine-induced atrophy
striae distensae
aplasia cutis
focal dermal hypoplasia (Goltz)
atrophoderma (Pasini and Pierini)
relapsing polychondritis (type II collagen degeneration of cartilage)

VF3. Fiber Disorders, Elastin Increased or Prominent

Abnormal elastic fibers are increased focally in the dermis and may become calcified as in pseudoxanthoma elasticum, or there is diffuse elastosis in the superficial reticular dermis of sun-exposed skin. Pseudoxanthoma elasticum is a good example (37).

Pseudoxanthoma Elasticum

CLINICAL SUMMARY. In this disorder, genetically abnormal elastic fibers with a tendency toward calcification occur in the skin and frequently also in the retina and within the walls of arteries, particularly the gastric mucosal arteries, coronary arteries, and large peripheral arteries. The inheritance is usually autosomal recessive but is occasionally autosomal dominant. The cutaneous lesions usually appear first in the second or third decade of life and are generally progressive in extent and severity. They consist of soft, yellowish, coalescing papules, and the affected skin appears loose and wrinkled. The sides of the neck, the axillae, and the groin are the most common sites of lesions. In the eyes, so-called angioid streaks of the fundi may cause progressive impairment of vision. Involvement of the arteries of the gastric mucosa may lead to gastric hemorrhage, coronary artery involvement may result in attacks of angina pectoris, and involvement of the large peripheral arteries may cause intermittent claudication. Radiologic examination in such cases reveals extensive calcification of the affected arteries.

HISTOPATHOLOGY. Histologic examination of the involved skin reveals in the middle and lower thirds of the dermis considerable accumulations of swollen and irregularly clumped fibers stain like elastic fibers with orcein or Verhoeff's stain. With routine hematoxylin-eosin, the altered elastic fibers stain faintly basophilic because of their calcium imbibition, and staining for calcium with the von Kossa method shows them well. In the vicinity of the altered elastic fibers, there may be accumulations of a slightly basophilic mucoid material, which stains strongly positive with the colloidal iron reaction or with Alcian blue. In some cases with pronounced elastic tissue calcification, a macrophage and giant cell reaction may be present.

The angioid streaks occur in Bruch's membrane, which is located between the retina and the choroid and possesses numerous elastic fibers in its outer portion, the lamina elastica. Calcification of these fibers causes fissures to form in the lamina elastica. These fissures result in repeated hemorrhages and exudates, which in turn cause scarring and pigment shifting in the retina. Gastric bleeding is the result of calcification of elastic fibers in the thin-walled arteries located immediately beneath the gastric mucosa. The internal elastic lamina is particularly affected. In muscular arteries, such as the coronary arteries and the large peripheral arteries, calcification begins in the internal and external elastic laminae, leading to their fragmentation, and subsequently extends to the media and intima.

Conditions to consider in the differential diagnosis:

pseudoxanthoma elasticum
penicillamine-induced elastosis perforans
solar elastosis
erythema ab igne
annular elastolytic giant cell granuloma (actinic granuloma)

VF4. Fiber Disorders, Elastin Reduced

Elastin may be reduced focally or diffusely as part of an inborn error of its metabolism or as an acquired phenomenon. These disorders are uncommon. Anetoderma is prototypic (38).

Macular Atrophy (Anetoderma)

CLINICAL SUMMARY. Macular atrophy, or anetoderma, is characterized by atrophic patches located mainly on the upper trunk. The skin of the patches is thin and blue-white and bulges slightly. The lesions may give the palpating finger the same sensation as a hernial orifice. In many patients, new lesions continue to appear over a period of several years.

HISTOPATHOLOGY (NOT SHOWN). Early, erythematous lesions usually show a moderate perivascular infiltrate of mononuclear cells. Occasionally, neutrophils and eosinophils predominate and nuclear dust is present, resulting in a histologic picture of leukocytoclastic vasculitis. The elastic tissue may still appear normal in an early lesion, but usually it is already decreased or even absent. Mononuclear cells may be seen adhering to elastic fibers. Longstanding lesions generally show a more or less complete loss of elastic tissue, either in the papillary and upper reticular dermis or in the upper reticular dermis only.

Conditions to consider in the differential diagnosis:

cutis laxa
anetoderma
middermal elastolysis

VF5. Fiber Disorders, Perforating

Abnormal elastin or collagen fibers may be extruded through the epidermis, which may form channels that extend down

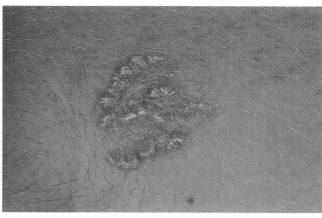

Clin. Fig. VF5

Clin. Fig. VF5. *Elastosis perforans serpiginosa.* Papules in an annular and serpiginous configuration appeared on the volar forearms in a healthy adult woman.

Fig. VF5.a. *Elastosis perforans serpiginosum, low power.* There is a narrow curved channel extending through an acanthotic epidermis. The upper portion of the channel contains basophilic degenerate material. The lower portion of the channel contains elastic fibers in addition to the degenerate material. (E. Heilman and R. Friedman)

Fig. VF5.b. *Elastosis perforans serpiginosum, high power.* There are thickened degenerated elastic fibers at the origin of the epidermal channel. (E. Heilman and R. Friedman)

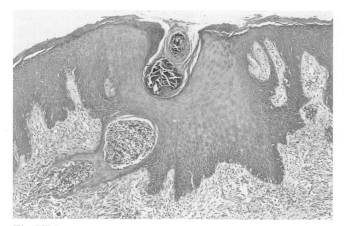

Fig. VF5.a

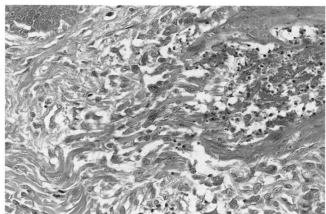

Fig. VF5.b

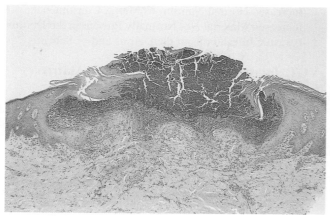

Fig. VF5.c

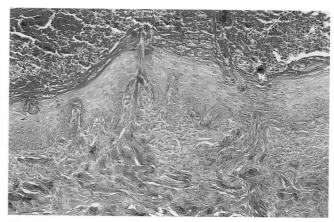

Fig. VF5.d

Fig. VF5.c. *Reactive perforating collagenosis, low power.* A cup-shaped channel containing degenerated collagen bundles and basophilic material.

Fig. VF5.d. *Reactive perforating collagenosis, trichrome stain, medium power.* Blue-stained collagen fibers perforating the channel and extending to the surface.

into the dermis. Elastosis perforans serpiginosum (EPS) is prototypic (39).

Elastosis Perforans Serpiginosum

CLINICAL SUMMARY. In EPS, increased numbers of thickened elastic fibers are present in the upper dermis and altered elastic fibers are extruded through the epidermis. It is a rare disorder that affects young individuals, men more often than women, with a peak incidence in the second decade. EPS is primarily a papular eruption localized to one anatomic site and most commonly affecting the nape of the neck, the face, or the upper extremities. The papules are typically 2 to 5 mm

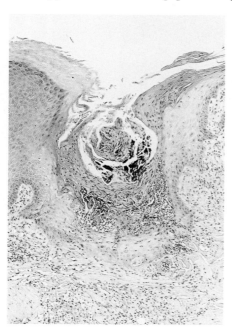

Fig. VF5.e. *Perforating folliculitis, medium power.* A dilated follicular unit contains a keratotic plug with an admixture of basophilic debris. The follicular epithelium is perforated, and there are degenerated collagen fibers in the adjacent dermis. (E. Heilman and R. Friedman)

Fig. VF5.e

in diameter and are arranged in arcuate or serpiginous groups and may coalesce.

Important associations of EPS with systemic diseases include Down syndrome, Ehlers–Danlos syndrome, osteogenesis imperfecta, pseudoxanthoma elasticum, and Marfan's syndrome. In addition, on rare occasions EPS is observed in association with Rothmund–Thompson syndrome or other connective tissue disorders, and it also may occur as a complication of penicillamine administration.

HISTOPATHOLOGY. The essential findings include a narrow transepidermal channel of acantholytic epidermis that may be straight, wavy, or of corkscrew shape containing thick, coarse, elastic fibers admixed with granular basophilic staining debris. A mixed inflammatory cell infiltrate accompanies the fibers in the channel. Abnormal elastic fibers are present in the upper dermis in the vicinity of the channel. In this zone, the elastic fibers are increased in size and number. As these fibers enter the lower portion of the channel, they maintain their normal staining characteristics, but as they approach the epidermal surface, they may not stain as expected with elastic stains.

Reactive Perforating Collagenosis

See Figs. VF5.c and VF5.d.

Perforating Folliculitis

See Fig. VF5.e.

Conditions to consider in the differential diagnosis:
elastosis perforans serpiginosum
Kyrle's disease
perforating folliculitis
reactive perforating collagenosis
perforating disorder of renal failure and diabetes
perforating calcific elastosis
perforating granuloma annulare

VG. DEPOSITION OF MATERIAL IN THE DERMIS

The dermis serves as a reaction site for a variety of inflammatory, infiltrative, and desmoplastic processes, which may include accumulations of matrix molecules that may be either indigenous to the normal dermis or foreign to it.

1. Increased Normal Nonfibrous Matrix Constituents
2. Increased Material Not Normally Present in the Dermis
3. Parasitic Infestations of the Dermis and/or Subcutis

VG1. Increased Normal Nonfibrous Matrix Constituents

Ground substance (hyaluronic acid) is increased, associated with a varying inflammatory infiltrate that can include lym-

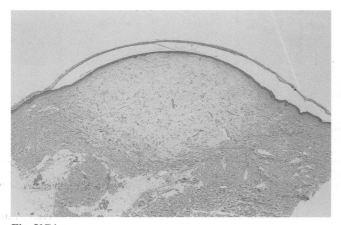

Fig. VG1.a

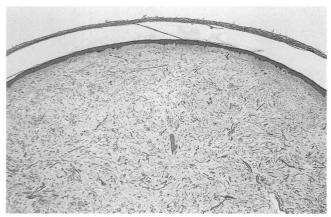

Fig. VG1.b

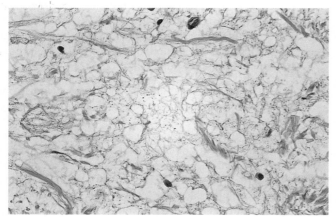

Fig. VG1.c

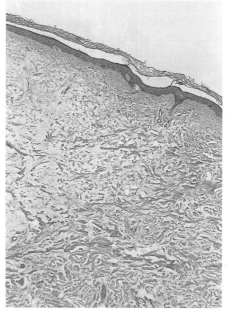

Fig. VG1.d

Fig. VG1.a. *Cutaneous focal mucinosis, low power.* There is a zone of pallor in the superficial dermis, extending up to the epidermis.

Fig. VG1.b. *Cutaneous focal mucinosis, medium power.* The collagen bundles are separated by ground substance (mucin) that can be shown by a colloidal iron stain to contain abundant hyaluronic acid.

Fig. VG1.c. *Cutaneous focal mucinosis, high power.* There is an increase in interstitial mucin, and an apparent diminution in collagen, but vessels are not increased.

Fig. VG1.d. *Cutaneous focal mucinosis, medium power.* At the edge of the lesion, the mucin gradually diminishes.

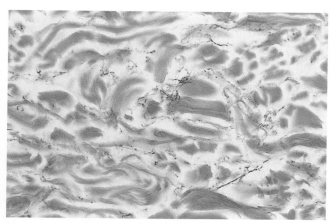

Fig. VG1.e. *Lupus erythematosus, high power.* Basophilic mucinous material is present diffusely between otherwise unaltered collagen bundles in a lesion from a patient with lupus.

phocytes, plasma cells, and eosinophils. Digital mucous cysts and focal mucinosis (40) are common examples.

Digital Mucous Cysts and Focal Mucinosis

CLINICAL SUMMARY. Two types of digital mucous cysts exist. One type presents as a pale papule, analogous to focal mucinosis. It differs from focal mucinosis only by its location near the proximal nail fold and by its greater tendency to fluctuation (41). The other type is located on the dorsum of a finger near the distal interphalangeal joint and is due to a herniation of the joint lining, thus representing a ganglion (42).

HISTOPATHOLOGY. The *myxomatous type* of digital mucous cyst in its early stage has the same histologic appearance as that seen in focal mucinosis, namely, an ill-defined area of

mucinous material. Subsequently, multiple clefts form and then coalesce into one large cystic space containing mucin composed largely of hyaluronic acid, which stains with Alcian blue and colloidal iron. The cystic space in early lesions is separated from the epidermis by mucinous stroma, but in older lesions is found in a subepidermal location with thinning of the overlying epidermis. The collagen at the periphery of the cyst appears compressed. No lining of the cyst wall is apparent. In the *ganglion type* of digital mucous cyst, the cyst shows an epithelial lining and evidence of a pedicle leading to the joint spaces on surgical exploration.

Mucinosis in Lupus Erythematosus

See Fig. VG1.e.

Myxedema

See Figs. VG1.f and VG1.g.

Scleredema

See Figs. VG1.h–VG1.j.

Scleromyxedema

See Figs. VG1.k–VG1.m.

   Conditions to consider in the differential diagnosis:
      granuloma annulare
      pretibial myxedema
      generalized myxedema
      juvenile cutaneous mucinosis
      papular mucinosis (lichen myxedematosus)
      scleromyxedema
      reticulated erythematous mucinosis
      scleredema
      focal dermal mucinosis
      digital mucous cyst/myxoid cyst

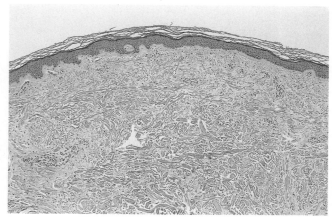

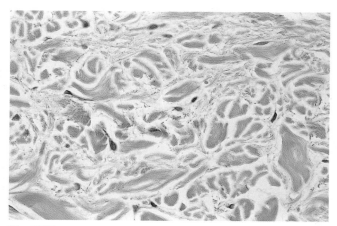

Fig. VG1.f

Fig. VG1.g

Fig. VG1.f. *Myxedema, low power.* Increased mucin is present in the dermis, particularly in the upper half. As a result, the dermis is greatly thickened.

Fig. VG1.g. *Myxedema, high power.* The mucin as threads and granules resulting in the splitting up of collagen bundles into fibers and wide separation of the fibers. As a result of shrinkage of the mucin during the process of fixation and dehydration, there are empty spaces within the mucin deposits. The number of fibroblasts is not increased.

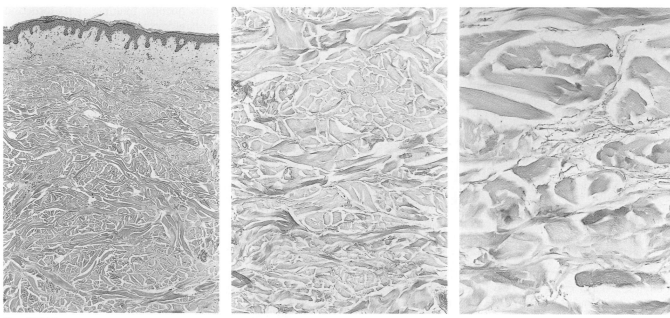

Fig. VG1.h   Fig. VG1.i   Fig. VG1.j

Fig. VG1.h. *Scleredema, low power.* The dermis is greatly thickened. The collagen bundles are thickened and separated by clear spaces, causing fenestration of the collagen.

Fig. VG1.i. *Scleredema, medium power, colloidal iron.* The separation of collagen bundles is not accompanied by an increase in cellularity.

Fig. VG1.j. *Scleredema, high power, colloidal iron.* In this and the previous figure, the separation is seen to be due to interstitial mucin, which is highlighted by the colloidal iron reaction.

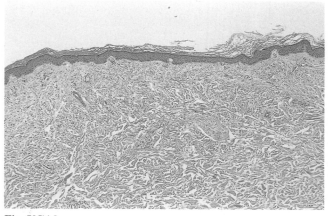
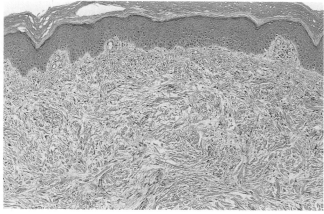

Fig. VG1.k   Fig. VG1.l

Fig. VG1.k. *Scleromyxedema, low power.* The skin is diffusely thickened, and there is an appearance of increased cellularity.

Fig. VG1.l. *Scleromyxedema, medium power.* The increased cellularity is due to extensive proliferation of fibroblasts throughout the dermis, associated with irregularly arranged bundles of collagen.

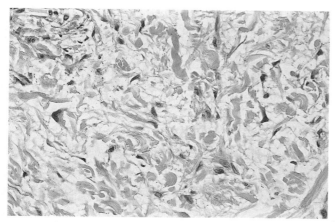

Fig. VG1.m. *Scleromyxedema, high power.* The collagen bundles tend to be split into individual fibers by mucin. As a rule, the amount of mucin is greater in the upper half than in the lower half of the dermis.

cutaneous myxoma
mucocoele, mucinous mucosal cyst
lupus erythematosus
hereditary progressive mucinous histiocytosis

VG2. Increased Material Not Normally Present in the Dermis

Materials not present in substantial amounts in the normal dermis are deposited, as crystals (gout), amorphous deposits (calcinosis), hyaline material (colloid milium, amyloidosis, porphyria), or as pigments. Gout is prototypic (43).

Gout

CLINICAL SUMMARY. In the early stage of gout, there are usually irregularly recurring attacks of acute arthritis. In the late stage, deposits of monosodium urate form within and around various joints, leading to chronic arthritis with de-

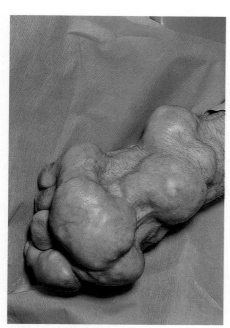

Clin. Fig. VG2.a

Clin. Fig. VG2.a. *Gout.* This elderly woman had a 17-year history of large globular tophi that become tender and required drainage.

Fig. VG2.a. *Gout, low power.* Irregular masses of pale material are present in the dermis.

Fig. VG2.b. *Gout, high power.* The material consists of narrow elongated crystals, best seen postfixation in alcohol. After aqueous fixation, a negative impression of the dissolved crystals can usually be discerned. There is a surrounding foreign-body giant cell reaction.

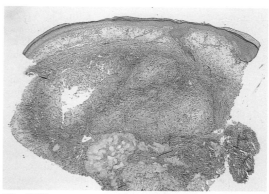

Fig. VG2.a

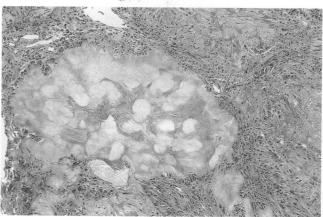

Fig. VG2.b

struction in the joints and the adjoining bone. During this late stage, urate deposits, called tophi, may occur in the dermis and subcutaneous tissue. Tophi are most commonly observed on the helix of the ears, over the bursae of the elbows, and on the fingers and toes. They may attain a diameter of several centimeters and when large may discharge a chalky material. In rare instances, gout may present as tophi on the fingertips or as panniculitis on the legs without the coexistence of a gouty arthritis.

HISTOPATHOLOGY.   For the histologic examination of tophi, fixation in absolute ethanol or an ethanol-based fixative, such as Carnoy's fluid, is preferable to fixation in formalin; aqueous fixatives such as formalin dissolve the characteristic urate crystals, leaving only amorphous material that, however, can usually be recognized as the residue of a tophus because of the characteristic rim of foreign-body giant cells and macrophages that surrounds the aggregates of amorphous material. Anhydrous tissue processing is also important to preserve the urate crystals. On fixation in alcohol, tophi can be seen to consist of variously sized sharply demarcated aggregates of needle-shaped urate crystals lying closely packed in the form of bundles or sheaves. The crystals often have a brownish color and are doubly refractile on polariscopic examination.

Colloid Milium

See Figs. VG2.c and VG2.d

Idiopathic Calcinosis Cutis

CLINICAL SUMMARY.   Even though the underlying connective tissue disease in some instances of dystrophic calcinosis cutis may be mild and can be overlooked unless specifically searched for, there remain cases of idiopathic calcinosis cutis that resemble dystrophic calcinosis cutis but show no underlying disease. Tumoral calcinosis is regarded as a special manifestation of idiopathic calcinosis cutis (44). It consists of numerous large, subcutaneous, calcified masses that may be associated with papular and nodular skin lesions of calcinosis. The disease usually is familial and is associated with hyperphosphatemia. Otherwise, the resemblance of tumoral calcinosis to the dystrophic calcinosis universalis observed with dermatomyositis is great.

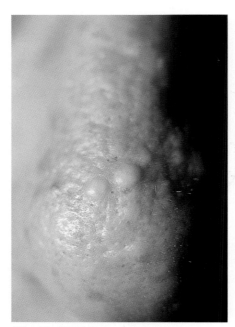

Clin. Fig. VG2.b

Clin. Fig. VG2.b. *Colloid milium.* These asymptomatic, whitish, soft papules on the nose were an incidental finding on examination.

Fig. VG2.c. *Colloid milium, low power.* A nodule of pink amorphous material is present in the papillary dermis.

Fig. VG2.d. *Colloid milium, medium power.* The papillary dermis adjacent to the nodule shows severe actinic elastosis.

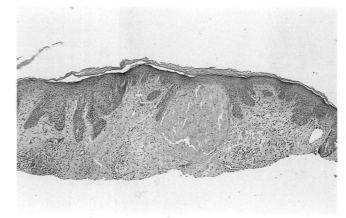

Fig. VG2.c

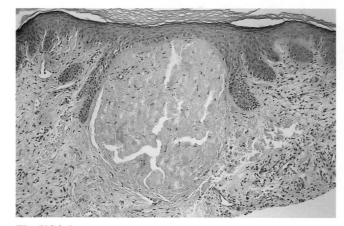

Fig. VG2.d

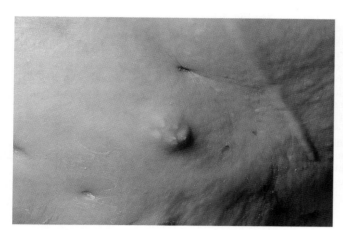

Clin. Fig. VG2.c

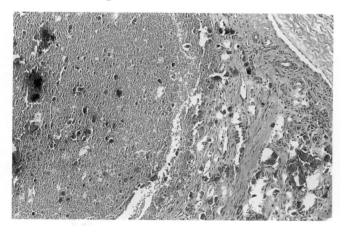

Fig. VG2.f

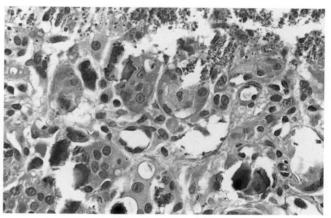

Fig. VG2.e

Fig. VG2.g

Clin. Fig. VG2.c. *Calcinosis cutis*. Firm, grouped, whitish papules on the trunk of an individual without obvious predisposing factors for calcification.

Fig. VG2.e. *Idiopathic calcinosis cutis, low power*. A tumoral mass of calcium is present in the dermis. There are no obvious changes of associated connective tissue disease, or other predisposing condition for dystrophic calcification.

Fig. VG2.f. *Idiopathic calcinosis cutis, medium power*. An amorphous mass of calcium in the dermis, with an adjacent reaction.

Fig. VG2.g. *Idiopathic calcinosis cutis, high power*. There is a brisk foreign-body reaction to the calcium deposits.

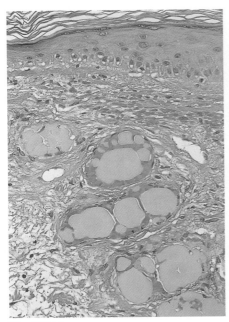

Fig. VG2.h. *Cryoglobulinemia, medium power.* In type I cryoglobulinemia, amorphous material (precipitated monoclonal cryoglobulins in this case of Waldenstrom's macroglobulinemia) is deposited subjacent to endothelium and throughout the vessel wall and within the vessel lumen, resulting in a noninflammatory thrombuslike appearance.

Fig. VG2.h

HISTOPATHOLOGY. Tumoral calcinosis shows in the subcutaneous tissue large masses of calcium surrounded by a foreign-body reaction. Intradermal aggregates are present in some cases. Discharge of calcium may take place through areas of ulceration or by means of transepidermal elimination.

Cryoglobulinemia
See Fig. VG2.h.

Keratin Granuloma
See Figs. VG2.i–VG2.k.

Suture Granuloma
See Figs. VG2.l–VG2.n.

Conditions to consider in the differential diagnosis:
    gout
    colloid milium
    calcinosis cutis
    calcinosis universalis, circumscripta (scleroderma)
    tumoral calcinosis
    idiopathic calcification of the scrotum
    subepidermal calcified nodule
    amyloidosis
    dermal pigments
    minocycline

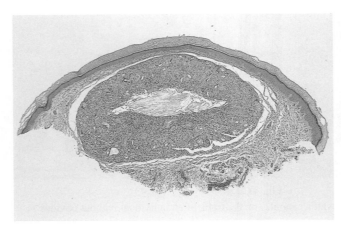

Fig. VG2.i.

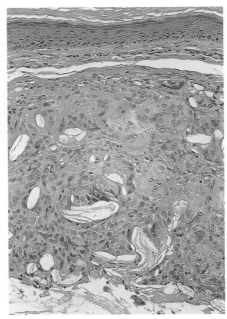

Fig. VG2.j

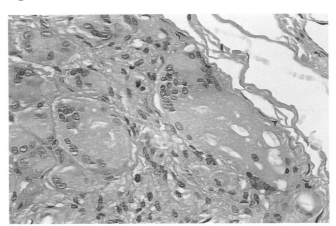

Fig. VG2.k

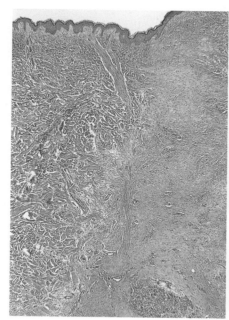

Fig. VG2.l

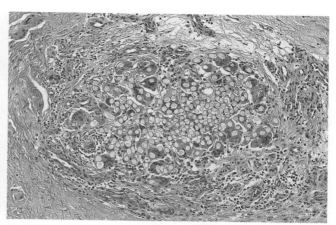

Fig. VG2.m

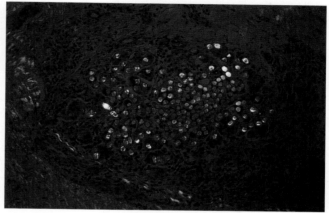

Fig. VG2.n

Fig. VG2.l. *Suture granuloma, low power.* At the base of a scar to the right, there is a cluster of pink cells and gray fibers.

Fig. VG2.m. *Suture granuloma, medium power.* The cells are foreign-body giant cells and the fibers are those of a suture cut in cross-section.

Fig. VG2.n. *Suture granuloma, high power.* Many manufactured fibers are birefringence as viewed here between crossed polarizing filters.

Fig. VG2.i. *Keratin granuloma, low power.* There is a collection of keratin in the dermis, representing the site of rupture of an epidermal cyst. There is a foreign-body giant cell reaction at the periphery.

Fig. VG2.j. *Keratin granuloma, medium power.* Gray-pink keratin flakes are present in the center of the lesion and in giant cells at its periphery.

Fig. VG2.k. *Keratin granuloma, high power.* In some lesions, the flakes of keratin may be difficult to appreciate, but may be found within the cytoplasm of giant cells. Their color is often gray rather than the expected pink.

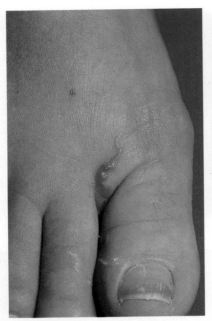

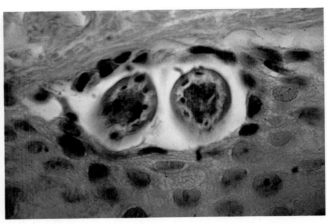

Fig. VG3.a

Clin. Fig. VG3

Clin. Fig. VG3. *Larva migrans.* Shortly after vacationing in Jamaica, a patient noticed a pruritic creeping movement that manifested as a serpiginous plaque. Aggressive cryotherapy resulted in resolution.

Fig. VG3.a *Larva migrans, high power.* Cross-section of larva of ancylostoma in the stratum corneum (periodic acid–Schiff stain). (From Johnson BJ Jr., Honig P, Jaworsky C, eds. *Pediatric dermatopathology.* Newton, MA: Butterworth-Heineman, 1994. Reprinted with permission.)

argyria
chrysiasis
mercury pigmentation
hemochromatosis
alkaptonuric ochronosis
calcaneal petechiae (hemoglobin)
lipoid proteinosis (hyalinosis cutis et mucosae,
   Urbach-Wiethe)
cryoglobulinemia
porphyria cutanea tarda
foreign material—dirt, glass, paraffin, grease
tattoo reactions
silicone, talc, starch
cactus, sea-urchin, hair granulomas
intralesional steroids
vaccines
Hunter's syndrome (lysosomal storage granules)

VG3. Parasitic Infestations of the Skin

Macroscopically visible parasitic agents may infest the dermis and subcutis. Creeping eruption (larva migrans) is a good example (45).

Larva Migrans Eruption

CLINICAL SUMMARY. Larva migrans eruption, commonly known as creeping eruption, is caused by filariform larvae of the dog and cat hookworms *Ancylostoma braziliensis* and *A. caninum.* Migration is manifested by an irregularly linear, thin, raised burrow, 2 to 3 mm wide. The larva moves a few millimeters per day. The eruption is self-limited because humans are abnormal hosts. The feet and buttocks are the areas most commonly involved.

HISTOPATHOLOGY. The larva is found in a specimen taken from just beyond the leading edge of the track. It is located in a burrow in the superficial epidermis. The lesion, aside from the larva, which is often not observed in the biopsies, shows spongiosis and intraepidermal vesicles containing necrotic keratinocytes. The epidermis and the upper dermis contain a chronic inflammatory infiltrate with many eosinophils.

Conditions to consider in the differential diagnosis:

Larva migrans (Ancylostoma)
subcutaneous dirofilariasis
onchocerciasis
strongyloidiasis
schistosomiasis
subcutaneous cysticercosis
myiasis

REFERENCES

1. Bressler GS, Jones RE Jr. Erythema annulare centrifugum. *J Am Acad Dermatol* 1981;4:597.
2. Shaffer B, Jacobsen C, Beerman H. Histopathologic correlation of lesions of papular urticaria and positive skin test reactions to insect antigens. *Arch Dermatol* 1954;70:437.
3. Cohen LM, Capeless EL, Krusinski PA, Maloney ME. Pruritic urticarial papules and plaques of pregnancy and its relationship to maternal-fetal weight gain and twin pregnancy. *Arch Dermatol* 1989;125:1534.
4. Jeerapaet P, Ackerman AS. Histologic patterns of secondary syphilis. *Arch Dermatol* 1973;107:373.
5. Berger BW. Erythema chronicum migrans of Lyme disease. *Arch Dermatol* 1984;120:1017.
6. Magrinat G, Kerwin KS, Gabriel DA. The clinical manifestations of Degos' syndrome. *Arch Pathol Lab Med* 1989;113:354.
7. Wall LM, Smith NP. Perniosis: a histopathological review. *Clin Exp Dermatol* 1981;6:263
8. Diaz-Perez JL, Winkelmann RK. Cutaneous polyarteritis nodosa. *Arch Dermatol* 1974;110:407.
9. Finan MC, Winkelman RK. The cutaneous extravascular necrotizing granuloma (Churg-Strauss granuloma) and systemic disease: a review of 27 cases. *Medicine (Baltimore)* 1983;62:142.
10. Fischer AH, Morris DJ. Pathogenesis of calciphylaxis: study of three cases with literature review. *Hum Pathol* 1995;26:1055.
11. Akasu R, Kahn HJ, From L. Lymphocyte markers on formalin-fixed tissue in Jessner's lymphocytic infiltrate and lupus erythematosus. *J Cutan Pathol* 1992;19:59.
12. Von Den Driesch P. Sweet's syndrome: acute febrile neutrophilic dermatosis. *J Am Acad Dermatol* 1994;31:535.
13. Bisno AL, Stevens DL. Streptococcal infections of skin and soft tissues. *N Engl J Med* 1996;334:240.
14. Ridley DS. Histological classification and the immunological spectrum of leprosy. *Bull World Health Organ* 1974;51:451.
15. Risdall RJ, Dehner LP, Duray P, et al. Histiocytosis X (Langerhans cell histiocytosis): prognostic role of histopathology. *Arch Pathol Lab Med* 1983;107:59.
16. Fisher GB, Greer KE, Copper PH. Eosinophilic cellulitis (Wells' syndrome). *Int J Dermatol* 1985;24:101.
17. Convit J, Ulrich M, Fernandez CT, et al. The clinical and immunological spectrum of American cutaneous leishmaniasis. *Trans R Soc Trop Med Hyg* 1993;87:444.
18. Kopf AW, Weidman AI. Nevus of Ota. *Arch Dermatol* 1962;85:195.
19. Tanabe JL, Huntley AC. Granulomatous tertiary syphilis. *J Am Acad Dermatol* 1986;15:341.
20. O'Brien TJ. Iodic eruptions. *Australas J Dermatol* 1987;28:119.
21. Mercurio MG, Elewski BE. Cutaneous blastomycosis. *Cutis* 1992;50:422.
22. Olive KE, Kataria YP. Cutaneous manifestations of sarcoidosis. *Arch Intern Med* 1985;145:1811.
23. Farina MC, Gegundez MI, Pique E, et al. Cutaneous tuberculosis: a clinical, histopathologic, and bacteriologic study. *J Am Acad Dermatol* 1995;33:433.
24. Umbert P, Winkelmann RK. Histologic, ultrastructural, and histochemical studies of granuloma annulare. *Arch Dermatol* 1977;113:1681.
25. Lowitt MH, Dover JS. Necrobiosis lipoidica. *J Am Acad Dermatol* 1991;25:735.
26. Mehregan DA, Winkelmann RK. Necrobiotic xanthogranuloma. *Arch Dermatol* 1992;128:94.
27. Veys EM, De Keyser F. Rheumatoid nodules: differential diagnosis and immunohistological findings. *Ann Rheum Dis* 1993;52:625.
28. Epstein WL, Shahen JR, Krasnobrod H. The organized epithelioid cell granuloma: differentiation of allergic (zirconium) from colloidal (silica) types. *Am J Pathol* 1963;43:391.
29. Olsen TG, Helwig EB. Angiolymphoid hyperplasia with eosinophilia: a clinicopathologic study of 116 patients. *J Am Acad Dermatol* 1985;12:781.
30. Urabe H, Honbo S. Sporotrichosis. *Int J Dermatol* 1986;25:255.
31. Hacker P. Botryomycosis. *Int J Dermatol* 1983;22:455.
32. Estes SE, Hendricks AA, Merz WG, Prystowsky SD. Primary cutaneous aspergillosis. *J Am Acad Dermatol* 1980;3:397.
33. Fiumara NJ, Rothman K, Tang S. The diagnosis and treatment of chancroid. *J Am Acad Dermatol* 1986;15:939.
34. Su WP, Schroeter AL, Perry HO, Powell FC. Histopathologic and immunopathologic study of pyoderma gangrenosum. *J Cutan Pathol* 1986;13:323.
35. Callen JP, Tuffanelli DL, Provost TT. Collagen-vascular disease: an update. *J Am Acad Dermatol* 1993;28:477.
36. Goltz RW, Henderson RR, Hitch JM et al. Focal dermal hypoplasia syndrome. *Arch Dermatol* 1970;101:1.
37. Danielsen L, Kohayasi T, Larsen HW, et al. Pseudoxanthoma elasticum. *Acta Derm Venereol (Stockh)* 1970;50:355.
38. Miller WM, Ruggles CW, Rist TE. Anetoderma. *Int J Dermatol* 1979;18:43.
39. Mehregan AH. Elastosis perforans serpiginosa: a review of the literature and report of 11 cases. *Arch Dermatol* 1968;97:381.
40. Wilk M, Schmoekel C. Cutaneous focal mucinosis: a histopathological and immunohistochemical analysis of 11 cases. *J Cutan Pathol* 1994;21:446.
41. Salasche SJ. Myxoid cysts of the proximal nail fold. *J Dermatol Surg Oncol* 1984;10:35.
42. Armijo M. Mucoid cysts of the fingers. *J Dermatol Surg Oncol* 1981;7:317.
43. Lichtenstein L, Scott HW, Levin MH. Pathologic changes in gout. *Am J Pathol* 1956;32:871.
44. Pursley TV, Prince MJ, Chausmer AB et al. Cutaneous manifestations of tumoral calcinosis. *Arch Dermatol* 1979;115:1100.
45. Sulica VJ, Berberian B, Kao GF. Histopathologic findings in cutaneous larva migrans [abstract]. *J Cutan Pathol* 1988;15:346.

VI

Tumors and Cysts of the Dermis and Subcutis

Neoplasms in the reticular dermis may arise from any of the tissues included in the dermis-lymphoreticular tissue, connective tissue, and epithelial tissue of the skin appendages. In addition, metastases are commonly present in the dermis and subcutis. A neoplastic nodule is a circumscribed collection of neoplastic cells in the dermis. Abscesses, granulomas, and cysts may also present as nodules. Cysts are considered separately. In general, neoplastic nodules can be differentiated from reactive and inflammatory nodules by the presence of a monotonous population of cells consistent with a clonal proliferation, whereas inflammatory nodules are composed of inflammatory cell types (lymphocytes, neutrophils, histiocytes), generally in a heterogeneous mixture.

VIA. SMALL CELL TUMORS

The cells of this group of tumors range in size from that of a small lymphocyte to approximately that of a histiocyte. These tumors are generally characterized by having very scant cytoplasm, so that the nuclei are closely apposed to one another and may even mold on one another, as is characteristic in small cell carcinomas of the lung. The nuclei, although larger than those of lymphocytes (except in the case of a well-differentiated small cell lymphoma), are relatively small by virtue of having compact hyperchromatic chromatin and, usually, absent or inconspicuous nucleoli.

1. Tumors of Lymphocytes or Hemopoietic Cells
2. Tumors of Lymphocytes and Mixed Cell Types
3. Tumors of Plasma Cells
4. Small Round Cell Tumors

VIA1. Tumors of Lymphocytes or Hemopoietic Cells

Nodular infiltrates or extensive diffuse infiltrates of normal and/or atypical lymphocytes are found in the dermis. Cutaneous follicular center cell lymphoma is prototypic (1).

Cutaneous B-Cell Lymphoma

CLINICAL SUMMARY. Primary cutaneous follicular center cell lymphoma (FL) was at first regarded as the cutaneous counterpart of nodal follicular center lymphoma. More recently, it has become apparent that these lymphomas resemble lymphomas of the "mucosal-associated lymphoid tissue" (MALToma) and the so-called "marginal zone" lymphomas of the spleen, and share the favorable prognosis of these extranodal neoplasms. Another form of lymphoma in which a follicular pattern is evident and that may occur in the skin is

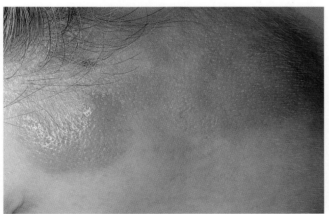

Clin. Fig. VIA1.a

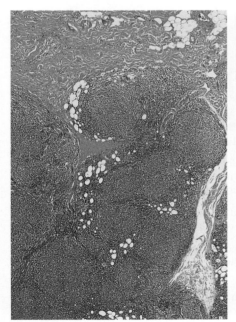

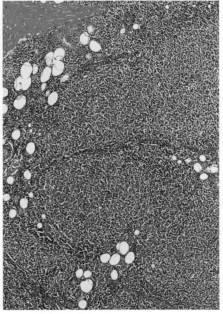

Fig. VIA1.a   Fig. VIA1.b

Clin. Fig. VIA1.a. *Cutaneous lymphoma.* A 57-year-old woman with B-cell lymphoma developed asymptomatic erythematous-lavender plaques and tumors on the face and scalp.

Fig. VIA1.a. *Cutaneous follicular B-cell lymphoma, low power.* A multinodular pattern is clearly evident in this lymphomatous infiltrate situated at the dermal–subcutaneous junction composed of small cleaved follicular center cells arranged as coalescing follicles. (P. LeBoit and T. McCalmont)

Fig. VIA1.b. *Cutaneous follicular B-cell lymphoma, medium power.* Note the absence of tingible-body macrophages. (P. LeBoit and T. McCalmont)

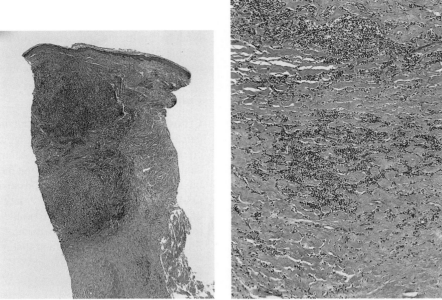

Fig. VIA1.c

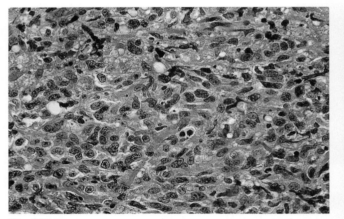

Fig. VIA1.e

Fig. VIA1.d

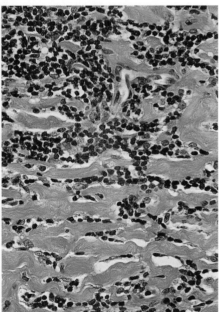

Fig. VIA1.f

Fig. VIA1.c. *Cutaneous diffuse B-cell lymphoma, low power.* There is a dense dermal infiltrate of basophilic cells that does not involve the overlying epidermis. Typically, in cutaneous B-cell lymphoma, the infiltrate is "bottom heavy," meaning that a significant portion of the infiltrate involves the lower dermis.

Fig. VIA1.d. *Cutaneous diffuse B-cell lymphoma, medium power.* The dermal infiltrate may be nodular in appearance, however, as seen here the cells frequently permeate between bundles of reticular dermal collagen.

Fig. VIA1.e. *Cutaneous diffuse B-cell lymphoma, high power.* High power reveals cytologically atypical lymphoid cells admixed with nuclear fragments. With little pressure from a punch biopsy, these cells frequently show crush artifact.

Fig. VIA1.f. *Cutaneous diffuse B-cell lymphoma, high power.* Not all cells in cutaneous B-cell lymphoma are large and atypical. In this example, the cells are small, hyperchromatic, and monotonous in appearance.

mantle zone lymphoma. In general, the prognosis of cutaneous B-cell lymphomas is fvorable if the disease is primary, and unfavorable if the skin is secondarily involved from a nodal lymphoma. Spreading to the skin is observed in about 4% of the cases of nodal FL. The clinical presentation of primary cutaneous FL stereotypically comprises one or several nodules situated in a single area, most often the skin of the scalp or forehead. The lesions are red to purple, and can have intact or ulcerated surfaces.

HISTOPATHOLOGY. The infiltrates of cutaneous follicular lymphoma are most easily diagnosed when they are "bottom heavy" (the larger proportion of the tumor is in the lower dermis or subcutaneous fat), but "top heavy" patterns also occur. The neoplastic follicles can be of uniform size, with mantles that are thin or absent, resulting in coalescence of follicles. Tingible body macrophages, which represent cells engulfing the remnants of apoptotic lymphocytes, are rare. In contrast, a heterogeneous composition of follicles, with many tingible body macrophages and well-formed mantles of small lymphocytes around them, would favor a benign interpretation. The mitotic rate is low in cases in which small cleaved cells (centrocytes) predominate and higher as the proportion of large noncleaved cells or centroblasts increases. Most many variations of FL that occur in lymph nodes, such as irregularly shaped follicles, follicles with serrated outlines, follicles with thick mantles, conspicuous follicular dendritic cells, many tingible body macrophages, and follicles with extracellular amorphous material, can also occur in cutaneous lesions. In lesions with an immunophenotype resembling MALToma, the cells can resemble centrocytes, which are small lymphocytes with indented nuclei and varying amounts of pale cytoplasm. Although cytologically normal follicular center cells can predominate in lymphoma, some examples of FL contain cytologically aberrant cells, such as "dysplastic" small cleaved cells that have remarkably attenuated nuclei.

By immunohistochemistry, the B cells of cutaneous FL may express monotypic cell surface immunoglobulin or may fail to express immunoglobulin at all ("immunoglobulin-negative" FL). Light chain restriction can be used to demonstrate clonality in problematic cases. Genotypic studies can detect clonal rearrangement of the immunoglobulin heavy or light chain genes, or both.

Cutaneous Diffuse B-Cell Lymphoma

See Figs. VIA1.c–VIA1.f.

Cutaneous T-Cell Lymphoma, Tumor Stage

See Figs. VIA1.g–VIA1.i.

Conditions to consider in the differential diagnosis:
cutaneous T-cell lymphoma

lymphoblastic lymphoma, T-cell type
tumor-stage mycosis fungoides
adult T cell/lymphoma
cutaneous B-cell lymphoma
lymphoblastic lymphoma, B-cell type
small lymphocytic lymphoma
immunocytoma (lymphoplasmacytoid lymphoma)
primary cutaneous follicular lymphoma
diffuse large B-cell lymphoma
  (centroblastic/immunoblastic)
drug-induced pseudolymphoma
aluminum granuloma
pseudolymphomatous tattoo reaction
leukemia cutis

VIA2. Tumors of Lymphocytes and Mixed Cell Types

Nodular infiltrates or extensive diffuse infiltrates of normal lymphocytes are found in the dermis. Other reactive cell types (plasma cells, histiocytes) are admixed. B-cell cutaneous lymphoid hyperplasia is prototypic (2).

B-Cell Cutaneous Lymphoid Hyperplasia (Pseudolymphoma, Lymphocytoma Cutis)

CLINICAL SUMMARY. The term "pseudolymphoma" loosely refers to a group of conditions in which the microscopic appearance of lymphocytic infiltrates in the skin resembles that of one of the cutaneous lymphomas. There are many cutaneous pseudolymphomas, including lymphoid proliferations of B-cell or T-cell composition. B-cell cutaneous lymphoid hyperplasia (B-CLH) is often referred to simply as pseudolymphoma, because it was the first simulant of cutaneous lymphoma to be studied comprehensively. In B-CLH, nodules or plaques result from the recapitulation in the skin of the elements found in the cortices of reactive lymph nodes. Clinically, B-CLH generally presents with red to purple nodules or plaques, usually on the face or scalp. Lesions are usually solitary but may be multiple. Patients with multiple lesions often have only a few lesions affecting a circumscribed area (most often the skin of the head or neck), but rare patients have generalized lesions. Most lesions persist for months or years, and some resolve spontaneously.

HISTOPATHOLOGY. The infiltrates of B-CLH are nodular or diffuse and involve the dermis and/or the subcutis. A top-heavy pattern is often observed at scanning magnification (i.e., the infiltrate is denser in the dermis than in the subcutis). Follicles may be distinct or inconspicuous. In the follicular pattern, distinct germinal centers are present, identical in composition to secondary follicles in reactive lymph nodes. These consist of follicular center cells, which include small cleaved and large lymphocytes, and tingible body macrophages surrounded by a mantle of small lymphocytes.

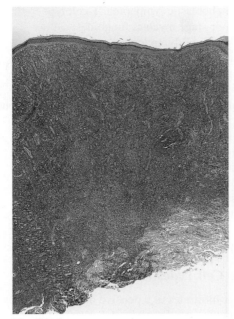

Fig. VIA1.g

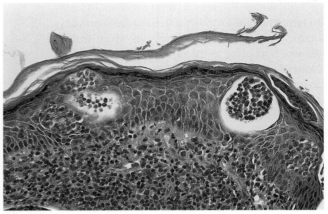

Fig. VIA1.h

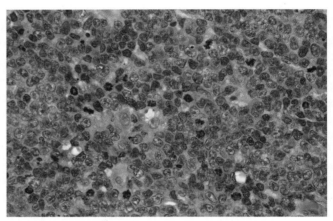

Fig. VIA1.i

Fig. VIA1.g. *Cutaneous T-cell lymphoma, tumor stage, low power.* In tumor stage mycosis fungoides there are dense aggregates of lymphoid cells filling the papillary and reticular dermis. The overlying epidermis may or may not be involved by these atypical cells.

Fig. VIA1.h. *Cutaneous T-cell lymphoma, tumor stage, medium power.* Focally, one may identify collections of epidermotropic T cells ("Pautrier microabscesses"), a feature that helps differentiate this lesion from cutaneous B-cell lymphoma.

Fig. VIA1.i. *Cutaneous T-cell lymphoma, tumor stage, high power.* Upon close inspection, the lymphoid cells show enlarged nuclei and there are numerous mitotic figures.

Mitotic figures are commonly found in these reactive follicles. The polarization seen in reactive lymph nodes is usually not evident. The mantle zone is composed of small lymphocytes. Peripheral to the follicles and their mantles is an admixture of cells that consist of T cells with small but irregularly shaped nuclei; immunoblasts (large cells with large vesicular nuclei and prominent, central nucleoli); histiocytes; and, rarely, histiocytic giant cells, eosinophils, polyclonal plasma cells, and plasmacytoid monocytes. The venules found in these interfollicular areas resemble the high endothelial venules of lymph nodes in that their endothelial cells have protuberant nuclei.

The nonfollicular pattern of B-CLH can present as a nodular or diffuse infiltrate with a mixture of cell types. A *sine qua non* is the presence of follicular center cells, but there are often eosinophils, macrophages, and plasma cells. Hints of follicles are sometimes apparent at scanning magnification as zones of pale-staining cells; the presence of follicular elements in such areas can be confirmed by immunostaining for antigens such as CD35 that recognize follicular dendritic cells, whose processes form a meshwork in lymphoid follicles.

Conditions to consider in the differential diagnosis:

    cutaneous lymphoid hyperplasia/lymphocytoma cutis
    Lennert's (lymphoepithelial) lymphoma
    angioimmunoblastic lymphadenopathy
    Borrelial lymphocytoma cutis
    chronic myelogenous leukemia

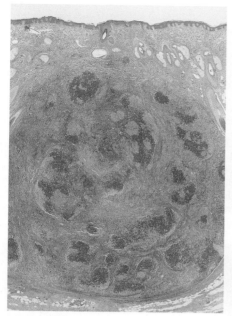

Fig. VIA2.a

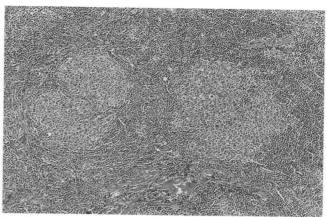

Fig. VIA2.b

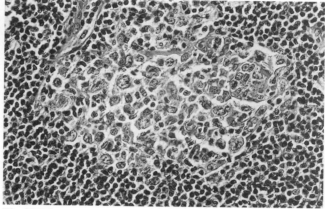

Fig. VIA2.c

Fig. VIA2.a. *Cutaneous lymphoid hyperplasia, low power.* In cutaneous lymphoid hyperplasia there are nodular aggregates of mononuclear cells within the dermis that may extend into the subcutaneous fat. The infiltrate may be diffuse, or as seen here, nodular in architecture.

Fig. VIA2.b. *Cutaneous lymphoid hyperplasia, medium power.* The lymphoid infiltrate mimics the pattern seen in lymph nodes with formation of germinal centers.

Fig. VIA2.c. *Cutaneous lymphoid hyperplasia, high power.* The germinal center consists of central large mononuclear cells with vesicular nuclei. These are surrounded by a mantle of small lymphocytes.

VIA3. Tumors of Plasma Cells

These are nodular plasma cell infiltrates, with scattered lymphocytes. Cutaneous plasmacytoma (3) and multiple myeloma (4) exemplify this reaction pattern.

Cutaneous Plasmacytoma and Multiple Myeloma

CLINICAL SUMMARY. Cutaneous lesions of multiple myeloma (MM) or plasmacytoma are usually circumscribed violaceous papules or nodules. Diffusely infiltrated plaques are occasionally observed. Cutaneous deposits of myeloma are rare, occurring in only about 2% of myeloma patients. Patients with myeloma can also develop a variety of nonspecific cutaneous complications, including deposits of light-chain–derived amyloid (primary systemic amyloidosis), pur-

puric lesions resulting from monoclonal cryoglobulinemia, diffuse normolipemic plane xanthoma, pyoderma gangrenosum, Sweet's syndrome, leukocytoclastic vasculitis, and erythema elevatum diutinum.

Monoclonal gammopathies can complicate a variety of other cutaneous diseases, such as scleromyxedema, necrobiotic xanthogranuloma with paraproteinemia, POEMS syndrome (polyneuropathy, organomegaly, endocrinopathy, M protein, and skin lesions), and scleredema. Myeloma supervenes in some patients with these disorders.

HISTOPATHOLOGY. In cutaneous lesions of MM and in plasmacytomas, there are monomorphous infiltrates of plasma cells, arrayed as densely cellular nodules or interstitially between collagen bundles. In the nodular pattern, clus-

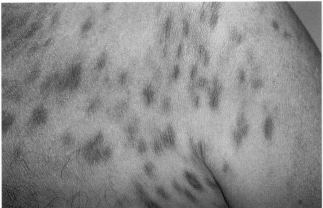

Clin. Fig. VIA3

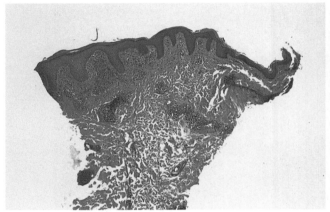

Fig. VIA3.a

Clin. Fig. VIA3. *Systemic plasmacytosis*. A middle-aged woman suddenly developed multiple nodules and papules.

Fig. VIA3.a. *Systemic plasmacytosis, low power*. Biopsy of a papule showed dense perivascular and partly interstitial infiltrates.

Fig. VIA3.b. *Systemic plasmacytosis, high power*. The infiltrates consisted of a monotonous population of histologically typical plasma cells. These appearances, taken in isolation, are suspicious but not diagnostic of an evolving myeloma. Demonstration of clonality would confirm the impression of a neoplastic rather than reactive infiltrate.

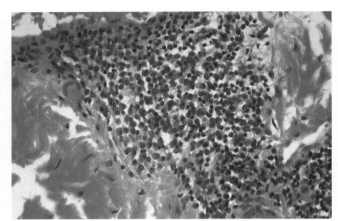

Fig. VIA3.b

ters of macrophages are sometimes present. Multinucleate plasma cells, plasmacytes with large atypical nuclei, and mitotic figures can be observed. Plasma cell bodies, round eosinophilic fragments of plasma cell cytoplasm, can be present in the background between intact cells but are not specific for MM. Intranuclear inclusions of immunoglobulin, known as Dutcher bodies, are rare in MM. Infiltrates that are composed of nuclei with a "clock-face" clumping of chromatin typical of mature, or Marshalko-type, plasma cells have been referred to as the *plasmacytic variant*. Infiltrates that are composed of cells with nuclei that resemble those of immunoblasts are sometimes referred to as *plasmablastic plasmacytoma*, whereas an even greater degree of nuclear atypia is observed in the anaplastic variant.

Conditions to consider in the differential diagnosis:

cutaneous plasmacytoma
multiple myeloma

VIA4. Small Round Cell Tumors

Tumors of small cells with scant cytoplasm and with small dark nuclei constitute a group of tumors that can usually be distinguished from one another with appropriate immuno-

histochemical investigations, in conjunction with light microscopic and clinical information. Some of these tumors arise in the deep soft tissue, but may rarely present in a deep skin biopsy. Merkel cell tumors are prototypic (5).

Cutaneous Small Cell Undifferentiated Carcinoma (Merkel Cell Tumor)

CLINICAL SUMMARY. Cutaneous small cell undifferentiated carcinoma (CSCUC) (Merkel cell, neuroendocrine, or trabecular carcinoma), an uncommon tumor, usually occurs as a solitary nodule on the head or on the extremities. The tumors are usually few in number, but occasionally are multiple. The lesions of Merkel cell tumors are firm, nodular, and red-pink in color. They usually are nonulcerated and range in size from 0.8 to 4.0 cm.

HISTOPATHOLOGY. Tumor cells with scanty cytoplasm and plump, round, or irregular nuclei are closely spaced in sheets and trabecular patterns and less commonly in ribbons and festoons. Pseudorosettes are an occasional feature. The nuclear chromatin is often dense and uniformly distributed. In some examples, nuclei focally or uniformly show margination of chromatin. Nucleoli generally are inconspicuous or absent. Nuclear molding may be a feature. Mitoses and nuclear fragments are regular features. In some tumors, the nests of cells are supported by scant, delicate, and paucicellular stroma. Lymphoid infiltrates are common at the margin and focally in the stroma. Contact with the epidermis is rare, but if a lesion invades the epidermis, the patterns may include rounded pagetoid defects in which tumor cells are collected. Keratinocytic dysplasia or carcinoma *in situ* in the overlying epidermis is not uncommon, and islands of squamous cell differentiation in the dermal nests occur uncommonly. Lymphatic invasion is commonly present.

The immunohistochemical profile is positive for neuron specific enolase (NSE+), protein gene product, chromogranins, Ber-EP4, and CD57. A single punctate zone of cytoplasmic immunoreactivity for cytokeratins, especially CK20, or neurofilaments is most characteristic. Epithelial membrane antigen (EMA) is expressed in 75% to 80% of

CSCUC. A reaction for cytokeratin 20 has been offered as a finding against the diagnosis of metastatic small cell carcinoma of the lung. Ultrastructurally, cytoplasmic, membrane-bound, round, dense-core granules of neuroendocrine type measure 100 to 200 nm in diameter. Perinuclear bundles or whorls of intermediate filaments 7 to 10 nm wide, and small desmosomes are regularly present. Tonofilaments attached to the desmosomes have been found in only a few cases.

Metastatic Small Cell Carcinoma

See Figs. VIA4.c–VIA4.e.

Conditions to consider in the differential diagnosis:
primitive neuroepithelial tumors
peripheral neuroblastoma/neuroepithelioma
Ewing's sarcoma
cutaneous small cell undifferentiated carcinoma
(Merkel cell tumor)

Clin. Fig. VIA4

Clin. Fig. VIA4. *Merkel cell tumor.* A smooth-topped erythematous nodule appeared suddenly and grew on the cheek of an elderly woman.

Fig. VIA4.a. *Merkel cell tumor, low power.* Scanning magnification reveals a dense dermal infiltrate of small basophilic cells. At this magnification the differential diagnosis includes cutaneous lymphoma and metastatic small cell carcinoma.

Fig. VIA4.b. *Merkel cell tumor, high power.* The individual cells are small, round, and have scant cytoplasm. The nuclei show a characteristic stippled appearance. Numerous mitoses are frequently seen.

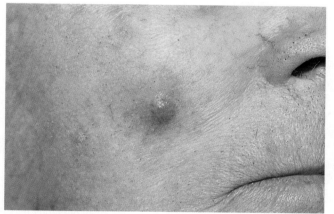

Fig. VIA4.a

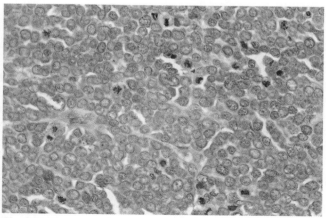

Fig. VIA4.b

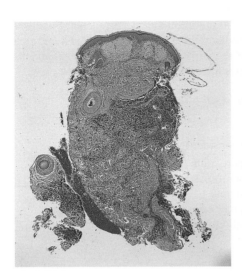

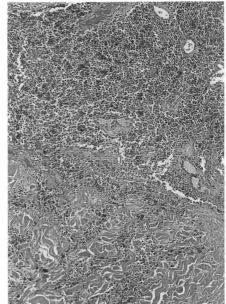

Fig. VIA4.c   **Fig. VIA4.d**

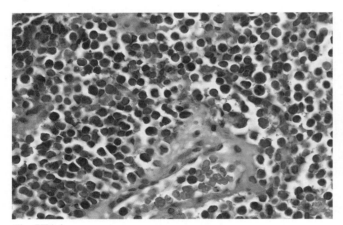

Fig. VIA4.e

Fig. VIA4.c. *Metastatic small cell carcinoma, low power*. There is an asymmetric nodular and diffuse collection of cells in the reticular dermis.

Fig. VIA4.d. *Metastatic small cell carcinoma, medium power*. The tumor consists of a monotonous population of small blue cells, infiltrating and disrupting the dermal architecture.

Fig. VIA4.e. *Metastatic small cell carcinoma, high power*. The small cells have scant cytoplasm, resulting in molding of nuclei against one another. The nuclei are small but larger than those of a lymphocyte. They have homogeneous chromatin and lack nucleoli. Immunohistochemistry may be needed to rule out a lymphoma in this case.

melanotic neuroepithelial tumor of infancy
lymphoma/leukemia
rhabdomyosarcoma
metastatic neuroendocrine carcinoma
small cell melanoma
small cell carcinoma (squamous or adenocarcinoma)
eccrine spiradenoma

VIB. LARGE POLYGONAL AND ROUND CELL TUMORS

Large polygonal and round cell tumors have large round to oval nuclei that often exhibit relatively open chromatin. There may be prominent nucleoli, especially in adenocarcinomas and in melanomas. The cytoplasm is abundant, and often amphophilic because of an abundant content of ribosomes.

1. Squamous Cell Tumors
2. Adenocarcinomas
3. Melanocytic Tumors
4. Eccrine Tumors
5. Apocrine Tumors
6. Pilar Tumors
7. Sebaceous Tumors
8. "Histiocytoid" Tumors
9. Tumors of Large Lymphoid Cells
10. Mast Cell Tumors
11. Tumors with Prominent Necrosis
12. Miscellaneous and Undifferentiated Epithelial Tumors

VIB1. Squamous Cell Tumors

Proliferations of large cells with more or less abundant cytoplasm, and with evidence of desmosome formation and/or keratin production occupy the dermis as nodular masses. Primary tumors may show evidence of origin from the epidermis in the form of a contiguous precursor (actinic keratosis) or, less specifically, of blending between the tumor cells and the epidermal cells. The possibility of metastatic squamous cell carcinoma must be considered and differentiated from the possibility of a primary cutaneous squamous cell carcinoma.

Squamous Cell Carcinoma, Deep

CLINICAL SUMMARY. Squamous cell carcinoma may occur anywhere on the skin and on mucous membranes with squamous epithelium. Clinically, squamous cell carcinoma of the skin most commonly consists of a shallow ulcer surrounded by a wide, elevated, indurated border and often covered by a crust that conceals a red granular base. Occasionally, raised, fungoid, verrucous lesions without ulceration occur. Most commonly, it arises in sun-damaged skin, either as such or

from an actinic keratosis. Next to sun-damaged skin, squamous cell carcinomas arise most commonly in scars from burns and in stasis ulcers, termed *Marjolin's ulcers*. Carcinomas arising in sun-damaged skin in general have a very low propensity to metastasize, except for carcinomas of the lower lip, even though in most cases these are also induced by exposure to the sun (6).

HISTOPATHOLOGY. The tumors consist of irregular masses of epidermal cells that proliferate downward into the dermis. The invading tumor masses are composed in varying proportions of more or less mature squamous cells and of atypical (anaplastic) squamous cells. The latter are characterized by such changes as great variation in the size and shape of the cells, hyperplasia and hyperchromasia of the nuclei, absence of intercellular bridges, keratinization of individual cells, and the presence of atypical mitotic figures. Differentiation in squamous cell carcinoma is in the direction of ker-

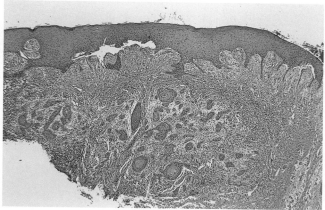

Fig. VIB1.a

Fig. VIB1.a. *Squamous cell carcinoma, invasive, low power.* Arising from the base of the epidermis there are endophytic proliferative lobules of atypical epithelium that are associated with a patchy lymphocytic infiltrate.

Fig. VIB1.b. *Squamous cell carcinoma, invasive, medium power.* Haphazardly oriented lobules are of varying shapes and sizes and show an infiltrative growth pattern within the dermis. The lobule at the top of this photomicrograph shows formation of a squamous pearl, a whorled aggregate of parakeratin within the epithelial island.

Fig. VIB1.c. *Squamous cell carcinoma, high power.* The atypical keratinocytes may show a spectrum of cytologic atypia, from mild to severe.

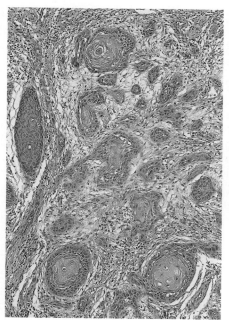

Fig. VIB1.b

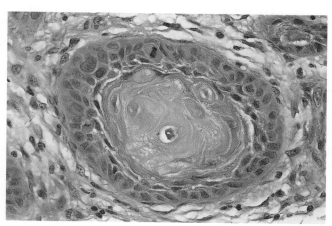

Fig. VIB1.c

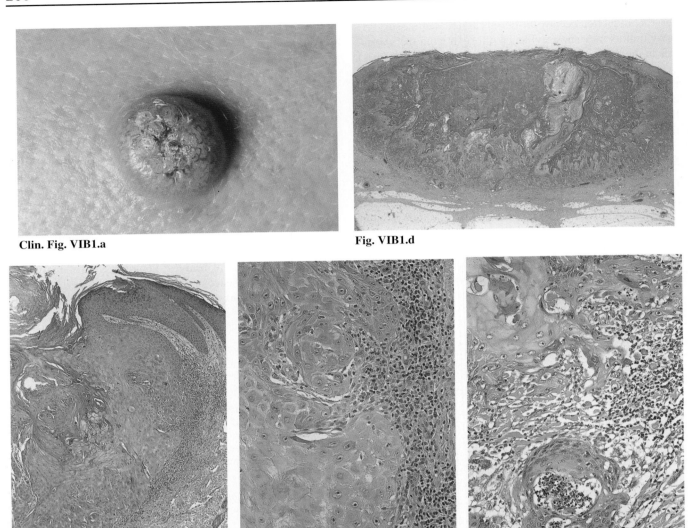

Clin. Fig. VIB1.a

Fig. VIB1.d

Fig. VIB1.e

Fig. VIB1.f

Fig. VIB1.g

Clin. Fig. VIB1.a. *Keratoacanthoma.* A symmetric tumor with a keratin-filled cup-shaped center developed suddenly in chronically sun-damaged skin of an elderly man.

Fig. VIB1.d. *Keratoacanthoma, low power.* The epidermis is invaginated forming a cup-like crater, which is filled with masses of keratin. There is an infiltrate of mononuclear cells at the dermal–epidermal junction.

Fig. VIB1.e. *Keratoacanthoma, medium power.* The epidermis shows an abrupt transition from relatively normal to a proliferation of eosinophilic hyalinized ground-glass–appearing atypical keratinocytes. At the dermal–epidermal junction, there is a brisk infiltrate of lymphocytes that are exocytotic to this proliferative atypical epithelium.

Fig. VIB1.f. *Keratoacanthoma, high power.* The dermal–tumor junction shows a dense infiltrate of mononuclear cells that are exocytotic to this proliferative, eosinophilic, hyalinized ground-glass–appearing tumor.

Fig. VIB1.g. *Keratoacanthoma, high power.* Within the proliferative epithelium of a cup-shaped tumor, there are intraepidermal collections of polymorphonuclear leukocytes.

atinization, which often takes place in the form of horn pearls. These are very characteristic structures composed of concentric layers of squamous cells showing gradually increasing, usually incomplete, keratinization toward the center. Keratohyaline granules within the horn pearls are sparse or absent.

Keratoacanthoma

CLINICAL SUMMARY.   Solitary keratoacanthoma, a common lesion, occurs in elderly persons, usually as a single lesion, and consists of a firm dome-shaped nodule 1.0 to 2.5 cm in diameter with a horn-filled crater in its center. The lesions may occur on any hairy cutaneous site, with a predilection for exposed areas. They usually reach their full size within 6 to 8 weeks and involute spontaneously, leaving a slightly depressed scar, generally in less than 6 months. Healing takes place. An increased incidence of keratoacanthoma is observed in immunosuppressed patients and in the Muir–Torre syndrome of sebaceous neoplasms and keratoacanthomas associated with visceral carcinomas. Giant and locally destructive forms of keratoacanthoma exist.

HISTOPATHOLOGY.   The architecture of the lesion is as important to the diagnosis as the cellular characteristics. Therefore, if the lesion cannot be excised in its entirety, it is ad-visable that a fusiform specimen is excised for biopsy from the center of the lesion and that this specimen include the edge at least of one side and preferably of both sides of the lesion. A shave biopsy is inadvisable, because the histologic changes at the base of the lesion are often of great importance in the differentiation from squamous cell carcinoma.

In the early proliferative stage, there is a horn-filled, cup-shaped invagination of the epidermis from which strands of epidermis protrude into the dermis. These strands are poorly demarcated from the surrounding stroma in many areas, and may contain cells showing nuclear atypia and many mitotic figures, occasionally including atypical mitoses. Perineural invasion is sometimes seen. A fully developed lesion shows a large, irregularly shaped crater filled with keratin in its center. The nondysplastic adjacent epidermis extends like a lip or a buttress over the sides of the crater. At the base of the crater, irregular epidermal proliferations extend downward. There are only one or two layers of basophilic nonkeratinized cells at the periphery of the proliferations, whereas the cells within this shell appear eosinophilic and glassy as a result of keratinization. There are many horn pearls, most of which show complete keratinization in their center. The base appears regular and well-demarcated and usually does not extend below the level of the sweat glands. In the involuting stage, proliferation has ceased and most cells at the base of the crater have undergone keratinization.

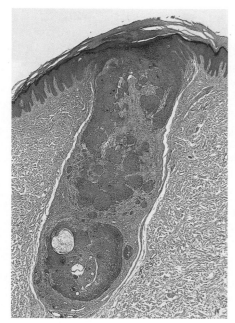
Fig. VIB1.h

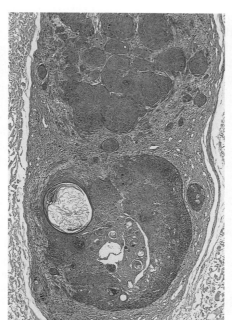
Fig. VIB1.i

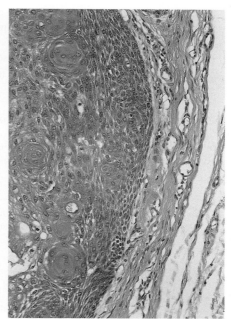
Fig. VIB1.j

Fig. VIB1.h. *Inverted follicular keratosis, low power.* This epithelial neoplasm arises from the epidermis and shows an endophytic architecture that vaguely resembles that of a hair follicle.

Fig. VIB1.i. *Inverted follicular keratosis, medium power.* This epithelial proliferation is embedded in a fibrotic stroma and is sharply separated from the adjacent reticular dermal collagen. Keratin-filled cystic structures are seen within it.

Fig. VIB1.j. *Inverted follicular keratosis, high power.* Numerous squamous eddies as depicted here are a characteristic feature of an inverted follicular keratosis.

Inverted Follicular Keratosis

Inverted follicular keratosis may be regarded as an endophytic form of the irritated, or activated, type of seborrheic keratosis in which the characteristic feature is the presence of numerous whorls or eddies composed of eosinophilic flattened squamous cells arranged in an onion-peel fashion, somewhat resembling poorly differentiated keratin pearls (7). These "squamous eddies" can be differentiated from the horn pearls of squamous cell carcinoma by their large number, small size, and circumscribed configuration. Frequently, some of these proliferations are seen to originate from the walls of keratin-filled invaginations. The combination of an inverted or invaginated architectural pattern and the squamous eddies can falsely suggest the possibility of squamous cell carcinoma.

Pseudoepitheliomatous Hyperplasia

Pseudoepitheliomatous hyperplasia (PEH) is a reaction pattern of squamous epithelium that usually occurs in association with certain neoplasms or over a chronic inflammatory process and may be regarded as reparative in nature. Conditions that may be associated with PEH are listed below in the differential diagnosis section. The reactive epithelium may extend into the superficial reticular dermis, simulating a carcinoma. However, the epithelium is typically very bland, with a single layer of basal cells maturing continuously to the surface. Although mitoses may be present, they are not abnormal. There may be evidence of the underlying stimulus in the dermis. Without such a finding, the distinction between PEH and well-differentiated invasive squamous cell carcinoma may be almost impossible to make on histologic grounds alone.

Proliferating Trichilemmal Cyst (Pilar Tumor)

CLINICAL SUMMARY. The proliferating trichilemmal cyst (8) is nearly always a single lesion, usually located on the scalp or on the back, most commonly in elderly women. Starting as a subcutaneous nodule suggestive of a wen, the tumor may grow into a large, elevated, lobulated mass that may undergo ulceration and thus greatly resemble a squamous cell carcinoma. Malignant transformation may occur.

HISTOPATHOLOGY. The lesion usually is well-demarcated from the surrounding tissue and is composed of variably sized lobules of squamous epithelium. Some lobules are surrounded by a vitreous layer and show palisading of their peripheral cell layer. Characteristically, the epithelium in the center of the lobules abruptly changes into eosinophilic amorphous keratin of the same type as that seen in the cavity of ordinary trichilemmal cysts. In addition to this trichilemmal pattern of keratinization, some proliferating trichilemmal cysts exhibit epidermoid changes, resembling that of the follicular infundibulum. This may result in horn pearls, some of which resemble squamous eddies. The tumor cells in many areas show some degree of nuclear atypia, as well as individual cell keratinization, which at first glance may suggest a squamous cell carcinoma. The tumor differs from a squamous cell carcinoma by its rather sharp demarcation from the surrounding stroma and by its abrupt mode of keratinization.

Prurigo Nodularis

See Figs. VIB1.r and VIB1.s.

Conditions to consider in the differential diagnosis:
  primary squamous cell carcinoma
  metastatic squamous cell carcinoma
  proliferating trichilemmal cyst
  inverted follicular keratosis
  keratoacanthoma
  inverted follicular keratosis
  prurigo nodularis

Clin. Fig. VIB1.b. *Pseudoepitheliomatous hyperplasia.* An elderly woman had an ulcer of 10 years' duration characterized by granulation tissue and a hypertrophic irregular border. Multiple biopsies ruled out squamous cell carcinoma.

Fig. VIB1.k. *Pseudoepitheliomatous hyperplasia, low power.* This reactive epithelial hyperplasia is present adjacent to a healing ulcer. Squamous cell carcinoma should always be considered in the differential diagnosis of this process, and a careful search for cytologic atypia and/or adjacent actinic keratosis or carcinoma *in situ* should be undertaken. The epidermis reveals marked irregular acanthosis with endophytic tongues extending into the superficial dermis. There is associated hyperkeratosis.

Fig. VIB1.l. *Pseudoepitheliomatous hyperplasia (PEH), medium power.* PEH can be difficult to differentiate from invasive squamous cell carcinoma. The presence of dermal fibrosis, as seen in this example, suggests a reactive process such as previous procedure at this site or a healing ulceration.

Fig. VIB1.m. *Pseudoepitheliomatous hyperplasia, high power.* Despite the irregular architecture and infiltrative pattern of the epithelial tongues, there is no high-grade atypia and the lesional cells appear to mature smoothly from a basal layer.

Fig. VIB1.n. *Pseudoepitheliomatous hyperplasia in North American blastomycosis, high power.* There is florid irregular epidermal hyperplasia extending deeply into the reticular dermis, associated with a mixed-cell inflammatory infiltrate and with multiple intraepithelial abscesses, a clue to the diagnosis of a deep fungal infection.

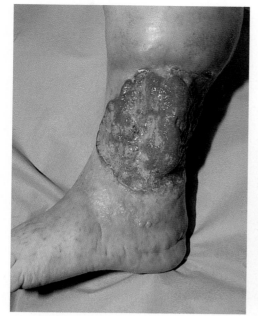

Clin. Fig. VIB1.b

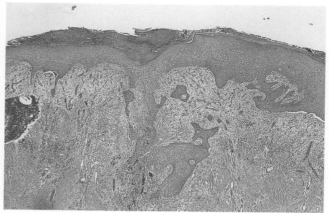

Fig. VIB1.k

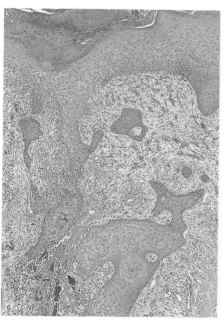

Fig. VIB1.l

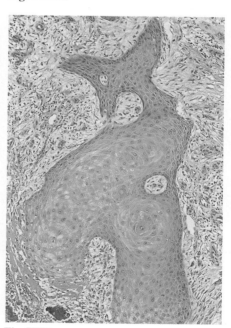

Fig. VIB1.m

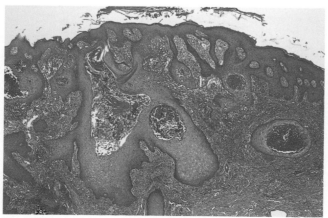

Fig. VIB1.n

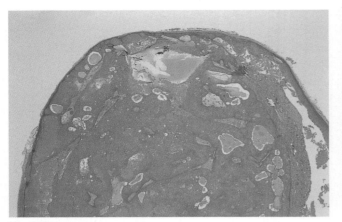

Fig. VIB1.o

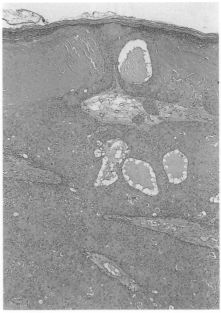

Fig. VIB1.p

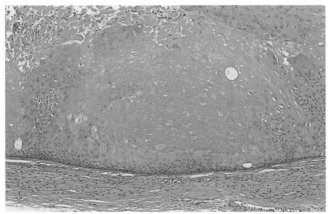

Fig. VIB1.q

Fig. VIB1.o. *Proliferating trichilemmal cyst, low power.* This photomicrograph shows the upper half of this neoplasm. It is composed of multiple lobules of interconnecting epithelium with multiple associated cystic spaces.

Fig. VIB1.p. *Proliferating trichilemmal cyst, medium power.* There are large bands of connected epithelial tissue with zones of keratinization.

Fig. VIB1.q. *Proliferating trichilemmal cyst, high power.* The wall of this proliferating cystic structure shows trichilemmal differentiation, that is, keratinization without formation of a granular cell layer. The epithelial cells may be large with an abundance of cytoplasm but fail to reveal high-grade cytologic atypia.

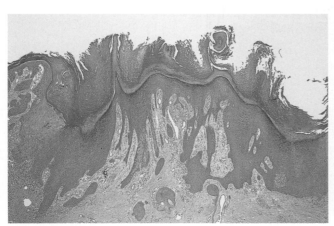

Fig. VIB1.r

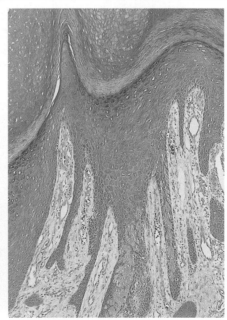

Fig. VIB1.s

VIB2. Adenocarcinomas

Proliferations of atypical cells with more or less abundant cytoplasm and with evidence of gland formation and/or mucin production occupy the dermis as nodular masses. The possibility of metastatic adenocarcinoma must be considered and differentiated from the possibility of a primary cutaneous adenocarcinoma of skin appendages (refer to eccrine, apocrine, pilar, sebaceous tumor sections, VIB4–VIB7).

Metastatic Adenocarcinoma

CLINICAL SUMMARY.   In women, most all cutaneous metastases are mammary or pulmonary adenocarcinomas. The latter are the most common in men. Colon metastases in both sexes and ovarian metastases in women account for most of the rest. Cutaneous metastatic disease as the first sign of internal cancer is most commonly seen with adenocarcinomas of the lung, kidney, and ovary. Inflammatory mammary carcinoma is a distinctive disorder that is characterized by an erythematous patch or plaque with an active spreading border that resembles erysipelas and usually affects the breast and nearby skin. The inflammatory appearance and warmth are attributed to capillary congestion. En cuirasse, or scirrhous, metastatic mammary carcinoma is characterized by a diffuse morphealike induration of the skin and rarely involves skin from other primary carcinomas. It usually begins as scattered papular lesions coalescing into a sclerodermoid plaque without inflammatory changes.

HISTOPATHOLOGY.   In scirrhous mammary carcinoma, the indurated areas are fibrotic and may contain only a few tumor cells. The tumor cells may be confused with fibroblasts. They have elongated nuclei similar to those of fibroblasts but larger, more angular, and more deeply basophilic. The tumor cells often lie singly, but in some areas they may form small groups or single rows between fibrotic and thickened collagen bundles. This latter feature of single filing is of diagnostic importance. In inflammatory carcinoma there is extensive invasion of the dermal and often the subcutaneous lymphatics by groups and cords of tumor cells. These cells are similar to those in the primary growth, and atypical in character with large, pleomorphic, hyperchromatic nuclei. Adenocarcinomas metastatic to skin from lung are often moderately differentiated, but some show well-formed, mucin-secreting, glandular structures. Individual tumor cells sometimes contain abundant cytoplasmic mucin, but usually lack large pools of mucin, which is more characteristically seen with gastrointestinal metastatic adenocarcinomas.

Metastatic Pulmonary Adenocarcinoma

See Figs. VIB2.a–VIB2.c.

Metastatic Mammary Carcinoma

See Figs. VIB2.d–VIB2.h.

Conditions to consider in the differential diagnosis:
   primary adenocarcinoma of skin adnexal origin
      (see below)
   mucin-producing squamous cell carcinoma
      (mucoepidermoid, adenosquamous carcinoma)
   metastatic adenocarcinoma

VIB3. Melanocytic Tumors

The proliferations in the dermis are melanocyte-derived, pigmented or amelanotic, benign, atypical, or malignant. Superficial lesions may involve the epidermis (junctional component). There may be a fibrous and inflammatory host response. S100 and HMB45 stains may be of value in recognizing melanocytic differentiation in amelanotic tumors. Intradermal melanocytic nevi, halo nevi, cellular blue nevi, Spitz nevi, primary melanomas of the nodular type, and metastatic melanomas are discussed here as examples of dermal melanocytic tumors (9). Nontumorigenic primary melanomas are discussed elsewhere (see sections IIB1 and IID2).

Melanocytic Nevi, Acquired and Congenital Types

CLINICAL SUMMARY.   Five types of melanocytic nevi can be distinguished: flat lesions, which are for the most part histologically junctional nevi; compound nevi, which include slightly elevated lesions often with raised centers and flat peripheries, many of which are histologically dysplastic nevi; papillomatous lesions; dome-shaped lesions; and pedunculated lesions (see section IIA2). Most nonpigmented, papillomatous, dome-shaped, and pedunculated nevi are intradermal nevi. Strictly defined congenital melanocytic nevi are by definition present at birth. They may be small (< 1.5 cm and especially when < 1 cm, generally indistinguishable from acquired nevi), intermediate (amenable to excision with primary closure), or large (not amenable to excision except with extraordinary measures). Pigment is variable in nevi and often absent in dermal nevi.

HISTOPATHOLOGY.   The lesional cells of nevi ("nevus cells") tend to be arranged in more or less well-defined nests and to contain variable pigment, especially superficially within the

---

Fig. VIB1.r. *Prurigo nodularis, low power.* There is hyperkeratosis and the epidermis is hyperplastic and highly irregular, with protrusion of tongues of cells well into the reticular dermis. The appearances, caused by chronic irritation, are reminiscent of pseudoepitheliomatous hyperplasia.

Fig. VIB1.s. *Prurigo nodularis, medium power.* The hyperplastic epithelium is well-differentiated, without substantial cytologic atypia.

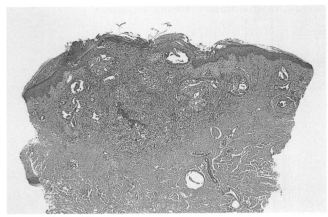

Fig. VIB2.a

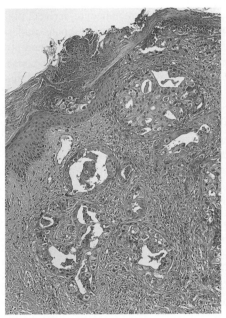

Fig. VIB2.b

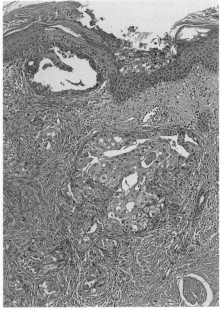

Fig. VIB2.c

Fig. VIB2.a. *Metastatic pulmonary adenocarcinoma, low power.* There are variably sized aggregates of tumor islands within the upper reticular dermis. This example shows secondary epidermal hyperplasia and hyperkeratosis.

Fig. VIB2.b. *Metastatic pulmonary adenocarcinoma, medium power.* Islands of atypical epithelial cells that form central lumina. The islands are of varying size and show mitotic activity.

Fig. VIB2.c. *Metastatic pulmonary adenocarcinoma, medium power.* The clear cell phenotype of this metastatic adenocarcinoma is fairly characteristic but not diagnostic of an adenocarcinoma primary in lung.

lesion. The most important architectural features that distinguish a dermal nevus from a melanoma are their overall smaller size and greater symmetry and the decrease in size of lesional cells from superficial to deep within the dermis, which is often referred to as "maturation." If dermal nevus cells are confined to the papillary dermis, they often retain a discrete or pushing border with the stroma. However, nevus cells that enter the reticular dermis tend to disperse among collagen fiber bundles as single cells or attenuated single files of cells, differing from melanomas, where groups rather than single cells tend to dissect and displace the collagen. Nevus cells

entering the reticular dermis are seen in many congenital nevi but also in acquired nevi, which may be termed "congenital pattern nevi." Relatively more specific indicators of congenital nevus include size greater than 1.5 cm and nevus cells within skin appendages, especially sebaceous units. Cytologically, nevus cells differ from melanoma cells by lacking high-grade and uniform cytologic atypia, and mitoses are totally absent in most benign nevi.

Lesions where nevus cells extend into the lower reticular dermis and the subcutaneous fat or are located within nerves, hair follicles, sweat ducts, and sebaceous glands are termed

Fig. VIB2.g. *Metastatic mammary carcinoma, low power.* In this example of breast carcinoma there are only a few scattered aggregates of tumor within the midreticular dermis.

Fig. VIB2.h. *Metastatic mammary carcinoma, high power.* Solid collections of malignant cells are seen within dilated lymphatics.

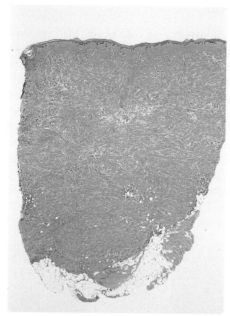

Fig. VIB2.d

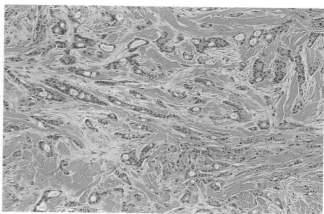

Fig. VIB2.e

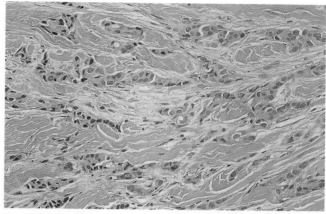

Fig. VIB2.f

Fig. VIB2.d. *Metastatic mammary carcinoma, infiltrating ductal type, low power.* The entire dermis is expanded and replaced by an infiltrative tumor. The tumor has replaced the adnexal structures.

Fig. VIB2.e. *Metastatic mammary carcinoma, infiltrating ductal type, medium power.* Throughout the dermis there are multiple small tumor aggregates permeating between bundles of reticular dermal collagen. Many of the tumor aggregates form small ducts.

Fig. VIB2.f. *Metastatic mammary carcinoma, infiltrating ductal type, high power.* The tumor cells show enlarged hyperchromatic nuclei and eosinophilic cytoplasm. The cytoplasm may show small clear vacuoles.

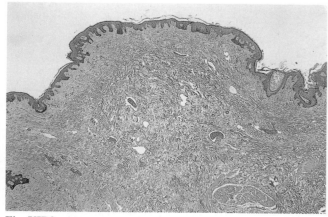

Fig. VIB2.g

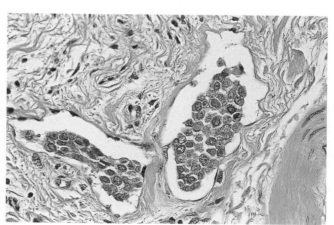

Fig. VIB2.h

"congenital pattern nevi" because these patterns may be seen, although not exclusively, in nevi that have been present since birth.

Acquired Nevi

See Figs. VIB3.a–VIB3.e.

Congenital Nevus

See Figs. VIB3.f and VIB3.g.

Acral Nevus

See Figs. VIB3.h and VIB3.i.

Balloon Cell Nevus

See Figs. VIB3.j–VIB3.l.

Halo Nevus

CLINICAL SUMMARY.   A halo nevus, also known as Sutton's nevus, nevus depigmentosa centrifugum, or leukoderma acquisitum centrifugum (10), represents a pigmented nevus surrounded by a depigmented zone. A similar halo reaction may be seen in relation to a primary or metastatic melanoma. In the common type of halo nevus, the central nevus gradually involutes over a period of several months. The area of depigmentation shows no clinical signs of inflammation and ultimately disappears in most cases, often after many months or even years. Most persons with halo nevi are children or young adults, and the back is the most common site. Not infrequently, halo nevi are multiple, occurring either simultaneously or successively.

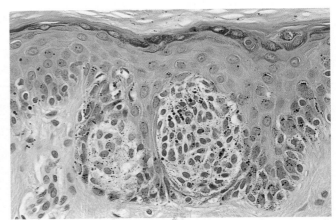

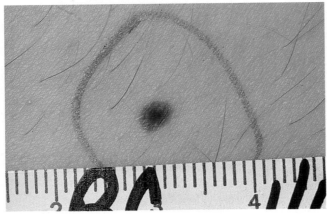

Clin. Fig. VIB3.a

Fig. VIB3.a

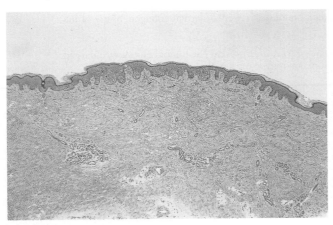

Fig. VIB3.b

Clin. Fig. VIB3.a. *Junctional nevus.* A small (<5 mm) symmetric, well-circumscribed, uniformly pigmented macule.

Fig. VIB3.a. *Junctional nevus, low power.* This is a relatively small and well-circumscribed nevus confined to the epidermis. No dermal component is seen.

Fig. VIB3.b. *Junctional nevus, high power.* The melanocytic proliferation is composed predominantly of nests of melanocytes with a few scattered single melanocytes at the dermal–epidermal junction. Significant atypia of these cells is not seen.

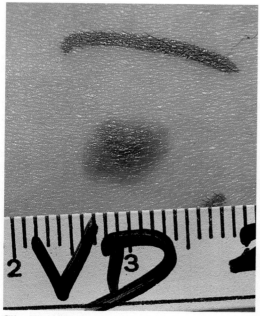

Clin. Fig. VIB3.b

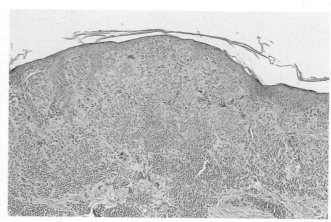

Fig. VIB3.c

Clin. Fig. VIB3.b. *Compound nevus.* An 8-mm, well-circumscribed, symmetric, and uniformly colored papule. A lesion of this size could be an acquired nevus or a small congenital pattern nevus.

Fig. VIB3.c. *Compound melanocytic nevus, medium power.* Nests of nevus cells in the epidermis overlying a dermal component of orderly nevus cells.

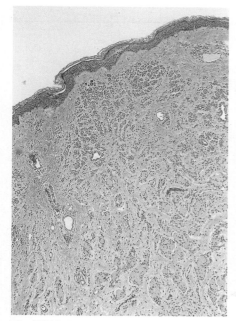

Fig. VIB3.d

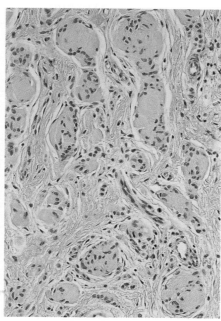

Fig. VIB3.e

Fig. VIB3.d. *Intradermal melanocytic nevus, medium power.* As in the junctional nevus, dermal nevi contain nevus cells that are recognized at this power chiefly by their tendency to be arranged in nests.

Fig. VIB3.e. *Intradermal melanocytic nevus, high power.* At the base of this dermal nevus the melanocytic cells resemble neural structures (neurotization).

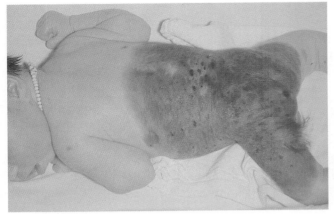

Clin. Fig. VIB3.c

Clin. Fig. VIB3.c. *Congenital nevus.* This giant hairy nevus was present at birth and covers a garment-like or bathing-trunk distribution.

Fig. VIB3.f. *Congenital nevus, low power.* This relatively large nevus is compound but is predominantly in the dermis. The lesion extends to the mid and deep reticular dermis.

Fig. VIB3.g. *Congenital nevus, medium power.* The dermal component is composed of bland uniform ovoid melanocytic cells. These cells extend into the reticular dermis and also around eccrine ducts and a hair follicle. This pattern may be seen in truly congenital nevi but may also be seen in some acquired nevi.

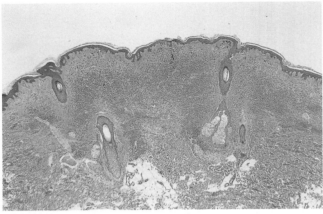

Fig. VIB3.f

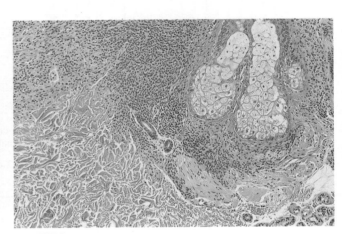

Fig. VIB3.g

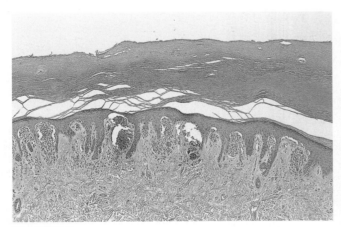

Fig. VIB3.h

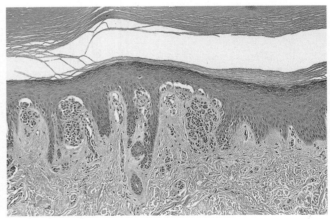

Fig. VIB3.i

Fig. VIB3.h. *Compound nevus, acral type, low power.* One can discern that this biopsy is from an acral site because of the thickened basket-weave stratum corneum. The nevus is small and symmetric, and shows both a junctional and superficial dermal component.

Fig. VIB3.i. *Compound nevus, acral type, medium power.* The nests in the papillary dermis are small, orderly, and lack atypia. The epidermal component may occasionally show a few pagetoid cells.

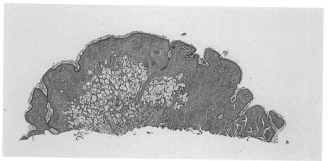

Fig. VIB3.j

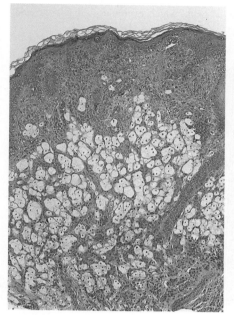

Fig. VIB3.k

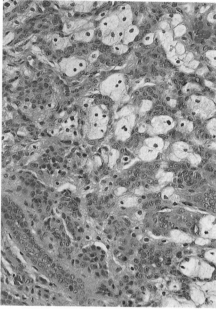

Fig. VIB3.l

Fig. VIB3.j. *Balloon cell nevus, low power.* This shave biopsy shows a compound nevus with a slightly papillomatous architecture. In the upper/mid-dermis there is a collection of clear cells.

Fig. VIB3.k. *Balloon cell nevus, medium power.* At the dermal–epidermal junction and within the superficial dermis there are nests of orderly pigmented melanocytic cells. These cells blend with larger melanocytic cells that show an abundance of clear cytoplasm.

Fig. VIB3.l. *Balloon cell nevus, high power.* Upon close inspection, the clear cells all show small, uniform, centrally placed nuclei. The lack of cytologic atypia and mitotic activity help differentiate this lesion from a balloon cell melanoma.

HISTOPATHOLOGY. In the early stage, nests of nevus cells are embedded in a dense inflammatory infiltrate, in the upper dermis and at the epidermal–dermal junction. Later, more scattered nevus cells than nests are observed. Even when melanin is still present in the nevus cells, these cells often show evidence of damage to their nuclei and cytoplasm, and some frankly apoptotic nevus cells are commonly observed. Some cells, especially superficially, may have enlarged ovoid nucleoli, changes that may be regarded as a form of reactive atypia, but high-grade and uniform nuclear atypia is not observed, and lesional cell mitoses are usually absent. Importantly, the lesional cells tend to show evidence of maturation, becoming smaller with descent from superficial to deep within the lesion. Most cells in the dense inflammatory infiltrate are lymphocytes. However, some are macrophages containing various amounts of melanin. As the infiltrate invades the nevus cell nests, it often is difficult to distinguish between the lymphoid cells of the infiltrate and the type B nevus cells in the middermis because they, too, have the appearance of lymphoid cells. At a later stage, only a few and finally no distinct nevus cells can be identified. Gradually, after all nevus cells have disappeared, the inflammatory infiltrate subsides. The epidermis of the halo, lateral to the dermal nevus cells, may show subtle lymphocytic inflammation with damage to melanocytes followed by their disappearance and a progressive absence of melanin.

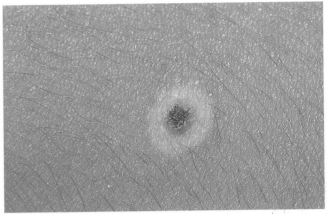

Clin. Fig. VIB3.d

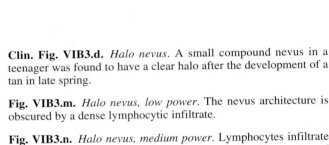

Clin. Fig. VIB3.d. *Halo nevus.* A small compound nevus in a teenager was found to have a clear halo after the development of a tan in late spring.

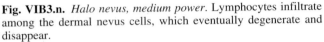

Fig. VIB3.m. *Halo nevus, low power.* The nevus architecture is obscured by a dense lymphocytic infiltrate.

Fig. VIB3.n. *Halo nevus, medium power.* Lymphocytes infiltrate among the dermal nevus cells, which eventually degenerate and disappear.

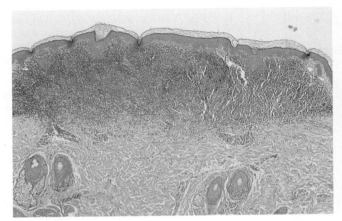

Fig. VIB3.m

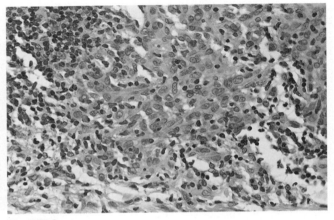

Fig. VIB3.n

Regressing Melanoma

See Figs. VIB3.o and VIB3.p.

Blue Nevus

See Figs. VIB3.q–VIB3.s.

Cellular Blue Nevus

CLINICAL SUMMARY.   A cellular blue nevus (11) presents as a blue nodule that is usually larger than the common blue nevus. It generally measures 1 to 3 cm in diameter but may be larger. It shows either a smooth or an irregular surface. About half of all cellular blue nevi have been located over the buttocks or in the sacrococcygeal region. Although rare, malignant degeneration of cellular blue nevi can occur (malignant blue nevus).

HISTOPATHOLOGY.   In the most common "mixed-biphasic" pattern, areas of deeply pigmented dendritic melanocytes, as observed also in common blue nevi, are admixed with cellular islands composed of closely aggregated rather large spindle-shaped cells with ovoid nuclei and abundant pale cytoplasm often containing little or no melanin. Not infrequently, the cellular islands penetrate into the subcutaneous fat, often forming a bulbous expansion there that is highly characteristic of cellular blue nevi. In some intersecting bundles, the cells appear rounded, perhaps as a result of cross-sectioning. Melanophages with abundant melanin may be present between the islands. The diagnosis of cellular blue nevus is generally easy in these "biphasic" lesions with both dendritic and spindle-shaped cells and with areas that resemble common blue nevi, but it can be difficult in occasional lesions without dendritic cells and in a few lesions that lack readily appreciable melanin. Larger islands composed of spindle-shaped cells may consist of many intersecting bundles of cells extending in various directions and resembling the storiform pattern observed in a neurofibroma. Some lesions consist entirely of pigmented spindle cells extending into the dermis. These lesions, referred to as the "monophasic spindle cell type" of cellular blue nevus, overlap histologically with Spitz nevi, deep penetrating nevi, and spindle cell melanomas. They tend to differ from the latter by overall architectural symmetry, by their monotony of cell type, and by lacking necrosis or frequent mitoses. Although frank anaplastic high-grade nuclear atypia is generally absent in cellular blue nevi, the nuclei may be large with prominent nucleoli. Although most of these lesions have a benign course, a few have been locally aggressive or have metastasized at least to regional lymph nodes, and a guarded prognosis is appropriate in the presence of more than a few mitoses (melanocytic tumor of uncertain malignant potential). The absence or scarcity of mitotic figures and the absence of areas of necrosis are evidence against a diagnosis of malignant blue nevus, and the presence of areas of dendritic cells elsewhere in the tumor, as well as the lack of a characteristic intraepidermal component, argue against a diagnosis of melanoma.

Deep Penetrating Nevus

See Figs. VIB3.w–VIB3.y.

Spitz Nevus

CLINICAL SUMMARY.   The importance of recognizing Spitz nevi is that the histology often resembles a nodular melanoma because of the large size of the lesional cells, often with considerable nuclear and cytoplasmic pleomorphism and an inflammatory infiltrate (12). This nevus, described by Sophie Spitz in 1948, is known also as spindle and epithelioid cell nevus. It occurs in children and in young to early middle-aged adults. Typically, it consists of a dome-shaped, hairless, pink nodule, usually smaller than 6 mm to 1 cm, and encountered most commonly on the lower extremities and face. The color is usually pink, and the nevus is then often diagnosed clinically as granuloma pyogenicum, angioma, or dermal nevus. However, it may be tan, brown, or even black. After an initial period of growth, most Spitz nevi are stable. In rare instances, there are multiple tumors, either agminated (grouped) in one area or widely disseminated.

HISTOPATHOLOGY.   In their overall architectural pattern, Spitz nevi resemble junctional or compound nevi. They are small, symmetric, and well-circumscribed. The epidermis is often hyperplastic with elongated rete ridges. The epidermal component is arranged in nests that tend to be oriented vertically and, although large, do not vary a great deal in size and shape or tend to become confluent. In Spitz nevi with junctional activity, there are often artifactual clefts between the nests of nevus cells and the surrounding keratinocytes, a feature that is less often seen in melanoma. Pagetoid permeation of the epidermis by tumor cells is usually slight, except occasionally and especially in young children.

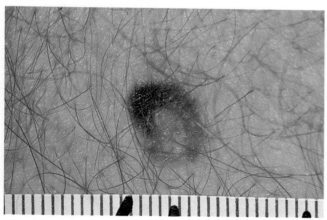

Clin. Fig. VIB3.e

Clin. Fig. VIB3.e. *Regressing melanoma.* The gray to skin-colored area in the center of this asymmetric variegated pigmented plaque is an area of partial regression. Note the lack of symmetry in this lesion compared with benign nevi including halo nevi.

Fig. VIB3.o. *Regression within a melanoma, low power.* In the right half of the image, there is a tumor in the dermis composed of large cells. In the left half, the papillary dermis is widened by fibroplasia that represents an area of regression of a portion of the radial growth phase of the tumor.

Fig. VIB3.p. *Regression within a melanoma, medium power.* Regression in melanoma is characterized by an expanded papillary dermis that shows delicate fibroplasia and edema. There is an increased number of small mature vascular channels, a lymphocytic infiltrate, and pigment-laden macrophages.

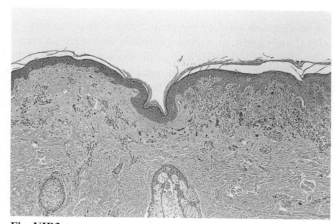

Fig. VIB3.o

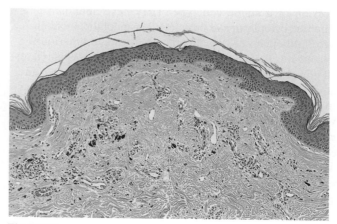

Fig. VIB3.p

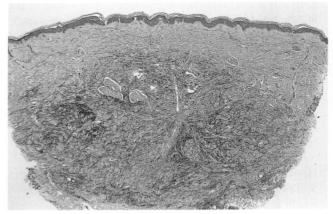

Fig. VIB3.q

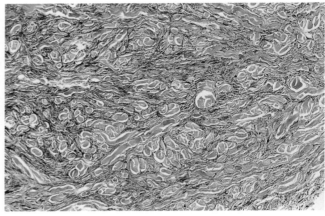

Fig. VIB3.r

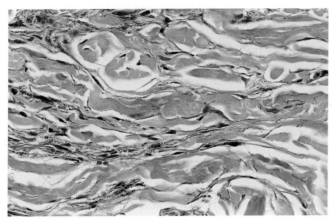

Fig. VIB3.s

Fig. VIB3.q. *Blue nevus, low power.* Within the dermis there is a poorly defined but symmetric spindle cell proliferation that is dark brown in color. There is no significant change in the overlying epidermis.

Fig. VIB3.r. *Blue nevus, medium power.* The spindled heavily pigmented cells encircle collagen bundles in the reticular dermis, a pattern also seen in dermatofibromas.

Fig. VIB3.s. *Blue nevus, high power.* The lesion is composed of elongate cells that are heavily pigmented and show prominent pigmented dendrites. The nuclei are small.

Important cytologic features of Spitz nevi include especially the large spindle and epithelioid cells, which define the lesion histologically. Apart from the shape of their cell bodies, the spindle cells and epithelioid cells in any given Spitz nevus resemble one another in nuclear and cytoplasmic consistency, suggesting that they may represent dimorphic expression of a single cell type. They have abundant amphophilic cytoplasm and prominent eosinophilic nucleoli. A useful although not pathognomonic cytologic criterion for Spitz nevi is the presence within the epidermis of coalescent red globular Kamino bodies. Of special importance is maturation of the cells with increasing depth, so that they become smaller and look more like the cells of a common nevus. Also important is the uniformity of the lesional cells from one side of the lesion to the other: At any given level of the lesion from the epidermis to its base, the lesional cells look the same. The small lesional cells at the base of most Spitz nevi tend to disperse as single cells or files of single cells among reticular dermis collagen bundles. Mitoses are found in about half of the cases, usually in small numbers ($< 2/mm^2$). Atypical mitoses are rare or absent. The com-

plete absence of mitoses in 50% of Spitz nevi is very helpful in ruling out melanoma in these cases.

Nodular Melanoma

CLINICAL SUMMARY. Nodular melanoma, by definition, contains only tumorigenic vertical growth. The lesion starts as an elevated variably pigmented papule that increases in size quite rapidly to become a nodule and often ulcerates. The ABCD criteria reviewed earlier do not apply to nodular melanomas, which are often quite small, symmetric, and well-circumscribed. They may be conspicuously pigmented, oligomelanotic, or amelanotic. When other risk factors such as thickness are controlled, the prognosis of nodular melanoma is not worse than that of other forms of melanoma.

HISTOPATHOLOGY. There is contiguous growth of uniformly atypical melanocytes in the dermis, forming an often asymmetric tumor mass. Asymmetry is often apparent at the cytologic level as variation in cell size, shape, and pigmen-

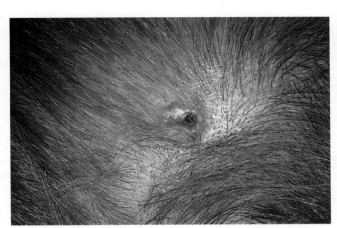

Clin. Fig. VIB3.f

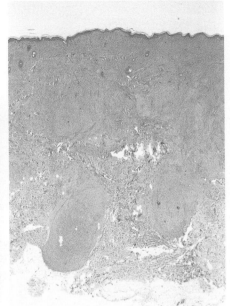

Fig. VIB3.t

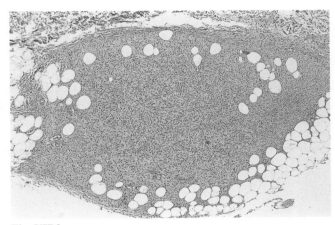

Fig. VIB3.u

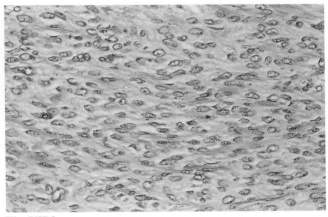

Fig. VIB3.v

Clin. Fig. VIB3.f. *Blue nodule in the scalp*. This blue nodule on clinical grounds could represent a cellular blue nevus, a malignant blue nevus, or malignant melanoma (primary or metastatic). Despite the symmetry of the lesion and its relatively small size, a malignant diagnosis is favored clinically by the presence of focal ulceration.

Fig. VIB3.t. *Cellular blue nevus, low power*. Cellular blue nevi are frequently relatively large, involving a good portion of the reticular dermis and extending deeply as tonguelike aggregates of tumor cells at the base of the lesion. The dendritic melanocytic component that resembles a common blue nevus can be seen at the periphery of the lesion.

Fig. VIB3.u. *Cellular blue nevus, medium power*. Involvement of the subcutaneous fat is common and does not imply a malignant diagnosis.

Fig. VIB3.v. *Cellular blue nevus, high power*. The cellular areas are composed of uniform spindled melanocytic cells with more cytoplasm and larger nuclei than what is seen in common blue nevus. There are irregularly distributed collections of coarse melanin pigment within the cells.

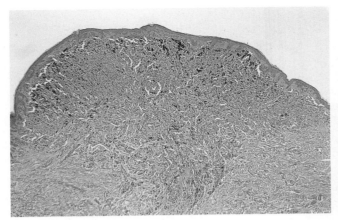

Fig. VIB3.w

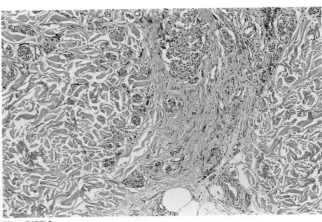

Fig. VIB3.x

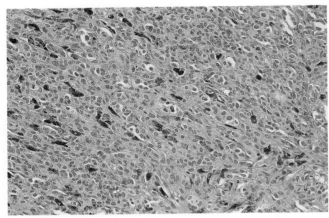

Fig. VIB3.y

Fig. VIB3.w. *Deep penetrating nevus, low power.* There is a relatively small and symmetric melanocytic lesion that is largely in the dermis, but has a junctional component. It shows a wedge-shaped architecture.

Fig. VIB3.x. *Deep penetrating nevus, medium power.* The lesion is largely within the dermis with very little intraepidermal component. It is composed of nests and fascicles of heavily pigmented melanocytic cells that extend deeply into the reticular dermis and also around follicular and neurovascular units.

Fig. VIB3.y. *Deep penetrating nevus, high power.* The tumor cells are epithelioid with an abundance of cytoplasm containing fine melanin pigment. Heavily pigmented melanophages are frequent. Most nuclei are small and uniform; however, mild random nuclear atypia may be seen in these lesions. Mitotic figures are absent or exceedingly rare.

Clin. Fig. VIB3.g. *Spitz nevus.* A symmetric pink nodule that appeared suddenly in a child, but then remained stable for several weeks before excision was arranged.

Fig. VIB3.z. *Spitz nevus, low power.* At scanning magnification there is a symmetric zone of epithelial hyperplasia. Because Spitz nevi are frequently amelanotic, the melanocytic component may be difficult to appreciate at low magnification.

Fig. VIB3.aa. *Spitz nevus, medium power.* At the dermal–epidermal interface there are large nests of spindled nonpigmented melanocytic cells described as "bunches of bananas." This pattern of irregular epidermal hyperplasia is a common finding in Spitz nevi.

Fig. VIB3.bb. *Spitz nevus, medium power.* In this example of a Spitz nevus, the nests of spindled melanocytes are predominantly within the dermis with little epidermal involvement. Eosinophilic globules (Kamino bodies) are seen in the upper left hand corner of this photomicrograph.

Fig. VIB3.cc. *Spitz nevus, medium power.* Higher magnification reveals the cytology of the cells to be both spindled in form and epithelioid with an abundance of cytoplasm. Eosinophilic nucleoli are frequently prominent.

Fig. VIB3.dd. *Spitz nevus, high power.* Single epithelioid cells permeate between bundles of reticular dermal collagen, a feature characteristically seen in Spitz nevi.

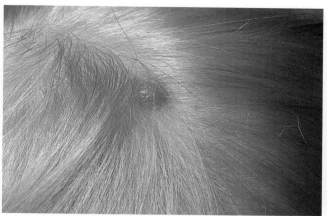

Clin. Fig. VIB3.g

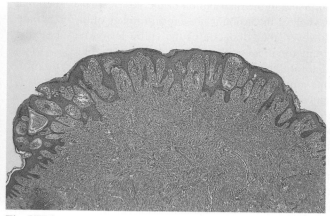

Fig. VIB3.z

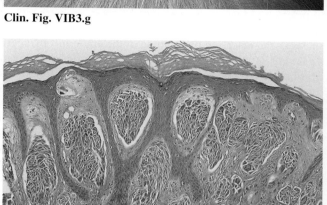

Fig. VIB3.aa

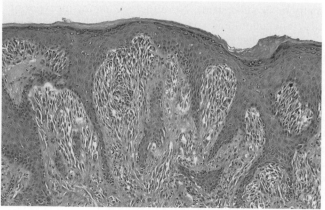

Fig. VIB3.bb

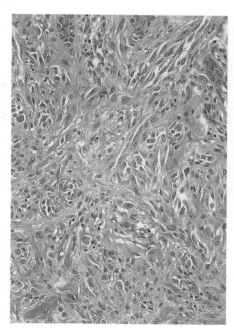

Fig. VIB3.cc

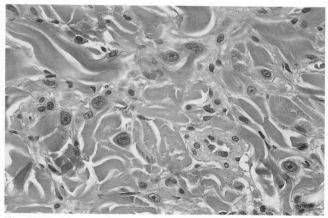

Fig. VIB3.dd

tation and in the distribution of the host response, such that one half of the lesion is not a mirror image of the other half. However, the silhouette of the entire lesion may be quite symmetric in a nodular melanoma because of the lack of an adjacent component. There is a variable lymphocytic infiltrate around the base or within the tumor. The epidermis is frequently ulcerated, or there is an adherent scale-crust. In a nodular melanoma, pagetoid permeation of the epidermis with tumor cells is limited to that portion overlying the dermal tumor, and in some cases, the epidermal involvement may be quite limited in degree. For this reason, nodular melanoma may be difficult or impossible to distinguish from a metastatic melanoma in the skin, and when the tumor is amelanotic, the distinction from other malignancies may require immunohistochemistry.

Cytologically, the tumor cells in the dermis tend to vary greatly in size and shape. Nevertheless, two major types of cells—epithelioid and spindle shaped—can be recognized. Usually one type predominates. The epithelioid cells tend to lie in nested or alveolar formations surrounded by delicate collagen fibers and the spindle-shaped cells in irregularly branching formations. Tumors in which spindle cells predominate may resemble sarcomas but in most cases differ from them by the presence of junctional melanocytic activity. The uniformly atypical nuclei of the melanoma cells are larger than those of melanocytes or nevus cells, with irregular nuclear membranes, hyperchromatic chromatin, and often prominent nucleoli that tend to be irregular in size, shape, and number. There is also a diagnostically important failure of the melanocytes in the deeper layers of the dermis to decrease in size (absence of "maturation"). Mitotic figures are usually present and often numerous in the lesional cells of the dermal and epidermal compartments of tumorigenic melanomas.

Metastatic Malignant Melanoma

CLINICAL SUMMARY.   Metastatic malignant melanoma most commonly presents as a firm red-purple to blue-black subcutaneous mass. Epidermotropic metastatic melanoma pre-

sents as small symmetric papules that may simulate a benign nevus (13).

HISTOPATHOLOGY.   The histologic appearance usually differs from that of a primary melanoma by the absence of an inflammatory infiltrate and of junctional activity. However, primary melanomas may occasionally fail to involve the epidermis and may also not show an inflammatory infiltrate, particularly when they are deeply invasive. Furthermore, some metastases exhibit a prominent lymphocytic infiltrate and can contact the overlying epidermis in a way that is suggestive of junctional activity. *Epidermotropic metastatic melanoma* refers to a metastatic deposit that is initially localized in the papillary dermis and involves the overlying epidermis. Most of these lesions occur in an extremity regional to a distal primary melanoma. Epidermotropic metastasis is characterized by thinning of the epidermis by aggregates of atypical melanocytes within the dermis, inward turning of the rete ridges at the periphery of the lesion, and usually no lateral extension of atypical melanocytes within the epidermis beyond the concentration of the metastasis in the dermis. However, this distinction can be very difficult in a few lesions where extension beyond the dermal component occurs. In some cases, the metastatic cells are small and nevoid, with few if any mitoses, and in these instances of *differentiated epidermotropic metastatic melanoma*, the lesions can be mistaken for compound nevi.

Metastatic Malignant Melanoma, Satellite Lesion

See Figs. VIB3.oo–VIB3.pp.

Epidermotropic Metastatic Melanoma

See Figs. VIB3.qq–VIB3.rr.

Conditions to consider in the differential diagnosis:
Superficial Melanocytic Nevi
compound melanocytic nevus
dermal melanocytic nevus, acquired type
dermal recurrent melanocytic nevus

Clin. Fig. VIB3.h. *Malignant melanoma, tumorigenic.* An elderly man presented with an asymmetric black tumor and cervical adenopathy.

Fig. VIB3.ee. *Nodular melanoma, low power.* This subtype of malignant melanoma frequently shows a dome-shaped or polypoid architecture. The asymmetric distribution of basophilic lymphoid cells in this lesion is a clue that the lesion is not benign.

Fig. VIB3.ff. *Nodular melanoma, medium power.* There is no radial growth phase to this lesion, the feature that distinguishes it from other forms of melanoma. Adjacent to the nodule seen on the left side of the photomicrograph, the epidermis fails to reveal changes of melanoma.

Fig. VIB3.gg. *Nodular melanoma, medium power.* The tumor shows its origination from the overlying epidermis that shows single and nested atypical melanocytes at the dermal–epidermal interface. In nodular melanoma, pagetoid spread may not be prominent.

Fig. VIB3.hh. *Nodular melanoma, high power.* The tumor cells are large with prominent nucleoli. Mitotic figures are generally identified and occasional cells show brown pigment within the cytoplasm.

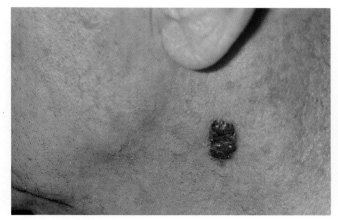

Clin. Fig. VIB3.h

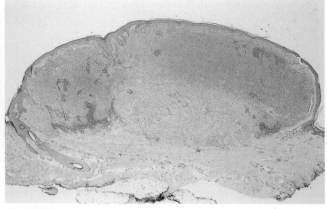

Fig. VIB3.ee

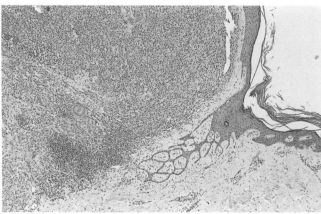

Fig. VIB3.ff

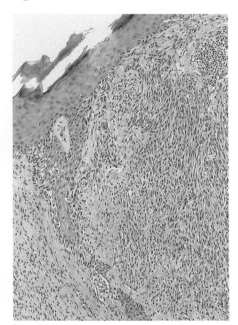

Fig. VIB3.gg

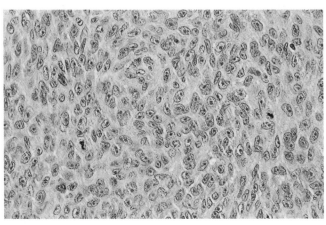

Fig. VIB3.hh

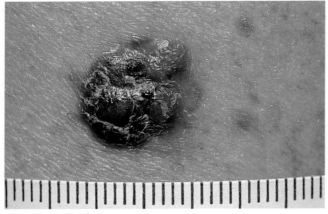

Clin. Fig. VIB3.i

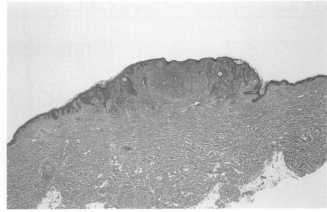

Fig. VIB3.ii

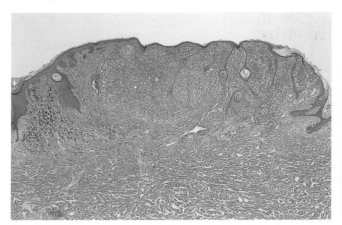

Fig. VIB3.jj

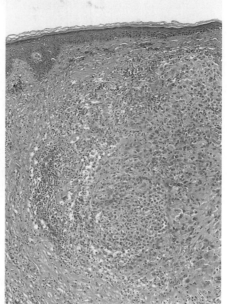

Fig. VIB3.kk

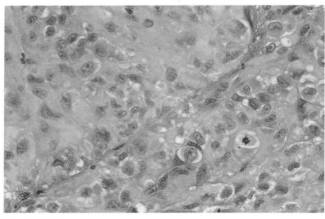

Fig. VIB3.ll

Clin. Fig. VIB3.i. *Malignant melanoma, superficial spreading type, tumorigenic.* This lesion has a prominent blue-black tumorigenic vertical growth phase nodule and an adjacent tan plaque component that represents an associated radial growth phase.

Fig. VIB3.ii. *Malignant melanoma, tumorigenic, low power.* Sections show a nodule of pale cells asymmetrically placed within a plaque lesion characterized at this magnification by epithelial hyperplasia and an infiltrate in the papillary dermis. This plaque represents a largely regressed radial growth phase component.

Fig. VIB3.jj. *Malignant melanoma, tumorigenic, medium power.* Around the nodule there are scattered lymphocytes and fairly numerous melanophages.

Fig. VIB3.kk. *Malignant melanoma, tumorigenic, medium power.* A moderately brisk tumor-infiltrating lymphocyte response is present around the nodule.

Fig. VIB3.ll. *Malignant melanoma, tumorigenic, high power.* The cells in the nodule are large epithelioid melanoma cells that have abundant cytoplasm and large irregular nuclei with prominent nucleoli. Mitoses are readily detected.

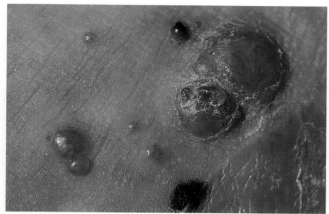

Clin. Fig. VIB3.j

Clin. Fig. VIB3.j. *Metastatic malignant melanoma.* A 69-year-old man presented with translucent erythematous and black nodules and papules surrounding the skin graft at the site of a previous melanoma of the foot.

Fig. VIB3.mm. *Metastatic malignant melanoma, low power.* In this example of metastatic melanoma there is a nodular tumor within the subcutaneous fat. There is no overlying tumor in the dermis or epidermis.

Fig. VIB3.nn. *Metastatic malignant melanoma, high power.* The tumor is composed of large atypical cells with an abundance of cytoplasm, large nuclei, and prominent nucleoli. Brown melanin pigment is seen within the cytoplasm of these cells. Mitotic figures, which may be few or numerous, and generally can be identified in metastatic lesions.

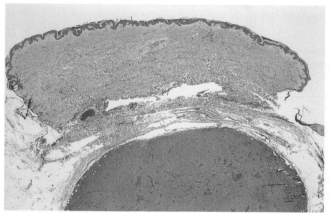

Fig. VIB3.mm

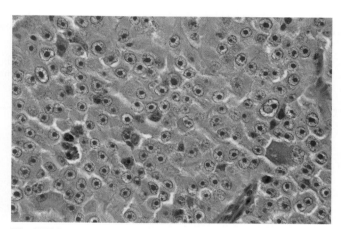

Fig. VIB3.nn

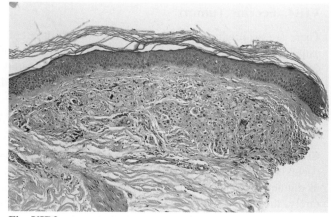

Fig. VIB3.oo

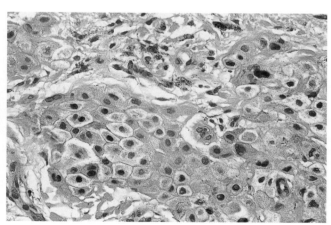

Fig. VIB3.pp

Fig. VIB3.oo. *Metastatic malignant melanoma, satellite lesion, low power.* This small black papule was present adjacent to a malignant melanoma. Within the upper dermis there are collections of heavily pigmented melanocytic cells without an overlying epidermal component.

Fig. VIB3.pp. *Malignant melanoma, satellite lesion, high power.* Small satellite lesions histologically may look very nevic. However, the aggregates are of various sizes, and the individual cells are large with hyperchromatic nuclei. The presence of mitotic figures, although not always numerous, is helpful in differentiating these lesions from nevi.

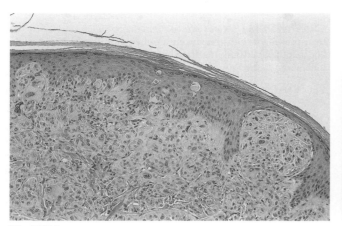

Fig. VIB3.qq

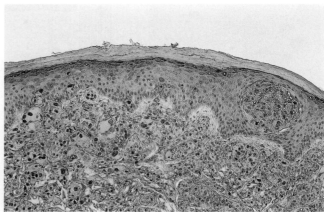

Fig. VIB3.rr

Fig. VIB3.qq. *Metastatic malignant melanoma, medium power.* In this example of epidermotropic metastatic melanoma, the cells lack melanin pigment and they show pagetoid spread, a pattern that mimics a primary malignant melanoma.

Fig. VIB3.rr. *Metastatic malignant melanoma, medium power, S100 stain.* This is an S100 stain of the lesion depicted in Fig. VIB3.qq. Tumor cells, both within the epidermis and dermis, are strongly positive both in primary and metastatic lesions of melanoma.

dysplastic nevi, compound
nevus of genital skin
nevus of acral skin
halo nevus
combined nevus
pigmented spindle cell nevus of Reed
balloon cell nevus
Superficial and Deep Melanocytic Nevi
small congenital nevus
intermediate and giant congenital nevi
deep penetrating nevus
spindle and epithelioid cell nevus (Spitz nevus)
Pigment-Synthesizing Dermal Neoplasms
metastatic melanoma
common blue nevus
cellular blue nevus
combined nevus
deep penetrating nevus
malignant blue nevus
proliferative nodules in congenital melanocytic nevi
malignant melanomas in congenital melanocytic nevi
malignant melanocytic schwannoma
dermal melanocytic tumors of uncertain malignant
  potential (MELTUMP)
nevus of Ota
melanotic neuroepithelial tumor of infancy
Tumorigenic Primary Melanomas
nodular melanomas
tumorigenic melanomas with radial and vertical
  growth phase
superficial spreading type
lentigo maligna type

acral lentiginous type
mucosal lentiginous type
desmoplastic melanoma
neurotropic melanoma
minimal deviation melanoma
Metastatic Malignant Melanoma
epidermotropic metastatic melanoma
satellites and in-transit metastatic melanoma
dermal and subcutaneous metastatic melanoma

VIB4. Eccrine Tumors

There are proliferations of eccrine ductal (small dark cells usually forming tubules at least focally) or glandular tissue or both in a hyalinized or sclerotic dermis. The inflammatory infiltrate is mainly lymphocytic. Eccrine spiradenoma and nodular hidradenoma are the prototypic examples.

Eccrine Spiradenoma

CLINICAL SUMMARY. As a rule, eccrine spiradenoma (14) occurs as a solitary intradermal nodule measuring 1 to 2 cm in diameter. Occasionally, there are several nodules, and rarely, there are numerous small nodules in a zosteriform pattern or large nodules in a linear arrangement. The nodules are often tender and occasionally painful.

HISTOPATHOLOGY. The tumor may consist of one large, sharply demarcated lobule, or of several such lobules located in the dermis without connections to the epidermis. There may be a fibrous capsule. The tumor lobules often appear deeply basophilic because of the close aggregation of the nuclei. The epithelial cells within the tumor lobules are arranged in intertwining cords, which may enclose small irregularly shaped islands of edematous connective tissue. Two types of epithelial cells are present in the cords, both with only scant cytoplasm. The cells of the first type have small dark nuclei; they are generally located at the periphery of the cellular aggregates. The cells of the second type have large pale nuclei; they are located in the center of the aggregates and may be arranged partially around small lumina observed in about half of the tumors or in a rosette arrangement. The lumina frequently contain small amounts of a periodic acid–Schiff- (PAS) positive, granular, eosinophilic material. In some cases, hyaline material is focally present in the stroma that surrounds the cords of tumor cells. A heavy diffuse lymphocytic infiltrate may be present.

Cylindroma

See Figs. VIB4.d–VIB4.f.

Poroma

See Figs. VIB4.g–VIB4.i.

Syringoma

See Figs. VIB4.j–VIB4.k.

Nodular Hidradenoma

CLINICAL SUMMARY. Nodular hidradenoma (15) is presently also called *clear cell hidradenoma* and *eccrine acrospiroma*. It is a fairly common tumor without a preferred site. The tumors present as intradermal nodules in most instances between 0.5 and 2.0 cm in diameter, although they may be larger. They are usually covered by intact skin, but some tumors show superficial ulceration and discharge serous material. Although the tumor only rarely gives the impression of being cystic clinically, gross examination of the specimen often reveals cysts.

HISTOPATHOLOGY. The tumor is well-circumscribed and may appear encapsulated. It is composed of lobulated masses located in the dermis and often extending into the subcutaneous fat, usually with no connection to the surface epidermis. The tumor nodules are frequently separated by a characteristic eosinophilic hyalinized stroma. Within the lobulated masses, tubular lumina of various sizes are often present. However, these may be absent or few in number. The tubular lumina may be branched or straight and are lined by cuboidal ductal cells or by columnar secretory cells, which may show evidence of decapitation secretion. There are often cystic spaces, which may be of considerable size and contain a faintly eosinophilic homogeneous material. In solid portions of the tumor, two types of cells can be recognized in varying proportions and with transitional forms. One type of cell is usually polyhedral or fusiform with a rounded nucleus and slightly basophilic cytoplasm. The second type of cell is usu-

ally round with very clear cytoplasm, so that the cell membrane is distinctly visible. Its nucleus appears small and dark. In some tumors, epidermoid differentiation is seen, with the cells appearing large and polyhedral and showing eosinophilic cytoplasm. There may even be keratinizing cells with formation of horn pearls. In other tumors, groups of squamous cells are arranged around small lumina that are lined with a well-defined eosinophilic cuticle and thus resemble the intraepidermal portion of the eccrine duct.

Clear Cell Syringoma

See Figs. VIB4.p and VIB4.q.

Chondroid Syringoma

See Figs. VIB4.r and VIB4.s.

Conditions to consider in the differential diagnosis:
eccrine nevus
papillary eccrine adenoma
clear cell (nodular) hidradenoma (eccrine acrospiroma)
syringoma
chondroid syringoma
eccrine spiradenoma
cylindroma (some consider apocrine)
eccrine syringofibroadenoma
mucinous syringometaplasia

Microcystic Adnexal Carcinoma

CLINICAL SUMMARY. Microcystic adnexal carcinoma (16), or sclerosing sweat duct carcinoma, may best be considered as a sclerosing variant of ductal eccrine carcinoma. This tumor, which is most commonly seen on the skin of the upper lip but occasionally also on the chin, nasolabial fold, or cheek, is an aggressive neoplasm that invades deeply. Local recurrence is common; however, metastases have not been reported.

HISTOPATHOLOGY. Microcystic adnexal carcinoma is a poorly circumscribed dermal tumor that may extend into the subcutis and skeletal muscle. Continuity with the epidermis or follicular epithelium may be seen. Two components within a desmoplastic stroma may be evident. In some areas, basaloid keratinocytes are seen, some of which contain horn cysts and abortive hair follicles; in other areas, ducts and glandlike structures lined by a two-cell layer predominate. The tumor islands typically reduce in size as the tumor extends deeper into the dermis. Cells with clear cytoplasm may be present, and sebaceous differentiation has been reported. Cytologically, the cells are bland without significant atypia; mitoses are rare or absent. Perineural invasion may be seen, a feature that may account for the high recurrence rate. Lack of circumscription, deep dermal involvement, and perineural involvement all aid in diagnosis because the cytology mimics benign adnexal neoplasms.

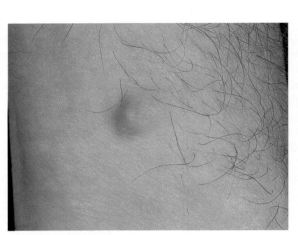

Clin. Fig. VIB4.a

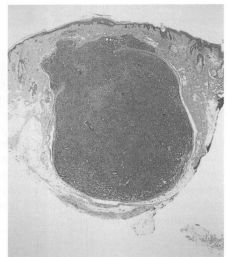

Fig. VIB4.a

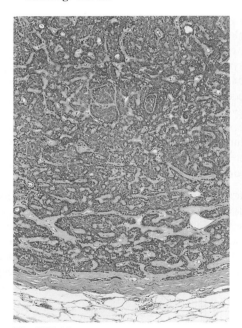

Fig. VIB4.b

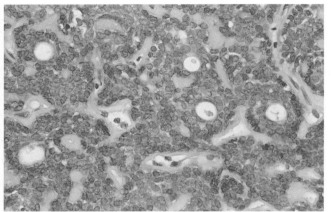

Fig. VIB4.c

Clin. Fig. VIB4.a. *Eccrine spiradenoma.* A 55-year-old man had a 30-year history of a bluish nodulocystic lesion of the wrist, with a history of recent enlargement and tenderness.

Fig. VIB4.a. *Eccrine spiradenoma, low power.* This adnexal neoplasm is a basaloid nodular tumor within the dermis. The lesion is sharply circumscribed and separated from the adjacent dermal collagen.

Fig. VIB4.b. *Eccrine spiradenoma, medium power.* This tumor may be separated from the surrounding dermis by a thin fibrous capsule. At this power, the tumor cells form an interlocking pattern.

Fig. VIB4.c. *Eccrine spiradenoma, high power.* The tumor is composed of small basaloid cells with small nuclei and scant cytoplasm. A second population of cells is also present with slightly larger, vesicular nuclei, and more cytoplasm. Seen here are small ductal lumina typical of eccrine differentiation. Also present are small collections of eosinophilic homogenous material, another typical feature of these tumors.

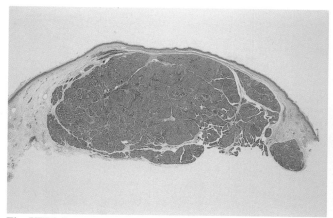

Fig. VIB4.d

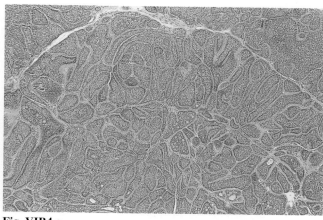

Fig. VIB4.e

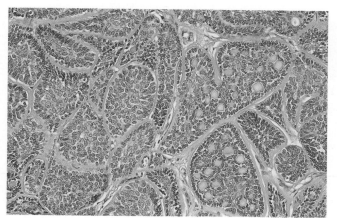

Fig. VIB4.f

Fig. VIB4.d. *Cylindroma, low power.* There is a relatively well-circumscribed basophilic tumor within the dermis. There is no association with the overlying epidermis that shows an effaced rete ridge pattern.

Fig. VIB4.e. *Cylindroma, medium power.* The tumor is composed of multiple islands of basaloid cells that fit neatly together, adjacent to one another; the close proximity and interdigitating nature resemble the pieces of a jigsaw puzzle.

Fig. VIB4.f. *Cylindroma, high power.* These tumors are composed of two populations of cells similar to what is seen in spiradenomas. The basaloid islands are surrounded by a homogenous eosinophilic basement membrane-like material. Round aggregates of similar eosinophilic material are also present within the islands.

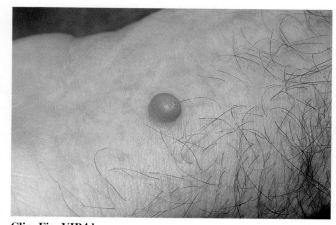

Clin. Fig. VIB4.b

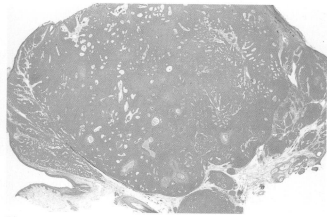

Fig. VIB4.g

Clin. Fig. VIB4.b. *Eccrine poroma.* A firm, slightly erythematous papule on the volar aspect of the wrist.

Fig. VIB4.g. *Eccrine poroma, low power.* A circumscribed proliferation of cells extending from the epidermis into the dermis. (*continues*)

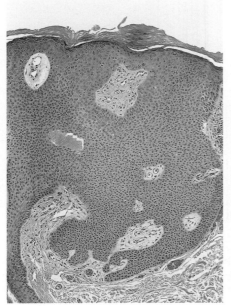

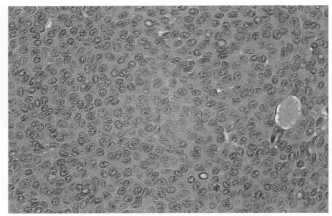

Fig. VIB4.h

Fig. VIB4.i

Fig. VIB4.h. *Eccrine poroma, medium power*. In another example, a polypoid tumor is formed.

Fig. VIB4.i. *Eccrine poroma, high power*. The legional cells form monotonous sheets. A structure within the tumor contains eosinophilic material, consistent with keratinization of an abortive duct. In other examples, ducts may be lined by an eosinophilic cuticle similar to that of an eccrine duct.

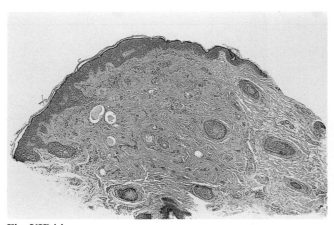

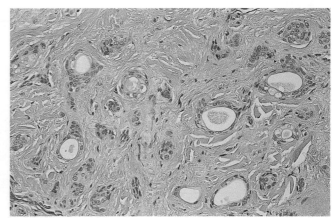

Fig. VIB4.j

Fig. VIB4.k

Fig. VIB4.j. *Syringoma, low power*. Within the upper half of the dermis there is a well-circumscribed adnexal tumor embedded in an eosinophilic stroma. Although this lesion has no capsule, the edge of the lesion is defined by the edge of the stroma.

Fig. VIB4.k. *Syringoma, medium power*. The tumor is composed of multiple small islands of bland-appearing epithelial cells. Many islands form small ducts lined by an eosinophilic cuticle. The islands may show a tadpole or comma-like appearance.

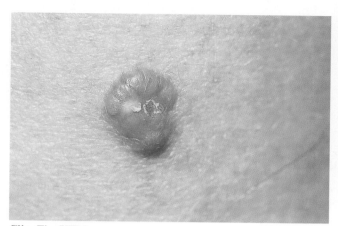

Clin. Fig. VIB4.c

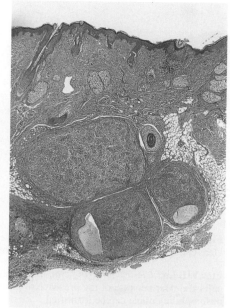

Fig. VIB4.l

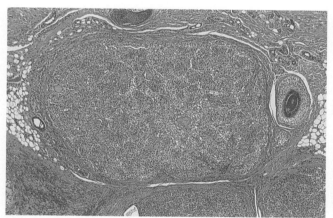

Fig. VIB4.m

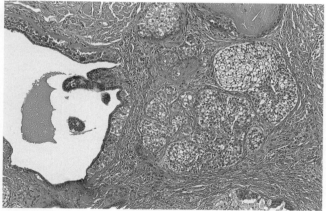

Fig. VIB4.n

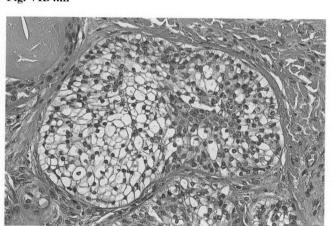

Fig. VIB4.o

Clin. Fig. VIB4.c. *Nodular hidradenoma.* A 55-year-old man presented with an asymptomatic, 1-cm, pink, telangiectatic, slightly scaly nodule on the lateral forearm. The lower pole was pigmented.

Fig. VIB4.l. *Nodular hidradenoma, low power.* Within the dermis, this neoplasm is composed of several well-circumscribed tumor lobules.

Fig. VIB4.m. *Nodular hidradenoma, medium power.* These tumor aggregates are well-circumscribed from the surrounding normal dermis and subcutaneous fat. The tumor islands may be surrounded by a thin fibrous capsule.

Fig. VIB4.n. *Nodular hidradenoma, medium power.* Within the tumor islands there may be small or large cystic spaces containing amorphous fluid. The spaces are lined by two rows of flattened epithelial cells.

Fig. VIB4.o. *Nodular hidradenoma, high power.* The epithelial cells frequently show clear cell change with the small basophilic nucleus pushed to the side of the cell. The clear cell change is secondary to glycogen deposition and stains positively with a periodic acid–Schiff test.

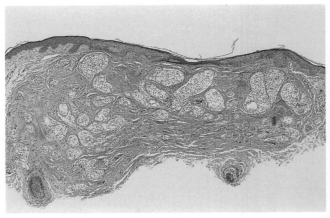

Fig. VIB4.p

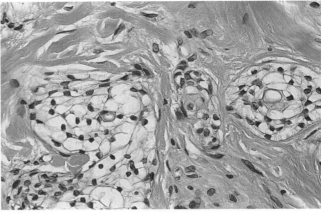

Fig. VIB4.q

Fig. VIB4.p. *Clear cell syringoma, low power.* Within the superficial dermis there are multiple small lobules of clear cells embedded in an eosinophilic sclerotic stroma.

Fig. VIB4.q. *Clear cell syringoma, high power.* Similar to the nodular (clear cell) hidradenoma, these epithelial cells are clear because of the presence of glycogen. In the center of these islands small eccrine ducts lined by an eosinophilic cuticle can be identified.

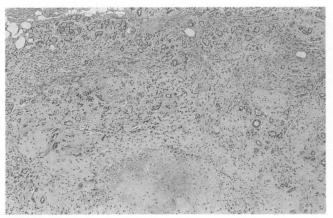

Fig. VIB4.r

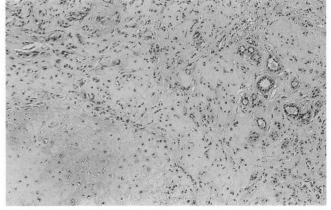

Fig. VIB4.s

Fig. VIB4.r. *Chondroid syringoma, low power.* This nodular tumor shows multiple tiny epithelial islands embedded in a bluish, myxoid matrix.

Fig. VIB4.s. *Chondroid syringoma, medium power.* The small epithelial islands form small ductal lumina typical of eccrine differentiation. The bluish chondroid matrix resembles cartilage.

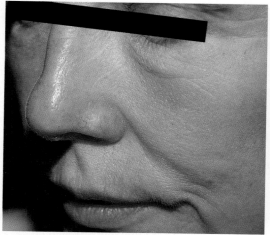

Clin. Fig. VIB4.d

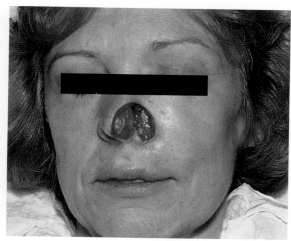

Clin. Fig. VIB4.e

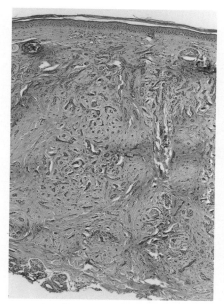

Fig. VIB4.t

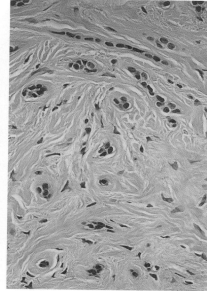

Fig. VIB4.u

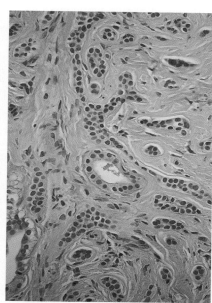

Fig. VIB4.v

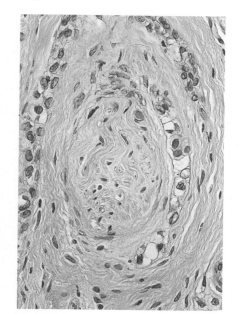

Fig. VIB4.w

Clin. Fig. VIB4.d. *Microcystic adnexal carcinoma.* A middle-aged woman developed a visually inconspicuous indurated swelling on the ala of the nose.

Clin. Fig. VIB4.e. *Microcystic adnexal carcinoma.* Moh's micrographic surgery was used to delineate the extent and to excise the tumor, resulting in the large defect seen here.

Fig. VIB4.t. *Microcystic adnexal carcinoma, low power.* A poorly circumscribed dermal tumor extends through the dermis to the base of the biopsy.

Fig. VIB4.u. *Microcystic adnexal carcinoma, medium power.* Ducts and solid cords of cells are present in a desmoplastic stroma.

Fig. VIB4.v. *Microcystic adnexal carcinoma, medium power.* Some of the ducts are lined by a single layer of cells; others may appear to have two layers.

Fig. VIB4.w. *Microcystic adnexal carcinoma, high power.* Perineural invasion is commonly seen in this neoplasm.

Mucinous Eccrine Carcinoma

See Figs. VIB4.x–VIB4.z.

   Conditions to consider in the differential diagnosis:
      sclerosing sweat duct carcinoma
      microcystic adnexal carcinoma
      malignant chondroid syringoma
      malignant clear cell (nodular) hidradenoma
      malignant eccrine spiradenoma
      malignant eccrine poroma (porocarcinoma)
      eccrine adenocarcinoma
      mucinous eccrine carcinoma
      adenoid cystic eccrine carcinoma
      aggressive digital papillary adenoma/adenocarcinoma
      syringoid eccrine carcinoma

VIB5. Apocrine Tumors

Tumors in the dermis are composed of proliferations of apocrine ductal and glandular epithelium (large pink cells with decapitation secretion). The stroma is sclerotic and well-vascularized, and the inflammatory cells are mainly lymphocytes.

Tubular Apocrine Adenoma

CLINICAL SUMMARY.   This tumor (17) consists of a well-defined nodule that is commonly located on the scalp. Most tumors have a smooth surface and are under 2 cm in diameter.

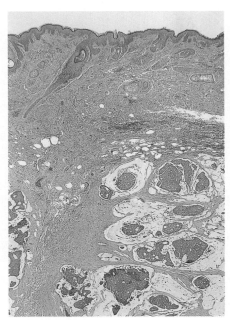

Fig. VIB4.x

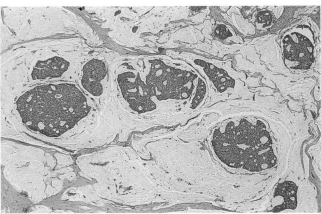

Fig. VIB4.y

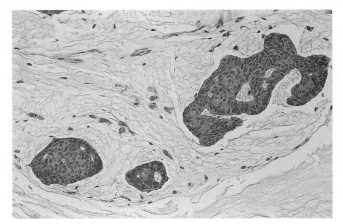

Fig. VIB4.z

Fig. VIB4.x. *Mucinous eccrine carcinoma, low power.* Within the deep dermis and subcutaneous fat there are basophilic islands of tumor cells embedded in a mucinous matrix. The islands are of various sizes. The overlying epidermis and superficial dermis are generally uninvolved.

Fig. VIB4.y. *Mucinous eccrine carcinoma, medium power.* These basaloid islands appear to be floating in the abundant hypocellular mucinous matrix.

Fig. VIB4.z. *Mucinous eccrine carcinoma, high power.* The epithelial islands are composed of crowded basaloid cells that focally show formation of small ducts. Cytologic atypia may be minimal.

HISTOPATHOLOGY. The characteristic feature of this tumor is the presence of numerous irregularly shaped tubular structures that are usually lined by two layers of epithelial cells. The peripheral layer consists of cuboidal or flattened cells, and the luminal layer is composed of columnar cells. Some tubules have a dilated lumen with papillary projections extending into it. Decapitation secretion of the luminal cells is seen in many areas, and cellular fragments are seen in some lumina.

Syringocystadenoma Papilliferum

CLINICAL SUMMARY. Syringocystadenoma papilliferum (18) occurs most commonly on the scalp or the face. It is usually first noted at birth or in early childhood and consists of either one papule or several papules in a linear arrangement or of a solitary plaque. The lesion increases in size at puberty, becoming papillomatous and often crusted. On the scalp, syringocystadenoma papilliferum frequently arises around puberty within a nevus sebaceus that has been present since birth.

HISTOPATHOLOGY. The epidermis shows varying degrees of papillomatosis. One or several cystic invaginations extend downward from the epidermis, lined in their upper portions by squamous keratinizing cells similar to those of the surface epidermis. In the lower portion of the cystic invaginations, numerous papillary projections extend into the lumina, lined by glandular epithelium often with two rows of cells. The luminal row of cells consists of high columnar cells with oval nuclei, faintly eosinophilic cytoplasm, and, occasionally, active decapitation secretion. The outer row consists of small cuboidal cells with round nuclei and scanty cytoplasm. Beneath the cystic invaginations, deep in the dermis, one can often find groups of tubular glands with large lumina, lined by apocrine cells with evidence of active decapitation secretion. A highly diagnostic feature is the almost invariable presence of a fairly dense cellular infiltrate composed nearly entirely of plasma cells in the stroma of this tumor, especially in the papillary projections. In about one third of the cases, syringocystadenoma papilliferum is associated with a nevus sebaceus.

Conditions to consider in the differential diagnosis:

Circumscribed Symmetric Apocrine Tumors
apocrine nevus
tubular apocrine adenoma ("tubulopapillary
    hidradenoma")
cylindroma (some consider eccrine)
hidradenoma papilliferum
syringocystadenoma papilliferum
apocrine hidrocystoma

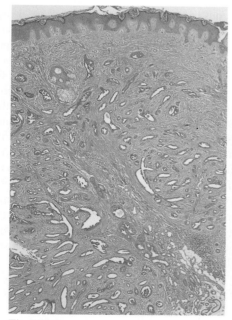

Fig. VIB5.a

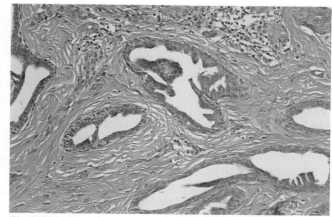

Fig. VIB5.b

Fig. VIB5.a. *Tubular apocrine adenoma, low power.* Irregularly shaped tubules lined by two layers of cells extend through the reticular dermis.

Fig. VIB5.b. *Tubular apocrine adenoma, medium power.* The double layer of cells and the presence of decapitation secretion differentiate this lesion from a microcystic adnexal carcinoma. The absence of high-grade atypia helps to eliminate a metastatic adenocarcinoma.

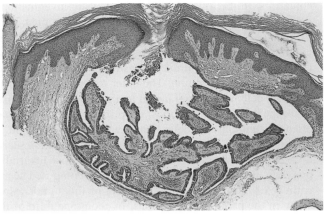

Fig. VIB5.c

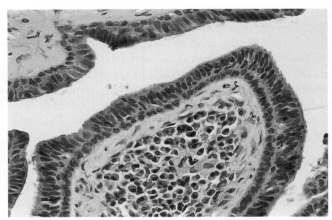

Fig. VIB5.d

Fig. VIB5.c. *Syringocystadenoma papilliferum, low power.* There is an endophytic epithelial neoplasm that arises from the surface epidermis. There are numerous papillary projections into the cystic lumen.

Fig. VIB5.d. *Syringocystadenoma papilliferum, high power.* The papillary projections are lined by two layers of cells: luminal columnar cells that show decapitation secretion and basilar cuboidal cells. The stroma contains numerous plasma cells.

Infiltrative Asymmetric Apocrine Tumors

apocrine adenocarcinoma

malignant cylindroma

erosive adenomatosis (florid papillomatosis of the nipple)

VIB6. Pilar Tumors

The dermal infiltrating tumor is composed of epithelium that differentiates toward hair or is a proliferation of portions of the follicular structure and its stroma. The inflammatory cell infiltrate is mainly lymphocytic, and the dermis is fibrocellular. Trichoepithelioma is prototypic (19).

Trichoepithelioma

CLINICAL SUMMARY.   The differentiation in this tumor is directed toward hair structures. It occurs either in multiple lesions or as a solitary lesion. Multiple trichoepithelioma is transmitted autosomal dominantly. Typically, the first lesions appear in childhood and gradually increase in number. There are numerous, rounded, skin-colored, firm papules and nodules located mainly in the nasolabial folds but also elsewhere on the face and occasionally also the scalp, neck, and upper trunk. Solitary trichoepithelioma is not inherited and consists of a firm, elevated, flesh-colored nodule usually less than 2 cm in diameter. Its onset usually is in childhood or early adult life, and it is commonly located in the anterior facial triangle.

HISTOPATHOLOGY.   As a rule, the lesions of multiple trichoepithelioma are superficial, well-circumscribed, small, and symmetric. Horn cysts are the most characteristic histologic feature, present in most lesions. They consist of a fully keratinized center surrounded by basophilic cells that lack high-grade atypia and mitoses. The keratinization is abrupt and complete, in the manner of so-called trichilemmal keratinization, not gradual and incomplete as in the horn pearls of squamous cell carcinoma. As a second major component, tumor islands composed of basophilic cells are arranged in a lacelike or adenoid network and occasionally also as solid aggregates. These tumor islands show peripheral palisading of their cells and are surrounded by a fibroblastic stroma. This stroma lacks the retraction artifact typical of basal cell carcinoma and frequently contains foci of granulomatous inflammation around fragments of keratin. The epithelial aggregates form invaginations, which contain numerous fibroblasts and thus resemble follicular papillae. Solitary trichoepithelioma is used as a histologic designation only for highly differentiated lesions. Solitary lesions with relatively little differentiation toward hair structures are best classified as keratotic basal cell carcinoma. If a lesion is to qualify for the diagnosis of solitary trichoepithelioma, it should contain numerous horn cysts and abortive hair papillae. Mitotic figures should be very rare or absent, and the lesion should not be unduly large, asymmetric, or infiltrative.

Dilated Pore of Winer

See Figs. VIB6.d and VIB6.e.

Pilar Sheath Acanthoma

See Figs. VIB6.f and VIB6.g.

Trichilemmoma

See Figs. VIB6.h–VIB6.j.

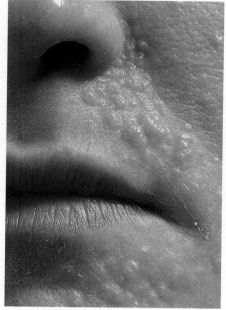

Clin. Fig. VIB6

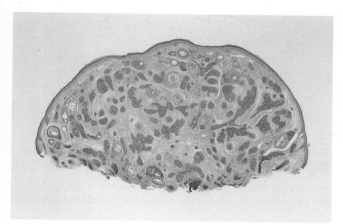

Fig. VIB6.a

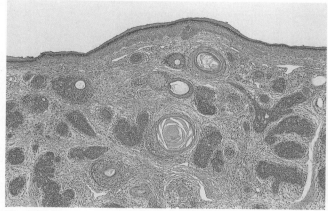

Fig. VIB6.b

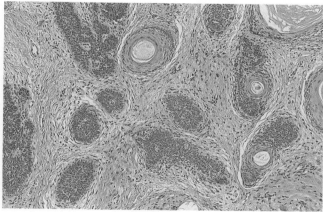

Fig. VIB6.c

Clin. Fig. VIB6. *Trichoepithelioma.* Since early childhood, a 22-year-old woman had developed firm, flesh-colored, discrete papules and nodules over the face around the nose and mouth.

Fig. VIB6.a. *Trichoepithelioma, low power.* At scanning magnification there is a dome-shaped epithelial neoplasm within the dermis. The epithelial islands do not connect to the overlying epidermis.

Fig. VIB6.b. *Trichoepithelioma, medium power.* These basaloid epithelial islands are associated with small cystic structures filled with laminated keratin.

Fig. VIB6.c. *Trichoepithelioma, medium power.* The epithelial islands show follicular differentiation mimicking the follicular bulb. The stroma is fibrotic and closely associated with these epithelial islands. Retraction artifact, as seen in basal cell carcinoma, is absent in these lesions.

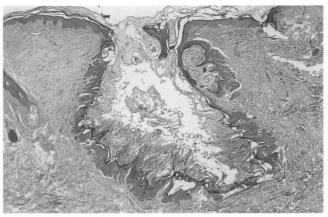

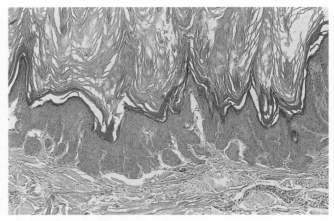

Fig. VIB6.d   **Fig. VIB6.e**

Fig. VIB6.d. *Dilated pore of Winer, low power.* There is a cystic structure that originates from the surface epidermis. The center of the lesion is filled with laminated keratin and there is a proliferative epithelial wall.

Fig. VIB6.e. *Dilated pore of Winer, medium power.* The epithelial wall shows a verrucous inner surface with elongation of rete ridges. There is infundibular keratinization with formation of a granular cell layer.

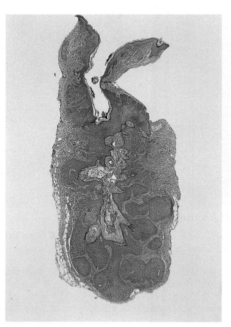

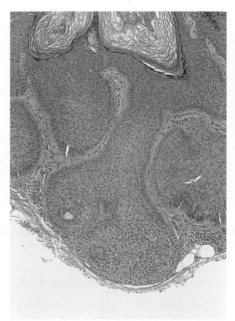

Fig. VIB6.f   **Fig. VIB6.g**

Fig. VIB6.f. *Pilar sheath acanthoma, low power.* This lesion shows the architecture of an epithelial cyst and that of a dilated pore of Winer. There is an invagination of epithelium filled with keratin opening to the skin surface. The wall of the cystic structure is, however, quite proliferative.

Fig. VIB6.g. *Pilar sheath acanthoma, medium power.* The wall of the cystic structure is composed of a proliferation of basaloid and squamous cells that focally show follicular differentiation mimicking the outer root sheath portion of the hair follicle in this image.

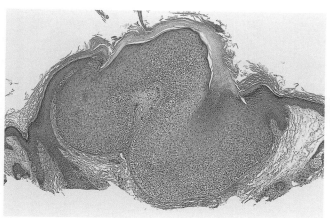

Fig. VIB6.h

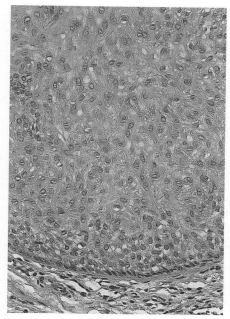

Fig. VIB6.i

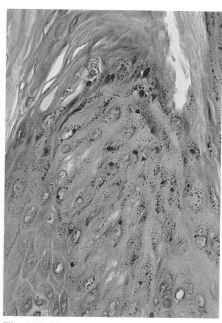

Fig. VIB6.j

Fig. VIB6.h. *Trichilemmoma, low power.* This epithelial neoplasm is well-circumscribed and shows both an endophytic architecture and a verrucous and hyperkeratotic surface.

Fig. VIB6.i. *Trichilemmoma, medium power.* The endophytic lobule is composed of bland-appearing epithelial cells that may show clear cell change. At the periphery the basal cells show a palisaded architecture and there may be a thickened basement membrane. These lesions do not have a mucinous stroma, a feature that helps differentiate them from basal cell carcinomas.

Fig. VIB6.j. *Trichilemmoma, high power.* At the edge of this lesion the verrucous surface may show hypergranulosis.

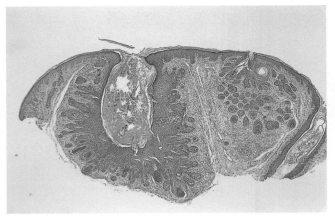

Fig. VIB6.k

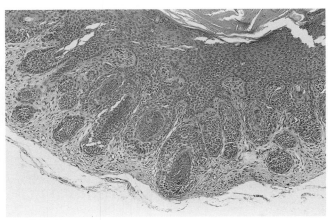

Fig. VIB6.l

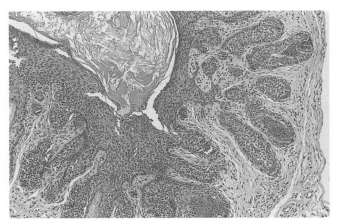

Fig. VIB6.m

Fig. VIB6.k. *Trichofolliculoma, low power.* A central cystic structure is filled with keratin and is associated with a hyperplastic wall, from which secondary hair follicles extend into the stroma.

Fig. VIB6.l. *Trichofolliculoma, medium power.* The secondary hair follicles arise from the central cystic structure. Tertiary follicles may also be present, branching from the secondary follicles.

Fig. VIB6.m. *Trichofolliculoma, medium power.* The secondary follicles produce hair shafts seen within the cystic canal.

Trichofolliculoma

See Figs. VIB6.k–VIB6.m.

Fibrofolliculoma

See Figs. VIB6.n–VIB6.p.

Trichoadenoma

See Figs. VIB6.q–VIB6.r.

Pilomatricoma

See Figs. VIB6.s–VIB6.v.

Conditions to consider in the differential diagnosis:
Follicular Infundibular Neoplasms
dilated pore of Winer
pilar sheath acanthoma
trichilemmoma
tumor of the follicular infundibulum
Branching and Lobular Pilosebaceous Neoplasms
trichofolliculoma
trichoepithelioma

tumor of follicular infundibulum
top of nevus sebaceus
Nodular Pilosebaceous Neoplasms
hair follicle nevus
keratoacanthoma
trichoepithelioma
desmoplastic trichoepithelioma
immature trichoepithelioma
hair follicle hamartoma
pilomatricoma
trichoblastoma
trichoblastic fibroma
trichoadenoma
proliferating trichilemmal cyst (pilar tumor)
inverted follicular keratosis
Tumors of Pilosebaceous Mesenchyme
trichodiscoma
fibrofolliculoma
tumors of the arrector pilae muscle
Infiltrative, Asymmetric
pilomatrix carcinoma (malignant pilomatricoma)
trichilemmal carcinoma
basal cell carcinoma with follicular differentiation

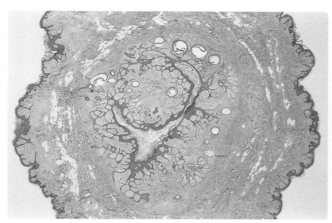

Fig. VIB6.n

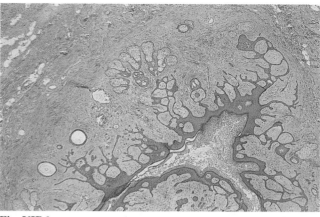

Fig. VIB6.o

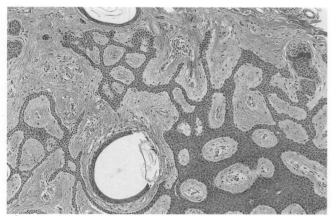

Fig. VIB6.p

Fig. VIB6.n. *Fibrofolliculoma, low power.* Although this specimen is tangentially oriented, one can still appreciate the central cystic cavity filled with keratin.

Fig. VIB6.o. *Fibrofolliculoma, medium power.* Arising from the central cystic structure are thin delicate strands of epithelium that show follicular differentiation, including formation of sebaceous lobules.

Fig. VIB6.p. *Fibrofolliculoma, medium power.* In the upper right-hand corner of this photomicrograph one can see the follicular differentiation mimicking a hair bulb, associated with the characteristic thin strands of epithelium ramifying in a fibrous stroma.

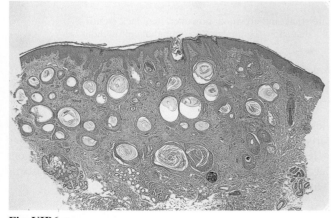

Fig. VIB6.q

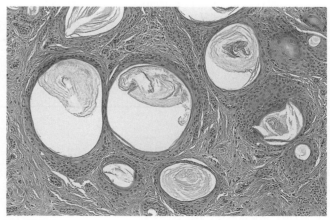

Fig. VIB6.r

Fig. VIB6.q. *Trichoadenoma, low power.* Within the upper two thirds of the dermis is a well-circumscribed lesion composed of multiple cystic structures embedded in a fibrotic stroma.

Fig. VIB6.r. *Trichoadenoma, medium power.* The cystic structures are formed by mature squamous epithelium that shows infundibular differentiation. They contain laminated keratin. Although not shown here, they may be associated with a granulomatous infiltrate secondary to rupture of these cysts.

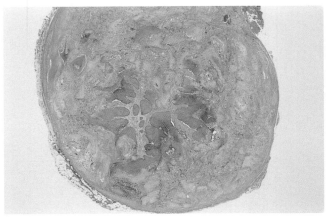

Fig. VIB6.s

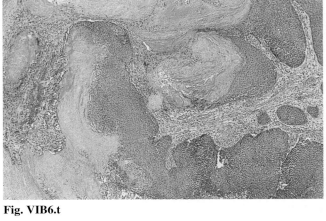

Fig. VIB6.t

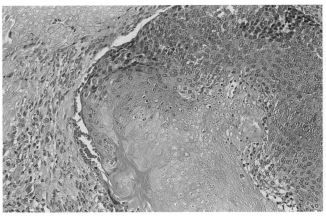

Fig. VIB6.u

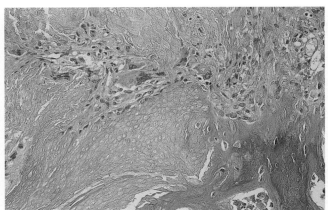

Fig. VIB6.v

Fig. VIB6.s. *Pilomatricoma, low power.* This well-circumscribed tumor shows both basophilic and eosinophilic elements.

Fig. VIB6.t. *Pilomatricoma, medium power.* The basophilic areas are composed of crowded areas of small basaloid cells that are in contiguity with the eosinophilic areas.

Fig. VIB6.u. *Pilomatricoma, high power.* The basaloid cells are small and crowded; however, they lack significant atypia. These cells blend with the eosinophilic shadow cells that show the ghost of an epithelial cell without viable basophilic staining.

Fig. VIB6.v. *Pilomatricoma, high power.* Adjacent to the shadow cells seen here are foreign-body–type giant cells, a frequent finding in these lesions.

VIB7. Sebaceous Tumors

The dermal masses are proliferations of the germinative epithelium and of mature sebocytes. The admixture of these cells varies from one tumor to the other. The dermis is fibrocellular. Sebaceous adenomas, epitheliomas, and carcinomas are the prototypes (20).

Sebaceous Adenoma and Sebaceous Epithelioma (Sebaceoma)

CLINICAL SUMMARY. Sebaceous adenoma presents as a yellow circumscribed nodule located on either the face or scalp. Sebaceous epithelioma, or sebaceoma, varies from a circumscribed nodule to that of an ill-defined plaque. Some of the lesions are yellow. Sebaceous epithelioma occasionally arises within a nevus sebaceus. Sebaceous epitheliomas and adenomas may also be found among the multiple sebaceous neoplasms that occur in association with multiple visceral carcinomas in the Muir–Torre syndrome.

HISTOPATHOLOGY. On histologic examination, sebaceous adenoma is sharply demarcated from the surrounding tissue. It is composed of incompletely differentiated sebaceous lobules that are irregular in size and shape. Two types of cells are present in the lobules. The first are undifferentiated basaloid cells identical to the cells at the periphery of normal sebaceous glands. The second are mature sebaceous cells. In most lobules, the two types of cells occur in approximately equal proportions, often arranged in such a way that groups of sebaceous cells are surrounded by basaloid cells. There may be foci of squamous epithelium with keratinization.

The histologic spectrum of sebaceous epithelioma (sebaceoma) extends from that in sebaceous adenoma to lesions that may be difficult to distinguish from sebaceous carcinoma. Generally, a sebaceoma shows irregularly shaped cell masses in which more than half of the cells are undifferentiated basaloid cells but in which there are significant aggregates of sebaceous cells and of transitional cells. Lesions verging on a sebaceous carcinoma show some degree of irregularity in the arrangement of the cell masses, and, although most cells are basaloid cells, many cells show differentiation toward sebaceous cells. Sebaceous adenoma and sebaceous epithelioma lack nuclear atypia and invasive asymmetric growth patterns, which are hallmarks of sebaceous carcinoma. Considerable mitotic activity in the basaloid regions may be present in either, however.

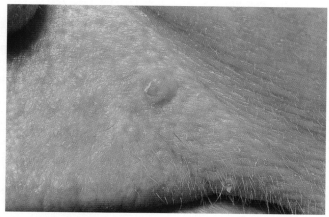

Clin. Fig. VIB7.a

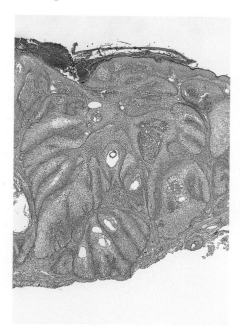

Fig. VIB7.a

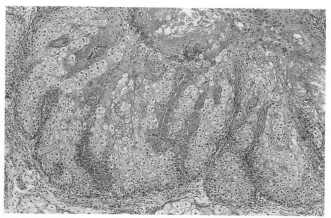

Fig. VIB7.b

Clin. Fig. VIB7.a. *Sebaceous adenoma.* A 67-year-old woman with bladder cancer and colon cancer and a history of keratoacanthoma and sebaceous adenoma (Muir–Torre syndrome) presented with an ill-defined, flesh-colored, yellowish papule on the upper lip.

Fig. VIB7.a. *Sebaceous adenoma, low power.* Arising from the surface epidermis is a multilobated epithelial neoplasm with clear cell change.

Fig. VIB7.b. *Sebaceous adenoma, medium power.* The clear cell change represents sebaceous differentiation manifested by vacuolated cytoplasm that indents the central nucleus. These cells compose at least 50% of the lesion. The second population of cells is composed of an increased number of basaloid cells at the periphery of the lobules.

Sebaceous Hyperplasia

See Figs. VIB7.c and VIB7.d.

Nevus Sebaceus of Jadassohn

See Figs. VIB7.e and VIB7.f.

Sebaceous Epithelioma

See Figs. VIB7.g and VIB7.h.

Sebaceous Carcinoma

See Figs. VIB7.i and VIB7.j.

CLINICAL SUMMARY. Carcinomas of the sebaceous glands occur most frequently on the eyelids but may occur elsewhere on the skin. The tumors usually manifests as a nodule that may or may not be ulcerated. Sebaceous carcinomas of the eyelids quite frequently cause death resulting from visceral metastases. Sebaceous carcinomas arising on the skin away from the eyelids may cause regional metastases, but visceral metastasis resulting in death is very rare.

HISTOPATHOLOGY. The tumors are characterized at scanning magnification by asymmetry and an infiltrative border formed by irregular lobular formations that vary greatly in size and shape. Although many cells are undifferentiated, distinct sebaceous cells showing a foamy cytoplasm are present in the center of most lobules. Many cells are atypical, showing considerable variation in the shape and size of their nuclei. Some large lobules contain areas composed of atypical keratinizing cells, as seen in squamous cell carcinoma. Sebaceous carcinomas of the eyelids often show pagetoid spread of malignant cells in the conjunctival or adjacent epithelium, a change that is seen very rarely in extraocular sebaceous carcinoma.

Conditions to consider in the differential diagnosis:

Symmetric Circumscribed Sebaceous Neoplasms
sebaceous hyperplasia
Fordyce's condition (ectopic sebaceous glands in
   mucosae)
rhinophyma
nevus sebaceus
sebaceous adenoma
sebaceous epithelioma
sebaceous trichofolliculoma
Infiltrative Asymmetric Sebaceous Neoplasms
sebaceous carcinoma
basal cell carcinoma with sebaceous differentiation

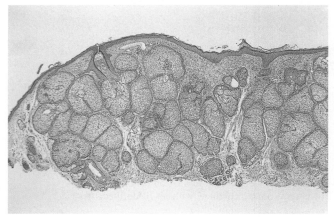

Fig. VIB7.c

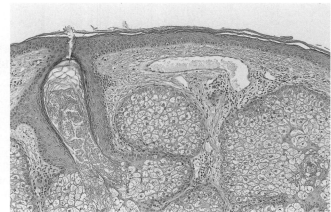

Fig. VIB7.d

Fig. VIB7.c. *Sebaceous hyperplasia, low power.* At scanning magnification there is an increased number of mature sebaceous lobules that are located superficially in the dermis, closer than normal to the overlying epidermis.

Fig. VIB7.d. *Sebaceous hyperplasia, medium power.* The sebaceous lobules are composed almost entirely of mature sebocytes with only a single row of undifferentiated basaloid cells at the periphery.

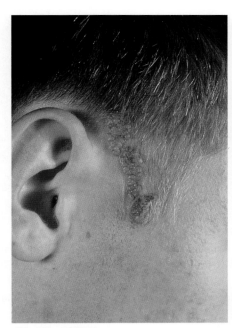

Clin. Fig. VIB7.b

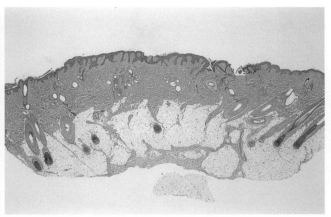

Fig. VIB7.e

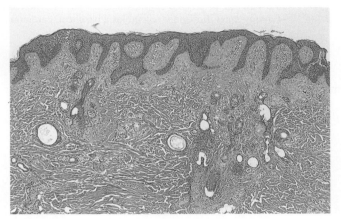

Fig. VIB7.f

Clin. Fig. VIB7.b. *Nevus sebaceus of Jadassohn.* A well-defined, yellow-brown verrucous plaque on the scalp that was present at birth.

Fig. VIB7.e. *Nevus sebaceus of Jadassohn, prepubertal, low power.* At scanning magnification there is an area in the center of this specimen that shows a decreased number of terminal hairs in the subcutaneous fat. This corresponds with the alopecia noted clinically.

Fig. VIB7.f. *Nevus sebaceus of Jadassohn, prepubertal, medium power.* In this area there are several abortive follicular structures in the superficial dermis that fail to produce a hair shaft. This nevus sebaceus is from a 1-year-old child. In this age group, the lesions do not show the characteristic verrucous epidermal hyperplasia and large mature sebaceous lobules that show direct association with the overlying epidermis.

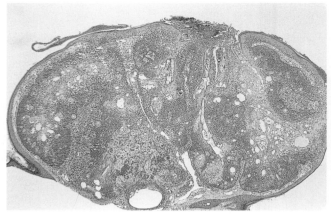

Fig. VIB7.g

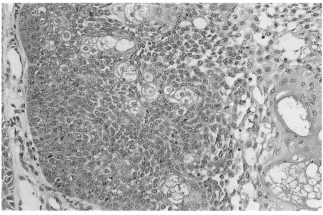

Fig. VIB7.h

Fig. VIB7.g. *Sebaceous epithelioma, low power.* There is a well-circumscribed neoplasm with a surface crust. At scanning magnification it resembles a basal cell carcinoma but lacks the typical mucinous stroma with retraction artifact.

Fig. VIB7.h. *Sebaceous epithelioma, medium power.* This lesion is composed of greater than 50% basaloid cells with a smaller population of mature sebaceous cells.

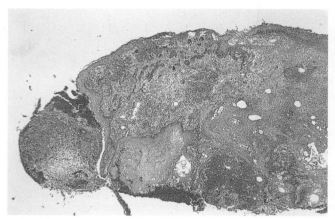

Fig. VIB7.i

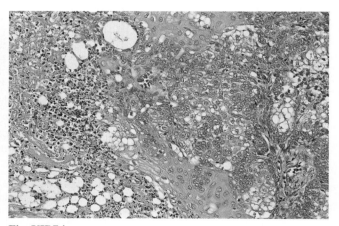

Fig. VIB7.j

Fig. VIB7.i. *Sebaceous carcinoma, low power.* This lesion shows focal ulceration, an infiltrative growth pattern, and an associated inflammatory reaction. At this magnification it has many features that resemble an invasive squamous cell carcinoma.

Fig. VIB7.j. *Sebaceous carcinoma, medium power.* Although in some areas the lesion may resemble squamous cell carcinoma, the characteristic feature is focal sebaceous differentiation characterized by vacuolated cytoplasm that indents the central nucleus.

VIB8. "Histiocytoid" Tumors

"Histiocytes" may have foamy cytoplasm reflecting the accumulation of lipids or may have eosinophilic or amphophilic cytoplasm surrounding an ovoid nucleus with open chromatin. Some nonhistiocytic lesions whose cells may simulate histiocytes are also included here. Xanthelasma and juvenile xanthogranuloma are prototypic. Reticulohistiocytoma is an important differential.

Xanthomas and Xanthelasma

CLINICAL SUMMARY. Tuberous and tuberoeruptive xanthomas are found predominantly in patients with an increase in chylomicron and very-low-density lipoprotein remnants. They are large nodes or plaques located most commonly on the elbows, knees, fingers, and buttocks. Most of the lipid in these xanthomas is in the form of cholesterol. Xanthelasmata consist of slightly raised, yellow, soft plaques on the eyelids.

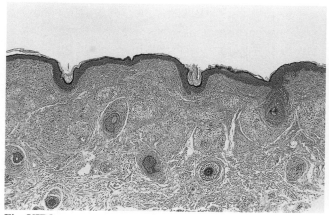

Fig. VIB8.a

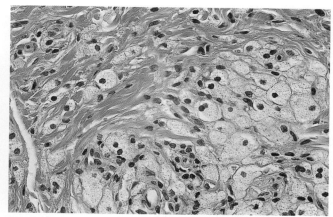

Fig. VIB8.b

Fig. VIB8.a. *Xanthelasma, low power.* Throughout the dermis there are poorly defined aggregates of pale-staining cells.

Fig. VIB8.b. *Xanthelasma, high power.* These foam cells are seen throughout the dermis without an organized pattern. They have small nuclei and prominent vacuolated cytoplasm.

Although xanthelasmata are the most common of the cutaneous xanthomas, they are also the least specific because they occur frequently in persons with normal lipoprotein levels. Plane xanthomas typically develop in skin folds and especially in the palmar creases. Diffuse plane xanthomas are typically seen as multiple grouped papules and poorly defined yellowish plaques in normolipemic patients, often with paraproteinemia, lymphoma, or leukemia.

HISTOPATHOLOGY. The histologic appearance of xanthomas of the skin and the tendons is characterized by foam cells, which are macrophages that have engulfed lipid droplets. There may be varying degrees of fibrosis, giant cells, and clefts, depending on the type and site of xanthoma sampled, but most are surprisingly similar. Most of these foam cells or xanthoma cells are mononuclear, but giant cells, especially of the Touton type with a wreath of nuclei, may be found. Larger extracellular deposits of cholesterol and other sterols leave behind clefts. Xanthelasmata located on the eyelids are characterized by the fairly superficial location of foam cells and the nearly complete absence of fibrosis. Superficial striated muscles, vellus hairs, small vessels, and a thinned epidermis all suggest location on the eyelid and serve as clues to the histologic diagnosis of xanthelasma.

Eruptive Xanthoma

See Figs. VIB8.c–VIB8.e.

Verruciform Xanthoma

See Figs. VIB8.f and VIB8.g.

Juvenile Xanthogranuloma

See Figs. VIB8.h–VIB8.j.

CLINICAL SUMMARY. Juvenile xanthogranuloma (JXG) (21) is a benign disorder in which one, several, or occasionally numerous red to yellow nodules are present. Despite the name, the lesions are also seen in adults but are most common in young children. In children, the lesions may grow rapidly but almost always regress within a year. Lesions in adults are not uncommon but are usually solitary and persistent. JXG has also been identified in many other organ systems, usually in association with macronodular lesions. A number of systemic complications are associated with JXG. Ocular involvement including glaucoma and bleeding into the anterior chamber is the most common, and bone involvement may occur.

HISTOPATHOLOGY. The typical JXG contains histiocytes with a variety of cellular features. Early lesions may show large accumulations of histiocytes without any lipid infiltration intermingled with only a few lymphoid cells and eosinophils. When no foam cells or giant cells are seen, the possibility of JXG is often overlooked. Usually some degree of lipidization is present, even in very early lesions, manifested by pale-staining histiocytes. In mature lesions, a granulomatous infiltrate is usually present containing foam cells, foreign-body giant cells, and Touton giant cells and histiocytes, lymphocytes, and eosinophils. Older regressing lesions show proliferation of fibroblasts and fibrosis replacing part of the infiltrate. The oncocytic or reticulohistiocytic type of histiocyte with an eosinophilic cytoplasm is uncommon in childhood lesions but may be seen in adult lesions. The spindle cell variant is also more common in adults. Here one sees predominantly a spindle cell proliferation, similar to blue nevus or dermatofibroma, with few foamy or giant cells.

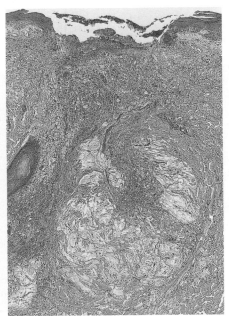

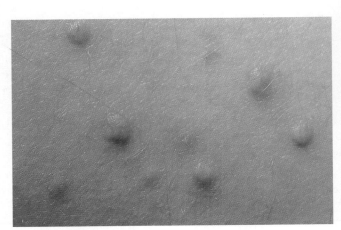

Clin. Fig. VIB8.a

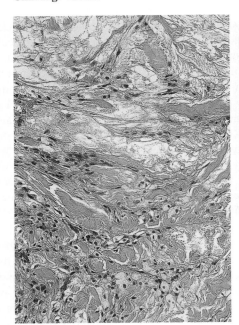

Fig. VIB8.c

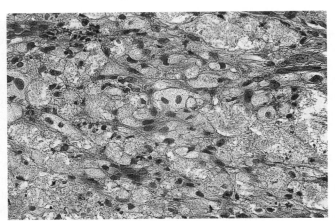

Fig. VIB8.e

Fig. VIB8.d

Clin. Fig. VIB8.a. *Eruptive xanthomas.* Multiple yellow-red papules and nodules developed suddenly on the buttock skin of a 35-year-old woman. Testing revealed markedly elevated triglycerides.

Fig. VIB8.c. *Eruptive xanthoma, low power.* Within the middermis there is an inflammatory infiltrate associated with clear spaces forming clefts.

Fig. VIB8.d. *Eruptive xanthoma, medium power.* These variably sized clefts represent the lipid deposition. In the lower half of this photomicrograph are foam cells (macrophages).

Fig. VIB8.e. *Eruptive xanthoma, high power.* Multiple foamy histiocytes are found throughout the dermis. In eruptive xanthomas, neutrophils, as seen here, are admixed with these histiocytes.

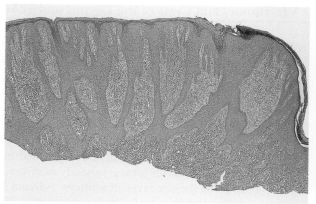

Fig. VIB8.f

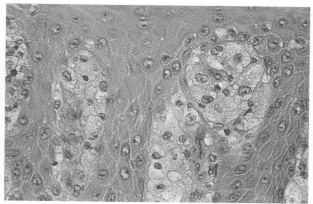

Fig. VIB8.g

Fig. VIB8.f. *Verruciform xanthoma, low power.* The epidermis shows prominent hyperplasia and hyperkeratosis. There is a mixed infiltrate in the papillary and superficial reticular dermis.

Fig. VIB8.g. *Verruciform xanthoma, high power.* Within the tips of the dermal papillae there are large histiocytes with an abundance of foamy cytoplasm.

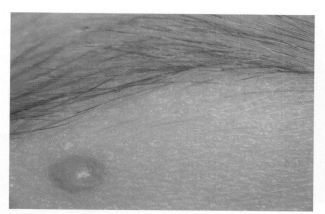

Clin. Fig. VIB8.b

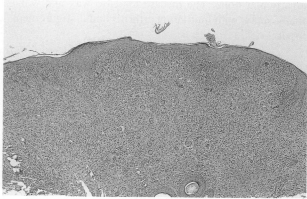

Fig. VIB8.h

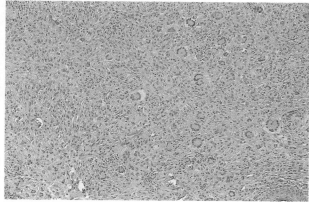

Fig. VIB8.i

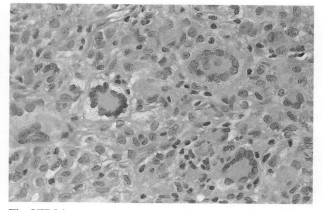

Fig. VIB8.j

Clin. Fig. VIB8.b. *Juvenile xanthogranuloma.* A 10-year-old girl developed several discrete red to yellow nodules and papules on the face and trunk that later resolved spontaneously.

Fig. VIB8.h. *Juvenile xanthogranuloma, low power.* In a xanthogranuloma there is a dense infiltrate forming a solid mass occupying nearly the entire thickness of the dermis.

Fig. VIB8.i. *Juvenile xanthogranuloma, medium power.* There is a dense mixed infiltrate composed predominantly of histiocytes. There may be few or multiple multinucleated giant cells. Eosinophils and neutrophils are frequently seen, especially in early lesions.

Fig. VIB8.j. *Juvenile xanthogranuloma, high power.* Characteristic Touton giant cells show a wreath of nuclei surrounded by vacuolated cytoplasm.

Reticulohistiocytosis

CLINICAL SUMMARY. Two types of reticulohistiocytosis (22) are recognized: giant cell reticulohistiocytoma (GCRH) and multicentric reticulohistiocytosis (MRH). Both types occur almost exclusively in adults. The histologic picture is very similar in the two types. In GCRH there is usually a single nodule ("solitary reticulohistiocytoma") but occasionally multiple lesions are seen, most commonly on the head and neck. The nodules are smooth and 0.5 to 2.0 cm in diameter. They may involute spontaneously. Even patients with multiple lesions show no sign of systemic involvement.

In MRH, the patients tend to be middle-aged women, with widespread cutaneous involvement and a destructive arthritis. Nodules ranging in size from a few millimeters to several centimeters are most common on the extremities. The polyarthritis may be mild or severe and may be mutilating, especially on the hands, through destruction of articular cartilage and subarticular bone. The disease tends to wax and wane over many years, with mutilating arthritis and disfigurement real possibilities.

HISTOPATHOLOGY. The characteristic histologic feature in both GCRH and MRH is the presence of numerous multinucleate giant cells and oncocytic histiocytes showing abundant eosinophilic, finely granular cytoplasm, often with a "ground glass" appearance. In older lesions, giant cells and fibrosis are more common. There may be subtle differences between the two lesions. For example, in MRH the giant cells are smaller (50–100 mm), have fewer nuclei (perhaps 10), and are almost always strikingly PAS positive. However, the two conditions often cannot be separated microscopically. The polyarthritis present in nearly all instances of MRH is caused by the same type of infiltrate as found in the cutaneous lesions, and similar infiltrates of uncertain clinical significance have been described in other organs.

Conditions to consider in the differential diagnosis:

Foamy Histiocytes
xanthomas (eruptive, plane, tuberous, tendon)
verruciform xanthoma
xanthelasma
cholestanolemia, phytosterolemia
xanthoma disseminatum
diffuse normolipemic plane xanthoma
papular xanthoma
eruptive normolipemic xanthoma
progressive nodular histiocytoma (superficial)

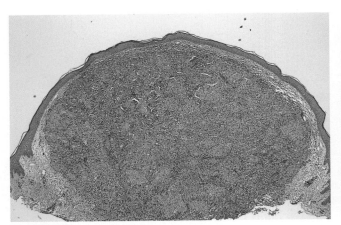

Fig. VIB8.k

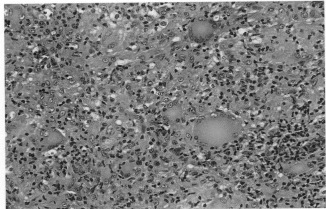

Fig. VIB8.l

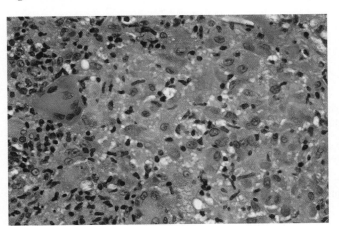

Fig. VIB8.m

Fig. VIB8.k. *Reticulohistiocytoma, low power.* At this magnification the lesion resembles a xanthogranuloma with a dense nodular infiltrate in the dermis; the overlying epidermis shows an effaced architecture.

Fig. VIB8.l. *Reticulohistiocytoma, medium power.* This dense infiltrate is mixed but there are scattered giant cells whose cytoplasm show an eosinophilic ground glass appearance. They may show a ring of nuclei but they lack the foamy cytoplasm typical of a Touton giant cell.

Fig. VIB8.m. *Reticulohistiocytoma, high power.* The infiltrate is mixed with numerous histiocytes and lymphocytes and eosinophils. One giant cell seen here shows an eosinophilic cytoplasm without a vacuolated periphery.

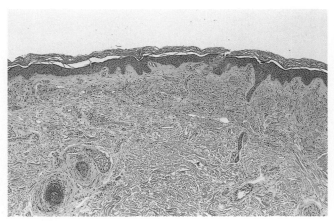

Fig. VIB8.n

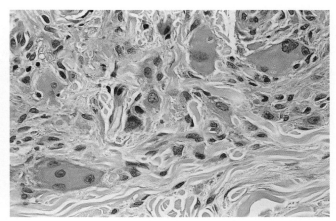

Fig. VIB8.o

Fig. VIB8.n. *Multicentric reticulohistiocytosis, low power.* There are poorly defined cellular aggregates in the upper third of the reticular dermis.

Fig. VIB8.o. *Multicentric reticulohistiocytosis, high power.* This infiltrate is mixed but contains large giant cells with one or more nuclei and eosinophilic "ground glass" cytoplasm.

Langerhans cell histiocytosis (rare xanthomatous type)
histoid leprosy
Nonfoamy Histiocytes
dermatofibroma/histiocytoma
Langerhans cell histiocytosis
congenital self-healing reticulohistiocytosis
indeterminate cell histiocytosis
granuloma annulare
eruptive histiocytomas
benign cephalic histiocytosis
sinus histiocytosis with massive lymphadenopathy
juvenile xanthogranuloma
Giant Cells Prominent
juvenile xanthogranuloma
multicentric reticulohistiocytosis
solitary reticulohistiocytoma
giant cell reticulohistiocytoma
necrobiotic xanthogranuloma with paraproteinemia
xanthoma disseminatum
Histiocytic Simulants
pleomorphic large cell lymphoma (Ki-1, usually T
  cells)
epithelioid sarcoma
leukemia cutis

VIB9. Tumors of Large Lymphoid Cells

Large lymphoid cells may be mistaken for carcinoma or melanoma cells, but may be distinguished morphologically by their tendency to less cohesive growth in large sheets, by the absence of epithelial or melanocytic differentiation, and by immunopathology. Anaplastic large-cell lymphoma is prototypic (23). Lymphomatoid papulosis (LyP) (24) and leukemia cutis are important differentials.

Cutaneous CD30+ (Ki-1+) Anaplastic Large Cell Lymphoma

CLINICAL SUMMARY. The entity historically described as Ki-1+ lymphoma was first recognized as a neoplasm manifested as cutaneous nodules composed of lymphocytes with large strikingly atypical nuclei. The neoplastic cells, usually of T-cell lineage, by definition expressed the Ki-1 (now known as CD30) antigen. The CD30 antigen is an inducible marker of lymphocyte activation that can be identified on either B or T cells. CD30 expression can also be observed in tumor stage MF, some pleomorphic T-cell lymphomas, and some nonneoplastic eruptions including LyP (see below). CD30+ anaplastic large cell lymphoma (ALCL) lesions typically present as a single or a few large nodules or tumors located on the extremities, and ulceration and crusting are common. The lymphoma can present at any age. Patients with cutaneous ALCL do not usually develop systemic symptoms, in contrast to patients with nodal involvement at presentation. CD30+ ALCL appears to be the most common cutaneous lymphoma in patients with human immunodeficiency virus (HIV). In contrast to immunocompetent individuals, HIV-seropositive patients with CD30+ ALCL have a dismal prognosis.

HISTOPATHOLOGY. It is now established that CD30+ lymphoma is not a single entity but comprises a spectrum of disorders linked by the presence of a common neoplastic cell type. The spectrum includes CD30+ ALCL and LyP. CD30+ ALCL is characterized by a nodular dermal and subcutaneous infiltrate of large lymphocytes with abundant faintly basophilic cytoplasm, large irregularly shaped vesicular nuclei with coarsely clumped chromatin along nuclear membranes, and large irregularly shaped nucleoli. Wreath-

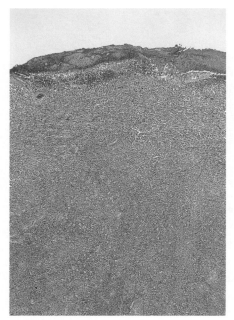

Fig. VIB9.a. *Cutaneous anaplastic large cell lymphoma, low power.* This relatively large tumor is composed of a dense infiltrate occupying the entire dermis. There is associated ulceration of the overlying epidermis.

Fig. VIB9.b. *Large cell anaplastic lymphoma, medium power.* There are dense sheets of atypical cells admixed with inflammatory cells, frequently eosinophils. A number of the atypical cells show more than one nucleus.

Fig. VIB9.c. *Large cell anaplastic lymphoma, high power.* Many cells are large, with large hyperchromatic nuclei; bizarre forms and mitotic figures are frequently seen.

Fig. VIB9.a

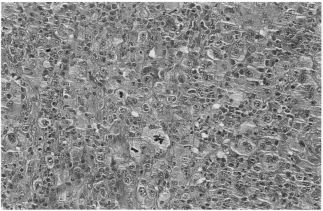

Fig. VIB9.b

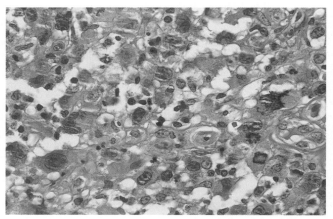

Fig. VIB9.c

shaped multinucleated cells are often present, as are embryo-shaped nuclei. Sarcomatoid (spindled) cellular morphology is encountered in rare cases. Epidermal hyperplasia or ulceration and an inflammatory infiltrate rich in neutrophils are commonly observed. Because of the abundant cytoplasm and the compact arrangement of the lesional cells, some examples may simulate a carcinoma or a sarcoma. Conversely, CD30 can be expressed by a variety of carcinomas, including embryonal carcinoma. Lesions of LyP are usually separable histologically in that atypical lymphocytes are arrayed in small numbers or in small clusters rather than sheets, within a heterogeneous infiltrate in which neutrophils and/or eosinophils are usually conspicuous.

Lymphomatoid Papulosis

CLINICAL SUMMARY. The atypical cells of LyP (24) and ALCL share similar cellular morphology, CD30 expression, and clonal rearrangement of the T-cell receptor gene. Thus, a strong case can be made that these conditions comprise a disease spectrum. Within this spectrum, the overall number of clinical lesions is roughly inversely proportional to the durability of the lesions. Thus, lesions of LyP tend to be numer-

ous, short-lived, and recurrent in most instances, whereas ALCL lesions tend to be few in number and persistent.

HISTOPATHOLOGY. Lesions of LyP are usually separable histologically from cutaneous anaplastic large cell lymphoma in that atypical lymphocytes are arrayed in small numbers or in small clusters rather than sheets, within a heterogeneous infiltrate in which neutrophils and/or eosinophils are usually conspicuous. The epidermis can show a variety of patterns in LyP biopsies, including infiltration by small to medium-sized convoluted lymphocytes, an interface reaction with necrotic keratinocytes, or necrosis and ulceration.

Leukemia Cutis

CLINICAL SUMMARY. Leukemias are neoplasms of hematolymphoid cells that usually present with prominent involvement of the peripheral blood. They can be broadly grouped into acute and chronic forms of either lymphoid or myeloid lineage. Cutaneous leukemic infiltrates present as macules, papules, plaques, nodules, and ulcers. Lesions can be erythematous or purpuric. Extramedullary deposits of acute myelogenous leukemia are commonly referred to as

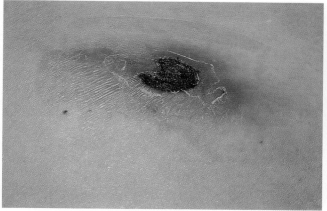

Clin. Fig. VIB9

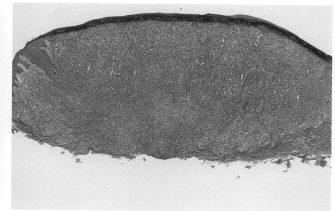

Fig. VIB9.d

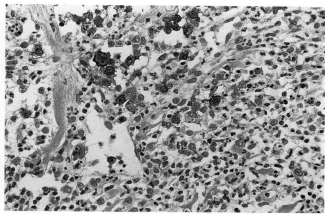

Fig. VIB9.e

Fig. VIB9.f

Clin. Fig. VIB9. *Lymphomatoid papulosis*. Indurated erythematous nodules, some with ulcerated centers, developed on a recurrent basis in this elderly man.

Fig. VIB9.d. *Lymphomatoid papulosis, low power*. There is a diffuse and vaguely wedge-shaped infiltrate in the reticular dermis. (P. LeBoit and T. McCalmont)

Fig. VIB9.e. *Lymphomatoid papulosis, high power*. The infiltrate is heterogeneous and includes neutrophils and eosinophils and small lymphocytes and a few large lymphoid cells. (P. LeBoit and T. McCalmont)

Fig. VIB9.f. *Lymphomatoid papulosis, high power*. As demonstrated in this CD30 immunostain, there are only a few large neoplastic CD30+ cells, which in contrast to anaplastic large cell lymphoma do not form large sheets or nodular clusters. (P. LeBoit and T. McCalmont)

granulocytic sarcomas or chloromas. In addition to these specific infiltrates of leukemia, there are various inflammatory skin diseases that occur in conjunction with leukemia, sometimes referred to as leukemids. These disorders include leukocytoclastic vasculitis, pyoderma gangrenosum, Sweet's syndrome, urticaria, erythroderma, erythema nodosum, and erythema multiforme.

HISTOPATHOLOGY. The most common pattern of skin involvement consists of an interstitial (reticular) infiltrate marked by diffuse permeation of the reticular dermis by leukemic cells in horizontal strands between collagen bundles. Nodular infiltrates of leukemic cells can also occur.

Dense bandlike infiltrates in the superficial dermis and sparse superficial and deep perivascular infiltrates are occasionally observed.

Acute myelogenous leukemia can assume either an interstitial or a nodular pattern. The epidermis is spared, but the subcutis is often involved. The diagnosis hinges in large part on the recognition of myeloblasts, which have scant cytoplasm, large vesicular nuclei, and nucleoli of variable size. Eosinophilic myelocytes or metamyelocytes are not pathognomonic of acute myelogenous leukemia but strongly favor that diagnosis in the proper context. These immature cells have the granules of mature eosinophils with monolobed nuclei. Cutaneous infiltrates of chronic myeloid leukemia are

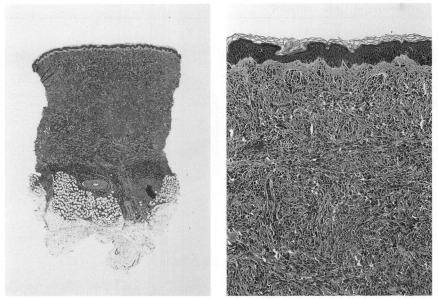

Fig. VIB9.g   Fig. VIB9.h

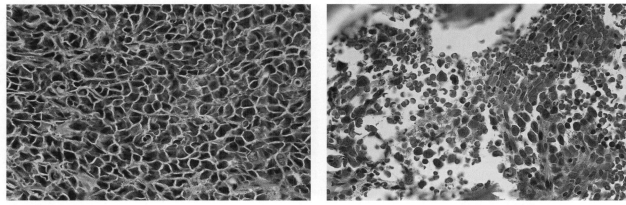

Fig. VIB9.i   Fig. VIB9.j

Fig. VIB9.g. *Leukemia cutis, acute myelogenous leukemia, low power.* There is a dense infiltrate occupying the entire dermis extending into the subcutaneous fat. At this magnification, the predominant differential diagnosis is lymphoma cutis.

Fig. VIB9.h. *Leukemia cutis, acute myelogenous leukemia, medium power.* This dense infiltrate is separated from the overlying normal appearing epidermis. The cells show an infiltrative pattern in between collagen bundles without organization.

Fig. VIB9.i. *Leukemia cutis, acute myelogenous leukemia, high power.* The infiltrate is composed entirely of atypical cells with hyperchromatic nuclei and eosinophilic cytoplasm.

Fig. VIB9.j. *Acute myelogenous leukemia, bone marrow biopsy.* The atypical cells seen in the skin biopsy resemble those seen here in the bone marrow biopsy.

Fig. VIB10.a. *Urticaria pigmentosa, low power.* There is a dense nodular infiltrate involving the upper half of the dermis. The overlying epidermis shows mild hyperplasia.

Fig. VIB10.b. *Urticaria pigmentosa, medium power.* The infiltrate is composed of uniform ovoid cells that are present densely in the reticular dermis but also fill the papillary dermis. The cells do not involve the overlying epidermis.

Fig. VIB10.c. *Urticaria pigmentosa, high power.* The individual cells have small uniform ovoid nuclei and an abundance of granular cytoplasm. Scattered eosinophils are frequently seen in all forms of mastocytosis, a clue to the diagnosis.

Fig. VIB10.d. *Urticaria pigmentosa. Giemsa stain.* The mast cell granules metachromatically stain purple with Giemsa stain.

less common than those of acute myelogenous leukemia. Similar diffuse or nodular patterns occur. The infiltrates contain a range of myelocytic differentiation from myeloblasts to segmented neutrophils. Acute lymphocytic (lymphoblastic) leukemia shares features with lymphoblastic lymphoma, presenting typically as diffuse or nodular monomorphous infiltrates of lymphoblasts, cells with scant cytoplasm, and round nuclei that are slightly to moderately convoluted with thin but well-defined nuclear membranes and finely dispersed chromatin. Histochemical and immunophenotypic studies can help in the identification of leukemic infiltrates. Reactions used to identify myeloblastic differentiation include histochemical studies such as those for myeloperoxidase, Sudan black B, and the chloroacetate esterase (Leder) stain, or immunoperoxidase stains including lysozyme, myeloperoxidase, CD33 (My-9), and neutrophil-specific elastase (25).

Conditions to consider in the differential diagnosis:
  pleomorphic peripheral T-cell lymphoma
  cutaneous anaplastic large cell lymphoma (CD30 (Ki-1) lymphoma (regressing atypical histiocytosis)
  leukemia cutis
  cutaneous Hodgkin's disease

VIB10. Mast Cell Tumors

Mast cells predominate in a nodular dermal infiltrate, with scattered eosinophils.

Urticaria Pigmentosa, Nodular Lesions

CLINICAL SUMMARY. Children or adults with urticaria pigmentosa may present with multiple brown nodules or plaques that, on stroking, show urtication and occasionally

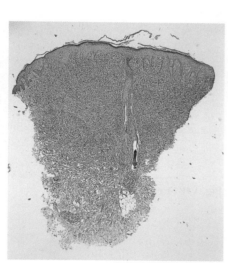

Fig. VIB10.a

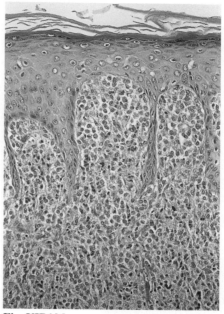

Fig. VIB10.b

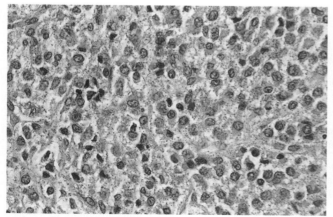

Fig. VIB10.c

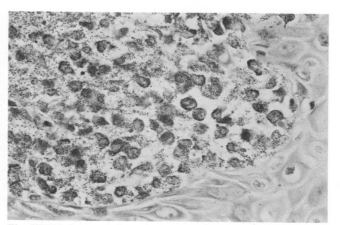

Fig. VIB10.d

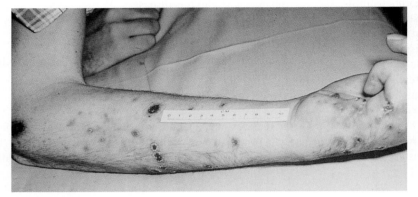

Clin. Fig. VIB11

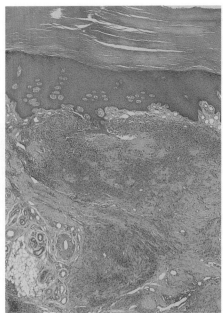

Fig. VIB11.a

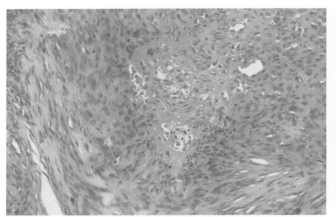

Fig. VIB11.b

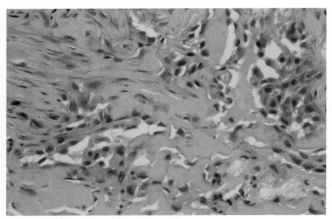

Fig. VIB11.c

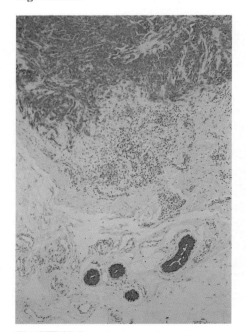

Fig. VIB11.d

Clin. Fig. VIB11. *Epithelioid sarcoma*. Flexion contractures of the fingers, with multiple ulcerating nodules of the hand and forearm. (P. Heenan)

Fig. VIB11.a. *Epithelioid sarcoma, low power*. The epidermis is hyperplastic and overlies several poorly defined nodules in the dermis with central foci of necrosis. (P. Heenan)

Fig. VIB11.b. *Epithelioid sarcoma, medium power*. Epithelioid cells with eosinophilic cytoplasm and pleomorphic nuclei surround a central zone of necrosis. (P. Heenan)

Fig. VIB11.c. *Epithelioid sarcoma, high power*. Atypical epithelioid cells line irregular spaces, producing an angiosarcoma-like pattern, with spindle cells in the intervening stroma. (P. Heenan)

Fig. VIB11.d. *Epithelioid sarcoma, low power*. Positive immunostaining for cytokeratins AE1 and AE3. Vimentin stain (not shown) was also positive. (P. Heenan)

blister formation. Infants, almost exclusively, may present with a usually solitary large cutaneous nodule, which on stroking often shows not only urtication but also large bullae. Adults with urticaria pigmentosa have macular lesions with telangiectasia; urtication on stroking is variable (see also section IIIA2).

HISTOPATHOLOGY. In these nodular or plaque lesions, the mast cells lie closely packed in tumorlike aggregates. The infiltrate may extend through the entire dermis and even into the subcutaneous fat. The mast cell nuclei in these tumors are cuboidal rather than spindle shaped, and the cells have ample eosinophilic cytoplasm and a well-defined cell border. In adults, the diagnosis can be difficult. An increase in interstitial mast cells is helpful in establishing the diagnosis.

Conditions to consider in the differential diagnosis:

mastocytosis (urticaria pigmentosa, nodular lesions)

VIB11. Tumors with Prominent Necrosis

Necrosis is a striking feature in epithelioid sarcoma, which may be in consequence mistaken for a granulomatous process. In addition, many advanced malignancies, often metastatic, have prominent necrosis (26).

Epithelioid Sarcoma

CLINICAL SUMMARY. This is a distinctive rare malignant soft tissue neoplasm of uncertain origin, occurring most commonly in the distal extremities of young adult males as a slowly growing dermal or subcutaneous nodule. However, the tumor has been reported in a wide range of anatomic sites. This aggressive neoplasm is characterized by multiple recurrences, often producing ulcerated nodules and plaques in the dermis and subcutis, and by regional and systemic metastases resulting in a poor prognosis.

HISTOPATHOLOGY. The tumors are composed of irregular nodules of atypical epithelioid cells with abundant eosinophilic cytoplasm and pleomorphic nuclei, merging with spindle cells. These aggregates are embedded in collagenous fibrous tissue in which there may be focal hemorrhage, hemosiderin, and mucin deposition with a patchy lymphocytic infiltrate. Mitoses are present in varied frequency, vascular invasion is a common feature, and foci of necrosis are present in the centers of tumor nodules. Ulceration follows epidermal involvement by the larger tumor nodules, and invasion extends diffusely into the subcutis and deeper soft tissues. A fibromalike variant of epithelioid sarcoma has also been reported in which the spindle cell pattern predominates without the characteristic epithelioid cells and nodularity. At low power, the neoplasm may suggest a granulomatous process such as granuloma annulare, necrobiosis lipoidica, or rheumatoid nodule. The cellular atypia, diffuse stromal invasion, and foci of necrosis involving tumor cells and not only stroma, as in the necrobiotic granulomatous processes, identify the process as malignant, and the diagnosis is supported by positive immunostaining for cytokeratin and vimentin, and negativity for leukocyte common antigen.

Conditions to consider in the differential diagnosis:

epithelioid sarcoma
metastatic carcinomas, sarcomas, melanomas
occasional advanced primary malignant tumors

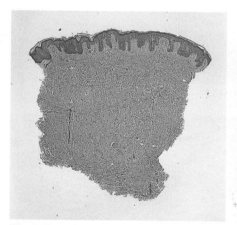

Fig. VIB12.a

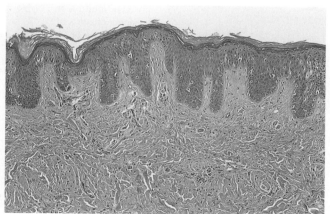

Fig. VIB12.b

Fig. VIB12.a. *Granular cell tumor, low power.* There is an eosinophilic infiltrative lesion within the dermis that is difficult to identify at low power. However, note the absence of adnexal structures in this punch biopsy.

Fig. VIB12.b. *Granular cell tumor, medium power.* Epidermal hyperplasia overlying a granular cell tumor may be mild as seen here, or it may be striking pseudoepitheliomatous hyperplasia resembling a squamous cell carcinoma.

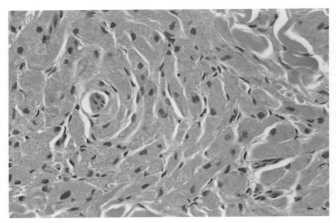

Fig. VIB12.c

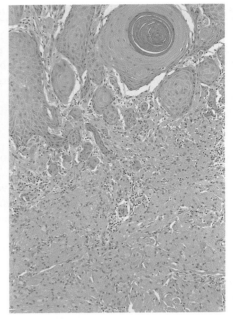

Fig. VIB12.d

Fig. VIB12.c. *Granular cell tumor, high power.* The individual cells are large with an abundance of eosinophilic granular cytoplasm. There are small nuclei without mitoses or cytologic atypia. These granules can be highlighted using the periodic acid–Schiff stain.

Fig. VIB12.d. *Granular cell tumor with pseudoepitheliomatous hyperplasia, medium power.* The highly irregular proliferation of the overlying epidermis seen here is a characteristic although not invariable feature of granular cell tumors and may be mistaken for squamous cell carcinoma in a superficial biopsy.

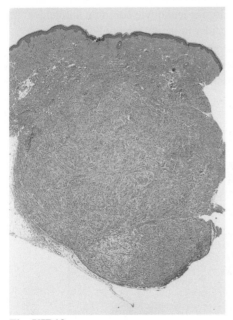

Fig. VIB12.e

Fig. VIB12.e. *Cellular neurothekeoma, low power.* There is a relatively well-circumscribed nodule within the dermis.

Fig. VIB12.f. *Cellular neurothekeoma, medium power.* The neoplasm is composed of multiple interlacing clusters of cells that may be reminiscent of a neuroma at this magnification.

Fig. VIB12.g. *Cellular neurothekeoma, high power.* The cells are spindle and epithelioid in form, some with an abundance of eosinophilic cytoplasm. The nuclei are relatively small and uniform with minimal atypia and minimal mitotic activity.

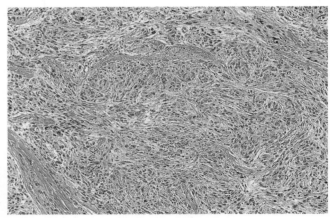

Fig. VIB12.f

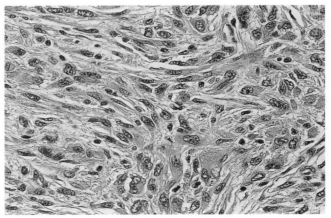

Fig. VIB12.g

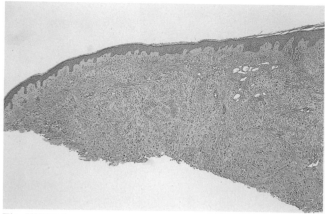

Fig. VIB12.h

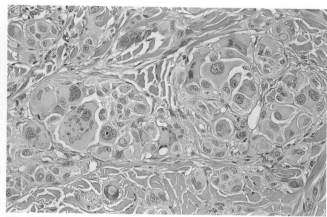

Fig. VIB12.i

Fig. VIB12.h. *Metastatic malignant melanoma, low power.* A pale staining, poorly defined tumor has replaced the reticular dermis.

Fig. VIB12.i. *Metastatic malignant melanoma, high power.* The tumor is composed of pleomorphic anaplastic cells. Many cells show multiple nuclei as well as atypical nuclei and prominent nucleoli. Because of the absence of melanin pigment, immunoperoxidase stains are necessary to definitively identify this as metastatic melanoma and not metastatic carcinoma.

VIB12. Miscellaneous and Undifferentiated Epithelial Tumors

Proliferations of atypical cells with more or less abundant cytoplasm and contiguous cell borders occupy the dermis as nodular masses.

Granular Cell Tumor

See Figs. VIB12.a–VIB12.d.

Cellular Neurothekeoma

See Figs. VIB12.e–VIB12.g.

Metastatic Malignant Melanoma

See Figs. VIB12.h and VIB12.i.

Conditions to consider in the differential diagnosis:
Epithelial Tumors
undifferentiated carcinoma (large cell, small cell)
neuroendocrine tumor
Epithelial Simulants
anaplastic large cell lymphoma (CD30/Ki-1, usually T cells)
epithelioid sarcoma
granular cell nerve sheath tumor (granular cell tumor/schwannoma)
plexiform granular cell nerve sheath tumor
malignant granular cell tumor
epithelioid angiosarcoma
cellular neurothekeoma (immature nerve sheath myxoma)
ganglioneuroma
cephalic brainlike hamartoma (nasal glioma)
encephalocele
cutaneous meningiomas

VIC. SPINDLE CELL, PLEOMORPHIC AND CONNECTIVE TISSUE TUMORS

In the dermis there is a proliferation of elongated tapered "spindle cells;" these may be of fibrohistiocytic, muscle, neural (Schwannian), melanocytic, or of unknown origin. Immunohistochemistry may be essential in making these distinctions.

1. Fibrohistiocytic Spindle Cell Tumors
2. Schwannian/Neural Spindle Cell Tumors
3. Spindle Cell Tumors of Muscle
4. Melanocytic Spindle Cell Tumors
5. Tumors and Proliferations of Angiogenic Cells
6. Tumors of Adipose Tissue
7. Tumors of Cartilaginous Tissue
8. Tumors of Osseous Tissue

VIC1. Fibrohistiocytic Spindle Cell Tumors

There is a proliferation of spindle to pleomorphic cells that may synthesize collagen or may be essentially undifferentiated. Because there are no useful specific markers for fibroblasts, immunohistochemistry is of little diagnostic utility except to rule out nonfibrous spindle cell tumors. Morphology is critical for accurate diagnosis.

Dermatofibroma

CLINICAL SUMMARY. Dermatofibromas (27) occur in the skin as firm, indolent, red to red-brown or occasionally blue-black, single or multiple nodules, usually only a few milli-

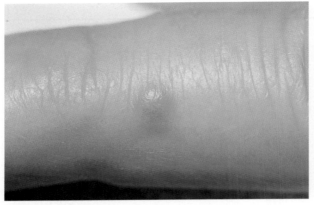

Clin. Fig. VIC1.a

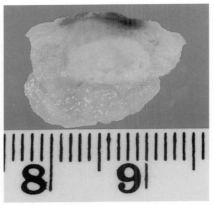

Clin. Fig. VIC1.b

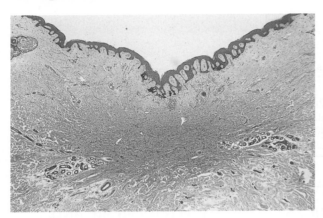

Fig. VIC1.a

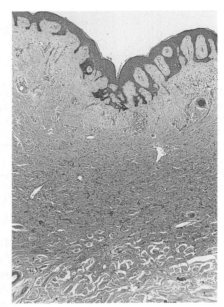

Fig. VIC1.b

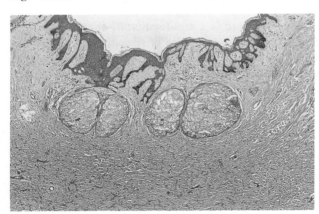

Fig. VIC1.c

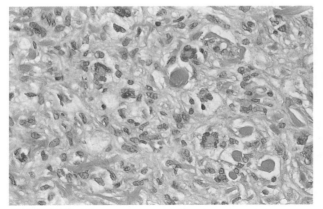

Fig. VIC1.d

Clin. Fig. VIC1.a. *Dermatofibroma*. A 47-year-old man presented with a 4 mm deep firm smooth red nodule on the extensor finger.

Clin. Fig. VIC1.b. *Dermatofibroma*. A sectioned gross specimen demonstrating a circumscribed yellowish nodule in the reticular dermis. The epidermis is hyperplastic and hyperpigmented, and is separated from the epidermis by a clear zone. (P. Heenan)

Fig. VIC1.a. *Dermatofibroma, low power*. There is a symmetrical but noncircumscribed area of hypercellularity in the middermis. This proliferation is associated with retraction of the overlying epidermis which produces the dimple sign which is seen clinically.

Fig. VIC1.b. *Dermatofibroma, medium power*. Within the mid dermis there is a proliferation of bland appearing spindled cells. As can be seen in the lower portion of this lesion, these cells encircle bundles of reticular dermal collagen.

Fig. VIC1.c. *Dermatofibroma, medium power*. The overlying epidermis becomes hyperplastic as well as hyperpigmented.

Fig. VIC1.d. *Dermatofibroma, high power*. Some dermatofibromas contain foamy and multinucleated histiocytes with peripheral foamy cytoplasm which represent Touton giant cells.

meters in diameter. The cut surface of the lesions varies in color from white to yellowish brown, depending on the proportions of fibrous tissue, lipid, and hemosiderin present. The lesions usually persist indefinitely.

HISTOPATHOLOGY. The epidermis is usually hyperplastic, with hyperpigmentation of the basal layer and elongation of the rete ridges, separated by a clear (Grenz) zone from a spindle cell tumor in the dermis. The highly characteristic hyperplasia of the overlying epidermis in the center of the lesion may mimic basal cell carcinoma and has considerable value in establishing the diagnosis of dermatofibroma. The dermal tumor is composed of fibroblast-like spindle cells, histiocytes, and blood vessels in varying proportions. Foamy histiocytes and multinucleated giant cells containing lipid or hemosiderin may be present, sometimes in large numbers, forming xanthomatous aggregates. Capillaries may be plentiful in the stroma, giving the lesion an angiomatous component; when associated with a sclerotic stroma, such lesions have been referred to as sclerosing hemangioma. In some small lesions, the spindle cells are distributed singly between the collagen bundles, forming a zone of subtly increased cellularity, whereas in larger tumors there is much denser cellularity and the spindle cells are arranged in sheets or interlocking strands in storiform pattern. The dermal tumor is poorly demarcated on both sides, so that the fibroblasts and the young basophilic collagen extend between the mature eosinophilic collagen bundles of the dermis and surround them, trapping normal collagen bundles at the periphery of the tumor nodule.

Cellular dermatofibroma is a very densely cellular tumor with fascicular and storiform growth patterns and frequent extension into the subcutis. The neoplasm shares some features, therefore, with dermatofibrosarcoma protuberans, from which it is distinguished by the overlying epidermal hyperplasia, polymorphism of the tumor cell population, extension of tumor cells at the edge of the lesion to surround individual hyalinized collagen bundles, and the absence of immunostaining for CD34. The cellular dermatofibroma also extends into the subcutis along the septa or in a bulging expansile pattern rather than in the more diffusely infiltrative pattern of dermatofibrosarcoma protuberans, which produces a typical honeycomb-like pattern and extends far along interlobular septa of the panniculus.

Cellular Dermatofibroma

See Figs. VIC1.e and VIC1.f.

Dermatofibrosarcoma Protuberans

CLINICAL SUMMARY. Dermatofibrosarcoma protuberans (DFSP) (28) is a slowly growing dermal spindle cell neoplasm of intermediate malignancy that usually forms an indurated plaque on which multiple reddish purple firm nodules subsequently arise, sometimes with ulceration. The tumors occur most frequently on the trunk or the proximal extremities of young adults and only rarely in the head and neck. A small proportion of cases have been reported in childhood and, rarely, as congenital lesions. Local recurrence is common but metastasis is rare.

HISTOPATHOLOGY. DFSP is composed of densely packed, monomorphous, plump spindle cells arranged in a storiform (matlike) pattern in the central areas of tumor nodules, whereas at the periphery there is diffuse infiltration of the

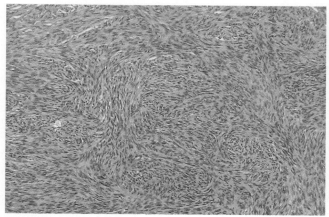

Fig. VIC1.e

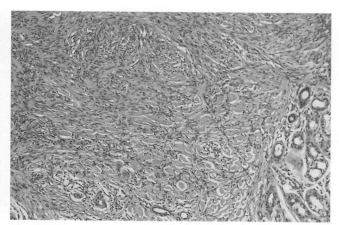

Fig. VIC1.f

Fig. VIC1.e. *Cellular dermatofibroma, medium power.* The tumor consists of spindle cells arranged in densely cellular fascicular and storiform patterns. (P. Heenan)

Fig. VIC1.f. *Cellular dermatofibroma, medium power.* At the periphery of the lesion, the spindle cells surround individual collagen bundles. A negative immunohistochemical stain for CD34 (not shown) assists in differentiating a cellular dermatofibroma from a dermatofibrosarcoma protuberans (see Figs. VIC1.g–VIC1.h). (P. Heenan)

dermal stroma, frequently extending into the subcutis and producing a characteristic honeycomb pattern. Infiltration into the underlying fascia and muscle is a late event. The peripheral elements of the tumor may have a deceptively bland appearance and may extend far along septa of the panniculus, which can cause difficulties in determining the true extent of the tumor. Myxoid areas, sometimes resembling liposarcoma, include a characteristic vascular component of

slitlike, anastomosing, thin-walled blood vessels presenting a crow's foot or chicken wire appearance. Melanin-containing cells may be present in a small proportion of tumors, so-called Bednar tumor (pigmented DFSP, storiform neurofibroma). Fibrosarcomatous areas are seen in a small proportion of DFSP, characterized by a fascicular or herringbone growth pattern of the spindle cells. This variant does not appear to have any greater propensity for local recur-

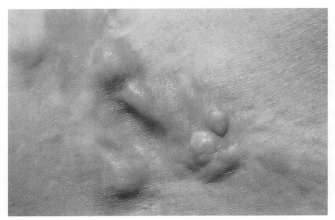

Clin. Fig. VIC1.c

Clin. Fig. VIC1.d

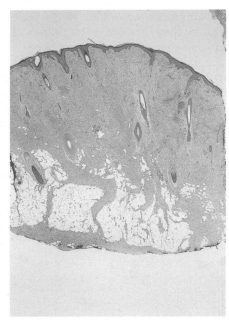

Fig. VIC1.g

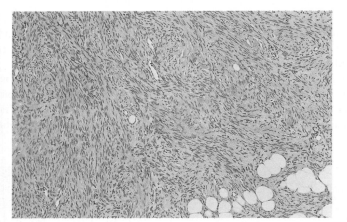

Fig. VIC1.h

Clin. Fig. VIC1.c. *Dermatofibrosarcoma protuberans, recurrent.* An elderly woman presented with multiple variably shaped flesh-colored nodules and papules in a chest wall excision scar.

Clin. Fig. VIC1.d. *Dermatofibrosarcoma protuberans.* A sectioned gross specimen reveals an asymmetric tumor spanning the dermis and infiltrating the subcutis. (P. Heenan)

Fig. VIC1.g. *Dermatofibrosarcoma protuberans, low power.* There is a tumor which occupies nearly the entire dermis and extends into the underlying subcutaneous fat.

Fig. VIC1.h. *Dermatofibrosarcoma protuberans, medium power.* A spindle cell proliferation shows a storiform or cartwheel pattern. (*continues*)

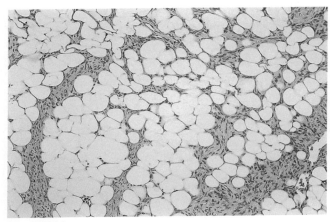

Fig. VIC1.i

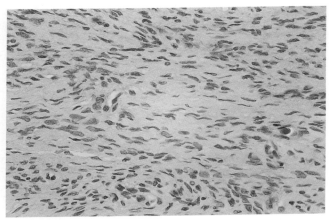

Fig. VIC1.j

Fig. VIC1.i. *Dermatofibrosarcoma protuberans, medium power.* This spindle cell proliferation characteristically infiltrates the subcutaneous fat, producing a honeycomb pattern.

Fig. VIC1.j. *Dermatofibrosarcoma protuberans, high power.* The neoplasm is composed of relatively uniform spindled cells whose nuclei are elongated with tapered ends. Mitoses may be identified but are usually few in number.

rence. Giant cells are seen in a small proportion of otherwise typical DFSP; it has been suggested that giant cell fibroblastoma is a juvenile variant of DFSP.

Atypical Fibroxanthoma

CLINICAL SUMMARY. Atypical fibroxanthoma (29) is a fairly common pleomorphic spindle cell neoplasm of the dermis that despite apparently malignant histologic features, usually follows an indolent or locally aggressive course. Because a small number of metastases have been reported, atypical fibroxanthoma has become regarded as a neoplasm of low-grade malignancy related to malignant fibrous histiocytoma, from which it is indistinguishable histologically. According to this view, the more favorable prognosis of atypical fibroxanthoma is related to its small size and superficial location. The disease usually presents as a solitary nodule less than 2 cm in diameter on the exposed skin of the head and neck or dorsum of the hand of elderly patients, often with a short history of rapid growth. The lesions are usually associated with severe actinic damage, and a few have arisen in areas treated by radiation.

HISTOPATHOLOGY. Atypical fibroxanthoma is an exophytic densely cellular neoplasm, unencapsulated but with only limited infiltration of the stroma, frequently with an epidermal collarette. The tumor may extend to the dermoepidermal junction,

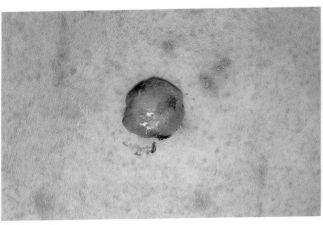

Clin. Fig. VIC1.e

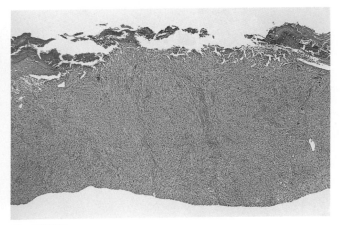

Fig. VIC1.k

Clin. Fig. VIC1.e. *Atypical fibroxanthoma.* A symmetrical nodule appeared suddenly and grew rapidly in the sun-damaged skin of an elderly man.

Fig. VIC1.k. *Atypical fibroxanthoma, high power.* The ulcerated tumor is composed of elongate spindle cells with a somewhat haphazard arrangement. *(continues)*

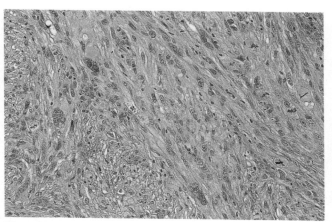

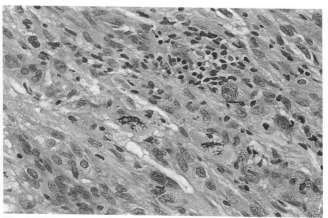

Fig. VIC1.l   **Fig. VIC1.m**

Fig. VIC1.l. *Atypical fibroxanthoma, medium power.* There is prominent nuclear pleomorphism and mitotic activity is striking.

Fig. VIC1.m. *Atypical fibroxanthoma, high power.* Atypical mitoses are frequently seen in these lesions.

but there is no direct continuity with the squamous epithelium, although ulceration is often present. Severe solar elastosis is present in the adjacent dermis. The classical tumor is composed of pleomorphic histiocyte-like cells and atypical giant cells, often with bizarre nuclei, prominent nucleoli, and numerous mitotic figures, including abnormal forms. The cells are arranged in a compact disorderly pattern, surrounding but not destroying adnexal structures. Fibroblast-like spindle cells are present in variable numbers; cells of morphology intermediate between

these spindle cells and histiocyte-like cells are also present. Scattered inflammatory cells and numerous small blood vessels are present, commonly with focal hemorrhage.

Malignant Fibrous Histiocytoma

See Figs. VIC1.n–VIC1.q.

Fibrous Papule (Angiofibroma)

See Figs. VIC1.r–VIC1.t.

(*Text continues on p. 332*)

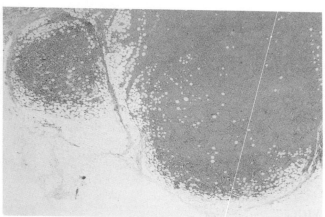

Fig. VIC1.n   **Fig. VIC1.o**

Fig. VIC1.n. *Malignant fibrous histiocytoma, low power.* Scanning magnification of a large spindle cell tumor shows extensive involvement of the subcutaneous fat and dermis.

Fig. VIC1.o. *Malignant fibrous histiocytoma, low power.* The size, location, and depth of involvement distinguish this lesion from an atypical fibroxanthoma, a smaller, more superficial lesion.

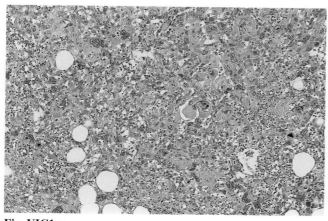

Fig. VIC1.p

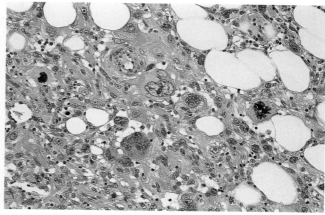

Fig. VIC1.q

Fig. VIC1.p. *Malignant fibrous histiocytoma, medium power.* This highly cellular tumor may show zones of spindled cells or, as seen here, large epithelioid cells with obvious nuclear atypia and pleomorphism.

Fig. VIC1.q. *Malignant fibrous histiocytoma, high power.* The atypical cells may have multiple nucleoli. Mitoses as well as atypical mitoses are easily identified.

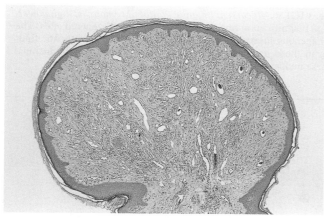

Fig. VIC1.r

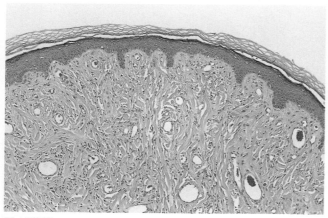

Fig. VIC1.s

Fig. VIC1.r. *Fibrous papule (angiofibroma), low power.* This dome-shaped neoplasm shows a normal overlying epidermis and a fibrovascular core.

Fig. VIC1.s. *Fibrous papule (angiofibroma), medium power.* The dermis is fibrotic and a distinction between papillary and reticular dermis cannot be made. There is an increased number of small, mature vascular channels which contain erythrocytes.

Fig. VIC1.t. *Fibrous papule (angiofibroma), high power.* The stroma is composed of collagen and stellate fibroblasts around the small vascular channels.

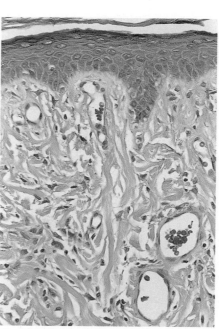

Fig. VIC1.t

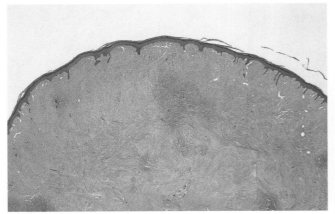

Fig. VIC1.u

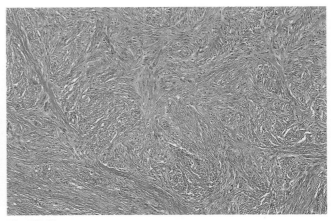

Fig. VIC1.v

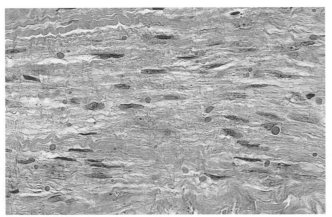

Fig. VIC1.w

Fig. VIC1.u. *Recurrent infantile digital fibromatosis, low power.* The dermis is replaced by a relatively uniform and symmetrical tumor.

Fig. VIC1.v. *Recurrent infantile digital fibromatosis, medium power.* The tumor is composed of uniform spindled cells embedded in a collagenous stroma. There is no atypia.

Fig. VIC1.w. *Recurrent infantile digital fibromatosis, high power.* High magnification reveals elongate nuclei with tapered ends. The collagenous stroma is wavy in appearance. The characteristic finding in these lesions is the eosinophilic cytoplasmic inclusions. These inclusions stain red using the Masson-Trichrome stain.

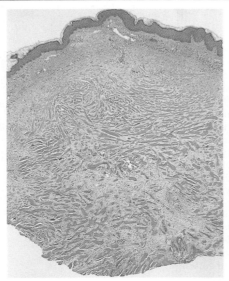

Fig. VIC1.x

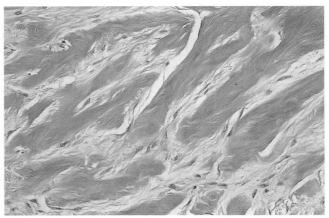

Fig. VIC1.y

Fig. VIC1.x. *Keloid, low power.* This lesion can be diagnosed at scanning magnification. No adnexal structures are seen within the dermis. Within the dermis, there are multiple bundles of thick eosinophilic collagen.

Fig. VIC1.y. *Keloid, high power.* The collagen bundles are markedly thickened and eosinophilic. Scattered small fibroblasts are seen between these hyalinized collagen bundles.

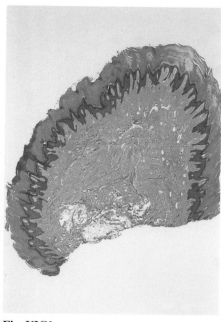

Fig. VIC1.z. *Acquired digital fibrokeratoma, low power.* This biopsy of acral skin shows a dome-shaped lesion which is hyperkeratotic. There is a fibrovascular core.

Fig. VIC1.aa. *Acquired digital fibrokeratoma, medium power.* The epidermis shows mild, uniform, verrucous hyperplasia. There are no viral cytopathic changes. The core shows fibrosis and a few small vascular channels.

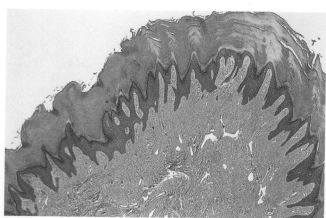

Fig. VIC1.aa

Fig. VIC1.z

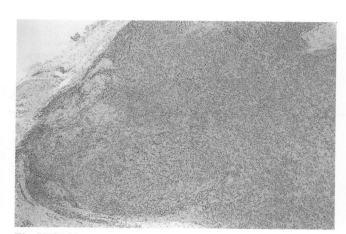

Fig. VIC1.bb

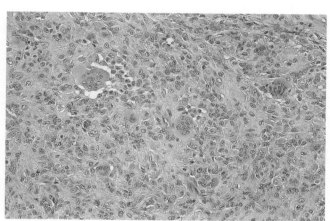

Fig. VIC1.cc

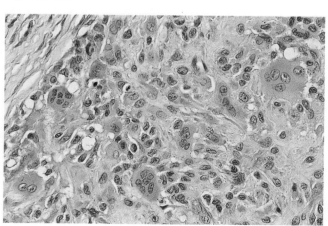

Fig. VIC1.dd

Fig. VIC1.bb. *Giant cell tumor of tendon sheath, low power.* Within the deep tissue there is a large, irregularly shaped nodular fibrohistiocytic proliferation.

Fig. VIC1.cc. *Giant cell tumor of tendon sheath, medium power.* The tumor is composed of plump histiocytes and numerous multinucleated giant cells.

Fig. VIC1.dd. *Giant cell tumor of tendon sheath, high power.* These osteoclast-like giant cells have multiple nuclei. There are also scattered lymphocytes throughout the lesion.

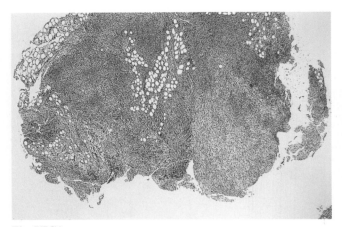

Fig. VIC1.ee

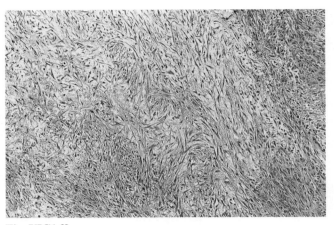

Fig. VIC1.ff

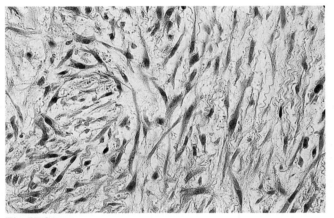

Fig. VIC1.gg

Fig. VIC1.ee. *Nodular fasciitis, low power.* There is a poorly defined hypercellular lesion which infiltrates the subcutaneous fat.

Fig. VIC1.ff. *Nodular fasciitis, medium power.* There are numerous haphazardly arranged spindled cells, some of which are embedded in a mucinous stroma.

Fig. VIC1.gg. *Nodular fasciitis, high power.* In the mucinous area there is a proliferation of plump, but cytologically bland appearing fibroblasts in a haphazard arrangement and a pale staining stroma. Mitotic figures may be frequent (not shown).

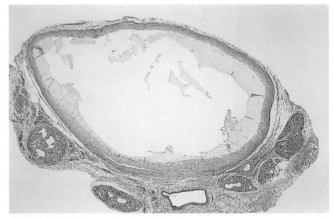

Fig. VIC1.hh

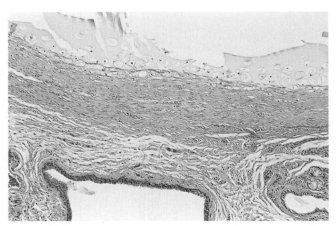

Fig. VIC1.ii

Fig. VIC1.hh. *Mucocele, low power.* Within the submucosa there is a cystic structure filled with amorphous material. Minor salivary glands are seen in the lower portion of this biopsy.

Fig. VIC1.ii. *Mucocele, medium power.* This lesion has no true cyst wall but the apparent wall is composed of a fibroblastic response. There are also numerous macrophages which have engulfed the mucinous material (muciphages). A dilated salivary duct is seen at the lower portion of this photomicrograph.

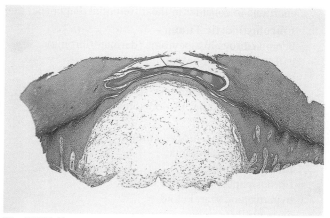

Fig. VIC1.jj

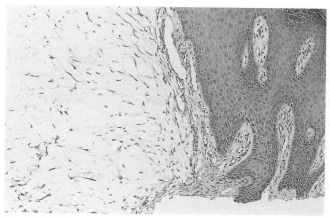

Fig. VIC1.kk

Fig. VIC1.jj. *Digital mucous cyst, low power.* This biopsy of acral skin shows a dome-shaped lesion created by an expanded papillary dermis. The overlying stratum corneum shows a focus of crusting.

Fig. VIC1.kk. *Digital mucous cyst, medium power.* The pale staining area is composed of glycosaminoglycans which can be highlighted using Alcian blue or colloidal iron stains. There are scattered small fibroblasts. The adjacent epidermis shows mild hyperplasia.

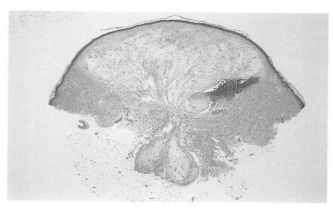

Fig. VIC1.ll

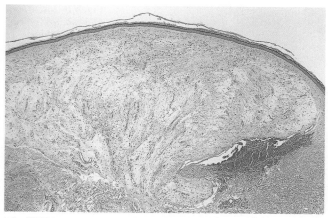

Fig. VIC1.mm

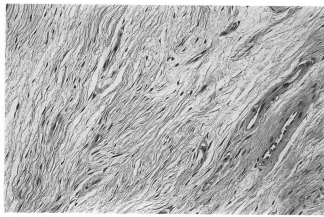

Fig. VIC1.nn

Fig. VIC1.ll. *Cutaneous myxoma, low power.* There is a symmetrical pale-staining area within the upper and mid dermis. The overlying epidermis shows an effaced rete ridge architecture.

Fig. VIC1.mm. *Cutaneous myxoma, medium power.* The nonencapsulated area within the dermis is hypocellular with a bluish, mucinous background representing the myxoid matrix.

Fig. VIC1.nn. *Cutaneous myxoma, high power.* There are scattered, bland-appearing fibroblasts and small mature vascular channels embedded in the bluish mucinous matrix.

Recurrent Infantile Digital Fibromatosis

See Figs. VIC1.u–VIC1.w.

Keloid

See Figs. VIC1.x and VIC1.y.

Acquired Digital Fibrokeratoma

See Figs. VIC1.z and VIC1.aa.

Giant Cell Tumor of Tendon Sheath

See Figs. VIC1.bb–VIC1.dd.

Nodular Fasciitis

See Figs. VIC1.ee–VIC1.gg.

Mucocele

See Figs. VIC1.hh and VIC1.ii.

Digital Mucous Cyst

See Figs. VIC1.jj and VIC1.kk.

Cutaneous Myxoma

See Figs. VIC1.ll–VIC1.nn.

Conditions to consider in the differential diagnosis:

Fibrohistiocytic Tumors
benign fibrous histiocytoma (dermatofibroma)
cellular dermatofibroma
aneurysmal fibrous histiocytoma
juvenile xanthogranuloma, spindle cell variant
progressive nodular histiocytoma (deep fibrous
  type)
plexiform fibrohistiocytic tumor
atypical fibroxanthoma
Fibrous Tumors
fibrous papule (angiofibroma)
hypertrophic scar, keloid
dermatofibrosarcoma protuberans
Sarcomas
malignant fibrous histiocytoma
angiomatoid fibrous histiocytoma
synovial sarcoma
Fibromatoses
desmoid tumor
recurrent infantile digital fibromatosis
juvenile hyaline fibromatosis

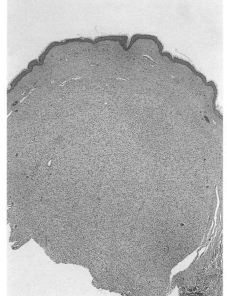

Fig. VIC2.a

Fig. VIC2.a. *Neurofibroma, low power.* There is a dome-shaped, nonencapsulated neoplasm within the dermis.

Fig. VIC2.b. *Neurofibroma, medium power.* The lesion is composed of elongate, wavy spindled cells which are embedded in an eosinophilic matrix. In the center of this photomicrograph there is a structure resembling a small cutaneous nerve.

Fig. VIC2.c. *Neurofibroma, high power.* The nuclei are elongated with tapered ends and they are embedded in an eosinophilic matrix. Mast cells, as seen in the center of this photomicrograph are frequently seen in neural tumors.

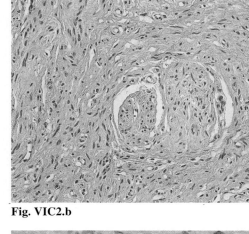

Fig. VIC2.b

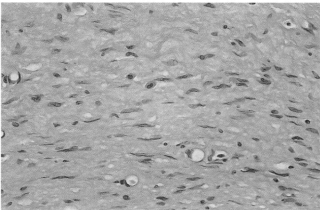

Fig. VIC2.c

Fibromas
fibroma of tendon sheath
follicular fibroma
acquired digital fibrokeratoma
elastofibroma
dermatomyofibroma
Giant Cell Tumors
giant cell fibroblastoma
giant cell tumor of tendon sheath
Proliferative Lesions of the Fascia
nodular fasciitis
cranial fasciitis of childhood
Myxoid Spindle Cell Lesions
cutaneous myxoma
digital mucous cyst
mucocele of oral mucosa

VIC2. Schwannian/Neural Spindle Cell Tumors

These tumors are composed of elongated narrow spindle cells that tend to have serpentine S-shaped nuclei and to be arranged in "wavy" fiber bundles. Immunohistochemistry for S100 is useful, but not specific.

Neurofibromas

CLINICAL SUMMARY. Extraneural sporadic cutaneous neurofibromas (ESCNs) (30) (the common sporadic neurofibromas) are soft, polypoid, skin-colored or slightly tan, and small (rarely larger than a centimeter in diameter). They usually arise in adulthood. The presence of more than a few cutaneous neurofibromas raises the possibility of neurofibromatosis and should prompt an evaluation for other confirmatory stigmata.

HISTOPATHOLOGY. Most examples of ESCN are faintly eosinophilic and are circumscribed but not encapsulated: they are extraneural. Thin spindle cells with elongated wavy nuclei are regularly spaced among thin wavy collagenous strands. The strands are either closely spaced (homogeneous pattern) or loosely spaced in a clear matrix (loose pattern). The two patterns are often intermixed in a single lesion. Rarely, ESCNs are composed of widely spaced spindle and stellate cells in a myxoid matrix. The regular spacing of adnexae is preserved in cutaneous neurofibromas. Entrapped small nerves occasionally are enlarged and hypercellular. Tactoid (tactile corpuscle-like) bodies and pigmented dendritic melanocytes are most uncommon. These tumors are

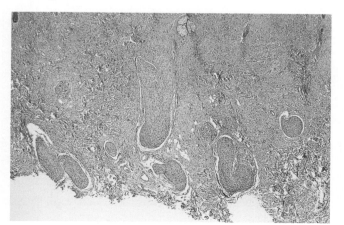

Clin. Fig. VIC2

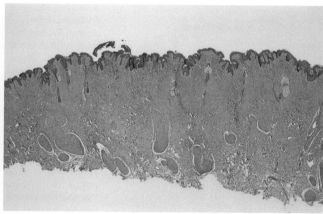

Fig. VIC2.d

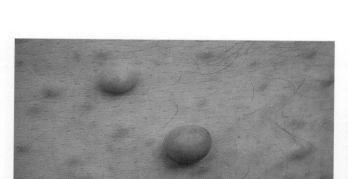

Fig. VIC2.e

Clin. Fig. VIC2. *Neurofibromatosis.* A 51-year-old man presented with axillary freckling, cafe au lait macules and generalized soft pigmented and flesh colored papules and nodules with button-hole compression (soft, compressible centers).

Fig. VIC2.d. *Plexiform neurofibroma, low power.* This plaque-like lesion shows multiple nodular aggregates embedded in an eosinophilic background.

Fig. VIC2.e. *Plexiform neurofibroma, medium power.* There are plexiform tangles of neural tissue with slight retraction from the background matrix. The background matrix shows typical changes of a neurofibroma. (*continues*)

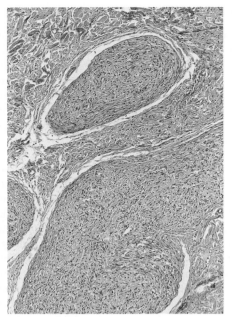

Fig. VIC2.f.
Plexiform neurofibroma, medium power. The plexiform tangles resemble large nerves. The background shows spindled cells in an eosinophilic matrix.

Fig. VIC2.g.
Plexiform neurofibroma, high power. Close inspection of the nodular aggregates reveal wavy spindled cells with small uniform nuclei. There are scattered mast cells.

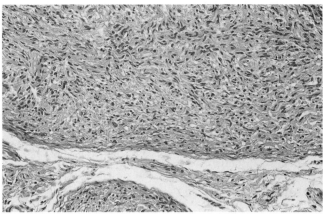

Fig. VIC2.g

Fig. VIC2.f

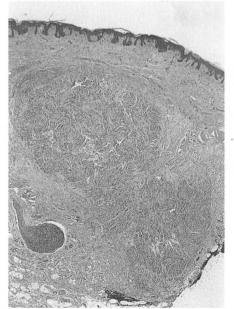

Fig. VIC2.h

Fig. VIC2.h.
Schwannoma (neurilemmoma), low power. Within the dermis there is a relatively well-circumscribed, but nonencapsulated cellular neoplasm. The overlying epidermis is unremarkable.

Fig. VIC2.i.
Schwannoma (neurilemmoma), medium power. In this area of the neurilemmoma the Antoni type A tissue shows Verocay body formation where the nuclei of the spindle cells are aligned in parallel arrays.

Fig. VIC2.j.
Schwannoma (neurilemmoma), medium power. In the Antoni type B tissue, Schwann cells are loosely spaced in a clear, watery matrix.

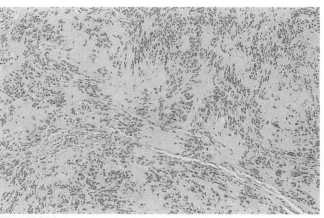

Fig. VIC2.i

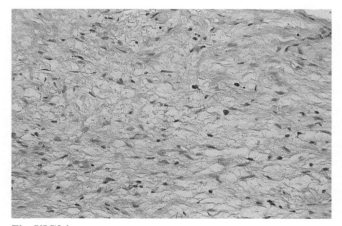

Fig. VIC2.j

essentially the same as those that occur in von Recklinghausen's neurofibromatosis.

Neurofibromatosis

See Figs. VIC2.d and VIC2.e.

Schwannoma (Neurilemmoma)

CLINICAL SUMMARY. These benign Schwann cell neoplasms present as solitary skin-colored tumors along the course of peripheral or cranial nerves (31). Their usual size is between 2 and 4 cm, and their usual location is the head or the flexor aspect of the extremities. When small, most schwannomas are asymptomatic, but pain, localized to the tumor or radiating along the nerve of origin, can be a complaint.

HISTOPATHOLOGY. Schwannomas are intraneural and symmetricly expansile. They are confined by the perineurium of the nerve of origin and displace and compress the endoneurial matrix. Most symmetrically bundled nerve fibers of the nerve of origin are displaced eccentrically between the tumor and the perineurium. Two variant patterns, namely Antoni A and Antoni B types, have been described. In the Antoni type A tissue, uniform spindle cells are arranged back to back and each cell is outlined by delicate rigid reticular fibers (basement membranes). The cells tend to cluster in stacks, and the respective nuclei tend to form palisades. Two neighboring palisades, the intervening cytoplasms of Schwann cells, and associated reticular fibers all constitute a Verocay body. In Antoni type B tissue, files of elongated Schwann cells, arranged end to end, and individual Schwann cells are loosely spaced in a clear watery matrix. Clusters of dilated congested vessels with hyalinized walls, thrombi, and subendothelial collections of foam cells are represented in both Antoni A and Antoni B tissue. Cystic changes, extravasated erythrocytes, and hemosiderin deposits are variable features.

Palisaded Encapsulated Neuroma

See Figs. VIC2.k–VIC2.m.

Accessory Digit

See Figs. VIC2.n and VIC2.o.

Conditions to consider in the differential diagnosis:
  Neurofibromas
    sporadic cutaneous neurofibroma (common neurofibroma)
    extraneural (common neurofibroma)
    intraneural neurofibroma
    pacinian neurofibroma

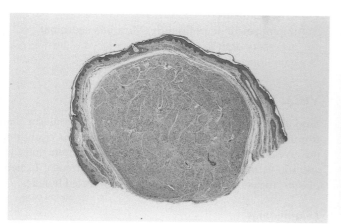

Fig. VIC2.k

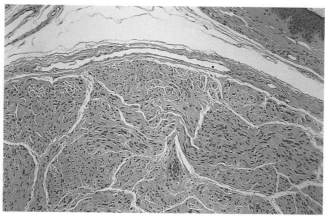

Fig. VIC2.l

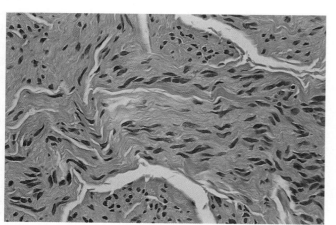

Fig. VIC2.m

Fig. VIC2.k. *Palisaded encapsulated neuroma, low power.* Within the superficial dermis, there is a well-circumscribed nodular tumor.

Fig. VIC2.l. *Palisaded encapsulated neuroma, medium power.* This well-circumscribed tumor is surrounded by a thin zone of fibrous connective tissue but despite its name does not always form a true capsule. The tumor is composed of interlacing bundles of neural tissue.

Fig. VIC2.m. *Palisaded encapsulated neuroma, high power.* These bundles are composed of elongate spindled cells which are wavy in appearance. Significant atypia or mitotic activity is not seen.

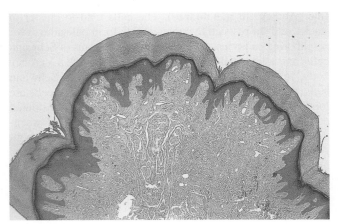

Fig. VIC2.n

Fig. VIC2.n. *Accessory digit, low power.* This dome shaped lesion of acral skin shows mild epidermal hyperplasia. There is increased cellularity in the dermis.

Fig. VIC2.o. *Accessory digit, medium power.* The dermal component of this lesion, which is nonencapsulated, is composed of haphazardly arranged bundles of neural tissue.

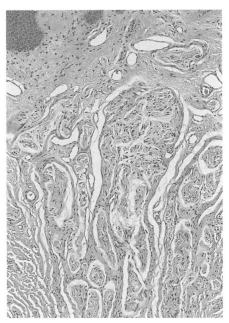

Fig. VIC2.o

Neurofibromatosis
plexiform neurofibroma
diffuse neurofibroma
Nerve Sheath Tumors
fibrolamellar nerve sheath tumor
storiform nerve sheath tumor (perineurioma)
mature (myxoid) neurothekeoma, nerve sheath
  myxoma
granular cell nerve sheath tumor (granular cell
  tumor/schwannoma)
plexiform granular cell nerve sheath tumor
malignant granular cell tumor
Extraneural Neuromas
traumatic neuroma
Intraneural Neuromas
palisaded and encapsulated neuroma
intraneural plexiform neuroma
mucosal neuroma syndrome
linear cutaneous neuroma
Neurilemmomas (Schwannomas)
typical schwannoma
cellular schwannoma
atypical schwannoma
transformed (borderline) schwannoma
epithelioid schwannoma
glandular schwannoma
plexiform schwannoma
infiltrating fascicular schwannoma of infancy
Malignant Schwannomas, Intraneural or Extraneural
malignant nerve sheath tumor
psammomatous malignant schwannoma
epithelioid malignant schwannoma

Miscellaneous
impingement neurofasciitis (Morton's neuroma)
accessory digit
ganglioneuroma

VIC3. Spindle Cell Tumors of Muscle

Smooth muscle cells have more abundant cytoplasm than fibroblasts or Schwann cells. The cytoplasm is trichrome positive and reacts with muscle markers-desmin, muscle-specific actin. The nuclei tend to have blunt ends. In neoplasms, the cells tend to be arranged in whorled bundles.

Leiomyomas

CLINICAL SUMMARY. Five types of leiomyomas of the skin (32) are multiple piloleiomyomas and solitary piloleiomyomas, both arising from arrectores pilorum muscles; solitary genital leiomyomas, arising from the dartoic, vulvar, or mammillary muscles; solitary angioleiomyomas, arising from the muscles of veins; and leiomyomas with additional mesenchymal elements.

Multiple piloleiomyomas, by far the most common type of leiomyoma, are small, firm, red or brown, intradermal nodules arranged in a group or in a linear pattern. Often, two or more areas are affected. Usually, but not always, the lesions are tender and give rise spontaneously to occasional attacks of pain. *Solitary piloleiomyomas* are intradermal nodules that are usually larger than those of multiple piloleiomyomas, measuring up to 2 cm in diameter. Most are tender and also occasionally painful. *Solitary genital leiomyomas* are located on the scrotum, the labia majora, or, rarely, the nipples. Their location is

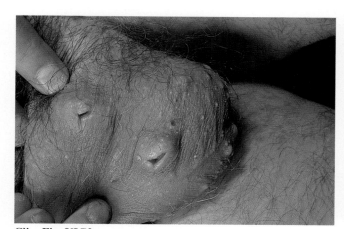

Clin. Fig. VIC3

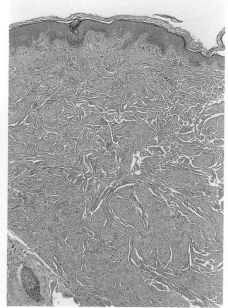

Fig. VIC3.a

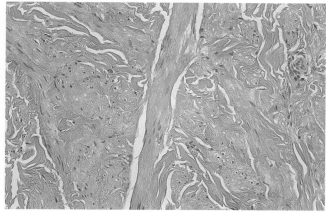

Fig. VIC3.b

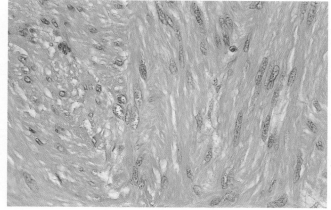

Fig. VIC3.c

Clin. Fig. VIC3. *Multiple scrotal leiomyomas*. A 60-year-old man presented with multiple asymptomatic flesh-colored nodules over the scrotum.

Fig. VIC3.a. *Leiomyoma, low power*. Within the dermis, there is a poorly circumscribed neoplasm which has replaced the preexisting adnexal structures. The neoplasm is composed of interlacing bundles of eosinophilic material.

Fig. VIC3.b. *Leiomyoma, medium power*. At this magnification, there are interwoven bundles of spindle cells, many perpendicular to one another. The nuclei are small and bland.

Fig. VIC3.c. *Leiomyoma, high power*. The nuclei of smooth muscle are elongate with blunt ends (cigar-shaped). Perinuclear vacuolization is frequently seen in smooth-muscle cells.

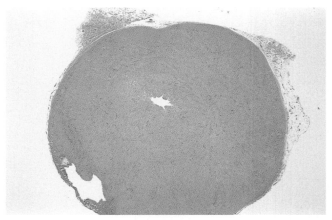

Fig. VIC3.d

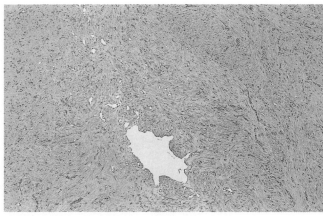

Fig. VIC3.e

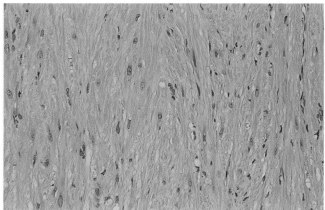

Fig. VIC3.f

Fig. VIC3.d. *Angioleiomyoma, low power.* There is a well-circumscribed nodule within the deep dermis or subcutaneous fat. Unlike piloleiomyoma, the lesion is sharply separated from the surrounding normal tissue.

Fig. VIC3.e. *Angioleiomyoma, medium power.* There are only a few dilated vascular channels within this proliferation of smooth muscle.

Fig. VIC3.f. *Angioleiomyoma, high power.* The nuclei are elongate with blunt ends and perinuclear vacuolization.

intradermal. In contrast to the other leiomyomas, most genital leiomyomas are asymptomatic. *Solitary angioleiomyomas* are usually subcutaneous. Pain and tenderness are evoked by most, but not all, angioleiomyomas.

HISTOPATHOLOGY. Piloleiomyomas, whether multiple or solitary, and genital leiomyomas are similar in histologic appearance. They are poorly demarcated and are composed of interlacing bundles of smooth muscle fibers with which varying amounts of collagen bundles are intermingled. The muscle fibers composing the smooth muscle bundles are generally straight, with little or no waviness; they contain centrally located, thin, very long, blunt-edged, "eel-like" nuclei. Angioleiomyomas differ from the other types of leiomyomas in that they are encapsulated and contain numerous vessels, with only small amounts of collagen as a rule. The numerous veins that are present vary in size and have muscular walls of varying thickness. On this basis, angioleiomyomas have been subdivided into a capillary or solid type, a cavernous type, and a venous type. In the capillary type, the vascular channels are numerous but small.

Angioleiomyoma

See Figs. VIC3.d–VIC3.f.

Smooth Muscle Hamartoma

See Figs. VIC3.g–VIC3.i.

Leiomyosarcoma

See Figs. VIC3.j–VIC3.n.

Conditions to consider in the differential diagnosis:
leiomyoma
angioleiomyoma
superficial leiomyosarcoma
infantile myofibromatosis
solitary myofibroma
dermatomyofibroma
benign mixed mesodermal proliferations
malignant mesenchymal tumors of uncertain
  origin
smooth muscle hamartoma
rhabdomyosarcoma

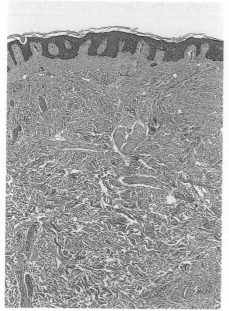

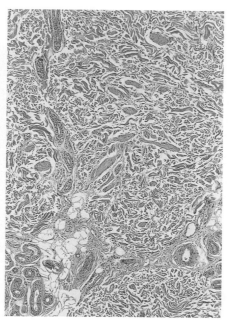

Fig. VIC3.g

Fig. VIC3.h

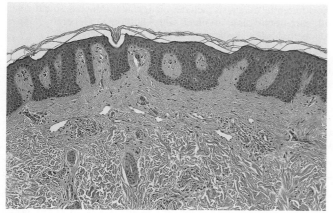

Fig. VIC3.g. *Becker's nevus/smooth muscle hamartoma, low power.* The epidermis is slightly hyperplastic. There is an increased number of smooth muscle bundles within the dermis. The smooth muscle bundles do not form a solid aggregate as they do in a leiomyoma.

Fig. VIC3.h. *Becker's nevus/smooth muscle hamartoma, medium power.* The bundles of smooth muscle are separated from one another by intervening normal collagen.

Fig. VIC3.i. *Becker's nevus /smooth muscle hamartoma, medium power.* The overlying epidermis shows slightly elongate rete ridges and diffuse basal layer hyperpigmentation. There are scattered small melanocytes without formation of nests.

Fig. VIC3.i

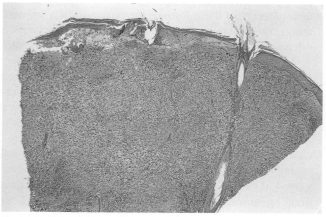

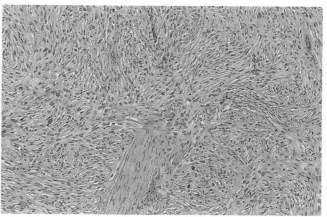

Fig. VIC3.j

Fig. VIC3.k

Fig. VIC3.j. *Leiomyosarcoma, low power.* The upper two-thirds of the dermis has been replaced by a highly cellular spindle cell neoplasm. There is no definitive association with the overlying epidermis.

Fig. VIC3.k. *Leiomyosarcoma, medium power.* The neoplasm is composed of spindled cells which form interlocking bundles, a similar pattern to what was seen in a leiomyoma. However, even at this power, the lesion is more cellular (more nuclei are visible). (*continues*)

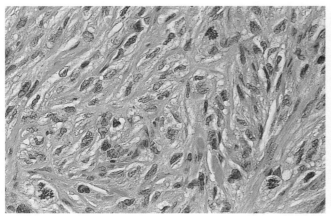

Fig. VIC3.l

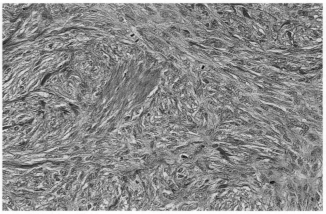

Fig. VIC3.m

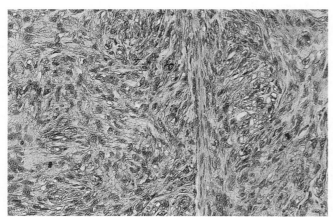

Fig. VIC3.n

Fig. VIC3.l. *Leiomyosarcoma, high power.* The individual cells are large and spindled in form. The nuclei are atypical and mitotic figures are requisite for the diagnosis. The nuclei may not always show the typical cigar shape that is seen in the benign leiomyoma. The differential diagnosis includes malignant melanoma, squamous cell carcinoma, and atypical fibroxanthoma. Generally, immunoperoxidase stains are required for definitive diagnosis.

Fig. VIC3.m. *Leiomyosarcoma. Trichrome stain.* The trichrome stain may be helpful in smooth muscle tumors staining the lesional cells red and the surrounding collagen blue.

Fig. VIC3.n. *Leiomyosarcoma. Smooth muscle actin stain.* This immunoperoxidase stain for smooth muscle actin shows positivity within tumor cells. Stains for S-100 protein, high and low molecular weight keratins, and histiocyte markers were negative in this tumor.

VIC4. Melanocytic Spindle Cell Tumors

Melanocytic spindle cell tumors may have many attributes of schwannian tumors described above. S100 is positive, and HMB45 is often negative in the spindle cell melanomas. Diagnosis of melanoma then depends on recognizing melanocytic differentiation—pigment synthesis or a characteristic intraepidermal *in situ* or microinvasive component.

Desmoplastic Melanoma

CLINICAL SUMMARY.   Desmoplastic melanoma (33) presents attributes of melanocytic, fibroblastic, and schwannian differentiation, often mixed within a single lesion. Desmoplasia is most often observed in a spindle cell vertical growth phase of lentigo maligna melanoma or acral lentiginous melanoma. The clinical presentation is therefore that of the *in situ* or microinvasive radial growth phase component. However, desmoplastic changes are occasionally seen in tumors with rounded or undifferentiated melanoma cells. Although the reported survival rate for desmoplastic melanoma is poor, this is because many of the cases reported in the earlier literature had already recurred at the time the diagnoses were

made. However, the probability of survival is relatively good for prospectively diagnosed and definitively treated desmoplastic melanoma, because, despite the considerable thickness of many of these lesions, the prognostically important mitotic rate and tumor-infiltrating lymphocyte responses are often favorable.

HISTOPATHOLOGY.   The collagen in desmoplastic melanoma is arranged as delicate fibrils that extend among the tumor cells and separate them from one another. The tumor cells are typically spindle shaped and tend not to exhibit high-grade nuclear atypia. The mitotic rate is often very low or even zero. A characteristic feature is the presence of clusters of tumor-infiltrating lymphocytes within the tumor. The cells tend to be arranged in "wavy" fiber bundles that may recall the "schwannian" patterns of neurofibromas, neurotized nevi, and malignant schwannomas and may lead to diagnostic error. Because the melanoma cells are usually elongated and amelanotic and are embedded in a markedly fibrotic stroma, the tumors may simulate a fibromatosis or a fibrohistiocytic lesion. Staining with S100 protein antibody usually marks many of the spindle-shaped cells, indicating that they are not fibroblastic. The HMB45 antigen is usually not demonstrable in these

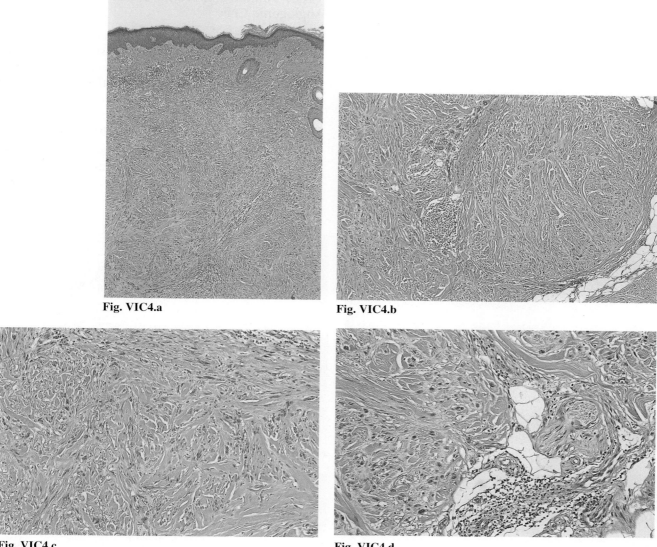

Fig. VIC4.a

Fig. VIC4.b

Fig. VIC4.c

Fig. VIC4.d

Fig. VIC4.a. *Desmoplastic melanoma, low power.* There is a spindle cell proliferation throughout the dermis. It is associated with increased collagen production, a feature which may suggest a diagnosis of a dermatofibroma or a fibromatosis.

Fig. VIC4.b. *Desmoplastic melanoma, medium power.* These lesions are generally not diagnosed early and therefore most lesions are relatively thick, extending to the deep reticular dermis or subcutaneous fat. The spindle cell proliferation is frequently associated with a patchy lymphoid infiltrate. Again, this photomicrograph demonstrates spindle cell proliferation associated with collagen production.

Fig. VIC4.c. *Desmoplastic melanoma, high power.* The spindle cells are haphazardly arranged and scattered cells show enlarged hyperchromatic nuclei.

Fig. VIC4.d. *Desmoplastic melanoma, high power.* Desmoplastic melanoma may mimic a neural tumor and it frequently shows neurotropism with spindle cells extending in and around small cutaneous nerves. The neurotropism is frequently associated with a lymphocytic infiltrate.

spindle-cell melanomas. The most convincing evidence that many of the tumors are melanomas may come from examination of the overlying intraepidermal component, where diagnostic changes of microinvasive or *in situ* melanoma may be seen, usually of the lentigo maligna, acral, or mucosal lentiginous types. Electron microscopy may or may not demonstrate melanosomes, often after prolonged searching.

Conditions to consider in the differential diagnosis:

desmoplastic melanoma, including amelanotic
cellular blue nevus, amelanotic
blue nevus, amelanotic
desmoplastic Spitz nevus
spindle cell metastatic melanoma

VIC5. Tumors and Proliferations of Angiogenic Cells

There is a dermal proliferation of vascular endothelium. Factor VIII staining may be helpful in demonstrating endothelial differentiation. The many variants of benign hemangiomas should be carefully considered in the differential diagnosis of Kaposi's sarcoma and angiosarcoma.

Pyogenic Granuloma (Lobular Capillary Hemangioma)

CLINICAL SUMMARY. Pyogenic granuloma (34) is a common proliferative lesion that often occurs shortly after a minor injury or infection of the skin. Typically, the lesion grows

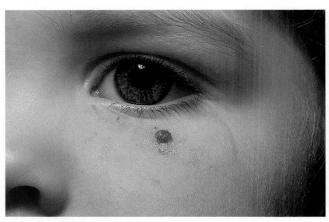

Clin. Fig. VIC5.a

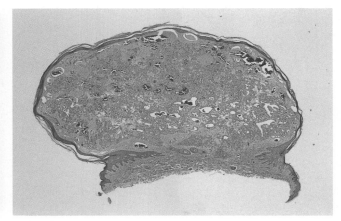

Fig. VIC5.a

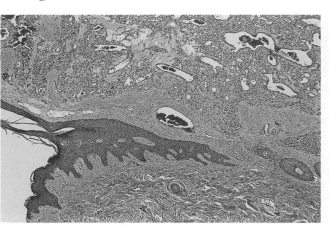

Fig. VIC5.b

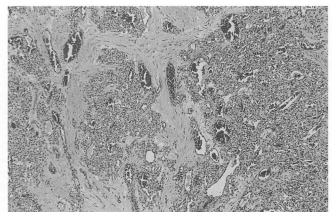

Fig. VIC5.c

Clin. Fig. VIC5.a. *Pyogenic granuloma*. This child suddenly developed a single dark red bleeding papule.

Fig. VIC5.a. *Pyogenic granuloma, low power*. Pyogenic granulomas show a dome shaped nodular architecture which sits above the level of the skin surface. The epidermis shows a flattened effaced rete ridge architecture.

Fig. VIC5.b. *Pyogenic granuloma, medium power*. At the edge of the neoplasm, the epidermis focally extends underneath the vascular proliferation forming a collarette.

Fig. VIC5.c. *Pyogenic granuloma, medium power*. There are lobular aggregates of small mature vascular channels filled with erythrocytes. These aggregates are separated by a fibrous stroma in long-standing lesions. This intervening stroma can be very edematous and mucinous in early lesions.

rapidly for a few weeks before stabilizing as an elevated bright red papule, usually not more than 1 to 2 cm in size; it then may persist indefinitely unless destroyed. Recurrence after surgery or cautery is not rare. Pyogenic granuloma most often affects children or young adults of either gender, but the age range is wide; the hands, fingers, and face, especially the lips and gums, are the most common sites. Pyogenic granuloma of the gingiva in pregnancy (epulis of pregnancy) is a special subgroup. A rare and alarming event is the development of multiple satellite angiomatous lesions at and around the site of a previously destroyed pyogenic granuloma.

HISTOPATHOLOGY. The typical lesion presents as a polypoid mass of angiomatous tissue protruding above the surrounding skin and often constricted at its base by a collarette of acanthotic epidermis. An intact flattened epidermis may cover the entire lesion, but surface erosions are common. In ulcerated lesions, a superficial inflammatory cell reaction can give rise to an appearance suggestive of granulation tissue, but inflammation is usually slight in the deeper part of the lesion and may be absent when the epidermis is intact. The angiomatous tissue tends to occur in discrete masses or lobules and is composed of a variably dilated network of blood-filled capillary vessels and groups of poorly canalized vascular tufts. Mitotic activity varies and can be prominent. Feeding vessels often extend into the adjacent dermis and rare lesions show a deep component in the reticular dermis.

Intravascular Papillary Endothelial Hyperplasia (Masson's Hemangio-Endotheliome Vegetant Intravasculaire)

CLINICAL SUMMARY. This not uncommon condition is an unusual endothelial proliferation in an organizing thrombus that can be misdiagnosed as angiosarcoma (35). The lesion arises primarily within a venous channel or secondarily within a preceding angioma or some type of vascular anomaly, including hemorrhoids, or extravascularly in association with a hematoma. The lesions are almost always solitary, arising in the skin, subcutaneous tissue, or even muscle with the head and neck region and the upper extremities, especially the fingers the most common sites. Primary lesions are usually tender nodules less than 2 cm in size, whereas secondary lesions occur because some preceding vascular abnormality increases in size.

HISTOPATHOLOGY. Often, low-power examination allows recognition of the intravascular nature of the process in a single thin-walled vein or as part of a preceding angiomatous condition. Extravascular lesions fail to reveal a blood vessel wall despite serial sectioning. The main lesion consists of a mass of anastomosing vascular channels with a variable degree of intraluminal papillary projections. The stroma consists of hyalinized eosinophilic material that may merge with uncanalized thrombus remnants. The infiltrating vascular channels show enlarged and prominent endothelial cells that may be heaped up to give rise to intraluminal prominences, but atypia and mitotic activity are slight.

Stasis Dermatitis with Vascular Proliferation (Acroangiodermatitis, Pseudo-Kaposi's Sarcoma)

CLINICAL SUMMARY. Patients with long-standing venous insufficiency and lower extremity edema may develop pruritic, erythematous, scaly papules and plaques on the lower legs, often in association with brown pigmentation and hair loss.

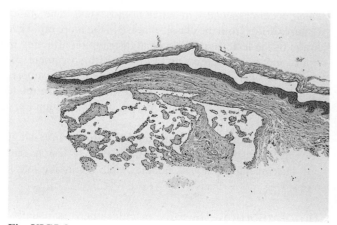

Fig. VIC5.d

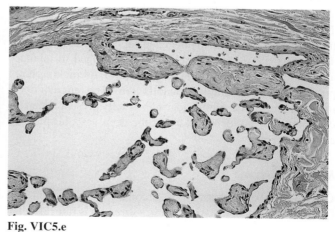

Fig. VIC5.e

Fig. VIC5.d. *Intravascular papillary endothelial hyperplasia, low power.* There are several dilated cystic spaces which show papillary fronds within the lumen of the channels.

Fig. VIC5.e. *Intravascular papillary endothelial hyperplasia, medium power.* The cystic spaces as well as the papillary fronds are all lined by a single layer of endothelial cells. Because of the papillary nature the fronds appear as small islands floating within a pond. The endothelial cells fail to reveal cytologic atypia.

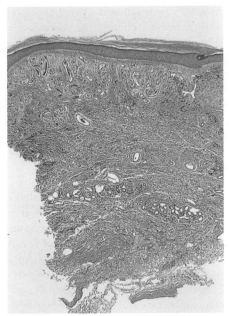

Fig. VIC5.f

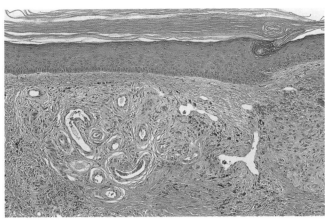

Fig. VIC5.g

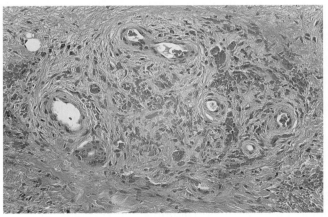

Fig. VIC5.h

Fig. VIC5.f. *Stasis dermatitis with vascular proliferation, low power.* Within the superficial dermis there is a proliferation of vascular channels associated with dermal pigment deposition.

Fig. VIC5.g. *Stasis dermatitis with vascular proliferation, medium power.* The vascular channels are mature and have thick walls. They form clusters within the superficial dermis. There is prominent pigment surrounding these vascular channels secondary to hemosiderin deposition. The overlying epidermis may or may not show spongiotic changes.

Fig. VIC5.h. *Stasis dermatitis with vascular proliferation, high power.* Surrounding the small vascular channels is extravasation of erythrocytes.

HISTOPATHOLOGY. The epidermis is hyperkeratotic with areas of parakeratosis, acanthosis, and focal spongiosis. There is a superficial perivascular lymphohistiocytic infiltrate that surrounds plump thickened capillaries and venules. The superficial dermal vessels may be arranged in lobular aggregates. The proliferation may be florid, mimicking Kaposi's sarcoma (acroangiodermatitis) (36). The reticular dermis is often fibrotic. Hemosiderin is usually present superficially but may be identified about the deep vascular plexus as well.

Kaposi's Sarcoma

CLINICAL SUMMARY. Kaposi's sarcoma (37) can be classified in four groups. *Classic Kaposi's sarcoma* is rare, affecting mainly patients of Eastern European and Mediterranean origin and occurs in male patients over the age of 50 with the slow development of angiomatous nodules and plaques on the lower extremities. *Kaposi's sarcoma in Africa* is very common, with a higher proportion of young people affected and with a more aggressive disease manifested by widespread tumors, deep infiltrative or elevated fungating le-

sions, and bone involvement. *AIDS-associated Kaposi's sarcoma* occurs especially in active homosexuals. The clinical features differ from the classic disease in the more rapid evolution of the lesions, their atypical distribution affecting the trunk, and a greater tendency to mucosal involvement. *Kaposi's sarcoma associated with iatrogenic immunosuppression* occurs in the context of organ transplantation-related immunosuppression and may regress on discontinuation of the therapy.

The histologic spectrum can be divided into stages roughly corresponding to the clinical type of lesion: early and late macules, plaques, nodules, and aggressive late lesions.

HISTOPATHOLOGY. In early macules there is usually a patchy, sparse, upper dermal perivascular infiltrate consisting of lymphocytes and plasma cells. Narrow cords of cells, with evidence of luminal differentiation, are insinuated between collagen bundles. Usually, a few dilated irregular or angulated lymphaticlike spaces lined by delicate endothelial cells are also present. Vessels with jagged outlines tending to separate collagen bundles are especially characteristic. Nor-

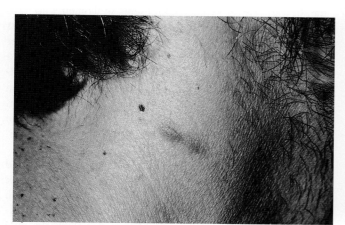

Clin. Fig. VIC5.b

Fig. VIC5.i

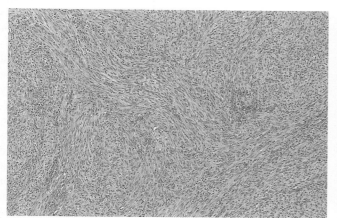

Fig. VIC5.j

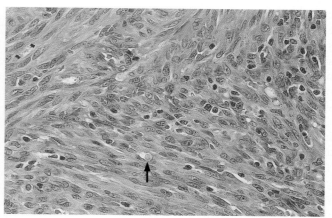

Fig. VIC5.k

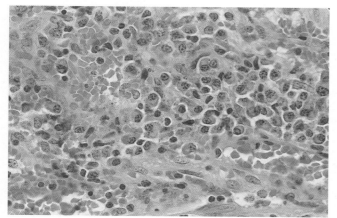

Fig. VIC5.l

Clin. Fig. VIC5.b. *Kaposi's sarcoma, plaque and early nodule.* An HIV positive man developed an elongated erythematous nodule.

Fig. VIC5.i. *Kaposi's sarcoma, nodular type, low power.* In nodular Kaposi's sarcoma there is a mass of spindle cells within the dermis. There is no association to the overlying epidermis.

Fig. VIC5.j. *Kaposi's sarcoma, medium power.* The spindle cells fail to reveal an organized pattern. The tumor is highly cellular, and occasionally the hemorrhage can be seen at scanning magnification.

Fig. VIC5.k. *Kaposi's sarcoma, high power.* The spindled cells show enlarged nuclei, and erythrocytes are seen between tumor cells. Occasionally, one can identify intracytoplasmic pink droplets (*arrow*).

Fig. VIC5.l. *Kaposi's sarcoma, high power.* An infiltrate of plasma cells is frequently seen in Kaposi's sarcoma.

mal adnexal structures and preexisting blood vessels often protrude into newly formed blood vessels, a finding known as the "promontory sign." In late macular lesions, there is a more extensive infiltrate of vessels in the dermis, with jagged vessels and with cords of thicker-walled vessels similar to those in granulation tissue. At this stage, red blood cell extravasation and siderophages may be encountered.

In the plaque stage, a diffuse infiltrate of small blood vessels extends through most parts of the dermis and tends to displace collagen. The vessels vary in morphology, some occurring as poorly canalized cords, some as blood containing ovoid vessels, and some having lymphatic-like features. Loosely distributed spindle cells, arranged in short fascicles, are also encountered. Intracytoplasmic hyaline globules, seen more often in lesions from patients with AIDS, may be found in areas of denser infiltrate.

In the tumor stage, well-defined nodules composed of vascular spaces and spindle cells replace dermal collagen. These tumor nodules tend to be compartmentalized by dense bands of fibrocollagenous tissue. Dilated lymphatic spaces can also be seen between tumor aggregates. The characteristic feature is a honeycomblike network of blood-filled spaces or slits, closely associated with interweaving spindle cells. The presence of a closely set honeycomblike pattern of back-to-back vascular spaces is an important diagnostic feature of Kaposi's sarcoma. In the vascular spaces of pyogenic granuloma and most angiomas, the endothelial cells of the capillary walls are more prominent and the vessels are set farther apart by intervening stroma. Blood pigment containing macrophages are nearly always prominent adjacent to the nodules, especially in lesions at dependent sites. The spindle cells in the nodules are elongated and fusiform with a well-defined cytoplasm. Their nuclei are ovoid and somewhat flattened with finely granular chromatin in the long axis of the cells. Nucleoli are generally inconspicuous, and nuclear atypia is absent or slight. Mitosis is infrequent. Prominent and consistent positivity for CD34 is seen in the spindle cell population.

Aggressive late-stage infiltrating lesions, mostly in African Kaposi's sarcoma, show a more obviously sarcomatous character with reduction or loss of the vascular component. The spindle cells demonstrate a greater degree of cytologic atypia with regard to size, shape, and nuclear features, with mitosis becoming frequent. In such lesions, phagocytozed erythrocytes and the presence of hyaline globules may provide clues about the tumor's origin.

Cutaneous Angiosarcoma

CLINICAL SUMMARY. Most angiosarcomas of the skin (38) arise in the following clinical settings: angiosarcoma of the face and scalp in the elderly, angiosarcoma (lymphangiosarcoma) secondary to chronic lymphedema, and angiosarcoma as a complication of chronic radiodermatitis or arising from the effects of severe skin trauma or ulceration.

Angiosarcoma of the scalp and face of the elderly is almost invariably a fatal tumor that usually arises as seemingly innoc-

uous erythematous or bruiselike lesions on the scalp or middle and upper face with predilection for men. Subsequent plaques, nodules, or ulcerations develop; metastasis to nodes or internal organs usually arises as a late complication, with many patients dying as a result of extensive local disease. Angiosarcoma after lymphedema (postmastectomy lymphangiosarcoma or the Stewart–Treves syndrome) presents in women who have had severe long-standing lymphedema of the arm after breast surgery but has also been described in men from causes other than cancer surgery, including congenital lymphedema and tropical lymphedema due to filaria. The prognosis despite radical surgery is extremely poor. Postirradiation angiosarcoma may arise in the skin after radiotherapy for internal cancer. The most common sites are the breast or chest wall and the lower abdomen after therapy for breast or gynecologic cancer.

HISTOPATHOLOGY. Usually, the tumor extends well beyond the limits of the apparent clinical lesion. As a rule, the tumor shows varied differentiation in different biopsies, even within different fields in a single biopsy. In well-differentiated areas, irregular anastomosing vascular channels lined by a single layer of somewhat enlarged endothelial cells permeate between collagen bundles. Isolation and enclosure of collagen bundles, figuratively referred to as "dissection of collagen," is a characteristic feature. Nuclear atypia is always present and may be slight to moderate, but occasional large hyperchromatic cells may be encountered. At this stage the vascular lumens are generally bloodless, but they may contain free-lying shed malignant cells. In less well-differentiated areas, endothelial cells increase in size and number, forming intraluminal papillary projections where there is enhanced mitotic activity. In poorly differentiated areas, solid sheets of large pleomorphic cells with little or no evidence of luminal differentiation can resemble metastatic carcinoma or melanoma. Focally, areas showing epithelioid cells are not uncommon. Other areas may simulate a poorly differentiated spindle cell sarcoma. Interstitial hemorrhage and widely dilated blood-filled spaces may sometimes develop.

Angiokeratoma

See Figs. VIC5.r and VIC5.s.

Arteriovenous Hemangioma

See Figs. VIC5.t and VIC5.u.

Cavernous Hemangioma

See Figs. VIC5.v and VIC5.w.

Cherry Hemangioma

See Figs. VIC5.x and VIC5.y.

Microvenular Hemangioma

See Figs. VIC5.z–VIC5.bb.

Cutaneous Lymphangioma

See Figs. VIC5.cc and VIC5.dd.

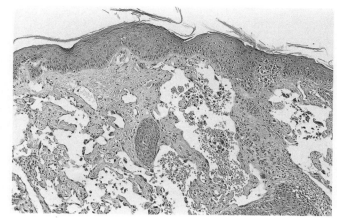

Fig. VIC5.m

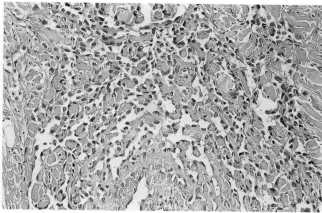

Fig. VIC5.n

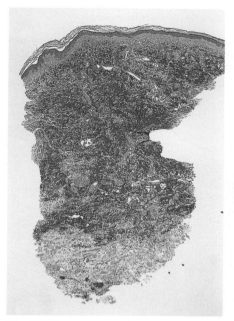

Fig. VIC5.o

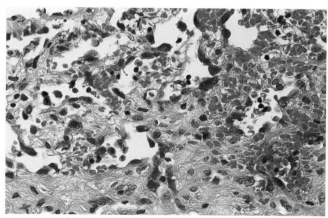

Fig. VIC5.p

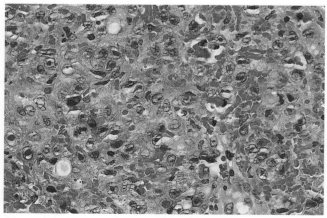

Fig. VIC5.q

Fig. VIC5.m. *Cutaneous angiosarcoma, low power.* Within the dermis there are multiple dilated cystic spaces lined by a prominent layer of single cells.

Fig. VIC5.n. *Cutaneous angiosarcoma, high power.* Other areas show poorly defined spaces lined by plump, hyperchromatic endothelial cells. This pattern of dissection throughout the reticular dermal collagen is typical of angiosarcoma.

Fig. VIC5.o. *Cutaneous angiosarcoma, low power.* In this example of angiosarcoma, scanning magnification only reveals extensive hemorrhage throughout the dermis.

Fig. VIC5.p. *Cutaneous angiosarcoma, high power.* Upon close inspection, there are vascular-like spaces lined by atypical, hyperchromatic endothelial cells.

Fig. VIC5.q. *Cutaneous angiosarcoma, high power.* In other areas, the proliferation of atypical cells may form solid sheets without formation of vascular spaces.

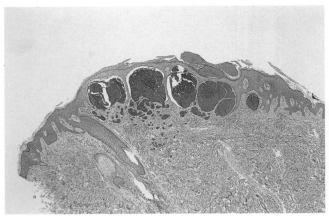

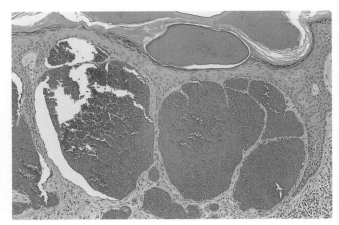

Fig. VIC5.r   Fig. VIC5.s

Fig. VIC5.r. *Angiokeratoma, low power.* There is a vascular proliferation predominantly within the papillary dermis. The associated epidermis is hyperplastic and appears to encircle the vascular channels.

Fig. VIC5.s. *Angiokeratoma, medium power.* The vascular channels are thin-walled and lined by mature endothelial cells. They are filled with erythrocytes. The hyperplastic epithelium surrounds these vascular channels, and occasionally it may appear that the vascular channels are within the epithelium.

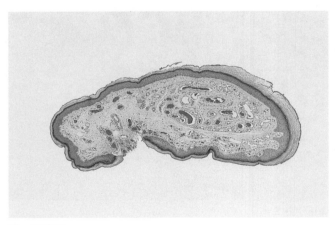

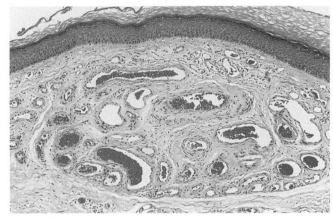

Fig. VIC5.t   Fig. VIC5.u

Fig. VIC5.t. *Arteriovenous hemangioma, low power.* There is a well-circumscribed vascular proliferation within the superficial dermis.

Fig. VIC5.u. *Arteriovenous hemangioma, medium power.* The vascular proliferation is composed of mature thick- and thin-walled vascular channels filled with erythrocytes.

Venous Lake

See Figs. VIC5.ee and VIC5.ff.

Epithelioid Hemangioendothelioma

See Figs. VIC5.gg–VIC5.ii.

Glomangioma

See Figs. VIC5.jj–VIC5.ll.

Subungual Glomus Tumor

See Figs. VIC5.mm and VIC5.nn.

Conditions to consider in the differential diagnosis:

Hyperplasias
intravascular papillary endothelial hyperplasia
reactive angioendotheliomatosis
angiolymphoid hyperplasia with eosinophilia
Angiomas
juvenile hemangioendothelioma (strawberry nevus)
cherry hemangioma
glomeruloid hemangioma
tufted angioma (angioblastoma)
angiokeratoma
cavernous hemangioma
sinusoidal hemangioma
verrucous hemangioma

(*text continues on p. 353*)

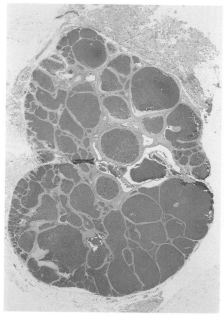

Fig. VIC5.v

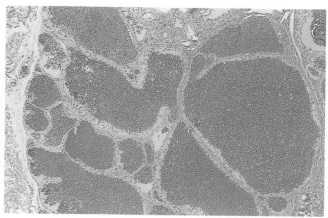

Fig. VIC5.w

Fig. VIC5.v. *Cavernous hemangioma, low power.* There is a proliferation of vascular channels filled with erythrocytes within the deep dermis and subcutaneous tissue. All cavernous hemangiomas are not as well-circumscribed as this example.

Fig. VIC5.w. *Cavernous hemangioma, medium power.* The vascular channels show thin-walled endothelial cells without atypia. The channels are filled with erythrocytes.

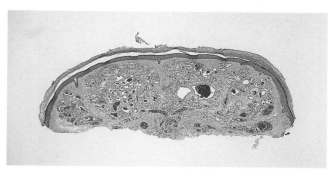

Fig. VIC5.x

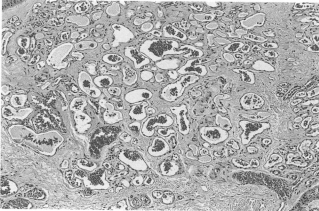

Fig. VIC5.y

Fig. VIC5.x. *Cherry hemangioma, low power.* This dome-shaped papular lesion shows a vascular proliferation within the superficial dermis.

Fig. VIC5.y. *Cherry hemangioma, medium power.* There is a proliferation of thin-walled mature vascular channels filled with erythrocytes. The associated stroma may be edematous or fibrotic.

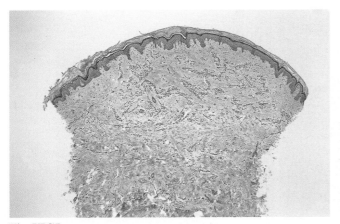

Fig. VIC5.z

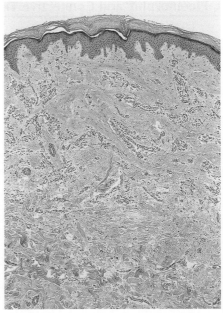

Fig. VIC5.aa

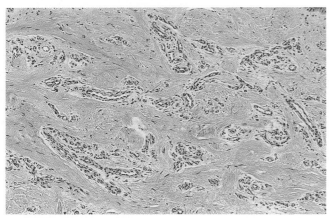

Fig. VIC5.bb

Fig. VIC5.z. *Microvenular hemangioma, low power*. At scanning magnification there is increased cellularity throughout the reticular dermis.

Fig. VIC5.aa. *Microvenular hemangioma, medium power*. There is a proliferation of small venules throughout the reticular dermis without formation of lobular aggregates. No large vascular spaces are seen.

Fig. VIC5.bb. *Microvenular hemangioma, high power*. The vessels are all mature small venules without atypia. There is an associated fibrotic stroma.

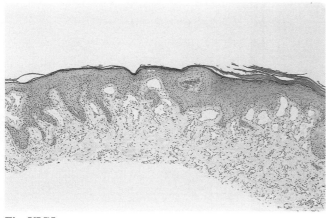

Fig. VIC5.cc

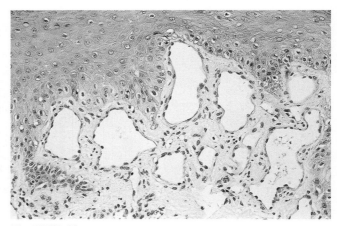

Fig. VIC5.dd

Fig. VIC5.cc. *Cutaneous lymphangioma, low power*. There are multiple dilated vascular channels within the papillary dermis extending into the superficial reticular dermis.

Fig. VIC5.dd. *Cutaneous lymphangioma, medium power*. In the papillary dermis, these vascular channels are lined by a thin wall consisting only of endothelial cells. Amorphous material may be seen within the lumen. Erythrocytes, however, are not present within the vascular channels.

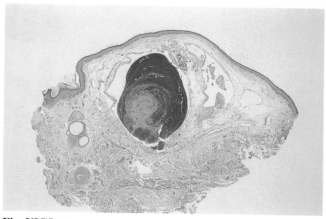

Fig. VIC5.ee

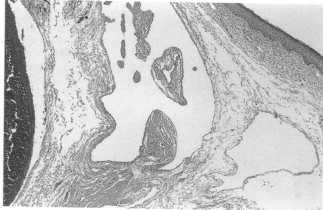

Fig. VIC5.ff

Fig. VIC5.ee. *Venous lake with thrombosis, low power.* In the superficial dermis there is a vascular dilatation composed of solitary or occasionally few dilated vascular spaces. In this example there is a relatively large organizing thrombus within the vascular channel.

Fig. VIC5.ff. *Venous lake with thrombosis, medium power.* The thrombosis is seen at the left hand side of this photomicrograph. In the superficial dermis the dilated vascular channel is lined by a thin endothelial wall.

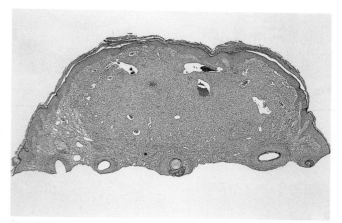

Fig. VIC5.gg

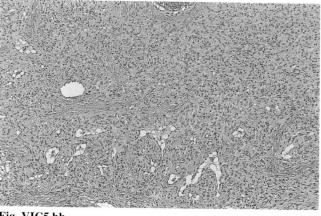

Fig. VIC5.hh

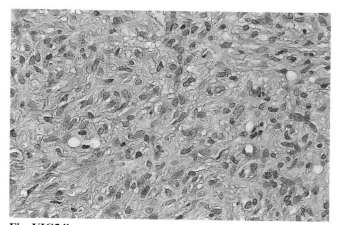

Fig. VIC5.ii

Fig. VIC5.gg. *Epithelioid hemangioendothelioma, low power.* There is a relatively well-circumscribed but nonencapsulated dome-shaped lesion within the dermis. The epidermis is uninvolved, and shows an effaced rete ridge pattern.

Fig. VIC5.hh. *Epithelioid hemangioendothelioma, medium power.* The neoplasm is composed of a solid sheet of uniform, bland appearing cells associated with small dilated vascular channels which contain erythrocytes.

Fig. VIC5.ii. *Epithelioid hemangioendothelioma, high power.* The cells contain an abundance of cytoplasm and show intracytoplasmic vacuoles. There are scattered erythrocytes between the cells. Significant cytologic atypia is not present.

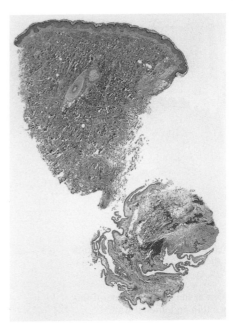

Fig. VIC5.jj

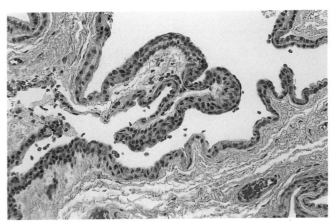

Fig. VIC5.kk

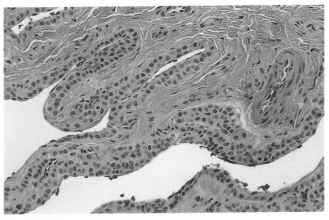

Fig. VIC5.ll

Fig. VIC5.jj. *Glomangioma, low power*. In the deep reticular dermis, there is a neoplasm composed of multiple cystic-like spaces lined by a thickened wall.

Fig. VIC5.kk. *Glomangioma, medium power*. The cystic spaces are lined by several layers of small cuboidal cells.

Fig. VIC5.ll. *Glomangioma, medium power*. Another area of the glomangioma showing cystic spaces lined by cuboidal glomus cells. The individual cells are monotonously bland and lack cytologic atypia. Erythrocytes may be seen in the cavernous spaces.

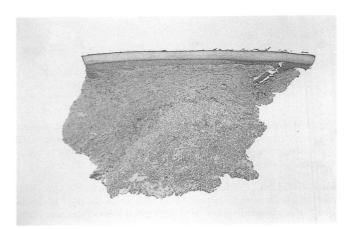

Fig. VIC5.mm

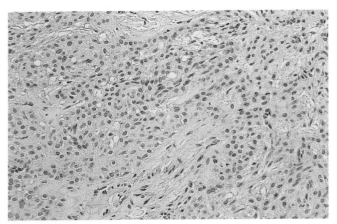

Fig. VIC5.nn

Fig. VIC5.mm. *Subungual glomus tumor, low power*. This nail bed biopsy shows a cellular tumor in the deep dermis. In contrast to a glomangioma, only rare vascular channels are seen.

Fig. VIC5.nn. *Subungual glomus tumor, high power*. There are both thin cords and solid areas of tumor composed of uniform cuboidal cells with small round nuclei.

microvenular hemangioma
targetoid hemosiderotic (hob-nail) hemangioma
cirsoid aneurysm (AV hemangioma)
epithelioid hemangioma
pyogenic granuloma
bacillary angiomatosis
Lymphangiomas
cavernous lymphangioma and cystic hygroma
lymphangioma circumscriptum
progressive lymphangioma (benign
   lymphangioendothelioma)
lymphangiomatosis
Telangiectases
hereditary hemorrhagic telangiectasia
spider nevus
venous lakes
Vascular Malformations
angioma serpiginosum
Glomus Tumors
glomus tumor, glomangioma, glomangiomyoma
infiltrating glomus tumor
glomangiosarcoma
Vascular Lipomas
angiomyolipoma
angiolipoma
Angiosarcomas
cutaneous angiosarcoma
epithelioid angiosarcoma
Kaposi's Sarcoma
Kaposi's Sarcoma Simulants (see also angiomas)
aneurysmal fibrous histiocytoma
spindle cell hemangioendothelioma

Kaposi-like infantile hemangioendothelioma
acroangiodermatitis (pseudo-Kaposi's sarcoma)
multinucleate cell angiohistiocytoma
Hemangioendotheliomas
epithelioid hemangioendothelioma
retiform hemangioendothelioma
malignant endovascular papillary angioendothelioma
   (Dabska's tumor)
spindle cell hemangioendothelioma
Kaposi-like infantile hemangioendothelioma
Other Vascular Tumors
angiomatosis
hemangiopericytoma
intravascular lymphoma (malignant
   angioendotheliomatosis)

VIC6. Tumors of Adipose Tissue

Most tumors of adipose tissue occur in the subcutis or deeper soft tissues, but some may involve the skin. The lesional cells may range from mature adipocytes indistinguishable from those of mature fat in typical lipomas to more or less undifferentiated round cells or pleomorphic cells in the high-grade liposarcomas. Nevus lipomatosus superficialis is a lipomatous neoplastic or hamartomatous disorder that primarily involves the skin (39).

Nevus Lipomatosus Superficialis

CLINICAL SUMMARY.   Nevus lipomatosus superficialis is a fairly uncommon lesion that may present as groups of soft flattened papules or nodules that have smooth or wrinkled

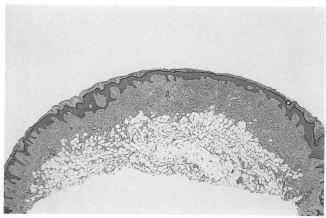

Fig. VIC6.a

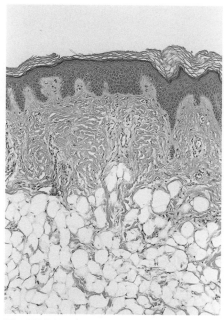

Fig. VIC6.a. *Nevus lipomatosus superficialis, low power.* Mature adipose tissue extends up into the reticular dermis. There is no associated inflammatory reaction.

Fig. VIC6.b. *Nevus lipomatosus superficialis, medium power.* Mature adipocytes are seen in the superficial and mid-reticular dermis.

Fig. VIC6.b

surfaces and are skin-colored or pale yellow. Characteristically, the lesions are linearly distributed on one hip or buttock (nevus lipomatosus superficialis of Hoffman and Zurhelle) from where they may overlap onto the adjacent skin of the back or the upper thigh. Other areas, such as the thorax or the abdomen, are only rarely affected. The lesions may be present at birth or may begin in infancy (nevus angiolipomatosus of Howell), in which case the replacement of hypoplastic dermis may cause pseudotumorous yellow protrusions and may be associated with skeletal and other malformations, but they develop most commonly during the first two decades of life and occasionally later. Multiple lesions may coalesce. Solitary lesions may be diagnosed as nevus lipomatosus superficialis or as solitary, baglike, soft fibromas or polypoid fibrolipomas. The rather common presence of fat cells within long-standing intradermal melanocytic nevi represents an involutionary phenomenon and not a nevus lipomatosus.

HISTOPATHOLOGY.   Groups and strands of fat cells are found embedded among the collagen bundles of the dermis, often as high as the papillary dermis. The proportion of fatty tissue varies greatly. In cases with only small deposits, the fat cells are apt to be situated in small foci around the subpapillary vessels. In instances with relatively large amounts of fat, the fat lobules are irregularly distributed throughout the dermis, and the boundary between the dermis and the hypoderm is ill defined or lost. The fat cells may all be mature, but in some instances an occasional small incompletely lipidized cell may be observed. Aside from the presence of fat cells, the dermis may be entirely normal, but in some instances the density of the collagen bundles, the number of fibroblasts, and the vascularity are greater than in normal skin.

Lipoma

By definition, lipomas contain mature adipocytes as a principal component. They tend to be surrounded by a thin connective tissue capsule and are composed, often entirely, of normal fat cells that are indistinguishable from the fat cells in the subcutaneous tissue.

Angiolipomas

Angiolipomas usually occur as encapsulated subcutaneous lesions. As a rule, they arise in young adults. The forearm is the single most common location for this tumor, which is more often multifocal than solitary. They are often tender or painful. Inapparent at the gross level, angiolipomas microscopically show sharp encapsulation, numerous, small-caliber vascular channels containing characteristic microthrombi and variable amounts of mature adipose tissue. The degree of vascularity is quite variable, ranging from only a few small angiomatous foci to lesions with a predominance of dense vascular and stromal tissue.

Spindle Cell Lipoma

Clinically, the tumor is a slowly growing painless nodule centered in the dermis or subcutis and exhibiting a predilection for the posterior neck and shoulder girdle region in men in their sixth decade. Although the lesion is well-circumscribed histologically, it is seldom encapsulated. It is comprised of mature fat cells and uniform slender spindle cells within a mucinous matrix. Spindle cell lipoma is polymorphous as a result of variations in cellularity, collagen content, and the ratio of spindle cells to mature adipocytes.

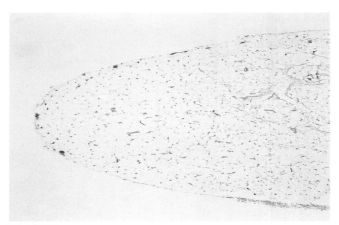

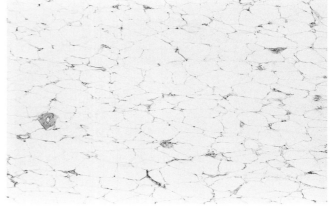

Fig. VIC6.c   **Fig. VIC6.d**

Fig. VIC6.c. *Lipoma, low power.* This circumscribed neoplasm shows a very thin fibrous capsule. Lipomas reside in the subcutaneous fat. At scanning magnification, the lesion is hypocellular.

Fig. VIC6.d. *Lipoma, high power.* A lipoma is composed of uniform adipocytes which are approximately of equal size. The small nucleus is pushed to the side of the cell and is barely visible.

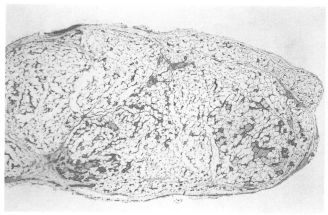

Fig. VIC6.e

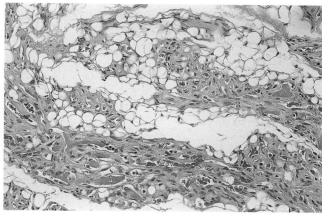

Fig. VIC6.f

Fig. VIC6.e. *Angiolipoma, low power.* Similar to a lipoma, an angiolipoma is a well-circumscribed subcutaneous mass with a very thin fibrous capsule. However, in contrast, this lesion is more cellular than the one in Fig. VIC6.c.

Fig. VIC6.f. *Angiolipoma, medium power.* The increased cellularity in angiolipomas is secondary to a proliferation of small mature vascular channels filled with erythrocytes and fibrin thrombi.

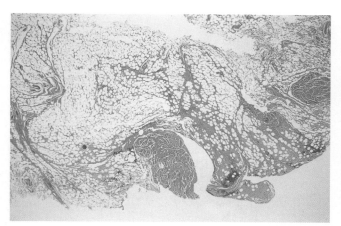

Fig. VIC6.g

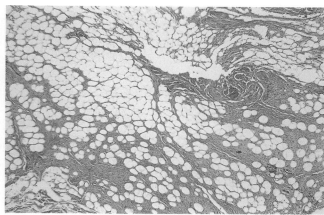

Fig. VIC6.h

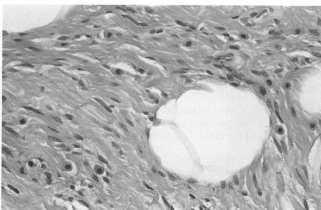

Fig. VIC6.g. *Spindle cell lipoma, low power.* At scanning magnification, this tumor is composed of cellular areas as well as hypocellular areas.

Fig. VIC6.h. *Spindle cell lipoma, medium power.* The hypocellular areas are mature adipocytes. In the hypercellular areas there is a proliferation of bland appearing spindle cells.

Fig. VIC6.i. *Spindle cell lipoma, high power.* The spindle cells are wavy in appearance but lack cytologic atypia. The associated stroma is frequently mucinous and there are scattered mast cells.

Fig. VIC6.i

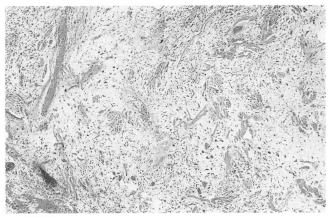

Fig. VIC6.j

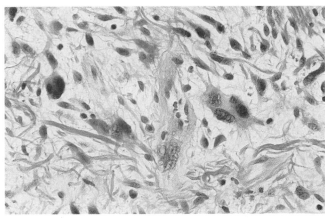

Fig. VIC6.k

Fig. VIC6.j. *Pleomorphic lipoma, low power.* Mature and immature fat cells are situated singly and in groups in a mucinous stroma traversed by dense collagen bundles.

Fig. VIC6.k. *Pleomorphic lipoma, high power.* Characteristic multinucleated giant cells, found in most but not all cases, exhibit multiple, marginally placed, often overlapping hyperchromatic nuclei within an eosinophilic cytoplasm. This peculiar arrangement is not unlike that of the petals of a small flower, and these giant cells are therefore referred to as floret-type giant cells.

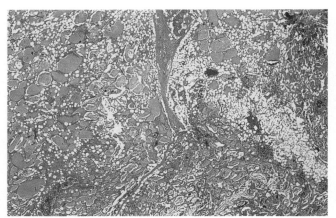

Fig. VIC6.l

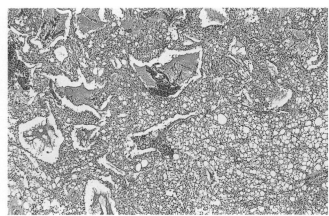

Fig. VIC6.m

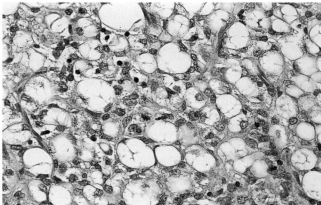

Fig. VIC6.n

Fig. VIC6.l. *Liposarcoma, round cell type, low power.* This is a large, poorly circumscribed tumor without a defined capsule. Although in some areas one can identify adipocytes, other areas are very cellular.

Fig. VIC6.m. *Liposarcoma, medium power.* In the lower right hand area of this photomicrograph are adipocytes. However, the vast majority of the tumor is hypercellular.

Fig. VIC6.n. *Liposarcoma, high power.* Admixed with the adipocytes are larger cells with large hyperchromatic nuclei, many of which contain vacuoles that indent the nucleus, creating a delicate scalloping of the nuclear membrane (monovacuolar and multivacuolar lipoblasts). Mitotic figures are also seen.

Pleomorphic Lipomas

CLINICAL SUMMARY. Like spindle cell lipomas, most pleomorphic lipomas are solitary tumors of the shoulder girdle and neck in men in the fifth to seventh decade. The lesion presents as a slowly growing well-circumscribed dermal or subcutaneous mass grossly resembling an ordinary lipoma. Despite occasional lipoblastlike cells and atypical mitotic figures, local excision should be curative.

DIFFERENTIAL DIAGNOSIS. No single feature confirms the diagnosis of pleomorphic lipoma and excludes liposarcoma. Only a multivariate analysis leads to the correct diagnosis, and such an analysis should consider the age and sex of the patient, anatomic location, size, epicenter of growth (deep or superficial), degree of local invasion, and histologic appearance. Liposarcomas differ from pleomorphic lipomas by their infiltrative growth, greater cellularity, more nuclear atypicality, including atypical mitoses; more numerous multivacuolated lipoblasts; prominent necrosis; and absence of thick collagen bundles. Floret-type giant cells are rarely seen in liposarcomas, and then only in small numbers.

Liposarcoma

Liposarcomas are large tumors of the deep subcutis or deeper soft tissue. As such, they rarely come to the attention of the dermatopathologist.
Conditions to consider in the differential diagnosis:

Lipomas
spindle cell lipoma
pleomorphic lipoma
chondroid lipoma
angiolipoma
Liposarcomas
well differentiated
atypical lipomatous tumor
myxoid
round cell
pleomorphic
Miscellaneous
hibernoma
benign lipoblastoma
nevus lipomatosus superficialis

VIC7. Tumors of Cartilaginous Tissue

Most tumors of cartilaginous tissue occur in the bones and joints or in the deep soft tissues, but some may involve the skin. The lesional cells may range from mature chondrocytes indistinguishable from those of mature cartilage in an enchondroma to more or less undifferentiated round cells or pleomorphic cells in a high-grade chondrosarcoma. Because of their location, these tumors come to the attention of the dermatopathologist only rarely.
Conditions to consider in the differential diagnosis:
chondroid lipoma
soft tissue chondroma
chondrosarcoma

VIC8. Tumors of Osseous Tissue

Metaplastic ossification, disturbances of calcium metabolism, and presumably other poorly understood mechanisms, including hereditary abnormalities, may lead to local areas of calcification and also to focal or diffuse ossification in the dermis.

Albright's Hereditary Osteodystrophy and Osteoma Cutis

CLINICAL SUMMARY. In Albright's hereditary osteodystrophy (AHO), multiple areas of subcutaneous or intracutaneous ossification are often encountered (40). These may be present at birth or may arise later in life and have no definite area of predilection. The areas may be small or large (5 cm). Those located in the skin may cause ulceration, and bony spicules may be extruded through the ulcer. In addition to cutaneous and subcutaneous osteomas, bone formation may be observed in some cases along fascial planes. AHO includes the syndromes of pseudohypoparathyroidism and pseudopseudohypoparathyroidism. Patients with AHO have short stature, round facies, and multiple skeletal abnormalities, such as curvature of the radius and shortening of some of the metacarpal bones. As a result of this shortening, some knuckles are absent when the fists are clenched, and depressions or dimples are apparent there instead. This important diagnostic sign is referred to as the Albright dimpling sign. Additional manifestations include basal ganglia calcification and mental retardation. The mode of inheritance is dominant, possibly X-linked dominant.

The term *osteoma cutis* is applied to cases of primary cutaneous ossification in which there is no evidence of AHO in either the patients or their families. The lesions may present as a solitary or even multiple tumorlike lesions. Clinically inapparent incidental small foci of ossification are commonly seen within the dermis or stroma in other lesions, such as melanocytic nevi or acne scars. The possibility of AHO should be seriously considered in patients with extensive foci of ossification.

HISTOPATHOLOGY. Spicules of bone of various sizes may be found within the dermis or in the subcutaneous tissue. The bone contains fairly numerous osteocytes and cement lines that may be accentuated in polarized light. In addition, there are osteoblasts along the surface of the spicules and often, osteoclasts in Howship's lacunae. The spicules of bone may enclose, either partially or completely, areas of mature fat cells, representing establishment of a medullary cavity. Hematopoietic elements are observed rarely among the fat cells. The histologic findings in osteoma cutis are the same as in primary cutaneous ossification occurring in conjunction with AHO.

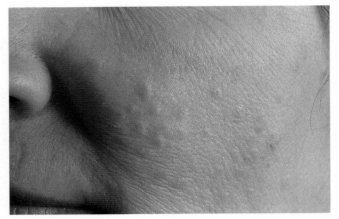

Clin. Fig. VIC8

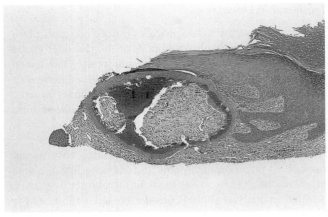

Fig. VIC8.a

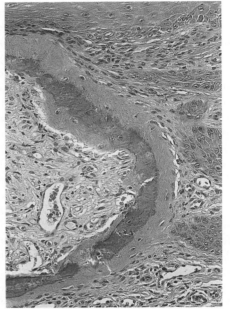

Fig. VIC8.b

Clin. Fig. VIC8. *Multiple cutaneous osteomas.* A 50-year-old woman developed multiple 2 to 3 mm flesh-colored and slightly erythematous firm papules on the cheeks.

Fig. VIC8.a. *Osteoma cutis, low power.* Within the superficial dermis there is a well-circumscribed zone of eosinophilic to purplish material.

Fig. VIC8.b. *Osteoma cutis, medium power.* Eosinophilic bone shows numerous osteocytes. There is an associated fibrovascular stroma.

Conditions to consider in the differential diagnosis:
  Albright's hereditary osteodystrophy
  osteoma cutis
  metaplastic ossification
  subungual exostosis

VID. CYSTS OF THE DERMIS AND SUBCUTIS

1. Pilar Differentiation
2. Eccrine and Similar Differentiation
3. Apocrine Differentiation

   A cyst is a space lined by epithelium; its contents are usually a product of its lining. Some cysts are inclusion or retention cysts of normal structures (hair follicle-related cysts). Others are benign neoplasms. Some malignant neoplasms may be cystic. These tend to be larger and asymmetric, with a poorly circumscribed and infiltrative border. Their epithelial lining is proliferative, with cytologic atypia.

VID1. Pilar Differentiation

Cystic proliferations are present in the dermis; these show spaces surrounded by epithelium of follicular origin and differentiation. Keratin is usually seen in the cystic cavity. Associated cells may be sparse or may include lymphocytes and plasma cells.

Epidermal or Infundibular Cyst

CLINICAL SUMMARY.   Epidermal cysts (41) are slowly growing, elevated, round, firm, intradermal or subcutaneous tumors that cease growing after having reached 1 to 5 cm in diameter. Most epidermal cysts arise spontaneously in hair-bearing areas, most commonly on the face, scalp, neck, and trunk but occasionally on the palms or soles and occasionally as a result of trauma. Usually, a patient has only one or a few epidermal cysts, rarely many. In Gardner's syndrome, numerous epidermal cysts occur, especially on the scalp and face.

HISTOPATHOLOGY. Epidermal cysts have a wall composed of true epidermis, as seen on the skin surface and in the infundibulum of hair follicles, the infundibulum being the uppermost part of the hair follicle that extends down to the entry of the sebaceous duct. In young epidermal cysts, several layers of squamous and granular cells can usually be recognized. In older epidermal cysts, the wall often is markedly atrophic, either in some areas or in the entire cyst, and may consist of only one or two rows of greatly flattened cells. The cyst is filled with horny material arranged in laminated layers. When an epidermal cyst ruptures and the contents of the cyst are released into the dermis, a considerable foreign-body reaction with numerous multinucleated giant cells results, forming a *keratin granuloma*. The foreign-body reaction usually causes disintegration of the cyst wall. However, it may lead to a pseudoepitheliomatous proliferation in remnants of the cyst wall, simulating a squamous cell carcinoma.

Trichilemmal (Pilar) Cyst

See Figs. VID1.c and VID1.d.

Steatocystoma

See Figs. VID1.e–VID1.g.

Vellus Hair Cyst

See Figs. VID1.h and VID1.i.

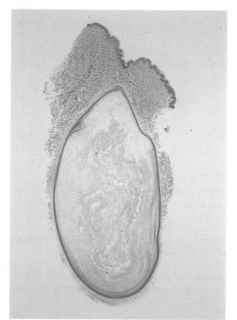

Clin. Fig. VID1

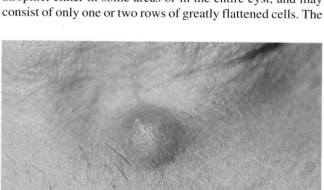

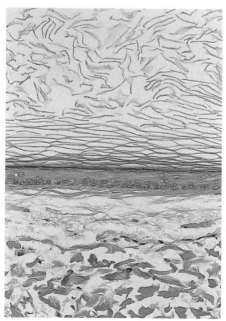

Fig. VID1.a **Fig. VID1.b**

Clin. Fig. VID1. *Epidermal cyst.* An elderly man presented with a firm, slowly enlarging, asymptomatic flesh-colored nodule on the cheek.

Fig. VID1.a. *Epidermal cyst, low power.* Within the dermis there is a well-circumscribed cystic structure filled with laminated keratin.

Fig. VID1.b. *Epidermal cyst, high power.* The wall of the cyst is composed of mature squamous epithelium with formation of a granular cell layer. The contents of the cyst are composed of laminated orthokeratin.

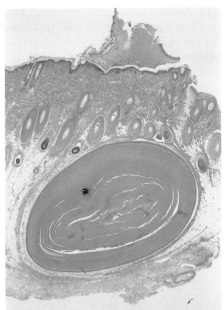

Fig. VID1.c. *Trichi-lemmal (pilar) cyst, low power.* In this scalp biopsy there is a well-circumscribed cystic structure in the subcutaneous fat.

Fig. VID1.d. *Trichi-lemmal (pilar) cyst, high power.* The wall of the cyst is com-posed of mature squamous epithelium which shows kera-tinization without formation of a granu-lar layer.

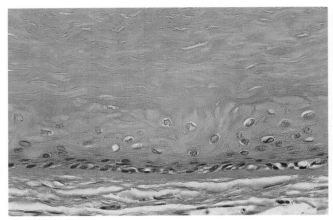

Fig. VID1.d

Fig. VID1.c

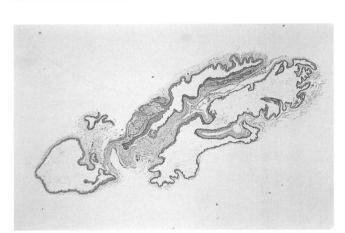

Fig. VID1.e

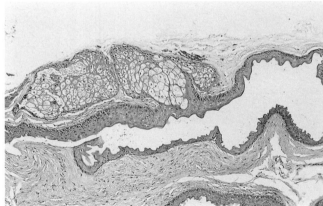

Fig. VID1.f

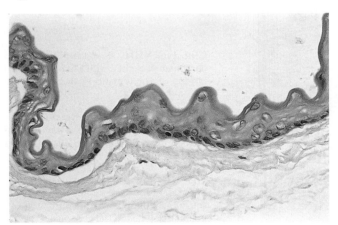

Fig. VID1.g

Fig. VID1.e. *Steatocystoma, low power.* Steatocystoma may show a solitary cystic space or a multiloculated appearance with numer-ous infoldings of the cyst wall.

Fig. VID1.f. *Steatocystoma, medium power.* Mature sebaceous lobules are seen arising from the wall of the cyst.

Fig. VID1.g. *Steatocystoma, high power.* The epithelial wall of the steatocystoma shows a corrugated luminal surface associated with an eosinophilic cuticle.

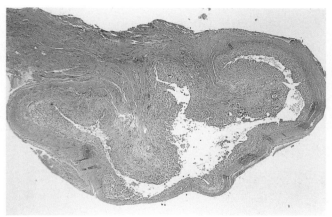

Fig. VID1.h

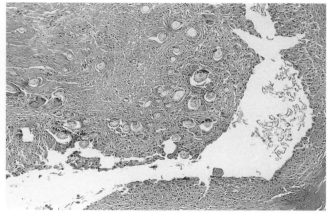

Fig. VID1.i

Fig. VID1.h. *Vellus hair cyst, low power.* The wall of this cyst is lined by granulation tissue as a result of rupture, followed by granulomatous inflammation. An early lesion would be lined by mature squamous epithelium with formation of a granular cell layer, changes indistinguishable from the lining of an epidermal inclusion cyst.

Fig. VID1.i. *Vellus hair cyst, medium power.* In the center of this cyst there are flecks of keratin as well as granulomatous inflammation. There are numerous small (vellus) hair shafts within the cavity of the cyst.

Conditions to consider in the differential diagnosis:

    epidermal cyst
    milia
    trichilemmal cyst
    steatocystoma multiplex
    pigmented follicular cyst
    dermoid cyst
    bronchogenic and thyroglossal duct cysts
    eruptive vellus hair cyst
    pilar sheath acanthoma
    dilated pore of Winer

VID2. Eccrine and Similar Differentiation

Cystic proliferations are present in the dermis; these show spaces surrounded by eccrine epithelium (small dark epithelial cells). The epithelium of ciliated and bronchogenic cysts is not eccrine but may resemble that of an eccrine cyst. Eccrine hidrocystoma is the prototype (42).

Eccrine Hidrocystoma

CLINICAL SUMMARY. In this condition, usually one lesion, but occasionally several and rarely numerous lesions, is present on the face. The lesions are small, translucent, cystic nodules 1 to 3 mm in diameter that often have a bluish hue. In some patients with numerous lesions, the number of cysts increases in warm weather and decreases during winter.

HISTOPATHOLOGY. Eccrine hidrocystoma shows a single cystic cavity located in the dermis. The cyst wall usually shows two layers of small cuboidal epithelial cells. In some areas, only a single layer of flattened epithelial cells can be seen, their flattened nuclei extending parallel to the cyst wall. Small papillary projections extending into the cavity of the cyst are observed only rarely. Eccrine secretory tubules and ducts are often located below the cyst and in close approximation to it, and, on serial sections, one may find an eccrine duct leading into the cyst from below. However, no connection can be found between the cyst and the epidermis.

Median Raphe Cyst

See Figs. VID2.c and VID2.d.

Bronchogenic Cyst

See Figs. VID2.e–VID2.g.

Cutaneous Endometriosis

See Figs. VID2.h–VID2.j.

    Conditions to consider in the differential diagnosis:

        eccrine hidrocystoma
        cutaneous ciliated cyst
        bronchogenic and thyroglossal duct cysts
        median raphe cyst of the penis
        cutaneous endometriosis

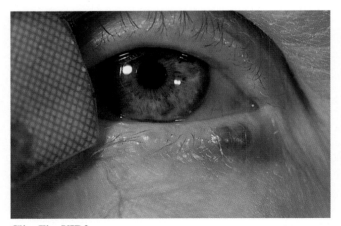

Clin. Fig. VID2

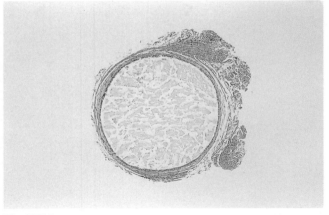

Fig. VID2.a

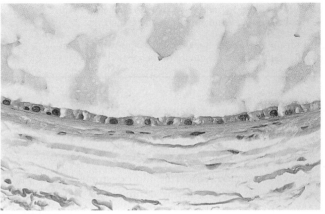

Fig. VID2.b

Clin. Fig. VID2. *Eccrine hidrocystoma.* An elderly woman developed compressible blue translucent papules on the lower eyelid.

Fig. VID2.a. *Eccrine hidrocystoma, low power.* Within the dermis there is a well-circumscribed solitary cystic structure filled with amorphous material.

Fig. VID2.b. *Eccrine hidrocystoma, high power.* The wall of the cystic structure is composed of cuboidal cells.

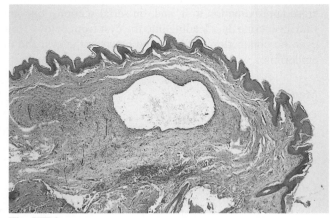

Fig. VID2.c

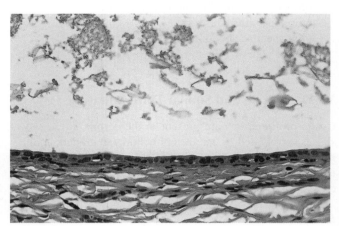

Fig. VID2.d

Fig. VID2.c. *Median raphe cyst of the penis, low power.* Within the superficial dermis there is a solitary cystic structure.

Fig. VID2.d. *Median raphe cyst of the penis, high power.* The wall of the cyst is frequently composed of pseudostratified columnar epithelium or, as seen here, only 1 to 2 layers of cells may be present, resembling an eccrine hidrocystoma.

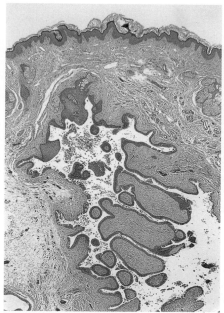

Fig. VID2.e

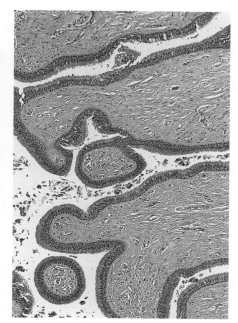

Fig. VID2.f

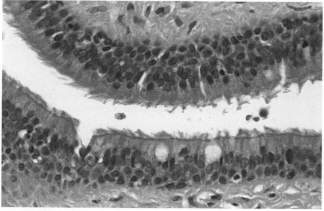

Fig. VID2.g

Fig. VID2.e. *Bronchogenic cyst, low power.* Within the dermis there is a solitary cyst with a slightly papilliferous wall.

Fig. VID2.f. *Bronchogenic cyst, medium power.* The projections are lined by pseudostratified columnar epithelium. There is a fibrotic stroma which may contain smooth muscle.

Fig. VID2.g. *Bronchogenic cyst, high power.* The pseudostratified columnar epithelial wall shows numerous cilia extending into the lumen. Goblet cells are also present.

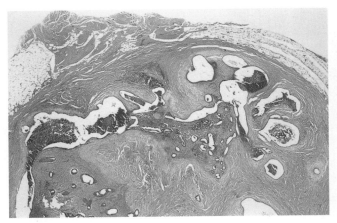

Fig. VID2.h

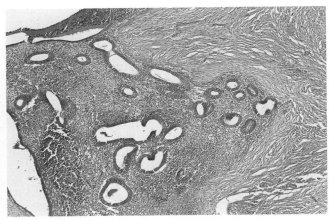

Fig. VID2.i

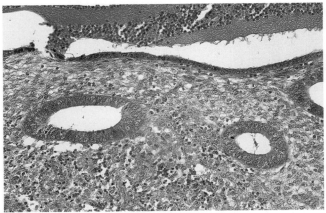

Fig. VID2.j

Fig. VID2.h. *Cutaneous endometriosis, low power.* This well-circumscribed nodular tumor is present in the deep dermis and subcutaneous fat. It is composed of two elements, glandular structures and a prominent stroma.

Fig. VID2.i. *Cutaneous endometriosis, medium power.* Numerous glandular structures are embedded in a well-vascularized and hypercellular stroma. In some areas, as on the right side of this photomicrograph, the stroma is fibrotic.

Fig. VID2.j. *Cutaneous endometriosis, high power.* The glandular component and the associated hemorrhagic stroma resemble uterine endometrium during the phases of the menstrual cycle.

VID3. Apocrine Differentiation

Cystic proliferations are present in the dermis; these show spaces surrounded by apocrine epithelium (large pink cells with decapitation secretion). There may be lymphocytes and plasma cells (syringocystadenoma). Apocrine hidrocystoma (43) and hidradenoma papilliferum are prototypic (44).

Apocrine Hidrocystoma

CLINICAL SUMMARY. Apocrine hidrocystoma presents as a solitary translucent cystic nodule, between 3 and 15 mm in diameter. The lesion may be skin colored or may have a blue hue resembling a blue nevus. The usual location is on the face but also on the ears, scalp, chest, or shoulders. Multiple apocrine hidrocystomas are rare.

HISTOPATHOLOGY. The dermis contains one or several large cystic spaces into which papillary projections often extend. The inner surface of the wall and the papillary projections are lined by a row of secretory cells of variable height showing decapitation secretion indicative of apocrine secretion. There is an outer layer of elongated myoepithelial cells, their long axes running parallel to the cyst wall.

Hidradenoma Papilliferum

CLINICAL SUMMARY. Hidradenoma papilliferum occurs only in women, usually on the labia majora or in the perineal or perianal region. The tumor is covered by normal skin and measures only a few millimeters in diameter. Malignant changes are extremely rare.

HISTOPATHOLOGY. The tumor represents an adenoma with apocrine differentiation. It is located in the dermis, is well-circumscribed, is surrounded by a fibrous capsule, and has no connection with the overlying epidermis. Some tumors have a peripheral epithelial wall with areas of keratinization. Within the tumor, there are tubular and cystic structures. Papillary folds project into the cystic spaces. Usually, the lumina are surrounded by a double layer of cells consisting of a luminal layer of secretory cells and of an outer layer of small cuboidal cells with deeply basophilic nuclei. These are myoepithelial cells. The lumina are lined occasionally with only a single row of columnar cells, which show an oval pale-staining nucleus located near the base, a faintly eosinophilic cytoplasm, and active decapitation secretion as seen in the secretory cells of apocrine glands.

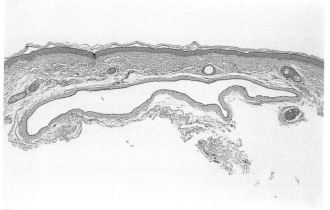

Fig. VID3.a

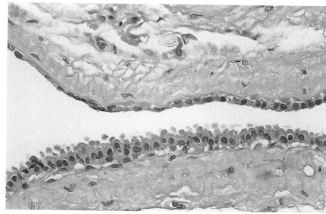

Fig. VID3.b

Fig. VID3.a. *Apocrine hidrocystoma, low power.* There is a well-circumscribed cystic structure within the dermis.

Fig. VID3.b. *Apocrine hidrocystoma, high power.* The wall of this cystic structure is composed of one or more layers of bland-appearing cuboidal cells. The cells show decapitation secretion manifested by small droplets of cytoplasm on their luminal surface.

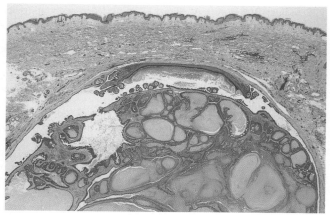

Fig. VID3.c

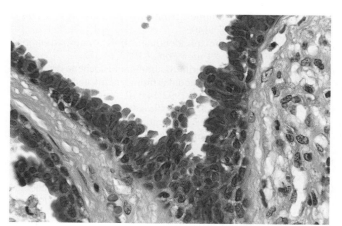

Fig. VID3.d

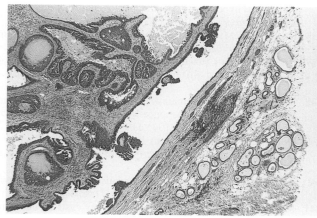

Fig. VID3.e

Fig. VID3.f

Fig. VID3.c. *Hidradenoma papilliferum, low power.* This well-circumscribed neoplasm has a thin surrounding fibrous capsule.

Fig. VID3.d. *Hidradenoma papilliferum, low power.* There are multiple papillary folds and cystic spaces.

Fig. VID3.e. *Hidradenoma papilliferum, medium power.* There are numerous papillary projections which extend into the cystic spaces.

Fig. VID3.f. *Hidradenoma papilliferum, high power.* The lesional cells facing the lumen show evidence of decapitation secretion.

Conditions to consider in the differential diagnosis:

hidradenoma papilliferum

syringocystadenoma papilliferum

apocrine hidrocystoma

REFERENCES

1. Garcia CF, Weiss LM, Warnke RA, Wood GS. Cutaneous follicular lymphoma. *Am J Surg Pathol* 1986;10:454.
2. Smolle J, Torne R, Soyer HP, Kerl H. Immunohistochemical classification of cutaneous pseudolymphomas: delineation of distinct patterns. *J Cutan Pathol* 1990;17:149.
3. Wong KF, Chan JK, Li LP, et al. Primary cutaneous plasmacytoma: report of two cases and review of the literature. *Am J Dermatopathol* 1994;16:392.
4. Kois JM, Sexton FM, Lookingbill DP. Cutaneous manifestations of multiple myeloma. *Arch Dermatol* 1991;127:69.
5. Ratner D, Nelson BR, Brown MD, Johnson TM. Merkel cell carcinoma. *J Am Acad Dermatol* 1993;29:143.
6. Frierson HF Jr, Cooper PH. Prognostic factors in squamous cell carcinoma of the lower lip. *Hum Pathol* 1986;17:346.
7. Lever WF. Inverted follicular keratosis is an irritated seborrheic keratosis. *Am J Dermatopathol* 1983;5:474.
8. Brownstein MH, Arluk DJ. Proliferating trichilemmal cyst. *Cancer* 1981;48:1207.
9. Murphy GF, Elder DE. Benign melanocytic tumors. In: Murphy GF, Elder DE, eds. *Non-melanocytic tumors of the skin.* Washington, DC: Armed Forces Institute of Pathology, 1990:9.
10. Kopf AW, Morrill SD, Silberberg I. Broad spectrum of leukoderma acquisitum centrifugum. *Arch Dermatol* 1965;92:14.
11. Rodriguez HA, Ackerman LV. Cellular blue nevus. *Cancer* 1968;21:393.
12. Paniago-Pereira C, Maize JC, Ackerman AB. Nevus of large spindle and/or epithelioid cells: Spitz's nevus. *Arch Dermatol* 1978;114:1811.
13. Abernethy JL, Soyer HP, Kerl H, et al. Epidermotropic metastatic malignant melanoma simulating melanoma in situ: a report of 10 examples from two patients. *Am J Dermatopathol* 1994;18:1140.
14. Mambo NC. Eccrine spiradenoma: clinical and pathologic study of 49 tumors. *J Cutan Pathol* 1983;10:312.
15. Haupt HM, Stern JB, Berlin SJ. Immunohistochemistry in the differential diagnosis of nodular hidradenoma and glomus tumor. *Am J Dermatopathol* 1992;14:310.
16. Leboit P, Sexton M. Microcystic adnexal carcinoma of the skin: a reappraisal of the differentiation and differential diagnosis of an under-recognized neoplasm. *J Am Acad Dermatol* 1993;29:609.
17. Umbert P, Winkelmann RK. Tubular apocrine adenoma. *J Cutan Pathol* 1976;3:75.
18. Vanatta PR, Bangert JL, Freeman RG. Syringocystadenoma papilliferum: a plasmacytotropic tumor. *Am J Surg Pathol* 1985;9:678.
19. Headington JT. Tumors of the hair follicle: a review. *Am J Pathol* 1976;85:479.
20. Prioleau PG, Santa Cruz DJ. Sebaceous gland neoplasia. *J Cutan Pathol* 1984;11:396.
21. Sangüeza OP, Salmon JK, White CR Jr, Beckstead JH. Juvenile xanthogranuloma: a clinical, histopathologic, and immunohistochemical study. *J Cutan Pathol* 1995;22:327.
22. Zelger B, Cerio R, Soyer HP, et al. Reticulohistiocytoma and multicentric reticulohistiocytosis: histopathologic and immunophenotypic distinct entities. *Am J Dermatopathol* 1994;16:577.
23. Paulli M, Berti E, Rosso R, et al. CD30/Ki-1 positive lymphoproliferative disorders of the skin: clinicopathologic correlation and statistical analysis of 86 cases. A multicentric study from the European Organization for Research and Treatment of Cancer Cutaneous Lymphoma Project Group. *J Clin Oncol* 1995;13:1343.
24. Karp DL, Horn TD. Lymphomatoid papulosis. *J Am Acad Dermatol* 1994;30:379.
25. Davey FR, Olson S, Kurec AS, et al. The immunophenotyping of extramedullary myeloid cell tumors in paraffin-embedded tissue sections. *Am J Surg Pathol* 1988;12:699.
26. Chase DR, Enzinger FM. Epithelioid sarcoma: diagnosis, prognostic indicators, and treatment. *Am J Surg Pathol* 1985;9:241.
27. Kanitakis J, Schmitt D, Thivolet J. Immunohistologic study of cellular populations of histiocytofibromas ("dermatofibromas"). *J Cutan Pathol* 1984;11:88.
28. Zelger B, Sidoroff A, Stanzl U, et al. Deep penetrating dermatofibroma versus dermatofibrosarcoma protuberans. *Am J Surg Pathol* 1994;18:677.
29. Fretzin DFJ, Helwig EB. Atypical fibroxanthoma of the skin. *Cancer* 1973;31:1541.
30. Reed RJ, Harkin JC. *Supplement: tumors of the peripheral nervous system.* 2nd series, Fasc. 3. Washington, DC: Armed Forces Institute of Pathology, 1983.
31. Hajdu SI. Schwannomas. *Mod Pathol* 1995;8:109.
32. Fisher WC, Helwig EB. Leiomyomas of the skin. *Arch Dermatol* 1963;88:510.
33. Carlson JA, Dickersin GR, Sober AJ, Barnhill RL. Desmoplastic neurotropic melanoma: a clinicopathologic analysis of 28 cases. *Cancer* 1995;75:478.
34. Patrice SJ, Wiss K, Mulliken JB. Pyogenic granuloma (lobular capillary hemangioma): a clinicopathologic study of 178 cases. *Pediatr Dermatol* 1994;8:267.
35. Hashimoto H, Daimaru Y, Enjoji M. Intravascular papillary endothelial hyperplasia. A clinicopathologic study of 91 cases. *Am J Dermatopathol* 1983;5:539.
36. Rao B, Unis M, Poulos E. Acroangiodermatitis: a study of ten cases. *Int J Dermatol* 1994;33:179.
37. Chor PJ, Santa Cruz DJ. Kaposi's sarcoma: a clinicopathologic review and differential diagnosis. *J Cutan Pathol* 1992;19:6.
38. Mark RJ, Tron LM, Sercarz J, et al. Angiosarcoma of the head and neck: the UCLA experience 1955 through 1990. *Arch Otolaryngol Head Neck Surg* 1993;119:973.
39. Dotz W, Prioleau PG. Nevus lipomatosus cutaneus superficialis: a light and electron microscopic study. *Arch Dermatol* 1984;120:376.
40. Brook CGD, Valman HG. Osteoma cutis and Albright's hereditary osteodystrophy. *Br J Dermatol* 1971;85:471.
41. McGavran MH, Binnington B. Keratinous cysts of the skin. *Arch Dermatol* 1966;94:499.
42. Sperling LC, Sakas EL. Eccrine hidrocystomas. *J Am Acad Dermatol* 1982;7:763.
43. Smith JD, Chernosky ME. Apocrine hidrocystoma (cystadenoma). *Arch Dermatol* 1974;109:700.
44. Meeker HJ, Neubecker RD, Helwig EG. Hidradenoma papilliferum. *Am J Clin Pathol* 1962;37:182.

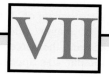

Inflammatory and Other Benign Disorders of Skin Appendages

The hair, sebaceous glands, eccrine glands, apocrine glands, and nails may be involved in inflammatory processes (hidradenitis, folliculitis). Some neoplasms may masquerade as inflammatory processes.

VIIA. PATHOLOGY INVOLVING HAIR FOLLICLES

Inflammatory processes may present as alopecia or as follicular localization of inflammatory rashes. Acne and related conditions present as dilatation of follicles that are filled with keratin.

1. Scant Inflammation
2. Lymphocytes Predominant
3. With Prominent Eosinophils
4. Neutrophils Prominent
5. Plasma Cells Prominent
6. Fibrosing and Suppurative Follicular Disorders

VIIA1. Scant Inflammation

There is follicular alteration with a sparse infiltrate of cells, mainly lymphocytes. Androgenic alopecia and trichotillomania are important examples.

Androgenetic Alopecia

CLINICAL SUMMARY. The expression of androgenetic alopecia frequently shows a familial and probably genetic inheritance pattern. Hair shafts become progressively finer and shorter, with true alopecia occurring only as a later event. This involutional process slowly evolves to become so severe that the scalp skin becomes exposed. This process can occur in women, although much less frequently than in men and with lesser severity, so that significant balding is quite unusual.

HISTOPATHOLOGY. Evaluation of this condition can be best achieved from transverse sectioning of punch biopsy material (1). Diminution of follicular size, most effectively measured by assessment of mean hair shaft diameter, can be obtained with relative simplicity using an optical micrometer. Because this approach allows assessment of all follicles in the specimen, direct counting of anagen, telogen, and catagen follicles can be undertaken and the percentages of each obtained. Reduction of follicular size appears to be randomized, so that, initially, normal-sized follicles coexist with an increased number of smaller ones, whereas ultimately, follicular reduction becomes more persistent and obvious. Associated with this reduction in follicular size, there is a progressive increase in the percentage of telogen follicles, both of normal club pattern and with increasing severity, diminutive or persistent telogen epithelial remnants (telogen germinal units). These structures appear to represent epithelial remnants of telogen follicles that no longer respond to the stimulus to return to anagen growth. Ultimately, there may be a reduction in the density of follicles. Periinfundibular fibroplasia ultimately leading to focal follicular scarring may be the explanation for the reduced follicular density. The diminution of follicles leads to a substantial increase in the number of empty follicular sheaths in the deeper dermis and subcutaneous tissue.

Trichotillomania

CLINICAL SUMMARY. Compulsive avulsion of hair shafts leads to zones of thin, ragged, broken stubble on the affected scalp. If the damage is done in localized fashion, it can mimic alopecia areata. Follicular breakage and loss may occasionally be associated with evidence of damage to the scalp by erosions or crusts.

HISTOPATHOLOGY. The most important findings in biopsy specimens are an increase in catagen hairs (up to

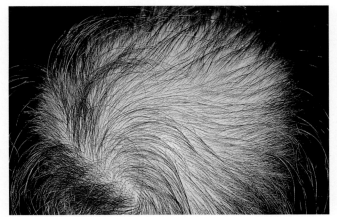

Clin. Fig. VIIA1.a

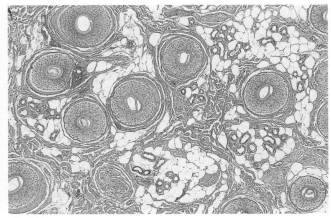

Fig. VIIA1.a

Clin. Fig. VIIA1.a. *Androgenetic alopecia.* Affected hairs, commonly seen on the vertex in males, undergo a shortened anagen phase resulting in a gradual transformation of terminal to velluslike hairs.

Fig. VIIA1.a. *Androgenetic alopecia, medium power, horizontal section.* Within the superficial subcutis, one sees the lower segment of terminal anagen follicles and an increased number of fibrous streamers. (*continues*)

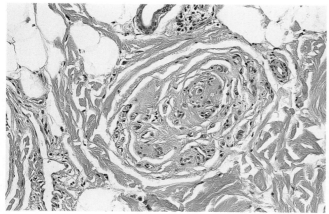

Fig. VIIA1.b

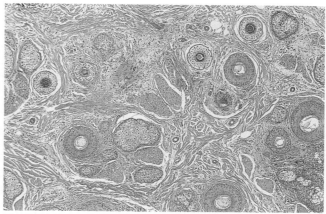

Fig. VIIA1.c

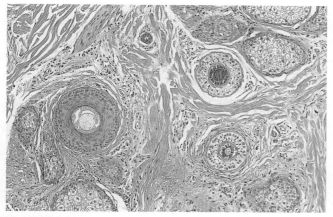

Fig. VIIA1.d

Fig. VIIA1.e

Fig. VIIA1.b. *Androgenetic alopecia, high power, horizontal section.* A streamer is characterized by a concentric arrangement of loose fibrovascular tissue resembling a collapsed fibrous sheath. Streamers result from shortening of follicles, either from follicular miniaturization or an increased percentage of follicles in the resting (telogen) phase.

Fig. VIIA1.c. *Androgenetic alopecia, medium power, horizontal section.* Early in the course of this disorder, the density of follicles remains normal. There is great variation in follicular size, with an increased number of indeterminate and vellus follicles. An increase in the percentage of catagen and telogen follicles can sometimes be seen.

Fig. VIIA1.d. *Androgenetic alopecia, medium power, horizontal section.* Higher magnification reveals hair shafts of varying diameter. Terminal hairs measure > 0.06 mm and vellus hairs measure < 0.03 mm, whereas the thickness of indeterminate hairs is between these two. All three are seen in this cross-section taken just below the level of the isthmus (the inner root sheath is fully keratinized but still intact).

Fig. VIIA1.e. *Androgenetic alopecia, high power, horizontal section.* A miniaturized hair resides next to a terminal hair at the level of the infundibulum.

75%), pigmentary defects and casts, evidence of traumatized hair bulbs, and trichomalacia (a complete but distorted fully developed terminal hair in its bulb). Occasionally, follicles may still be identified in anagen, but empty because of hair shaft avulsion. Follicles can show considerable distortion of the bulbar epithelium and sometimes conspicuous hemorrhage. Hair shaft avulsion may deposit melanin pigment in the hair papilla and peribulbar connective tissue. Pigment casts are also frequently identified in the isthmus or infundibulum. Trichomalacia if present is specific for trichotillomania. These various injuries to the bulbar portions of follicles are not accompanied by significant inflammatory infiltrates. Trichotillomania is not associated with miniaturization of follicles or with deep perifollicular infiltrates, features that usually serve to differentiate it from alopecia areata. Histologic findings in early traction alopecia are said to be identical with those of trichotillomania, but fewer follicles are involved, the changes are less dramatic, and vellus hairs are preserved.

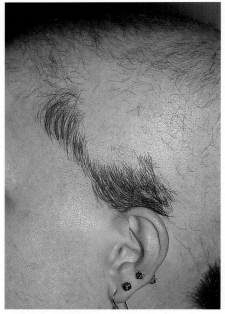

Clin. Fig. VIIA1.b

Clin. Fig. VIIA1.b. *Trichotillomania.* Plucking of hairs by a middle-aged woman with a delusional disorder resulted in well-demarcated patches of alopecia in a diffuse distribution.

Fig. VIIA1.f. *Trichotillomania, low power.* At scanning magnification there is a normal number of hair follicles per cross-section. There is a mild predominantly superficial inflammatory infiltrate.

Fig. VIIA1.g. *Trichotillomania, medium power.* One frequently sees distortion of the hair follicle, as manifested here by the twisted contour of the follicular canal.

Fig. VIIA1.h. *Trichotillomania, high power.* A characteristic finding in trichotillomania is the presence of pigment casts (clumps of pigment) that are present in the follicular canal.

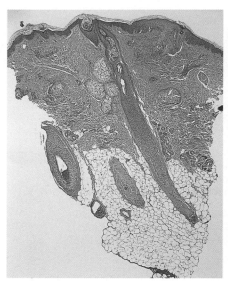

Fig. VIIA1.f

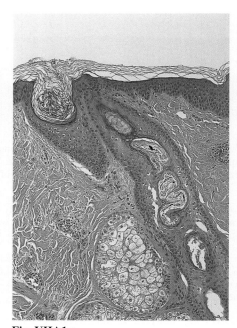

Fig. VIIA1.g

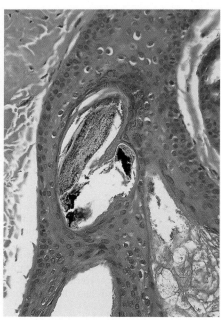

Fig. VIIA1.h

Telogen Effluvium

CLINICAL SUMMARY. Telogen effluvium represents the increased or excessive shedding of hair in the telogen phase of the growth cycle. This condition has several precipitating causes or associated conditions, including chemotherapy and debilitating diseases of various kinds, which may cause alopecia by eliciting changes in the length of the anagen period of growth and in the active process of release of hair shafts in telogen. Plucked or shed telogen hairs have a clublike appearance at the bottom of the shaft and are therefore often known as "club hairs."

HISTOPATHOLOGY. Telogen effluvium does not show significant dermal inflammatory infiltrates or evidence of diminution of follicular and hair shaft size, unless telogen effluvium occurs in patients with established androgenetic or another form of involutional alopecia. Proportions of normal

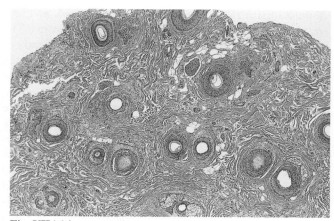

Fig. VIIA1.i

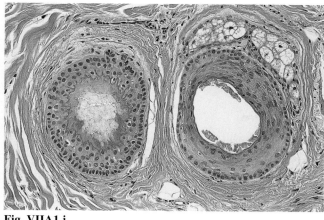

Fig. VIIA1.j

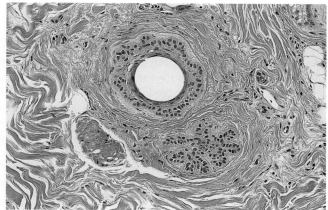

Fig. VIIA1.k

Fig. VIIA1.i. *Telogen effluvium, low power, horizontal section.* At scanning magnification there is a normal density of follicles with uniform diameters. An increased percentage of catagen and telogen follicles, as is seen in the early phases, is best appreciated at or just below the level of the isthmus. Inflammation is not seen here or in deeper levels within the fat.

Fig. VIIA1.j. *Telogen effluvium, high power, horizontal section.* A telogen (club) hair, on the left, is readily identifiable by a hair shaft that fills the follicular canal and merges with the outer root sheath via an eosinophilic zone, a consequence of trichilemmal keratinization.

Fig. VIIA1.k. *Telogen effluvium, medium power, horizontal section.* The irregular island of basaloid epithelium represents a telogen germinal unit, an epithelial remnant of a telogen follicle. Such structures may be increased in telogen effluvium.

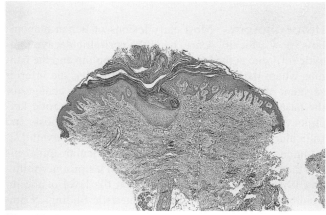

Fig. VIIA1.l

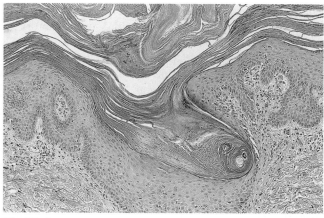

Fig. VIIA1.m

Fig. VIIA1.l. *Keratosis pilaris, low power.* In the center of this biopsy is the edge of a hair follicle that is manifested by an invagination of epithelium. This is associated with marked hyperkeratosis of the follicular orifice.

Fig. VIIA1.m. *Keratosis pilaris, medium power.* The follicular epithelium and the adjacent epidermis are mildly acanthotic. The characteristic hyperkeratotic scale is both ortho- and parakeratotic. There is only minimal inflammation in the surrounding dermis.

telogen follicles in excess of 15% to 25% are considered to be abnormal and suggest the likely presence of telogen. If a biopsy is obtained in the very early stages of recovery, early anagen regeneration follicles will also be present, whereas if recovery is substantial, the appearances may be entirely normal.

Keratosis Pilaris

Conditions to consider in the differential diagnosis:

Follicular Maturation Disorders
androgenetic alopecia
telogen effluvium
trichotillomania
scurvy
vitamin A deficiency (phrynoderma)
Follicular Keratinization Disorders
keratosis pilaris
lichen spinulosus
trichorrhexis invaginata (Netherton's syndrome)
trichostasis spinulosa
acne vulgaris
Favre–Racouchot syndrome (nodular elastosis with cysts and comedones)
nevus comedonicus
Bazex syndrome (follicular atrophoderma)

VIIA2. Lymphocytes Predominant

There is follicular alteration with an inflammatory infiltrate of mainly lymphocytes.

Alopecia Areata

CLINICAL SUMMARY.   Alopecia areata (2) is characterized by complete or nearly complete absence of hair in one or more circumscribed areas of the scalp. Inflammatory change is not clinically obvious, and the follicular openings are preserved. Complete scalp involvement (alopecia totalis) or complete or nearly complete loss of the entire body hair (alopecia universalis) can occur. Involvement of the eyebrows and eyelashes and a pitted defect in the nail plates are additional features of this condition. Most patients undergo spontaneous resolution, but a few patients have permanent hair loss. In the areas of active hair shedding, a short fractured hair shaft may be identified—the characteristic "exclamation point" hair.

HISTOPATHOLOGY.   The critical diagnostic pathologic sign is lymphocytic infiltrates in the peribulbar area of anagen follicles or follicles in early catagen. The lymphocytic infiltrates are present around the receding epithelial remnant, but also in the area of the collapsing follicular sheaths. While still in anagen, lymphocytes may be seen sparsely infiltrating the matrix epithelium. Follicular structures di-

minish in size rapidly and become miniaturized, and as a result are identified more superficially in the dermis. The diminutive follicles are observed predominantly in early or late catagen. During the recovery phase, diminutive anagen follicles may be quite numerous, many showing some peribulbar lymphocytic infiltrates. In long-standing cases, the inflammatory infiltrates appear to diminish. In severe alopecia universalis and totalis of long duration (a decade or more), functional follicular structures may be diminished in number and some scarring of the follicular sheaths may be identified. When biopsy specimens are sectioned transversely early in the disease, it can be demonstrated that the number of follicles is not diminished, but that follicles enter a persistent phase of telogen (telogen germinal units) and that there is a diminution of normal club telogen follicles.

Lichen Planopilaris

CLINICAL SUMMARY.   Lichen planopilaris (3) is lichen planus with follicular involvement in some or all lesions. This type of lichen planus predominantly affects the scalp. Initially, there may be only follicular papules or perifollicular erythema; however, with progressive hair loss, irregularly shaped atrophic patches of scarring alopecia develop on the scalp. The axillae and the pubic region may also be affected, and the alopecia in these areas may be cicatricial. Hyperkeratotic follicular papules may also be seen on glabrous skin. The association of scarring alopecia of hairbearing areas and hyperkeratotic follicular papules on glabrous skin is known as *Graham Little syndrome*. Lichen planopilaris may also coexist with typical lichen planus lesions on skin, mucous membranes, or nails. Linear lichen planopilaris of the face resolving with scarring has also been described.

HISTOPATHOLOGY.   Most early lesions of lichen planopilaris show a focally dense, bandlike perifollicular lymphocytic infiltrate at the level of the infundibulum and the isthmus where the hair bulge is located. Initially, the inferior segment of the hair follicle is spared. Vacuolar changes of the basal layer of the outer root sheath and necrotic keratinocytes are often seen. In addition, orthokeratosis and follicular plugging are observed. A few biopsies exhibit simultaneous involvement of the interfollicular epidermis and the hair follicles. In more developed lesions, perifollicular fibrosis and epithelial atrophy at the level of the infundibulum and isthmus are characteristic findings. Damage to the hair bulge, the site where stem cells of the hair follicle reside, results in permanent scarring alopecia. Advanced cases show alopecia with vertically oriented fibrotic tracts containing clumps of degenerated elastic fibers replacing the destroyed hair follicles. This end-stage scarring alopecia in which no visible hair follicles remain has been designated by some as pseudopelade of Brocq.

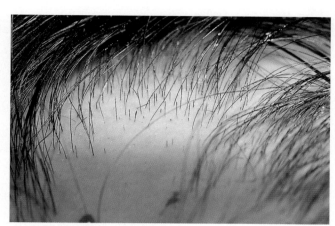

Clin. Fig. VIIA2.a

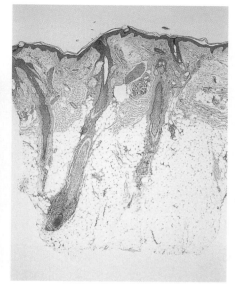

Fig. VIIA2.a

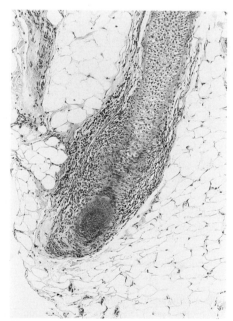

Fig. VIIA2.b

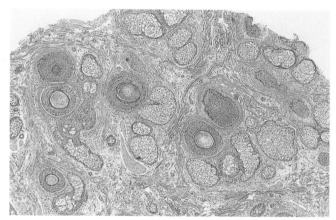

Fig. VIIA2.c

Clin. Fig. VIIA2.a. *Alopecia areata.* Well-circumscribed patch of alopecia with "exclamation point" hairs (tapering at proximal end) at the periphery typically respond to intralesional corticosteroids.

Fig. VIIA2.a. *Alopecia areata, low power, vertical section.* There are three catagen follicles, as indicated by a prominent eosinophilic cuticle. Beneath one of the catagen follicles there is a terminal anagen follicle with perifollicular inflammation within the subcutis. Catagen follicles are infrequently seen on vertical sectioning unless increased in number.

Fig. VIIA2.b. *Alopecia areata, high power, vertical section.* A dense lymphocytic infiltrate ("swarm of bees") hugs the bulb of the terminal anagen follicle seen in the previous figure.

Fig. VIIA2.c. *Alopecia areata, low power, horizontal section.* Most hairs present in this figure show varying degrees of eosinophilic change of the hair shaft, indicating various stages of transition from catagen to telogen hairs. At this level of sectioning, the differential diagnosis would include telogen effluvium.

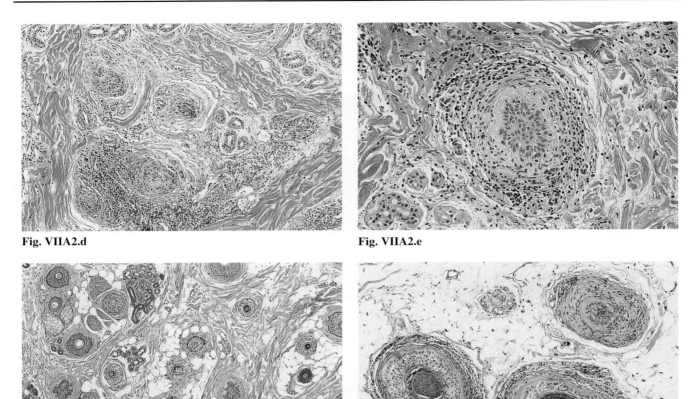

Fig. VIIA2.d

Fig. VIIA2.e

Fig. VIIA2.f

Fig. VIIA2.g

Fig. VIIA2.d. *Alopecia areata, medium power, horizontal section.* The increased percentage of resting follicles is reflected by the numerous streamers seen near the dermal–subcutaneous junction. A lymphoid infiltrate is apparent concentrated around the streamers.

Fig. VIIA2.e. *Alopecia areata, high power, horizontal section.* Perifollicular lymphocytes can be seen affecting catagen and telogen follicles as they retreat upward into the dermis. The eosinophilic vitreous membrane is characteristic of this catagen follicle.

Fig. VIIA2.f. *Alopecia areata, low power, horizontal section.* In long-standing alopecia areata, there is an increased number of catagen and telogen follicles. In addition, follicular miniaturization begins to occur.

Fig. VIIA2.g. *Alopecia areata, medium power, horizontal section.* Peribulbar lymphocytic inflammation is easily seen on horizontal sections within the subcutis. Because all follicles in the biopsy specimen can be visualized on horizontal sections, an increased number of streamers and catagen follicles can be easily assessed.

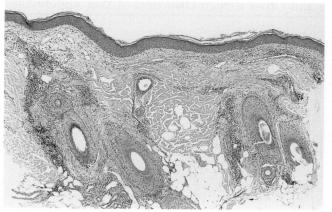

Fig. VIIA2.h

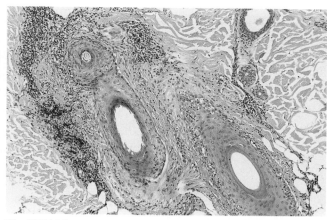

Fig. VIIA2.i

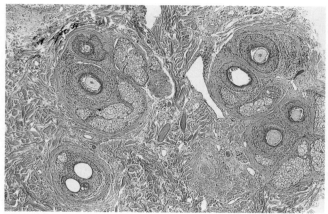

Fig. VIIA2.j

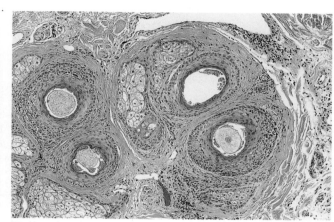

Fig. VIIA2.k

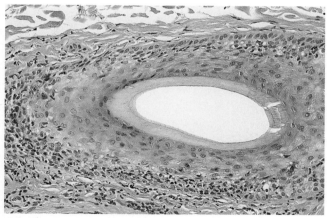

Fig. VIIA2.l

Fig. VIIA2.h. *Lichen planopilaris, low power, vertical section.* A dense mostly perifollicular lymphoid infiltrate affecting predominantly the isthmus and infundibulum is seen on scanning magnification. The interfollicular epidermis, which is best visualized on vertical sections, is largely unaffected.

Fig. VIIA2.i. *Lichen planopilaris, medium power, vertical section.* The lymphocytic infiltrate is associated with vacuolar alteration of the outer layers of the follicular epithelium.

Fig. VIIA2.j. *Lichen planopilaris, low power, horizontal section.* Follicular loss (i.e., scarring) is best identified on horizontal sections. A perifollicular lymphoid infiltrate is also apparent.

Fig. VIIA2.k. *Lichen planopilaris, medium power, horizontal section.* At the level of the isthmus, perifollicular fibrosis and inflammation are most prominent.

Fig. VIIA2.l. *Lichen planopilaris, high power, horizontal section.* The lymphocytic infiltrate is associated with blurring of the interface between the follicular epithelium and dermis, keratinocyte vacuolization, and dyskeratosis.

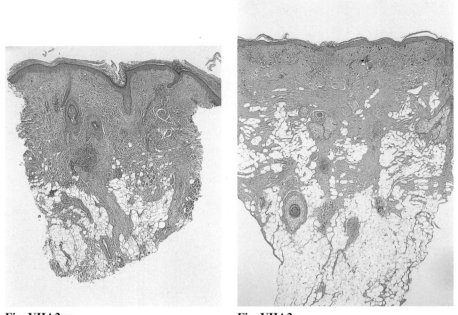

Fig. VIIA2.m   Fig. VIIA2.n

Fig. VIIA2.m. *Discoid lupus erythematosus of the scalp, low power.* A superficial and deep often quite prominent perivascular and perifollicular inflammatory infiltrate is seen at low magnification.

Fig. VIIA2.n. *Discoid lupus erythematosus, low power.* In some examples, as here, the infiltrate can be quite sparse. The number of hair follicles is diminished at scanning magnification.

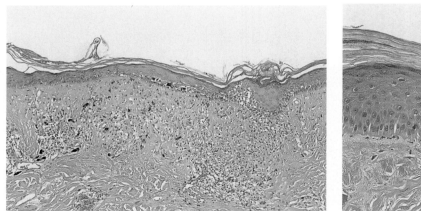
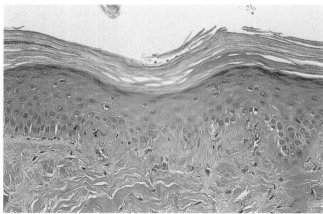

Fig. VIIA2.o   Fig. VIIA2.p

Fig. VIIA2.o. *Discoid lupus erythematosus, medium power.* As in other forms of lupus erythematosus, the epidermis reveals atrophy, vacuolar alteration, and an interface dermatitis. This superficial infiltrate is composed primarily of lymphocytes and there is prominent pigment incontinence.

Fig. VIIA2.p. *Discoid lupus erythematosus, high power.* Close examination of the epidermis reveals hyperkeratosis and thickening of the basement membrane zone. Pigment laden macrophages are seen in the papillary dermis.

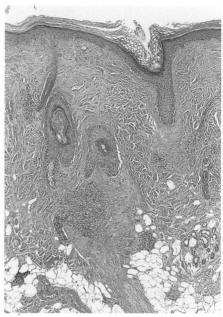

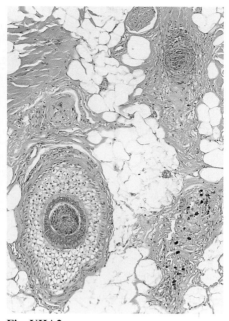

Fig. VIIA2.q. *Discoid lupus erythematosus, medium power.* The perifollicular infiltrate is associated with eventual scarring and fibrosis at the site of hair follicles.

Fig. VIIA2.r. *Discoid lupus erythematosus, medium power.* Pigment laden macrophages may be seen in the subcutaneous fat at the site of previous hair follicles. However, this finding is not specific to this diagnosis and can be seen in other forms of alopecia.

Fig. VIIA2.q

Fig. VIIA2.r

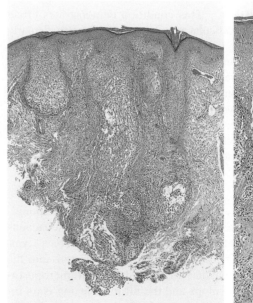

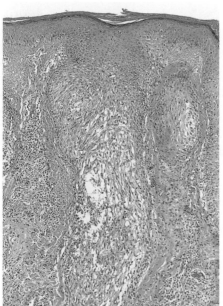

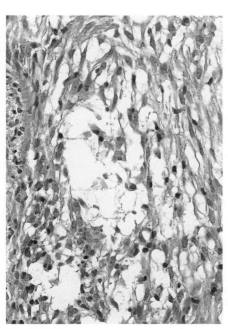

Fig. VIIA2.s

Fig. VIIA2.t

Fig. VIIA2.u

Fig. VIIA2.s. *Alopecia mucinosa, low power.* At scanning magnification, the follicular epithelium appears widened by multiple clear spaces. The overlying epidermis is uninvolved.

Fig. VIIA2.t. *Alopecia mucinosa, medium power.* The follicular keratinocytes are pale and in many areas are separated from adjacent keratinocytes. There is a surrounding perivascular and perifollicular lymphoid infiltrate.

Fig. VIIA2.u. *Alopecia mucinosa, high power.* The follicular epithelium appears clear because of extensive deposition of acid mucopolysaccharide. The epithelium is also infiltrated by small lymphoid cells that lack significant cytologic atypia. The acid mucopolysaccharide can be demonstrated using Alcian blue or colloidal iron stains. The predominant component is hyaluronic acid, which can be removed with digestion with hyaluronidase.

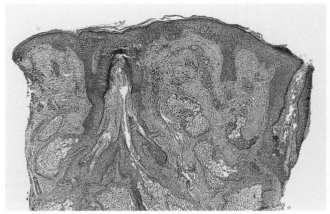

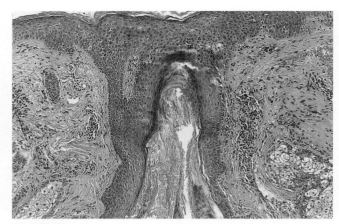

Fig. VIIA2.v   **Fig. VIIA2.w**

Fig. VIIA2.v. *Rosacea, low power.* This biopsy from facial skin reveals prominent sebaceous glands, a lymphoid infiltrate, and telangiectasia.

Fig. VIIA2.w. *Rosacea, high power.* The infiltrate may be perivascular, interstitial, and perifollicular.

Discoid Lupus Erythematosus of the Scalp

See Figs. VIIA2.m and VIIA2.n.

Alopecia Mucinosa

See Figs. VIIA2.s–VIIA2.u.

Rosacea

See Figs. VIIA2.v and VIIA2.w.

Conditions to consider in the differential diagnosis:
  alopecia areata
  discoid lupus erythematosus
  alopecia mucinosa/follicular mucinosis
  folliculotropic mycosis fungoides
  lichen planopilaris
  Fox-Fordyce disease
  syringolymphoid hyperplasia with alopecia
  lichen striatus
  chronic folliculitis
  rosacea
  perioral dermatitis
  disseminate and recurrent infundibular folliculitis
  acne varioliformis (acne necrotica)

VIIA3. Eosinophils Prominent

Eosinophils are prominent in the infiltrate and may infiltrate the follicular structures. Eosinophilic pustular folliculitis is prototypic (4).

Eosinophilic Pustular Folliculitis

CLINICAL SUMMARY. This condition demonstrates broad patches of itchy follicular papules and pustules particularly involving the face, trunk, and arms. The involved areas may take on various configurations; there may be central healing and peripheral spread. The condition occurs also in patients with human immunodeficiency virus (HIV) infection. Extrafollicular lesions with involvement of both palms and soles and scarring alopecia through scalp involvement may occur. Moderate leukocytosis and eosinophilia in the peripheral blood are also present.

HISTOPATHOLOGY. · Involved follicles may show spongiotic change with exocytosis extending from the sebaceous gland and its duct throughout the infundibular zone. Lymphocytes with some eosinophils initially migrate into the epidermis in a somewhat diffuse pattern, but micropustular aggregation develops and the ultimate lesion is an infundibular eosinophilic pustule. The epidermis adjacent to the follicle may be involved with eosinophilic microabscess formation. In the adjacent dermis, there are perivascular infiltrates of lymphocytes and numerous eosinophils.

Conditions to consider in the differential diagnosis:
  eosinophilic pustular folliculitis
  erythema toxicum neonatorum
  Ofuji's syndrome
  fungal folliculitis

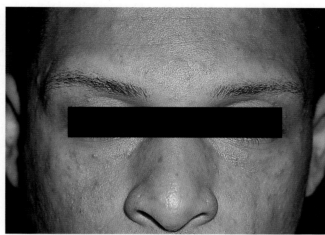

Clin. Fig. VIIA3

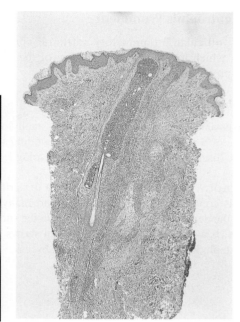

Fig. VIIA3.a

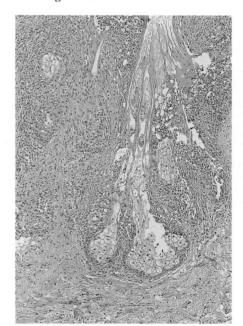

Fig. VIIA3.b

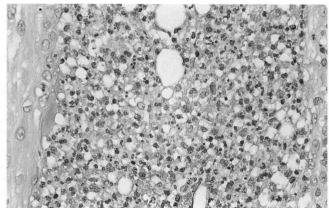

Fig. VIIA3.c

Clin. Fig. VIIA3. *Eosinophilic pustular folliculitis.* Pruritic erythematous papules commonly seen on the face of HIV-infected patients characterize this recalcitrant condition.

Fig. VIIA3.a. *Eosinophilic pustular folliculitis, low power.* In the center of this punch biopsy, a hair follicle shows an intense inflammatory infiltrate involving the upper half of the follicular epithelium.

Fig. VIIA3.b. *Eosinophilic pustular folliculitis, medium power.* The infiltrate involves the follicular epithelium, sebaceous ducts and lobules, and the surrounding dermis.

Fig. VIIA3.c. *Eosinophilic pustular folliculitis, high power.* The infiltrate is composed predominantly of neutrophils and numerous eosinophils.

VIIA4. Neutrophils Prominent

There is a follicular inflammatory infiltrate containing neutrophils, which may result in disruption of the follicle. Furuncle is prototypic (5).

Acute Deep Folliculitis (Furuncle)

CLINICAL SUMMARY. A furuncle is caused by staphylococci and consists of a tender, red, perifollicular swelling terminating in the discharge of pus and of a necrotic plug.

HISTOPATHOLOGY. A furuncle shows an area of perifollicular necrosis containing fibrinoid material and many neutrophils. At the deep end of the necrotic plug, in the subcutaneous tissue, is a large abscess. A Gram stain shows small clusters of staphylococci in the center of the abscess.

Tinea Capitis

See Figs. VIIA4.c–VIIA4.e.

Majocchi's Granuloma

CLINICAL SUMMARY. Occasionally, *Trichophyton rubrum* causes an asymptomatic nodular perifolliculitis in circumscribed areas, often called *Majocchi's granuloma*. It was first described as a scalp infection seen in children, but is seen most commonly on the legs in association with an infection of the soles, particularly in women who shave their legs (6).

HISTOPATHOLOGY. Sections show a nodular folliculitis and perifolliculitis forming an abscess in the dermis. On staining with periodic acid–Schiff (PAS) or methenamine silver, nu-

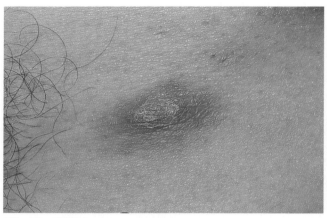

Clin. Fig. VIIA4

Clin. Fig. VIIA4. *Furuncle.* An inflamed tender nodule represents the acute stage of a furuncle caused by *Staphylococcal aureus*.

Fig. VIIA4.a. *Acute folliculitis.* Scanning magnification is essentially indistinguishable from eosinophilic pustular folliculitis. The hair follicle shows intense infiltration of its epithelium by an inflammatory cell reaction. There is a surrounding perivascular infiltrate.

Fig. VIIA4.b. *Acute folliculitis, high power.* The infiltrate within the follicular epithelium is composed predominantly of neutrophils. Eosinophils may be seen but not to the extent that they are present in eosinophilic pustular folliculitis.

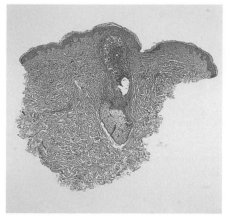

Fig. VIIA4.a

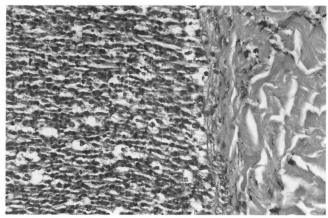

Fig. VIIA4.b

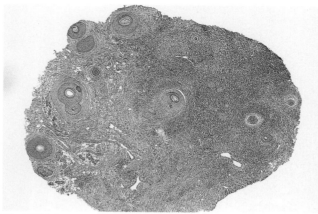

Fig. VIIA4.c

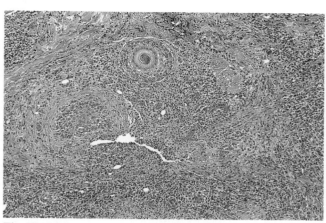

Fig. VIIA4.d

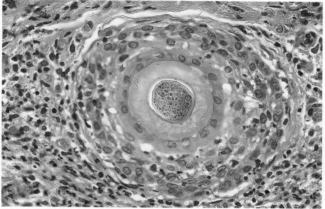

Fig. VIIA4.e

Fig. VIIA4.c. *Tinea capitis, low power, horizontal section.* The extensive inflammation in this case has led to follicular destruction and scarring.

Fig. VIIA4.d. *Tinea capitis, medium power, horizontal section.* The dense inflammatory infiltrate contains mixed cell types.

Fig. VIIA4.e. *Tinea capitis, high power, horizontal section.* Neutrophils and other inflammatory cells surround this small follicle. Fungal elements are present within the hair shaft.

merous hyphae and spores are seen within hairs and hair follicles and in the inflammatory infiltrate of the dermis. The fungal elements reach the dermis through a break in the follicular wall. The dermal infiltrate shows lymphoid cells, macrophages, epithelioid cells, and scattered multinucleated giant cells around and within an area of central necrosis, and often suppuration.

Herpes Simplex Viral Folliculitis

Conditions to consider in the differential diagnosis:

Superficial Folliculitis
acute bacterial folliculitis
impetigo Bockhart
Pseudomonas folliculitis
acne vulgaris
alopecia of secondary syphilis

Deep Folliculitis
furuncle, carbuncle
folliculitis barbae, decalvans
pseudofolliculitis of the beard
pyoderma gangrenosum

Follicular Occlusion Disorders
dissecting cellulitis/perifolliculitis capitis abscedens
  et suffodens
hidradenitis suppurativa
acne conglobata

Fungal Folliculitis
Majocchi granuloma (*T. rubrum*)
favus (*T. schoenleinii*)
Pityrosporum folliculitis
viral folliculitis
acne fulminans

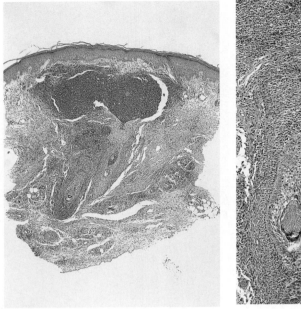

Fig. VIIA4.f

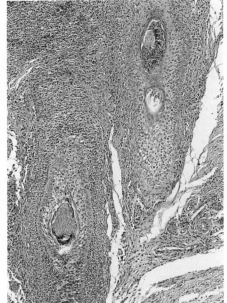

Fig. VIIA4.g

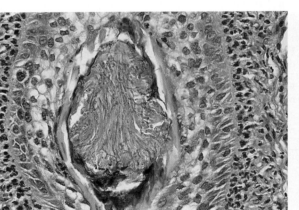

Fig. VIIA4.h

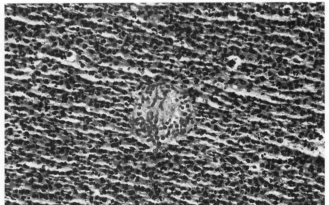

Fig. VIIA4.i

Fig. VIIA4.f. *Majocchi's granuloma, low power.* Scanning magnification reveals an abscess in the superficial dermis.

Fig. VIIA4.g. *Majocchi's granuloma, medium power.* Beneath this abscess, the hair follicles show an intense inflammatory reaction.

Fig. VIIA4.h. *Majocchi's granuloma, high power.* Upon close examination of the hair shaft on the H&E stained sections, one can identify pale blue-staining fungal hyphae within the hair shaft.

Fig. VIIA4.i. *Majocchi's granuloma, high power.* PAS stains reveal multiple organisms that have replaced a fragment of hair shaft embedded in a sea of neutrophils (abscess).

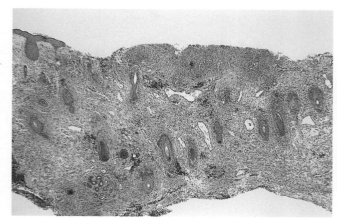

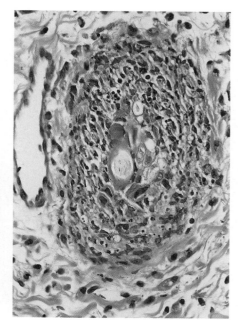

Fig. VIIA4.j   **Fig. VIIA4.k**

Fig. VIIA4.j. *Herpes simplex viral folliculitis, low power.* Viral folliculitis can be caused by both herpes simplex virus and varicella-zoster virus. Scanning magnification reveals epidermal ulceration and a perivascular and perifollicular inflammatory infiltrate that is generally mixed, including both acute and chronic inflammatory cells.

Fig. VIIA4.k. *Herpes simplex viral folliculitis, high power.* The follicular epithelium shows extensive necrosis and destruction associated with the inflammatory infiltrate that contains many neutrophils. Follicular keratinocytes show peripheral rimming of nuclear chromatin and may show multinucleation. These changes may also be seen in the epidermis.

VIIA5. Plasma Cells Prominent

Plasma cells are seen in abundance in the infiltrate. In most instances they are admixed with lymphocytes. Acne keloidalis is prototypic.

Folliculitis (Acne) Keloidalis Nuchae

CLINICAL SUMMARY. Folliculitis keloidalis nuchae represents a chronic folliculitis on the nape of the neck in men that causes hypertrophic scarring. In early cases, there are follicular papules, pustules, and occasionally abscesses. The lesions are replaced gradually by indurated fibrous nodules.

HISTOPATHOLOGY. Deep folliculitis progresses to follicular destruction and dermal fibrosis. Late-stage lesions show extensive fibrosis and scarring, sometimes with keloidal collagen.

Tinea Capitis

See Figs. VIIA5.e and VIIA5.f.

   Conditions to consider in the differential diagnosis:
      acne keloidalis nuchae
      fungal folliculitis
      alopecia of secondary syphilis

VIIA6. Fibrosing and Suppurative Follicular Disorders

There is extensive fibrosis of the dermis, often with keratin tunnels of follicular origin and with embedded hairs with associated foreign-body inflammation. Neutrophils and plasma cells are seen in abundance in the infiltrate, in addition to lymphocytes.

Follicular Occlusion Triad (Hidradenitis Suppurativa, Acne Conglobata, and Perifolliculitis Capitis Abscedens et Suffodiens)

CLINICAL SUMMARY. The three diseases included in the follicular occlusion triad are similar. Quite frequently, two or three of the diseases are encountered in the same patient. All three diseases represent a chronic, recurrent, deep-seated folliculitis resulting in abscesses and followed by the formation of sinus tracts and scarring. In *hidradenitis suppurativa*, the axillary and anogenital regions are affected. In acute lesions there are red tender nodules that become fluctuant and heal after discharging pus. In chronic cases, deep-seated abscesses lead to the discharge of pus through sinus tracts, resulting in severe scarring. *Acne conglobata* occurs mainly on the back, buttocks, and

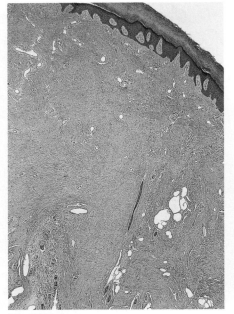

Fig. VIIA5.a

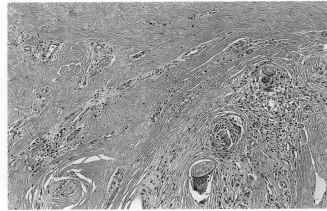

Fig. VIIA5.b

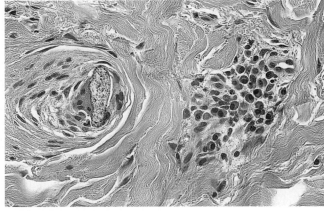

Fig. VIIA5.c

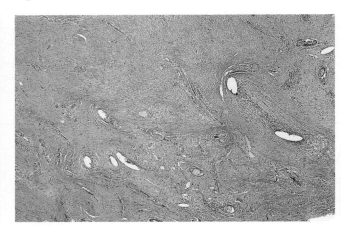

Fig. VIIA5.d

Fig. VIIA5.a. *Acne keloidalis nuchae, low power.* Several hair shafts are seen within the deep dermis surrounded by chronic inflammation and extensive scarring.

Fig. VIIA5.b. *Acne keloidalis nuchae, medium power.* The dermis becomes fibrotic secondary to chronic inflammation. Free hair shafts are surrounded by granulomatous inflammation.

Fig. VIIA5.c. *Acne keloidalis nuchae, high power.* A portion of a hair shaft is being engulfed by a multinucleated giant cell. The infiltrate also contains numerous plasma cells.

Fig. VIIA5.d. *Acne keloidalis nuchae, medium power.* In a late lesion, free hair shafts have incited chronic inflammation leading to dense fibrosis in the dermis.

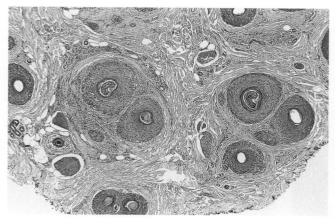

Fig. VIIA5.e

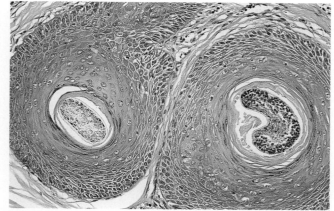

Fig. VIIA5.f

Fig. VIIA5.e. *Tinea capitis, low power, horizontal section.* The infiltrate in this example is perifollicular and interstitial and is composed predominantly of lymphocytes and plasma cells.

Fig. VIIA5.f. *Tinea capitis, high power, horizontal section.* This PAS-stained section highlights the fungal spores and hyphae in cross-section that characterize this endothrix infection with *Trichophyton tonsurans*. Horizontal sections demonstrate that not every follicle is involved.

chest, and only rarely on the face or the extremities. In addition to comedones, fluctuant nodules discharging pus or a mucoid material and deep-seated abscesses that discharge through interconnecting sinus tracts occur. In *perifolliculitis capitis abscedens et suffodiens*, which involves the scalp and neck, nodules and abscesses as described above occur in the scalp, also known as dissecting cellulitis of the scalp. *Pilonidal sinus* is often also considered to be a part of this group of disorders (the "follicular occlusion tetrad").

HISTOPATHOLOGY. Early lesions show follicular hyperkeratosis with plugging and dilatation of the follicle. The follicular epithelium may proliferate or may be destroyed. At first there is little inflammation, but eventually a perifolliculitis develops with an extensive infiltrate composed of neutrophils, lymphocytes, and histiocytes. Abscess formation results and leads to the destruction first of the pilosebaceous structures and later also of the other cutaneous appendages. Apocrine glands in hidradenitis suppurativa of the axillae or groin regions may be secondarily involved by the inflammatory process. In response to this destruction, granulation tissue containing lymphoid and plasma cells and foreign-body giant cells related to fragments of keratin and to embedded hairs infiltrate the area near the remnants of hair follicles. As the abscesses extend deeper into the subcutaneous tissue, draining sinus tracts develop that are lined with epidermis. In areas of healing, there is extensive fibrosis.

Folliculitis Decalvans

CLINICAL SUMMARY. Folliculitis decalvans occurs predominantly in men. Scattered through the scalp are slowly enlarging, bald, atrophic areas with follicular pustules at their peripheries. In some instances, other hairy areas, such as the bearded and pubic regions and the axillae and the eyebrows and eyelashes, are also involved (7).

HISTOPATHOLOGY. As in the other forms of chronic deep folliculitis, such as folliculitis keloidalis nuchae, in early lesions there is a perifollicular infiltrate composed largely of neutrophils but also containing lymphoid cells, histiocytes, and plasma cells. The infiltrate develops into a perifollicular abscess, leading to destruction of the hair and hair follicles. Older lesions show chronic granulation tissue containing numerous plasma cells and lymphoid cells and fibroblasts. Often, foreign-body giant cells are present around remnants of hair follicles, and particles of keratin may be located near the giant cells. As healing takes place, fibrosis is observed. If there is hypertrophic scar formation, as in folliculitis keloidalis nuchae, numerous thick bundles of sclerotic collagen are present.

Conditions to consider in the differential diagnosis:

acne keloidalis
pilonidal sinus
hidradenitis suppurativa
acne conglobata
perifolliculitis capitis abscedens et suffodens
  (dissecting cellulitis of the scalp)
folliculitis barbae, decalvans

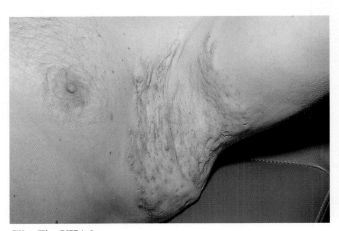

Clin. Fig. VIIA6.a

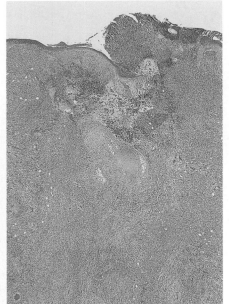

Fig. VIIA6.a

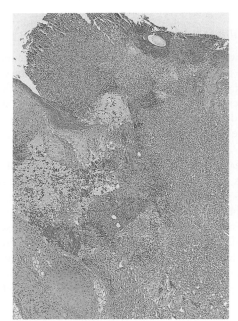

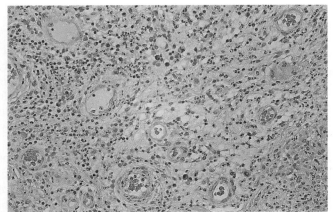

Fig. VIIA6.c

Fig. VIIA6.b

Clin. Fig. VIIA6.a. *Hidradenitis suppurativa.* Draining sinus tracts were present in the axillae, characteristic of hidradenitis suppurativa.

Fig. VIIA6.a. *Hidradenitis suppurativa, low power.* There is an area of epidermal ulceration associated with an invagination of epithelium. There is a dense inflammatory reaction throughout the dermis.

Fig. VIIA6.b. *Hidradenitis suppurativa, medium power.* At the edge of the ulceration, the epithelium shows hyperplasia. The infiltrate is intense and frequently forms abscesses composed of neutrophils.

Fig. VIIA6.c. *Hidradenitis suppurativa, high power.* The dermis, as seen here, may show granulation tissuelike changes with a mixed acute and chronic inflammatory infiltrate. One may also see extensive fibrosis and granulomatous inflammation, changes that may be indistinguishable from a ruptured epidermal cyst.

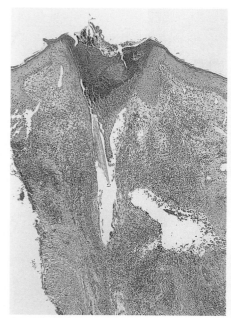

Fig. VIIA6.d

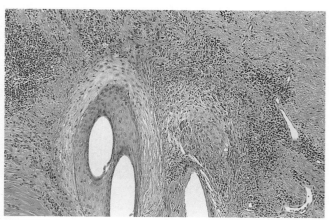

Fig. VIIA6.e

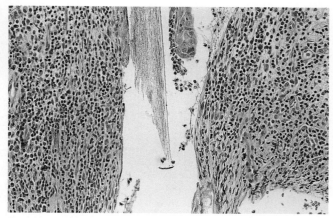

Fig. VIIA6.f

Fig. VIIA6.d. *Dissecting cellulitis of the scalp, low power*. Early lesions may show follicular plugging with acute perifollicular inflammation. Eventually the follicle is destroyed and replaced by dense mixed inflammation. The appearances are indistinguishable from hidradenitis suppurativa.

Fig. VIIA6.e. *Dissecting cellulitis of the scalp, medium power*. Perifollicular fibrosis ensues and is accompanied by granulomatous inflammation to follicular contents. Advanced lesions may show sinus tract formation.

Fig. VIIA6.f. *Dissecting cellulitis of the scalp, high power*. The follicular epithelium is almost completely destroyed, leaving the hair shaft exposed to the dermis and a mixed infiltrate of neutrophils, lymphocytes, histiocytes, and plasma cells.

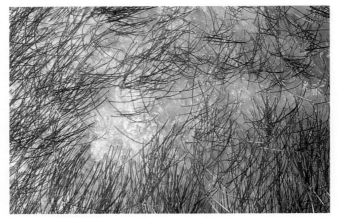

Clin. Fig. VIIA6.b

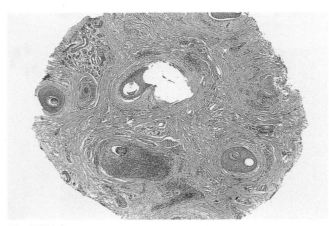

Fig. VIIA6.g

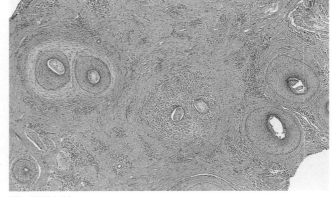

Fig. VIIA6.h

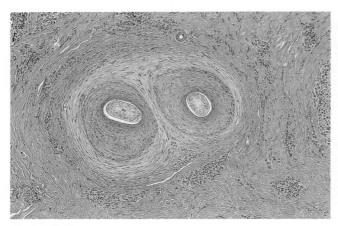

Fig. VIIA6.i

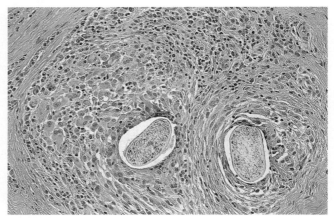

Fig. VIIA6.j

Clin. Fig. VIIA6.b. *Folliculitis decalvans.* An area of scarring alopecia in a middle-aged man, associated with a hyperkeratotic scale-crust with follicular hyperkeratosis and erythema.

Fig. VIIA6.g. *Folliculitis decalvans, low power, horizontal section.* Early lesions show perifollicular inflammation composed of acute and chronic inflammatory cells.

Fig. VIIA6.h. *Folliculitis decalvans, low power, horizontal section.* Later lesion shows destruction of follicular epithelium, dense interstitial inflammation, and perifollicular fibrosis, with free hairs in the tissue.

Fig. VIIA6.i. *Folliculitis decalvans, medium power, horizontal section.* There is perifollicular and interstitial fibrosis accompanied by an interstitial infiltrate of lymphocytes and plasma cells.

Fig. VIIA6.j. *Folliculitis decalvans, high power, horizontal section.* The eventual loss of follicular epithelium leads to a granulomatous response triggered by free hair shafts.

VIIB. PATHOLOGY INVOLVING SWEAT GLANDS

The eccrine glands and apocrine glands may be involved in inflammatory processes (hidradenitis).

1. Scant Inflammation
2. Lymphocytes Predominant
2a. With Plasma Cells
2b. With Eosinophils
2c. With Neutrophils

VIIB1. Scant Inflammation

Sweat glands are abnormal in color or size and number, but there is little or no inflammation.

Eccrine Nevus

CLINICAL SUMMARY.   Eccrine nevi (8) are very rare. They may show a circumscribed area of hyperhidrosis, a solitary sweat-discharging pore, or papular lesions in a linear arrangement. In the so-called eccrine angiomatous hamartoma, there may be one or several nodules or a solitary large plaque. The lesions are generally present on an extremity at birth. Hyperhidrosis and/or pain may be apparent.

HISTOPATHOLOGY.   Eccrine nevi show an increase in the size of the eccrine coil or in both the size and the number of coils. In other cases there is ductal hyperplasia consisting of thickening of the walls and dilatation of the lumina. Eccrine angiomatous hamartomas show increased numbers of eccrine structures and numerous capillary channels surrounding or intermingled with the eccrine structures. These hamartomas may also contain fatty tissue and pilar structures.

Conditions to consider in the differential diagnosis:

argyria
syringosquamous metaplasia
eccrine nevus
eccrine angiomatous hamartoma
coma blister

VIIB2. Lymphocytes Predominant

There is a predominantly lymphocytic infiltrate in and around the sweat glands. Lichen striatus is a prototypic example (9).

Lichen Striatus

CLINICAL SUMMARY.   This fairly uncommon dermatitis occurs as a rule in children. It presents as a unilateral eruption along Blaschko's lines on the extremities, trunk, or neck as either a continuous or an interrupted band composed of minute, slightly raised, erythematous papules, which may have a scaly surface. The lesions appear suddenly and usually involute within a year. They are occasionally pruritic.

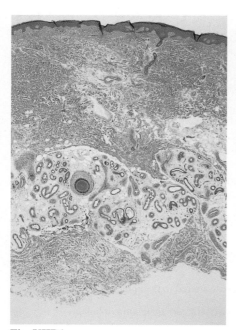

Fig. VIIB1.a

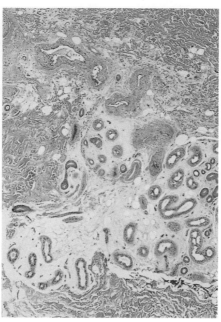

Fig. VIIB1.b

Fig. VIIB1.a. *Eccrine angiomatous hamartoma, low power.* In the deep dermis, there is an increased number of eccrine glands in a mucinous stroma.

Fig. VIIB1.b. *Eccrine angiomatous hamartoma, medium power.* The eccrine glands may be dilated, as seen here; there is an increased number of mature vascular channels (upper half of photomicrograph).

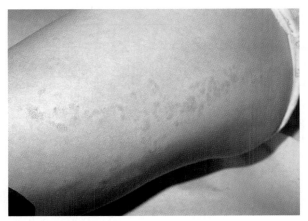

Clin. Fig. VIIB2

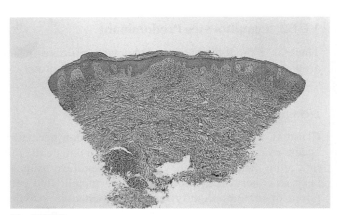

Fig. VIIB2.a

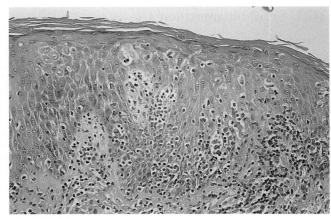

Fig. VIIB2.b

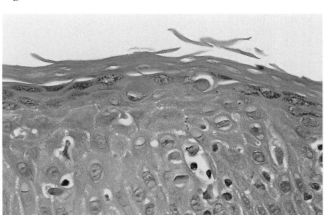

Fig. VIIB2.c

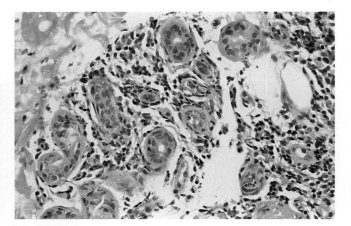

Fig. VIIB2.d

Clin. Fig. VIIB2. *Lichen striatus.* A linear eruption of erythematous papules suddenly appeared on the thigh of a girl.

Fig. VIIB2.a. *Lichen striatus, low power.* There is a patchy bandlike infiltrate in the papillary dermis. A sweat gland unit in the lower left is infiltrated by inflammatory cells.

Fig. VIIB2.b. *Lichen striatus, medium power.* There is lymphocytic exocytosis into the epidermis, associated with only mild spongiosis.

Fig. VIIB2.c. *Lichen striatus, high power.* Occasional apoptotic keratinocytes are scattered in the epidermis.

Fig. VIIB2.d. *Lichen striatus, high power.* A perieccrine lymphocytic infiltrate is a characteristic feature of lichen striatus.

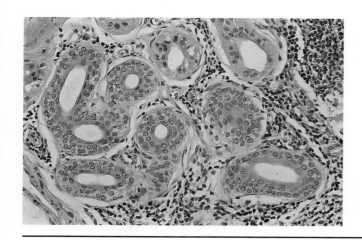

Fig. VIIB2a.a. *Lupus erythematosus, high power.* A perieccrine infiltrate composed predominantly of lymphocytes with or without a few plasma cells suggests a diagnosis of lupus erythematosus. Annular erythemas may also produce a perieccrine lymphocytic infiltrate.

HISTOPATHOLOGY. Although the histologic picture is highly variable, there is usually a superficial perivascular inflammatory infiltrate of lymphocytes admixed with a variable number of histiocytes. Plasma cells and eosinophils are rare. Focally, in the papillary dermis, the infiltrate may have a bandlike distribution with extension into the lower portion of the epidermis, with vacuolar alteration of the basal layer and necrotic keratinocytes. Additional epidermal changes consist of spongiosis and intracellular edema often associated with exocytosis of lymphocytes and focal parakeratosis. Less frequently, there are scattered necrotic keratinocytes in the spinous layer and subcorneal spongiotic vesicles filled with Langerhans cells. A very distinctive feature is the presence of an inflammatory infiltrate in the reticular dermis around hair follicles and eccrine glands.

Conditions to consider in the differential diagnosis:

lupus erythematosus
syringolymphoid hyperplasia with alopecia
lichen striatus
erythema annulare centrifigum
erythema chronicum migrans

VIIB2a. With Plasma Cells

There is a predominantly lymphocytic infiltrate in and around the sweat glands. Plasma cells are also present as a minority population.

Lupus Erythematosus

HISTOPATHOLOGY. In lupus, the inflammatory infiltrate in the dermis is usually lymphocytic, with or without an admixture of plasma cells (see also section IIIH4). Its distribution is a clue to the diagnosis of lupus. Lymphocytic and plasmacytic inflammation around eccrine coils is a characteristic finding. In hair-bearing areas, there is a similar infiltrate located around hair follicles and the sebaceous glands. Frequently, there are hydropic changes in the basal layer of the hair follicles, which may be of diagnostic value in the absence of dermal–epidermal changes. By impinging on pilosebaceous units, the infiltrate causes their gradual atrophy

and disappearance. A patchy inflammatory infiltrate also may be present in the upper dermis in an interstitial pattern, and occasionally, the infiltrate extends into the subcutaneous fat.

Conditions to consider in the differential diagnosis:

lupus erythematosus
secondary syphilis
cheilitis glandularis
erythema chronicum migrans

VIIB2b. With Eosinophils

There is an inflammatory infiltrate with eosinophils in and around the sweat glands.

Arthropod Bite

See Figs. VIIB2b.a and VIIB2b.b.

Conditions to consider in the differential diagnosis:
insect bite reactions
drug reaction

VIIB2c. With Neutrophils

There is an inflammatory infiltrate with neutrophils in and around the sweat glands.

Neutrophilic Eccrine Hidradenitis

This condition may present with erythematous, often acral, plaques several days after cytoreductive chemotherapy (10).

HISTOPATHOLOGY. There is variable infiltration of the eccrine coil by neutrophils and lymphocytes with necrosis of secretory epithelium. Individual cells or whole coils show increased cytoplasmic eosinophilia, degeneration of nuclei, and loss of integrity of cell walls.

Conditions to consider in the differential diagnosis:
insect bite reactions
neutrophilic eccrine hidradenitis
secondary syphilis

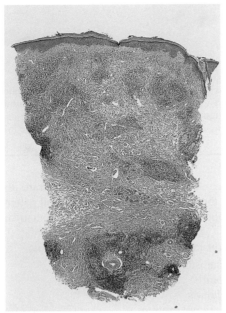

Fig. VIIB2b.a.
Arthropod bite, low power. Bite reactions reveal a superficial and deep inflammatory reaction that is perivascular, periadnexal, and interstitial.

Fig. VIIB2b.b.
Arthropod bite, high power. The inflammatory reaction is present around eccrine glands; however, generally there are numerous eosinophils, a clue to the diagnosis.

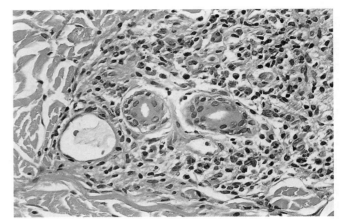

Fig. VIIB2b.b

Fig. VIIB2b.a

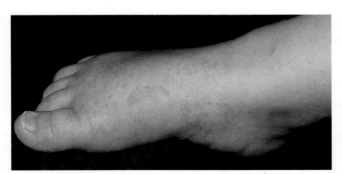

Clin. Fig. VIIB2c

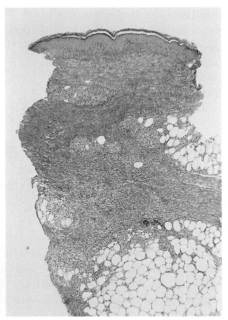

Fig. VIIB2c.a

Clin. Fig. VIIB2c. *Neutrophilic eccrine hidradenitis.* A young child with acute lymphocytic leukemia developed erythematous papules and plaques while on maintenance chemotherapy.

Fig. VIIB2c.a. *Neutrophilic eccrine hidradenitis, low power.* There is a sparse, perivascular, and perieccrine infiltrate seen predominantly at the dermal–subcutaneous junction. (*continues*)

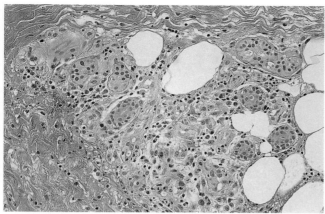

Fig. VIIB2c.b

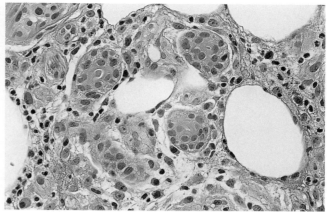

Fig. VIIB2c.c

Fig. VIIB2c.b. *Neutrophilic eccrine hidradenitis, medium power.* Upon closer inspection the inflammatory infiltrate is found to be predominantly around eccrine coils at the dermal–subcutaneous junction.

Fig. VIIB2c.c. *Neutrophilic eccrine hidradenitis, high power.* The infiltrate is mixed but contains neutrophils. The eccrine ducts show focal pallor consistent with early necrosis.

VIIC. PATHOLOGY INVOLVING NERVES

Specific inflammatory involvement of nerves is uncommon in dermatopathology.

1. Lymphocytic Infiltrates
2. Mixed Inflammatory Infiltrates
3. Neoplastic Infiltrates

VIIC1. Lymphocytic Infiltrates

Neurotropic spread of neoplasms, especially neurotropic melanoma, may be associated with a dense lymphocytic infiltrate that may tend to obscure a subtle infiltrate of neoplastic spindle cells.

Conditions to consider in the differential diagnosis:

neurotropic melanoma
leprosy (see sections VIIB2 and VIIB3)

VIIC2. Mixed Inflammatory Infiltrates

There is a mixed inflammatory infiltrate involving nerves.

Nerve Involvement in Leprosy

CLINICAL SUMMARY. Nerve involvement can be demonstrated in most lesions of leprosy (11) but is most prominent

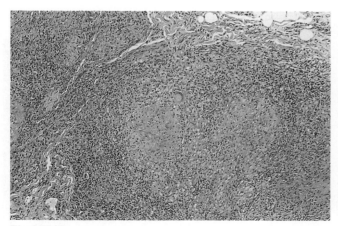

Fig. VIIC2.a

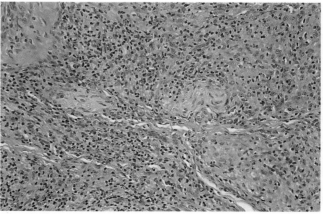

Fig. VIIC2.b

Fig. VIIC2.a. *Tuberculoid leprosy, medium power.* Within the dermis there is an intense granulomatous infiltrate.

Fig. VIIC2.b. *Tuberculoid leprosy, high power.* This granulomatous inflammation surrounds small cutaneous nerves.

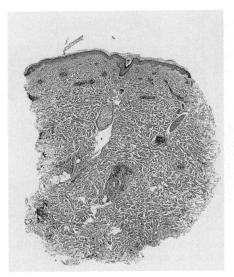

Fig. VIIC2.c

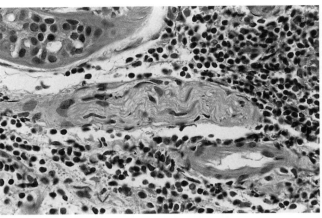

Fig. VIIC2.d

Fig. VIIC2.c. *Erythema chronicum migrans, low power*. There is a superficial and deep perivascular and periadnexal infiltrate without a significant interstitial component.

Fig. VIIC2.d. *Erythema chronicum migrans, high power*. This infiltrate, which is composed predominantly of lymphocytes and occasional plasma cells, may surround small nerves and eccrine units.

in the tuberculoid type (TT). In the various patterns of leprosy, the major peripheral nerves often undergo parallel pathologies. The inflammation is similar, and the same classification system is applied. However, the density of acid-fast bacilli is often a logarithm higher than in the nearby skin. The skin lesions of TT leprosy are scanty, dry, erythematous, hypopigmented papules or plaques with sharply defined edges. Anesthesia is prominent (except on the face). Thickened local peripheral nerves may be found. The lesions heal rapidly on chemotherapy.

HISTOPATHOLOGY. Primary TT leprosy has large epithelioid cells arranged in compact granulomas along with neurovascular bundles, with dense peripheral lymphocyte accumulation. Langhans giant cells are typically absent. Dermal nerves may be absent (obliterated) or surrounded and eroded by dense lymphocyte cuffs. Acid-fast bacilli are rarely found, even in nerves. A second pattern of TT leprosy is found in certain reactional states (see below).

Erythema Chronicum Migrans with Nerve Involvement

See Figs. VIIC2.c and VIIC2.d.

Arthropod Bite Reaction with Nerve Involvement

See Fig. VIIC2.e.

    Conditions to consider in the differential diagnosis:
      leprosy
      erythema chronicum migrans
      arthropod bite reaction

VIIC3. Neoplastic Infiltrates

Many neoplasms may occasionally involve nerves. The involvement by carcinomas (basal cell, squamous cell, metastatic) is commonly in the perineural space, whereas involvement by neurotropic melanoma tends to occupy the endoneurium and to be associated with a dense lymphocytic infiltrate that may tend to obscure a subtle infiltrate of neoplastic spindle cells. Thus, inflammatory neuropathy may be simulated.

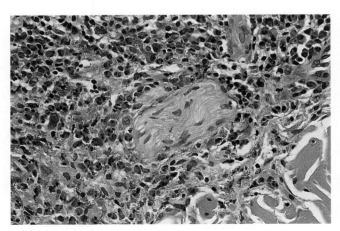

Fig. VIIC2.e. *Arthropod bite reaction, high power*. The inflammatory infiltrate of a bite reaction, which is rich in eosinophils, may also show perineural involvement.

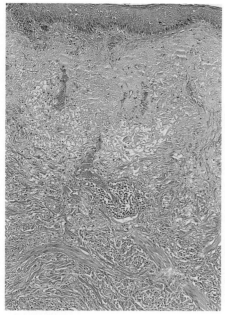

Fig. VIIC3.a

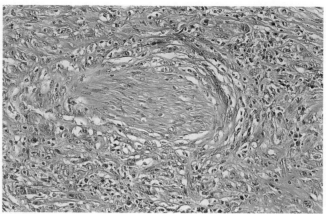

Fig. VIIC3.b

Fig. VIIC3.a. *Desmoplastic and neurotropic melanoma, medium power.* In the middermis there is a subtle proliferation of spindle cells associated with a lymphoid infiltrate.

Fig. VIIC3.b. *Neurotropic melanoma, high power.* The malignant nonpigmented melanoma cells surround this cutaneous nerve. These lesions have a higher incidence of local recurrence because of the perineural involvement.

Neurotropic Melanoma

CLINICAL SUMMARY. Neurotropic melanoma (12) is defined as a melanoma that invades nerves. Usually, there are no specific clinical stigmata of nerve involvement, but occasionally pain or paresthesias may be reported by the patient. Neurotropism in a primary melanoma is associated with increased risk for local recurrence, even after standard "definitive" therapy, and also with increased mortality.

HISTOPATHOLOGY. Neurotropism is often seen in a desmoplastic melanoma. Fascicles of neoplastic spindle cells invade cutaneous nerves, usually in a spindle-cell vertical component with fibrosis. However, some neurotropic melanomas lack these latter features of desmoplastic melanoma. Many of these are spindle-cell tumorigenic melanomas of acral lentiginous or lentigo maligna type, but some are composed of epithelioid cells. Although the neoplastic cells in the nerves are often highly atypical, in some cases the involvement may be subtle because the malignant cells may be sparsely distributed within the endoneurium of the nerve. In some cases, the presence of a lymphocytic infiltrate in the nerve may draw attention to the neoplastic involvement.

Conditions to consider in the differential diagnosis:

    neurotropic melanoma
    neurotropic carcinomas and other tumors

VIID. PATHOLOGY OF THE NAILS

Several inflammatory dermatoses more often seen elsewhere in the skin may present incidentally or exclusively in the nails. The reaction patterns may vary from those seen elsewhere, because of the unique responses of the nail plate to injury.

1. Lymphocytic Infiltrates
2. Lymphocytes with Neutrophils
3. Vesiculobullous Diseases
4. Parasitic Infestations

VIID1. Lymphocytic Infiltrates

There is an increased number of lymphocytes in the nail bed and matrix. They may be arranged in a perivascular or diffuse pattern and may be confined to the dermis or may involve the epidermis in a lichenoid, spongiotic, or other pattern.

Acral Lentiginous Melanoma

The periphery of an *in situ* component of acral lentiginous melanoma may mimic a lymphocytic infiltrate, because brisk infiltrating lymphocytes in a lichenoid pattern may obscure the lesional neoplastic melanocytes in focal areas of the lesion, especially when viewed at low power.

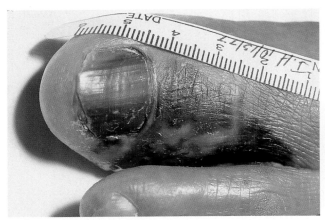

Clin. Fig. VIID1

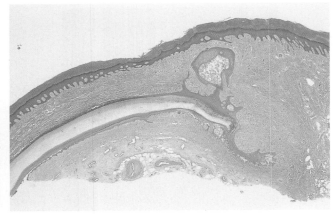

Fig. VIID1.a

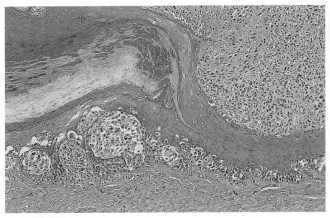

Fig. VIID1.b

Fig. VIID1.c

Clin. Fig. VIID1. *Subungual acral lentiginous melanoma.* There is a very broad and variegated pigmented lesion that extends from the nail to the surrounding skin. This extension of pigmentation from the nail to the skin is termed Hutchinson's sign. A subungual hematoma or benign nevus would remain confined to the nail bed.

Fig. VIID1.a. *Subungual acral lentiginous melanoma, low power.* This excisional biopsy of the proximal nail fold shows only subtle changes at the dermal–epidermal junction of the nail matrix at scanning magnification.

Fig. VIID1.b. *Subungual acral lentiginous melanoma, medium power.* At this magnification, one can identify variably sized collections of atypical melanocytes at the dermal–epidermal interface of the nail matrix, focally forming dermal collections in the upper right corner of this photomicrograph. There is an associated mild lymphoid infiltrate.

Fig. VIID1.c. *Acral lentiginous melanoma, high power.* In this field, the predominant feature is a diffuse lymphocytic infiltrate in the papillary dermis and basal epidermis, obscuring the subtle involvement of the epidermis by *in situ* melanoma.

Conditions to consider in the differential diagnosis:
  spongiotic dermatitis
  lichen planus
  acral lentiginous melanoma

VIID2. Lymphocytes with Neutrophils

Neutrophils may be present in the dermis in acute infections and in gangrenous necrosis. As in the skin proper, neutrophils in the skin of a nail suggest fungus infection, or may be indicative of psoriasis or a related condition (13).

Onychomycosis

CLINICAL SUMMARY. Fungal infection of the nails may be the most common nail disorder. There are four main types: distal subungual onychomycosis, proximal subungual onychomycosis, white superficial onychomycosis, and candidal onychomycosis. Distal subungual onychomycosis is the most common form and is usually caused by *Trichophyton rubrum*. The fungus initially invades the hyponychium and lateral nail folds, causing yellowing, onycholysis, and eventual subungual hyperkeratosis.

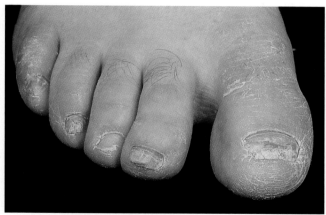

Clin. Fig. VIID2

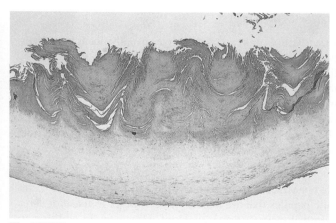

Fig. VIID2.a

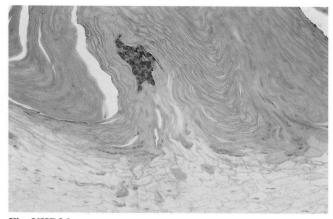

Fig. VIID2.b

Fig. VIID2.c

Clin. Fig. VIID2. *Onychomycosis*. Chronic infection with *Trichophyton rubrum* resulted in thickened yellowish nails with subungual debris.

Fig. VIID2.a. *Onychomycosis, low power*. This photomicrograph shows a nail plate composed of laminated keratin. One surface shows a papillomatous architecture with parakeratin. No nail bed or nail matrix is seen in this biopsy.

Fig. VIID2.b. *Onychomycosis, high power*. Within the orthokeratotic and parakeratotic scale there are focal collections of neutrophils. Hyphae can be seen on H&E stained sections, but this is quite difficult without special stains.

Fig. VIID2.c. *Onychomycosis, high power, PAS stain*. PAS stains reveal septate hyphae within the thickened keratin layer.

HISTOPATHOLOGY. Biopsy of the nail bed shows hyperkeratosis. A PAS stain should be performed on all nail biopsies. This stain reveals fungal organisms that are usually located in the lower stratum corneum near the nail bed epidermis and on the nail plate. The nail bed epidermis shows acanthosis, spongiosis, and exocytosis of lymphocytes and histiocytes. In proximal subungual onychomycosis, infection initially involves the area of the proximal nail fold. Superficial white onychomycosis is caused by *Trichophyton mentagrophytes*, located on the superficial nail plate only. The nail must be damaged for this to occur. In HIV-infected persons, superficial white onychomycosis is usually caused by *T. rubrum*. Candida may involve the nail plate and nail bed in patients with chronic mucocutaneous candidiasis and in HIV-infected patients.

Conditions to consider in the differential diagnosis:

  psoriasis
  tinea unguium, onychomycosis

VIID3. Vesiculobullous Diseases

Vesiculobullous disease more commonly seen elsewhere in the skin may also involve the nails. Darier's disease commonly involves the nail with characteristic clinical findings that are not often biopsied.

Darier's Disease

CLINICAL SUMMARY. Nail changes usually occur in association with other clinical findings. Rarely, involvement may be limited to the nail alone. Nail changes may occur in the proximal nail fold, matrix, nail bed, and hyponychium. Involvement of the nail matrix in Darier–White disease is usually located in the distal lunula. The nails show characteristic changes of V-shaped nicking, linear striations, onycholysis, and subungual keratotic reaction (see Clin. Fig. IVD1.b).

HISTOPATHOLOGY. The proximal nail fold may show keratotic papules that are histologically similar to those of acrokeratosis verruciformis of Hopf. However, in addition to papillary epidermal hyperplasia, focal areas of suprabasilar acantholysis may be seen. Histologically, this leukonychia is due to foci of persistent parakeratosis in the lower nail plate related to the usual histology of Darier–White disease of the distal matrix (14).

Conditions to consider in the differential diagnosis:

Darier's disease
pemphigus
erythema multiforme
toxic epidermal necrolysis
epidermolysis bullosa
bullous pemphigoid

VIID4. Parasitic Infestations

Scabies is an example of a parasitic infection that may involve the nails (15).

Scabies

CLINICAL SUMMARY AND HISTOPATHOLOGY. *Sarcoptes scabiei* may involve the nail unit. Organisms are often present in distal subungual hyperkeratotic debris found in the hypony-

chium and may be a cause of persistent epidemics of scabies. Norwegian scabies may cause severe involvement of the nail folds.

Conditions to consider in the differential diagnosis:

scabies
Norwegian scabies

REFERENCES

1. Whiting DA. Diagnostic and predictive value of horizontal sections of scalp biopsy specimens in male pattern androgenetic alopecia. *J Am Acad Dermatol* 1993;28:755.
2. Headington JT. The histopathology of alopecia areata. *J Invest Dermatol* 1991;96:69S.
3. Waldorf DS. Lichen planopilaris. *Arch Dermatol* 1966;93:684.
4. Buchness MR, Lim HW, Hatcher VA, et al. Eosinophilic pustular folliculitis in the acquired immunodeficiency syndrome. *N Engl J Med* 1988;318:1183.
5. Pinkus H. Furuncle. *J Cutan Pathol* 1979;6:517.
6. Mikhail GR. *Trichophyton rubrum* granuloma. *Int J Dermatol* 1970;9:41.
7. Suter L. Folliculitis decalvans. *Hautarzt* 1981;32:429.
8. Imai S, Nitto H. Eccrine nevus with epidermal changes. *Dermatologica* 1983;166:84.
9. Gianotti R, Restano L, Grimalt R, et al. Lichen striatus a chameleon: an histopathological and immunohistological study of forty-one cases. *J Cutan Pathol* 1995;22:18.
10. Harrist TJ, Fine JD, Berman RS, et al. Neutrophilic hidradenitis: a distinctive type of neutrophilic dermatosis associated with myelogenous leukemia and chemotherapy. *Arch Dermatol* 1982;118:263.
11. Ridley DS, Ridley MJ. The classification of nerves is modified by delayed recognition of *M leprae*. *Int J Lepr* 1986;54:596.
12. Smithers BM, McLeod GR, Little JH. Desmoplastic, neural transforming and neurotropic melanoma: a review of 45 cases. *Aust N Z J Surg* 1990;60:967.
13. Kouskoukis CE, Scher RK, Ackerman AB. What histologic finding distinguishes onychomycosis and psoriasis? *Am J Dermatopathol* 1983;5:501.
14. Zaias N, Ackerman AB. The nail in Darier-White disease. *Arch Dermatol* 1973;107:193.
15. Scher RK. Subungual scabies. *Am J Dermatopathol* 1983;5:187.

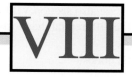

VIII

Disorders of the Subcutis

The reactions in the subcutis are mostly inflammatory, although tumors (proliferations) of the subcutis do occur (lipoma). Pathologic conditions arising in the dermis may infiltrate the subcutis.

VIIIA. SUBCUTANEOUS VASCULITIS AND VASCULOPATHY (SEPTAL OR LOBULAR)

True vasculitis is defined by the presence of necrosis and inflammation in vessel walls. Other forms of vasculopathy include thrombosis and thrombophlebitis, fibrointimal hyperplasia, and neoplastic infiltration of vessel walls.

1. Neutrophilic Vasculitis
2. Lymphocytic Vasculitis
3. Granulomatous Vasculitis

VIIIA1. Neutrophilic Vasculitis

Neutrophils and disrupted nuclei are present in the wall of the vessel, with associated eosinophilic "fibrinoid" necrosis.

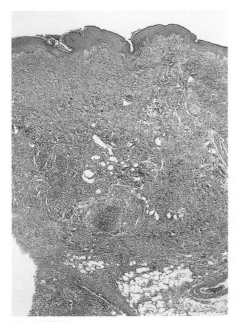

Fig. VIIIA1.a

Subcutaneous Polyarteritis Nodosa

See Figs. VIIIA1.a–VIIIA1.c. See also section VB3.
  Conditions to consider in the differential diagnosis:
    leukocytoclastic vasculitis
    subcutaneous polyarteritis nodosa
    superficial migratory thrombophlebitis
    erythema nodosum leprosum

VIIIA2. Lymphocytic Vasculitis

The concept of "lymphocytic vasculitis" is a controversial one. Many disorders characterized by lymphocytes within the walls of vessels are best classified as lymphocytic infiltrates. The term "vasculitis" may be appropriate when there is vessel wall damage, as in nodular vasculitis, even in the absence of neutrophils and "fibrinoid."

Fig. VIIIA1.a. *Subcutaneous polyarteritis nodosa, low power.* In the deep reticular dermis extending into the superficial subcutaneous tissue there is an intense perivascular inflammatory reaction. Even at scanning magnification, one can identify an intense infiltrate of a medium-sized vessel.

Fig. VIIIA1.b. *Subcutaneous polyarteritis nodosa, medium power.* This medium-sized artery shows extensive infiltration and destruction of the vessel by a neutrophilic infiltrate.

Fig. VIIIA1.c. *Subcutaneous polyarteritis nodosa, medium power.* Another medium-sized artery in the subcutaneous fat shows luminal obliteration, a mixed acute and chronic inflammatory infiltrate within the wall, and hemorrhage surrounding the vessel.

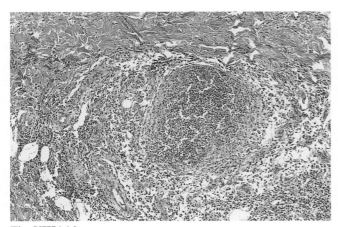

Fig. VIIIA1.b

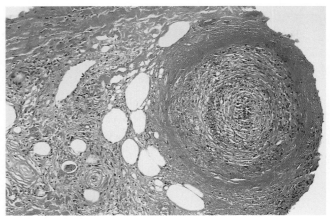

Fig. VIIIA1.c

Conditions to consider in the differential diagnosis:
nodular vasculitis
perniosis (see section VB2)
angiocentric lymphomas

VIIIA3. Granulomatous Vasculitis

The inflammatory infiltrate in the vessel walls is composed of mixed cells, including more or less epithelioid histiocytes, and giant cells. Other cell types, including lymphocytes and plasma cells and sometimes neutrophils and eosinophils, are commonly present also.

Erythema Induratum (Nodular Vasculitis)

CLINICAL SUMMARY. The lesions of erythema induratum (1), also known as "nodular vasculitis," consist of painless but somewhat tender, deep-seated, circumscribed, nodular, subcutaneous infiltrations of the lower legs, especially on the calves. Gradually, the infiltrations extend toward the surface, forming blue-red plaques that can ulcerate before healing with atrophy and scarring. Recurrences are common and are often precipitated by the onset of cold weather. Women are more commonly affected than men. "Nodular vasculitis" has been proposed as a term for those cases with erythema induratumlike lesions that are not associated with tuberculosis.

HISTOPATHOLOGY. In contrast to erythema nodosum, which is mainly a septal panniculitis, erythema induratum (nodular vasculitis) is initially mainly a lobular panniculitis due to vasculitis that produces ischemic necrosis of the fat lobule with relatively little involvement of the structures of the septa. The fat necrosis elicits granulomatous inflammation. Epithelioid cells and giant cells and/or lymphocytes and plasma cells form broad zones of inflammation surrounding the necrosis and extending between the fat cells, but can also form well-delimited granulomas of the tuberculoid type. Ziehl–Neelsen stains are negative for mycobacteria. Vascular changes are extensive and severe. The walls of small and medium-sized arteries and veins are infiltrated by a dense lymphoid or granulomatous inflammatory infiltrate, associated with endothelial swelling and edema of the vessel walls, fibrous thickening of the intima, and, often, thrombosis of the lumen. Compromise of the lumen produces ischemic and caseous fat necrosis, which when extensive may lead to involvement of the overlying dermis and ulceration. In the necrotic fat there are fat cysts, with surrounding amorphous, finely granular, eosinophilic material containing some pyknotic nuclei. Later lesions contain many foamy histiocytes surrounding the areas of fat necrosis.

Conditions to consider in the differential diagnosis:
erythema induratum/nodular vasculitis
erythema nodosum leprosum (type 2 leprosy reaction)
Wegener's granulomatosis
Churg–Strauss vasculitis

Crohn's disease
giant cell arteritis

VIIIB. SEPTAL PANNICULITIS WITHOUT VASCULITIS

The inflammation is mainly confined to the septa, although there may be some lobular involvement.

1. Septal Panniculitis, Lymphocytes and Mixed Infiltrates
2. Septal Panniculitis, Granulomatous
3. Septal Panniculitis, Sclerotic

VIIIB1. Septal Panniculitis, Lymphocytes and Mixed Infiltrates

The inflammation predominantly involves the subcutaneous septa, although there may be "spillover" into the fat lobules. The infiltrate is mainly lymphocytic, although other cells can be found, including plasma cells and acute inflammatory cells.

Erythema Nodosum

CLINICAL SUMMARY. Although the causes of erythema nodosum (2) are legion and cannot always be determined, streptococcal infection is the most common. In the *acute form* of erythema nodosum, there is a sudden appearance of tender bright red or dusky red-purple nodules that only slightly elevate the level of the skin surface and have a strong predilection for the anterior surfaces of the lower legs, although they also may occur elsewhere, but mostly on dependent regions. The lesions do not ulcerate and generally involute within a few weeks, whereas new lesions may intermittently appear for several months. The lesions are tender and warm, and the acute disease often is accompanied by fever, malaise, leukocytosis, and arthropathy. Focal hemorrhages are common and can cause the lesions to resemble bruises (*erythema contusiforme*). The *chronic form* of erythema nodosum may last from a few months to a few years and is also known as *erythema nodosum migrans* or subacute nodular migratory panniculitis. There are one or several red, slightly tender subcutaneous nodules that are found, usually unilaterally, on the lower leg. Most patients are women with a solitary lesion and a recent history of sore throat and arthralgia. The nodules enlarge by peripheral extension into plaques, often with central clearing.

HISTOPATHOLOGY. In early acute lesions there is edema of the subcutaneous septa with a lymphohistiocytic infiltrate, having a slight admixture of neutrophils and eosinophils. Focal fibrin deposition and extravasation of erythrocytes occur frequently. Often the inflammation is most intense at the periphery of the edematous septa and extends into the periphery of the fat lobules between individual fat cells in a lacelike fashion without prominent necrosis of the fat. Clusters of

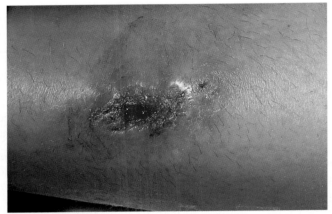

Clin. Fig. VIIIA3

Clin. Fig. VIIIA3. *Erythema induratum.* A young female presented with a tender ulcerated nodule in the left pretibial area. Cultures for tuberculosis were negative.

Fig. VIIIA3.a. *Erythema induratum/nodular vasculitis, low power*. There is inflammation involving the subcutaneous lobules with little or no inflammation in the overlying epidermis and dermis.

Fig. VIIIA3.b. *Erythema induratum/nodular vasculitis, medium power*. This is a predominantly lobular panniculitis with less intense involvement of the subcutaneous septae.

Fig. VIIIA3.c. *Erythema induratum/nodular vasculitis, high power*. This vein shows a moderately intense lymphoid infiltrate surrounding the vessel and also involving the wall of the vessel. Thickening of the intima and luminal thrombosis (not seen here) may also be present.

Fig. VIIIA3.d. *Erythema induratum/nodular vasculitis, high power*. The infiltrate in the subcutaneous fat is frequently granulomatous composed of histiocytes and giant cells and a mixed inflammatory infiltrate.

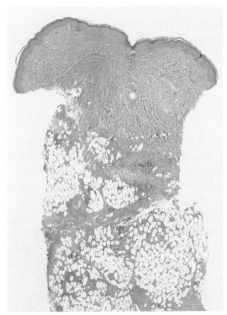

Fig. VIIIA3.a

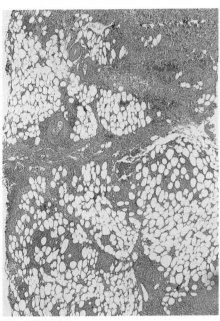

Fig. VIIIA3.b

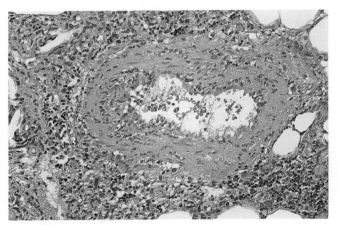

Fig. VIIIA3.c

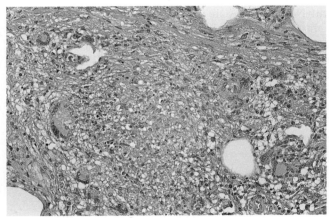

Fig. VIIIA3.d

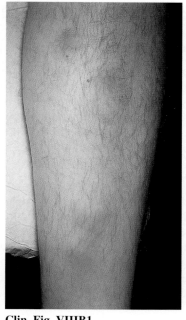

Clin. Fig. VIIIB1

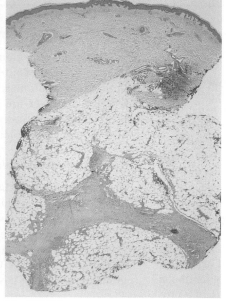

Fig. VIIIB1.a

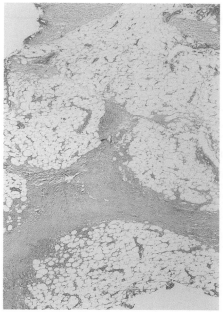

Fig. VIIIB1.b

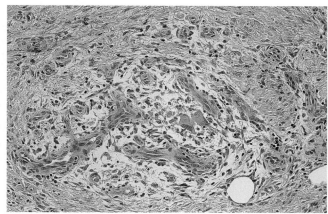

Fig. VIIIB1.c

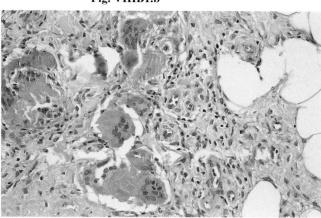

Fig. VIIIB1.d

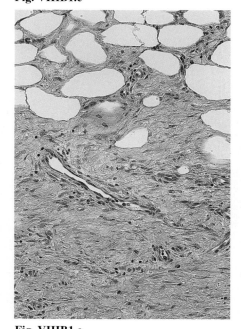

Fig. VIIIB1.e

Clin. Fig. VIIIB1. *Erythema nodosum.* Tender erythematous nodules on the shins is a classic presentation.

Fig. VIIIB1.a. *Erythema nodosum, low power.* Scanning magnification reveals thickening of the fibrous septa.

Fig. VIIIB1.b. *Erythema nodosum, medium power.* The septa are edematous and fibrotic. There is a mixed inflammatory infiltrate in this midstage lesion, which begins to extend into the adjacent fat lobules.

Fig. VIIIB1.c. *Erythema nodosum, high power.* The mixed nature of the infiltrate is apparent in this edematous focus that shows lymphocytes, histiocytes, scattered eosinophils, and multinucleated giant cells.

Fig. VIIIB1.d. *Erythema nodosum, high power.* Giant cells, eosinophils, and lymphocytes are present in the expanded septa.

Fig. VIIIB1.e. *Erythema nodosum, high power.* Vasculitis is absent. The septa are fibrotic.

macrophages around small blood vessels, or a slitlike space, occur in early lesions and are known as Miescher's radial nodules. The degree of vascular involvement is variable, but usually falls short of true vasculitis. Later, acute lesions show widening of the septa, often with fibrosis and with inflammation at the periphery of the fat lobules. Neutrophils usually are absent and there are more macrophages in the infiltrate. Macrophages at the edges of the fat lobules have a foam-cell appearance from phagocytized lipid. Loosely formed granulomas comprised of macrophages and giant cells, without lipid deposition, are more frequent in late lesions than in early ones. The oldest lesions have septal widening and fibrosis with a decrease in all inflammatory cells, except for a few persisting at the periphery of the fat lobules.

In chronic erythema nodosum, the histologic findings are generally the same as those of the late stages of acute erythema nodosum. However, granuloma and lipogranuloma formation often is more pronounced. There is vascular proliferation and thickening of the endothelium with extravasation of erythrocytes.

Conditions to consider in the differential diagnosis:

erythema nodosum and variants
Crohn's disease
morphea

VIIIB2. Septal Panniculitis, Granulomatous

Subcutaneous granulomas may present as ill-defined collections of epithelioid histiocytes, as well-formed epithelioid-cell granulomas, and as palisading granulomas in which histiocytes are radially arranged around areas of necrosis or necrobiosis. Most conditions in this list may also present as mixed lobular/septal panniculitis.

Subcutaneous Granuloma Annulare

CLINICAL SUMMARY.   In this disorder, subcutaneous nodules occur, especially in children, either alone or in association with intradermal lesions (3). The subcutaneous nodules clinically resemble rheumatoid nodules, although there is a greater tendency to occur on the legs and feet, and there is no history of arthritis. A very rare, deep, destructive form of granuloma annulare has also been described.

HISTOPATHOLOGY.   The subcutaneous nodules of granuloma annulare usually show large foci of palisaded histiocytes surrounding areas of degenerated collagen and prominent mucin with a pale appearance; however, biopsies in which mucin was not apparent or the central area appeared more fibrinoid have also been reported.

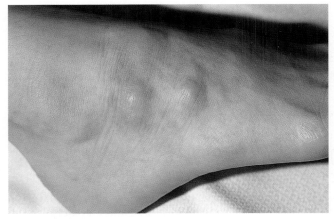

Clin. Fig. VIIIB2

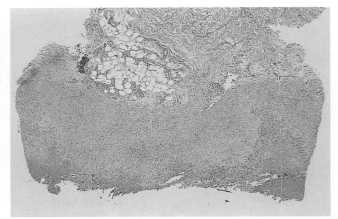

Fig. VIIIB2.a

Clin. Fig. VIIIB2. *Subcutaneous granuloma annulare.* Subcutaneous nodules in an annular distribution developed on a child's dorsal foot.

Fig. VIIIB2.a. *Subcutaneous granuloma annulare, low power.* The septum of the subcutaneous fat has been replaced by inflammation and altered connective tissue. (*continues*)

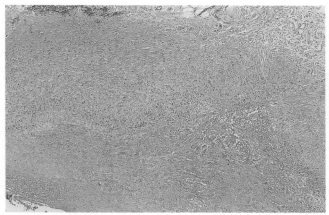

Fig. VIIIB2.b

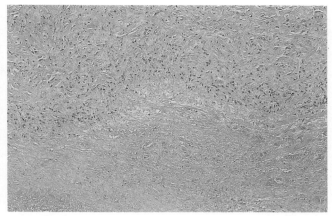

Fig. VIIIB2.c

Fig. VIIIB2.b. *Subcutaneous granuloma annulare, medium power.* In the subcutaneous septum, there is palisaded granulomatous inflammation surrounding a zone of altered collagen.

Fig. VIIIB2.c. *Subcutaneous granuloma annulare, high power.* The altered (necrobiotic) collagen seen in the lower half of this field is surrounded by a palisade of histiocytes and fibrosis.

Conditions to consider in the differential diagnosis:

    palisaded granulomas
    subcutaneous granuloma annulare
    rheumatoid nodules
    sarcoidosis
    lichen scrofulosorum
    Crohn's disease
    subcutaneous infections
    syphilis
    tuberculosis

VIIIB3. Septal Panniculitis, Sclerotic

Sclerosis of the panniculus may begin as a septal process and extend into the lobules.

Scleroderma and Morphea

HISTOPATHOLOGY. Changes in the subcutis are prominent in both scleroderma and morphea (4) (see also section VF1). The inflammatory infiltrate involving the subcutaneous fat in morphea is often much more pronounced than that in the dermis. It consists of lymphocytes and plasma cells and extends upward toward the eccrine glands. Trabeculae subdividing the subcutaneous fat are thickened by an inflammatory infiltrate and deposition of new collagen. Large areas of subcutaneous fat are replaced by newly formed collagen composed of fine wavy fibers. Vascular changes in the early inflammatory stage may consist of endothelial swelling and edema of the walls of the vessels. In the late sclerotic stage, as seen in the center of old morphea lesions, the inflammatory infiltrate has disappeared almost completely, except in some areas of the subcutis. The fascia and striated muscles underlying lesions of morphea may be affected in the linear, segmental, subcutaneous, and generalized types, showing fibrosis and sclerosis similar to that seen in subcutaneous tissue. The muscle fibers appear vacuolated and separated from one another by edema and focal collections of inflammatory cells. Aggregates of calcium may also be seen in the late stage within areas of sclerotic homogeneous collagen of the subcutaneous tissue.

In early lesions of systemic scleroderma, the inflammatory reaction is less pronounced than in morphea. The vascular changes in early lesions are slight, as in morphea. In contrast, in the late stage, systemic scleroderma shows more pronounced vascular changes than morphea, particularly in the subcutis. These changes include a paucity of blood vessels, thickening and hyalinization of their walls, and narrowing of the lumen.

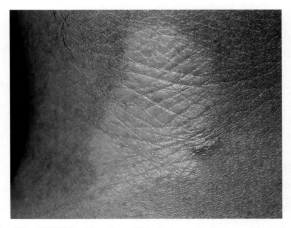

Clin. Fig. VIIIB3. *Morphea.* This indurated plaque with an ivory color represents the plaque type of this disease.

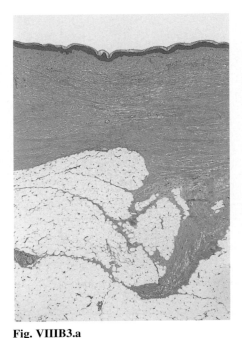

Fig. VIIIB3.a

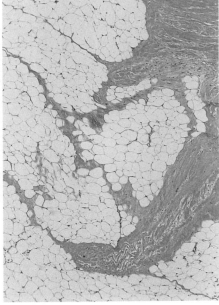

Fig. VIIIB3.b

Fig. VIIIB3.a. *Scleroderma/morphea, low power.* In the later stage of this disease, adnexal structures are absent and inflammation is minimal. The reticular dermal collagen is sclerotic and extends into the subcutaneous fat forming thickened hyalinized collagen within the septae. At this later stage, there is little or no inflammation.

Fig. VIIIB3.b. *Scleroderma/morphea, medium power.* The sclerotic subcutaneous septae lack the granulomatous inflammation, which is seen in later stages of erythema nodosum.

Conditions to consider in the differential diagnosis:

scleroderma, morphea
eosinophilic fasciitis
ischemic liposclerosis
toxins

VIIIC. LOBULAR PANNICULITIS WITHOUT VASCULITIS

The inflammation is mainly confined to the lobules, although there may be some septal involvement.

1. Lobular Panniculitis, Lymphocytes Predominant
2. Lobular Panniculitis, Lymphocytes and Plasma Cells
3. Lobular Panniculitis, Neutrophilic
4. Lobular Panniculitis, Eosinophils Prominent
5. Lobular Panniculitis, Histiocytes Prominent
6. Lobular Panniculitis, Mixed with Foam Cells
7. Lobular Panniculitis, Granulomatous
8. Lobular Panniculitis, Crystal Deposits, Calcifications
9. Lobular Panniculitis, Necrosis Prominent
10. Lobular Panniculitis, Embryonic Fat Pattern
11. Lobular Panniculitis, Miscellaneous

VIIIC1. Lobular Panniculitis, Lymphocytes Predominant

Lymphocytes are the primary infiltrating cells.

Lupus Erythematosus Panniculitis

CLINICAL SUMMARY. In patients with chronic cutaneous lupus erythematosus, the lesions can be deep and can involve the panniculus either alone or accompanied by dermal lesions (5). Patients can have either chronic discoid lupus erythematosus or systemic lupus erythematosus. Most commonly, the skin lesions are firm indurated subcutaneous nodules and plaques that tend to involve the skin of the trunk and proximal extremities, particularly the lateral aspects of the upper arms, thighs, and buttocks. The overlying skin shows no specific changes. The lesions are painful and have a tendency to ulcerate and to heal, leaving depressed scars. When the overlying skin is involved there is a loss of hair, erythema, poikiloderma, and epidermal atrophy. Patients may present with localized depressions of lipoatrophy alone. The term "lupus profundus" has been used both for lupus panniculitis and also for discoid lupus erythematosus lesions that involve the dermis and extend deeply into the subcutis.

HISTOPATHOLOGY. The histologic sections show a deep lymphocytic infiltrate in the fat lobules and in the septa. Lymphoid aggregates, nodules, and germinal centers are common. Usually there is mucinous edema of the septa and of the overlying dermis. The dermis can have a superficial and deep perivascular lymphocytic infiltrate with plasma cells or can have all changes of lesions of discoid lupus erythematosus. A distinctive feature is the so-called hyaline necrosis of the fat, in which portions of the fat lobule have lost nuclear staining of the fat cells and there is an accumulation of fibrin and other proteins in a homogeneous eosinophilic matrix between residual fat cells and extracellular fat globules. Blood vessels are infiltrated by lymphoid cells and can have restriction of their lumen diameter. Calcification may be present in older lesions.

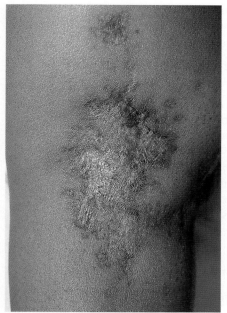

Clin. Fig. VIIIC1

Clin. Fig. VIIIC1. *Lupus panniculitis*. A patient with discoid lupus erythematosus developed an indurated subcutaneous area with postinflammatory hyper/hypopigmentation on the lateral thigh.

Fig. VIIIC1.a. *Lupus panniculitis, low power*. An intense inflammatory infiltrate is present at the dermal–subcutaneous junction, extending into the adipose tissue in an interstitial pattern. (C. Jaworsky)

Fig. VIIIC1.b. *Lupus panniculitis, medium power*. The inflammatory infiltrate outlines individual adipocytes, creating a lacelike pattern. (C. Jaworsky)

Fig. VIIIC1.c. *Lupus panniculitis, high power*. Foam cells indicate adipocyte injury. Note also the hyaline matrix between adipocytes. (C. Jaworsky)

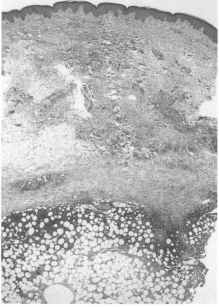

Fig. VIIIC1.a

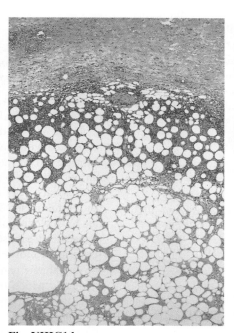

Fig. VIIIC1.b

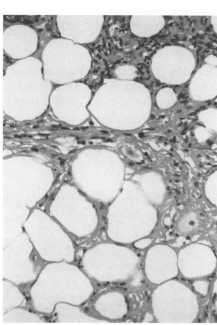

Fig. VIIIC1.c

Conditions to consider in the differential diagnosis:
  lupus panniculitis lupus profundus
  nodular vasculitis/erythema induratum, inapparent
    vasculitis
  poststeroid panniculitis
  subcutaneous lymphoma-leukemia

VIIIC2. Lobular Panniculitis, Lymphocytes and Plasma Cells

Lymphocytes and plasma cells are the primary infiltrating cells. These conditions are more likely to present as primarily septal or as mixed panniculitis (see sections VIIIB3 and VIIIC1).
  Conditions to consider in the differential diagnosis:
    lupus profundus
    scleroderma

VIIIC3. Lobular Panniculitis, Neutrophilic

Lymphocytes and neutrophils are the primary infiltrating cells. The conditions listed below are more likely to present as a mixed lobular and septal panniculitis (see section VIIID1). In some cases with pancreatic enzyme panniculitis, possibly with early lesions, biopsies of subcutaneous nodules show only a nonspecific pattern of a necrotizing panniculitis with a neutrophilic inflammatory response.
  Conditions to consider in the differential diagnosis:
    infection (cellulitis)
    necrotizing fasciitis
    ruptured follicles and cysts

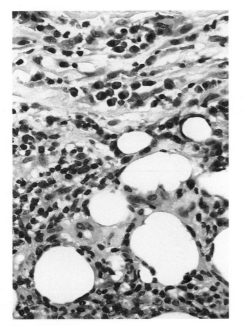

Fig. VIIIC2.a.
Lupus panniculitis, high power. A lymphoplasmacytic infiltrate splays collagen bundles and adipocytes (see also section VIIIC1). (C. Jaworsky)

Fig. VIIIC2.a

pancreatic fat necrosis
traumatic panniculitis

VIIIC4. Lobular Panniculitis, Eosinophils Prominent

Lymphocytes and eosinophils are the primary infiltrating cells. The conditions listed below are more likely to present as a mixed lobular and septal panniculitis (see section VIIID3).
  Conditions to consider in the differential diagnosis:
    eosinophilic fasciitis
    eosinophilic panniculitis
    arthropod bites
    parasites

VIIIC5. Lobular Panniculitis, Histiocytes Prominent

Lymphocytes and histiocytes are the primary infiltrating cells. The conditions listed below are more likely to present as a mixed lobular and septal panniculitis (see also section VIIID4).

Histiocytic Cytophagic Panniculitis (Subcutaneous T-Cell Lymphoma with Hemophagocytic Syndrome)

CLINICAL SUMMARY. Histiocytic cytophagic panniculitis (6) is a frequently fatal systemic disease that is characterized by recurrent, widely distributed, painful subcutaneous nodules associated with malaise and fever. The nodules can be hemorrhagic and may ulcerate. Hepatosplenomegaly, pancytopenia, and progressive liver dysfunction develop in most cases. The patients may follow a long chronic course, or the disease can be fulminant. Patients usually die a hemorrhagic death due to depletion of blood coagulation factors. In some patients, the disease seems limited to the skin and subcutaneous tissue and follows a more benign course. In most instances, the cytophagic panniculitis is the result of a malignant lymphoma in which the abnormal lymphocyte population has stimulated benign macrophages to engage in fulminant hemophagocytosis. Lymphoma may or may not be evident in any given biopsy of skin and/or subcutaneous tissue.

HISTOPATHOLOGY. A deep biopsy usually shows both subcutaneous and dermal nodules composed of macrophages and a mixed inflammatory infiltrate. In the subcutis, the inflammation is both septal and lobular. Often there is necrosis and hemorrhage. The nuclei of the macrophages are without significant atypia. In some areas the macrophages become so engorged by phagocytosis of erythrocytes, lymphocytes, and cell fragments that they have been named "bean bag cells." In some patients, early lesions contain a rather dense infiltrate of small lymphocytes and only focal areas with cytophagic histiocytes. The involvement of other organs by similar cytophagic macrophages leads to diffuse infiltration of liver, bone marrow, spleen, lymph nodes, myocardium, lungs, and gastrointestinal tract. The cytophagic macrophages can deplete almost all of the bone marrow elements.

Conditions to consider in the differential diagnosis:

cytophagic histiocytic panniculitis
Rosai–Dorfman disease

VIIIC6. Lobular Panniculitis, Mixed with Foam Cells

Lymphocytes, plasma cells, and a variety of infiltrating cells can be seen, including giant cells and foamy histiocytes.

Relapsing Febrile Nodular Nonsuppurative Panniculitis (Weber–Christian Disease)

CLINICAL SUMMARY. The diagnosis of Weber–Christian disease (7) is a diagnosis of exclusion. It is made much less frequently now than it was in the past, probably because of the greater power of current laboratory testing to reveal lupus erythematosus panniculitis, alpha-1-antitrypsin (AAT) deficiency panniculitis, or histiocytic cytophagic panniculitis in cases that might previously have been classified as Weber–Christian disease. The classic clinical description is of a disease characterized by the appearance of crops of tender nodules and plaques in the subcutaneous fat, usually in association with mild fever. The lower extremities are fa-

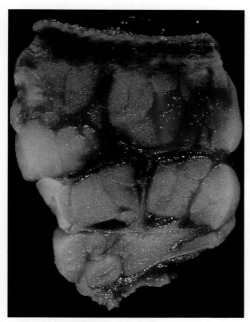

Clin. Fig. VIIIC5

Clin. Fig. VIIIC5. *Histiocytic cytophagic panniculitis.* This cross-sectioned skin nodule shows both septal and lobular infiltration and hemorrhage. Note also the dermal hemorrhage. (N.S. McNutt, A. Moreno, F. Contreras)

Fig. VIIIC5.a. *Histiocytic cytophagic panniculitis, medium power.* There is hemorrhagic necrosis of the fat, with an infiltrate of lymphocytes and macrophages. (N.S. McNutt, A. Moreno, F. Contreras)

Fig. VIIIC5.b. *Histiocytic cytophagic panniculitis, high power.* Macrophages and multinucleated cells ingest lymphocytes and erythrocytes to form "bean bag cells." (N.S. McNutt, A. Moreno, F. Contreras)

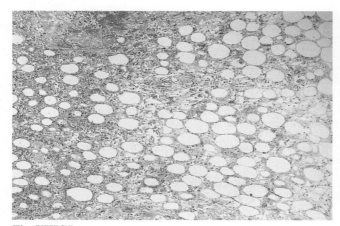

Fig. VIIIC5.a

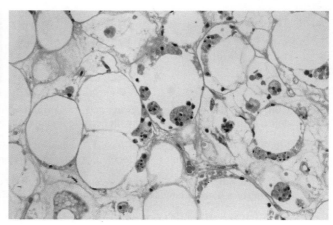

Fig. VIIIC5.b

vored sites, but lesions can occur also on the trunk, the upper extremities, and rarely on the face. The lesions may ulcerate; as they involute, they leave depressions in the skin surface. The overlying skin usually shows no involvement other than mild erythema. In general, the prognosis is good, with the attacks gradually becoming less severe and ultimately ceasing. The name Weber–Christian disease has been used in such a general fashion by some authors that the term loses meaning beyond being a clinical syndrome with nodular panniculitis for which the etiology has not yet been determined.

HISTOPATHOLOGY.   The histopathologic appearance itself is not sufficiently specific to exclude the other diseases mentioned above. The classic description is that of a lobular pan-

niculitis that evolves through three phases. The first phase is acute inflammation of the fat lobules with degeneration of fat cells accompanied by an infiltrate of neutrophils, lymphocytes, and macrophages. Neutrophils may predominate, but abscesses do not occur. In the second phase, after the lesions have been present for several days, the infiltrate is discretely localized to the fat lobules and consists mainly of foamy macrophages, usually also with a few lymphocytes and plasma cells. The foam cells can be large, and often some of them are multinucleated. Foamy macrophages replace the fat lobules and extracellular lipid masses ("microcysts") result from lysis of the fat. In some cases, the lesions perforate the skin surface and discharge a sterile, oily liquid. The third phase shows many fibroblasts and scattered lymphocytes and

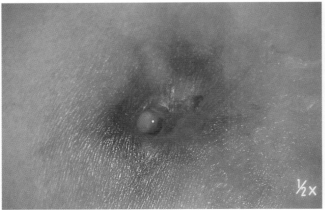

Clin. Fig. VIIIC6

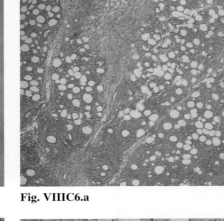

Fig. VIIIC6.a

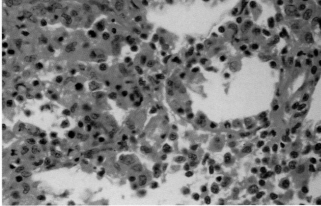

Fig. VIIIC6.b

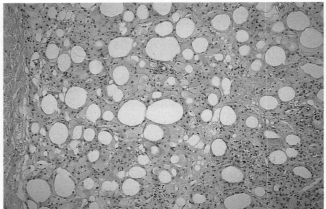

Fig. VIIIC6.c

Clin. Fig. VIIIC6. *Weber–Christian disease.* An indurated nodule on the leg has developed a perforation and drains a turbid, sterile, oily fluid with necrotic tissue. (N.S. McNutt, A. Moreno, F. Contreras)

Fig. VIIIC6.a. *Weber–Christian disease, low power.* A dense lymphocytic infiltrate is sharply localized to the fat lobules without vasculitis. (N.S. McNutt, A. Moreno, F. Contreras)

Fig. VIIIC6.b. *Weber–Christian disease, high power.* The infiltrate is composed mainly of lymphocytes and macrophages with variable numbers of neutrophils. (N.S. McNutt, A. Moreno, F. Contreras)

Fig. VIIIC6.c. *Weber–Christian disease, later lesion, medium power.* The fat is necrotic and has been extensively replaced by lipid-laden macrophages or foam cells. (N.S. McNutt, A. Moreno, F. Contreras)

a few plasma cells that have replaced the fat in clinical lesions that are depressed and indurated. Dense fibrosis results.

Systemic lesions that may be seen in Weber–Christian disease include involvement of the mesenteric and omental fat, involvement of intravisceral adipose tissue, causing focal necroses in liver or spleen, involvement of the bone marrow, and accumulation of large amounts of oily fluid in either the peritoneal or pleural cavity.

Conditions to consider in the differential diagnosis:

alpha-1-antitrypsin deficiency panniculitis
Weber–Christian disease
traumatic fat necrosis
cold panniculitis
injection granuloma
factitious panniculitis
necrobiotic xanthogranuloma with paraproteinemia

VIIIC7. Lobular Panniculitis, Granulomatous

Lymphocytes and histiocytes are the primary infiltrating cells. Except for erythema induratum, which was discussed in section VIIIA3 because it is usually associated with evident vasculitis, most conditions in this list may more usually present as mixed lobular/septal panniculitis.

Subcutaneous Sarcoidosis

See Figs. VIIC7.a and VIIC7.b.

Conditions to consider in the differential diagnosis:

erythema induratum/nodular vasculitis (if vasculitis is inapparent)
palisaded granulomas
subcutaneous granuloma annulare/pseudorheumatoid nodule
rheumatoid nodules

subcutaneous sarcoidosis
tuberculosis
Crohn's disease

VIIIC8. Lobular Panniculitis, Crystal Deposits, Calcifications

Crystalline deposits derived from free fatty acids or other precipitated salts are present in the fat lobules.

Subcutaneous Fat Necrosis of the Newborn

CLINICAL FEATURES.   Subcutaneous fat necrosis of the newborn usually occurs in premature or full-term infants, often after delivery with forceps (8). Indurated nodules and plaques appear in the subcutis a few days after birth. Rarely, in cases with numerous nodules, the lesions may discharge a caseous material. The patient's health generally is good, and the nodules resolve spontaneously after a few weeks or months. Rarely, infants become severely ill and die.

HISTOPATHOLOGY.   Focal areas of fat necrosis are present in the fat lobules and are infiltrated by macrophages and foreign-body giant cells. The fat deposits in the macrophages and giant cells contain crystalline fat, which forms needle-shaped clefts in a radial arrangement. Calcium deposits usually are scattered in the necrotic fat.

Calcifying Panniculitis (Calciphylaxis)

See Figs. VIIIC8.d and VIIIC8.e.

Conditions to consider in the differential diagnosis:

sclerema neonatorum
subcutaneous fat necrosis of the newborn
gout
oxalosis
calcifying panniculitis

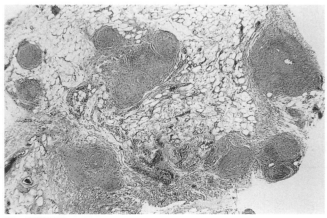

Fig. VIIIC7.a

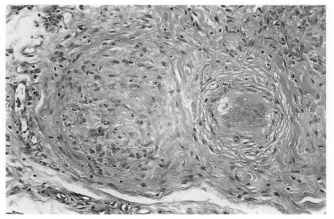

Fig. VIIIC7.b

Fig. VIIIC7.a. *Subcutaneous sarcoidosis, low power.* Within the subcutaneous fat, there are multiple granulomas with minimal necrosis.

Fig. VIIIC7.b. *Subcutaneous sarcoidosis, medium power.* The granulomas are well formed, composed of epithelioid histiocytes and giant cells with a sprinkling of lymphocytes. An asteroid body is present in one giant cell.

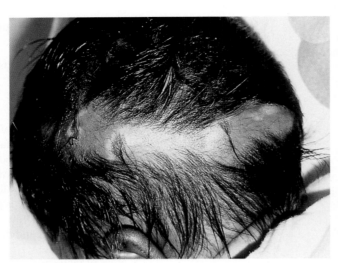

Clin. Fig. VIIIC8.a

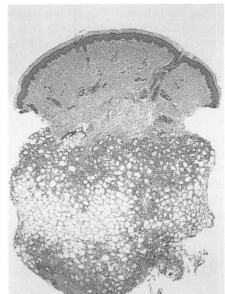

Fig. VIIIC8.a

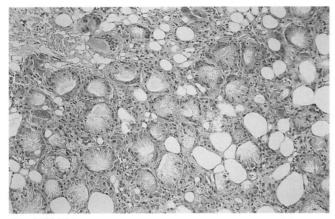

Fig. VIIIC8.b

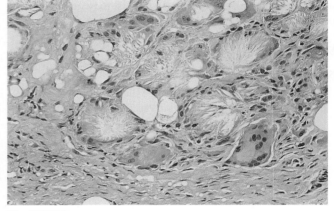

Fig. VIIIC8.c

Clin. Fig. VIIIC8.a. *Subcutaneous fat necrosis of the newborn.* A healthy full-term infant developed an indurated plaque with alopecia on the scalp, an unusual presentation. (P. Honig)

Fig. VIIIC8.a. *Subcutaneous fat necrosis of the newborn, low power.* Scanning magnification reveals a predominantly lobular panniculitis. The overlying epidermis and dermis show almost no inflammation.

Fig. VIIIC8.b. *Subcutaneous fat necrosis of the newborn, medium power.* Within the subcutaneous lobules there is a lymphoid infiltrate associated with large giant cells. Occasionally, as seen here, they may be numerous.

Fig. VIIIC8.c. *Subcutaneous fat necrosis of the newborn, high power.* The giant cells show numerous needle-shaped clefts in a radial array, a characteristic finding in this disease.

Fig. VIIIC8.f. *Calcifying panniculitis, medium power, von Kossa stain.* The material stains positive for calcium and is localized primarily to the walls of small vessels in the subcutis.

Fig. VIIIC8.g. *Calcifying panniculitis, high power, von Kossa stain.* Granular amorphous material characteristic of calcium is primarily deposited within the media of small vessels between individual adipocytes.

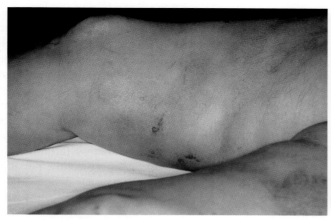

Clin. Fig. VIIIC8.b

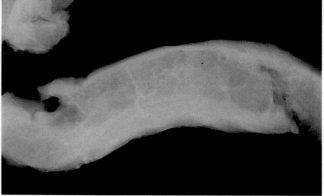

Clin. Fig. VIIIC8.c

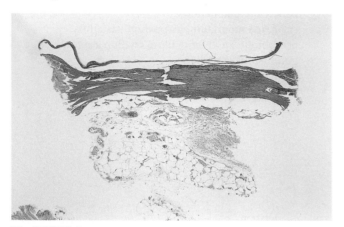

Fig. VIIIC8.d

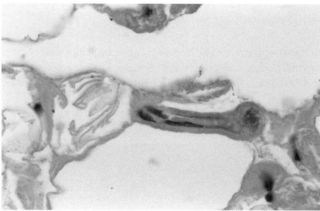

Fig. VIIIC8.e

Clin. Fig. VIIIC8.b. *Calcifying panniculitis*. This patient with hyperparathyroidism developed erythematous, hemorrhagic, indurated plaques that were cold to touch. (N.S. McNutt, A. Moreno, F. Contreras)

Clin. Fig. VIIIC8.c. *Calciphylaxis*. An x-ray of a skin biopsy from a patient with calciphylaxis reveals linear calcifications in vessel walls.

Fig. VIIIC8.d. *Calcifying panniculitis, low power*. Although the subcutis appears relatively unaffected at low power, gangrenous necrosis of the epidermis and dermis suggests vascular injury at a deeper level.

Fig. VIIIC8.e. *Calcifying panniculitis, high power*. In addition to lipomembranous change, small vessels within the subcutis are seen to contain basophilic granular material within their walls.

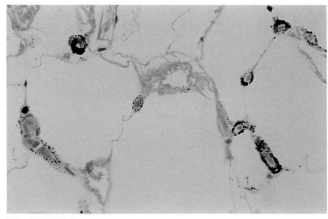

Fig. VIIIC8.f

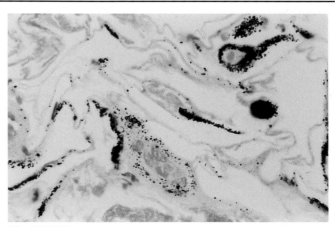

Fig. VIIIC8.g

VIIIC9. Lobular Panniculitis, Necrosis Prominent

There is fat necrosis with a resulting infiltrate that is mixed.

Subcutaneous Nodular Fat Necrosis in Pancreatic Disease

CLINICAL SUMMARY. In patients with pancreatitis or pancreatic neoplasms, the release of lipase enzymes into the blood can lead to nodules of fat necrosis in the subcutis (9). The pretibial region is the most common site of the nodules, but they may occur on the thighs, buttocks, and elsewhere. The nodules usually are tender and red and may be fluctuant, but they only rarely discharge oily fluid through fistulae. Abdominal pain is present in most cases of pancreatitis but may be absent in pancreatic carcinoma when the nodules appear. Arthralgia in the ankles is a common early symptom.

HISTOPATHOLOGY. The histologic appearance of the subcutaneous nodules in pancreatic disease is characteristic in most instances. In the foci of fat necrosis, there are ghostlike fat cells having thick faintly stained cell peripheries and no nuclear staining. Calcification forms basophilic granules in the cytoplasm of the necrotic fat cells and sometimes lamellar deposits around individual fat cells or patchy basophilic deposits at the periphery of the fat necrosis. A polymorphous infiltrate surrounds the foci of fat necrosis and consists of neutrophils, lymphoid cells, macrophages, foam cells, and foreign-body giant cells. There can be extensive hemorrhage into the lesions. Older lesions have fibrosis and hemosiderin deposition in addition to the inflammatory infiltrates. In some cases with pancreatic enzyme panniculitis, possibly with early lesions, biopsies of subcutaneous nodules show only a nonspecific pattern of a necrotizing panniculitis with a neutrophilic inflammatory response.

Conditions to consider in the differential diagnosis:

> pancreatic panniculitis
> erythema induratum, inapparent vasculitis
> necrobiotic xanthogranuloma with paraproteinemia
> gummatous syphilis
> infarct
> abscess

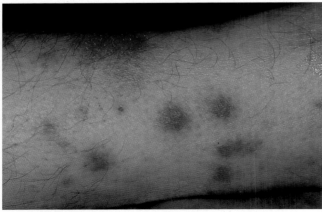

Clin. Fig. VIIIC9

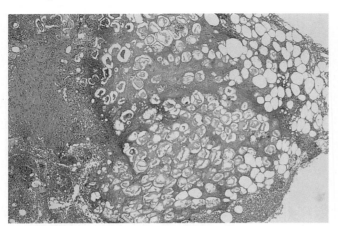

Fig. VIIIC9.a

Clin. Fig. VIIIC9. *Pancreatic panniculitis.* Erythematous nodules appear most commonly on the lower legs. (N.S. McNutt, A. Moreno, F. Contreras)

Fig. VIIIC9.a. *Pancreatic panniculitis, low power.* Necrotic fat cells contain eosinophilic deposits of partially hydrolyzed fat. Calcification forms granular basophilic material. Focal hemorrhage is frequent. (N.S. McNutt, A. Moreno, F. Contreras)

Fig. VIIIC9.b. *Pancreatic panniculitis, high power.* Many neutrophils are present at the margin of the zone of calcification and fat necrosis. (N.S. McNutt, A. Moreno, F. Contreras)

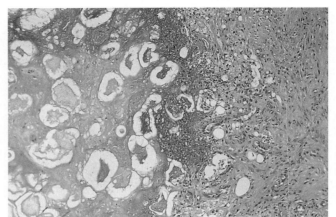

Fig. VIIIC9.b

VIIIC10. Lobular Panniculitis, Embryonic Fat Pattern

Because of atrophy or of failure of normal morphogenesis, immature small fat cells are present in the lobules.

Localized Lipoatrophy and Lipodystrophy

CLINICAL SUMMARY. Both localized lipoatrophy (10) and lipodystrophy can have lesions with a similar clinical appearance; however, lipoatrophy usually involves one or several circumscribed, round, depressed areas from one to several centimeters in diameter. In contrast, lipodystrophy produces the loss of large areas of subcutaneous fat. Most cases of lipodystrophy are of the cephalothoracic type and involve the face, neck, upper extremities, and upper trunk. Lipodystrophy may occur with diabetes and with glomerulonephritis (11). Lipoatrophic panniculitis also occurs in connective tissue panniculitis.

HISTOPATHOLOGY. Lesions of lipodystrophy are described with total loss of the subcutaneous fat producing dermis adjacent to fascia. However, localized lipoatrophy has been described as having two types: inflammatory and noninflam-

matory or involutional types. In the inflammatory type, multiple lesions are common and have a lymphocytic infiltrate around the blood vessels and scattered diffusely in the fat lobules. Areas of fat necrosis can be present with infiltration by macrophages. In the involutional type, usually there is only a solitary lesion that exhibits a decrease in size of the individual adipocytes. They are separated from each other by abundant eosinophilic, hyaline material, or in some instances by mucoid material.

Conditions to consider in the differential diagnosis:

> lipoatrophy
> lipodystrophy

VIIIC11. Lobular Panniculitis, Miscellaneous

Lymphocytes, plasma cells, and a variety of infiltrating cells can be seen, including giant cells and histiocytes.

Lipomembranous Change or Lipomembranous Panniculitis

CLINICAL SUMMARY. Patients with severe stasis, diabetes, and other causes of arterial vascular insufficiency to the

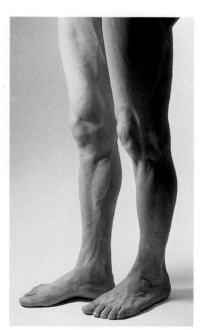

Clin. Fig. VIIIC10

Clin. Fig. VIIIC10. *Lipoatrophy.* Insulin resistance and hypertriglyceridemia were present in this middle-aged man who presented with loss of subcutaneous fat leading to the appearance of hypertrophic muscles.

Fig. VIIIC10.a. *Lipoatrophy secondary to intralesional corticosteroid, low power.* At this magnification the subcutaneous fat appears fibrotic and the lobules appear hypercellular.

Fig. VIIIC10.b. *Lipoatrophy secondary to intralesional corticosteroid, high power.* The individual adipocytes are small and the fat is not truly hypercellular but appears such because the individual nuclei are closer to one another.

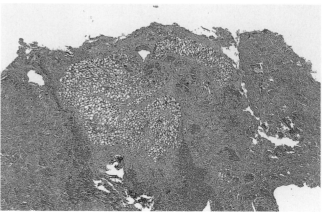

Fig. VIIIC10.a

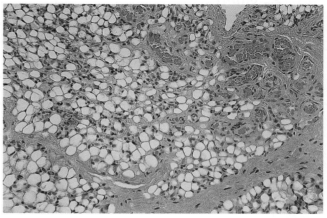

Fig. VIIIC10.b

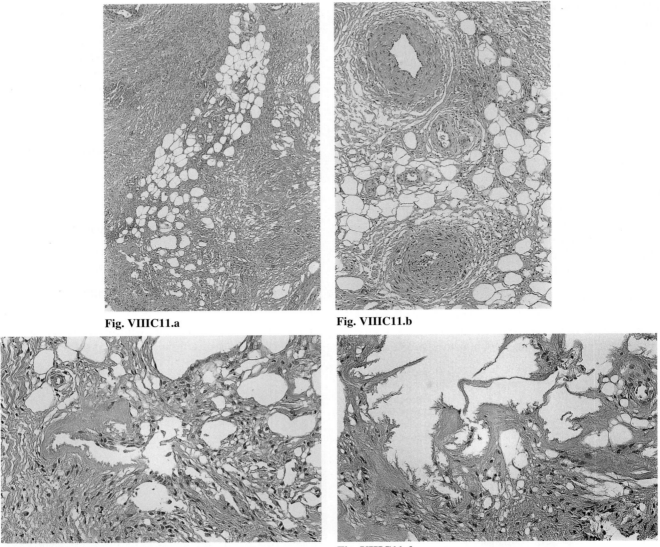

Fig. VIIIC11.a

Fig. VIIIC11.b

Fig. VIIIC11.c

Fig. VIIIC11.d

Fig. VIIIC11.a. *Lipomembranous panniculitis, low power.* This photomicrograph reveals deep dermis and subcutaneous fat. The subcutaneous tissue shows fibrosis of both septae and lobules associated with a mild chronic inflammatory infiltrate.

Fig. VIIIC11.b. *Lipomembranous panniculitis, medium power.* The adipocytes within the subcutaneous fat are of varying sizes.

Fig. VIIIC11.c. *Lipomembranous panniculitis, medium power.* Within the fat one can see variably sized cystic structures surrounded by eosinophilic material.

Fig. VIIIC11.d. *Lipomembranous panniculitis, high power.* These cysts are surrounded by feathery eosinophilic material that is frequently positive with periodic acid–Schiff stains.

lower legs can develop indurated plaques in the subcutis. They are depressed and painful but rarely ulcerate.

HISTOPATHOLOGY. The lesions are defined microscopically by the presence of lipomembranes around fat deposits or "cysts" (12). Biopsies deep into the fat show a lobular panniculitis with focal macrophage infiltration and fibrosis around the shrunken lobules. At the border of the lobules with the septa there are fat cysts that are lined by a thin eosinophilic layer of protein that has fine feathery projections into the fat cavity. This layer is called a lipomembrane and is positive on periodic acid–Schiff (PAS) and elastic-tissue stains. Early lesions have focal areas of fat necrosis, such as those produced by partial ischemia. Lipomembranous change has been found also in lupus erythematosus panniculitis and in morphea.

Conditions to consider in the differential diagnosis:

lipomembranous panniculitis
lipogranulomatosis of Rothmann–Makai
granulomatous panniculitis in light-chain disease
early stages of pyoderma gangrenosum
necrobiotic xanthogranuloma

VIIID. MIXED LOBULAR AND SEPTAL PANNICULITIS

Neoplastic infiltrates and inflammation due to trauma or infection do not respect anatomic compartments of the subcutis.

1. With Hemorrhage or Sclerosis
2. With Many Neutrophils
3. With Many Eosinophils
4. With Many Lymphocytes
5. With Cytophagic Histiocytes
6. With Granulomas

VIIID1. With Hemorrhage or Sclerosis

Inflammation due to trauma is likely to be associated with hemorrhage, neutrophilic inflammation, and sclerosis in late lesions.

Panniculitis Due to Physical or Chemical Agents

CLINICAL SUMMARY. Trauma may be due to physical injury or chemical injury, such as that produced by injection of noxious substances. Physical injury can be produced by blunt pressure or impact, cold (13) or excessive heat, or electrical injury. All of these factors can produce firm nodules in the subcutaneous fat. Surreptitious injections of noxious substances can produce bizarre clinical and histologic patterns of lesions. Insulin injections, often on the thigh and lower abdomen, can result in subcutaneous lesions. Meperidine hydrochloride or Demerol and pentazocine or Talwin injections are known to produce traumatic panniculitis. The introduction of oily substances such as paraffin or silicone for cosmetic effects can produce a panniculitis (14). Mentally ill persons and drug addicts may purposely or inadvertently inject themselves with foreign substances, such as feces or milk, sometimes used to dilute or cut narcotics (15). These various physical or chemical traumas lead to indurated subcutaneous nodules that may undergo liquefaction, ulcerate, and discharge pus or a thick oily fluid. Healing leaves depressed scars. Lesions produced by extreme cold may include nodules or plaques that appear from 1 to 3 days after exposure and subside spontaneously within 2 weeks. Excessive heat and electrical injury usually are accompanied by ulceration and eschar formation.

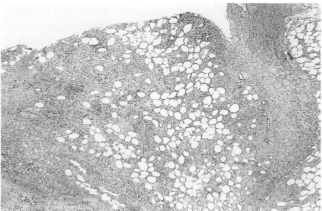

Fig. VIIID1.a

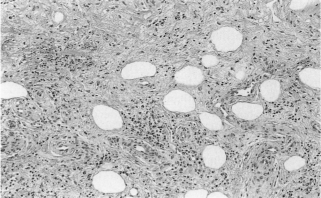

Fig. VIIID1.b

Fig. VIIID1.a. *Traumatic panniculitis, low power.* There is extensive fibrosis of the fat lobule with patchy inflammation.

Fig. VIIID1.b. *Traumatic panniculitis, medium power.* In addition to fibrosis between adipocytes, there is a mild mixed infiltrate composed of lymphocytes, histiocytes, and plasma cells. A focus of hemorrhage with a small cluster of neutrophils is present.

HISTOPATHOLOGY.   The injection of various toxic agents will produce a variable histologic picture of acute inflammation, with aggregation of neutrophils and focal fat necrosis with hemorrhage. Older lesions have infiltrates of lymphocytes and macrophages with fibrosis. Vasculitis usually is absent. Polarized light may reveal foreign material in injection sites. The injection of oily liquids leads to the formation of many pockets of fatty material fat cysts, often with a surrounding fibrous reaction containing foamy macrophages, which produces a "Swiss-cheese" appearance after the fat is extracted during routine histologic processing. Trauma due to cold injury initially has an infiltrate of lymphocytes and macrophages near the blood vessels of the deep plexus at the junction of dermis and subcutis. Such changes have also been described in perniosis. Biopsies at the third day, the height of the reaction, show rupture of the fat cells with fat pockets in the tissue surrounded by an infiltrate of lymphocytes, macrophages, neutrophils, and occasional eosinophils.

Conditions to consider in the differential diagnosis:

    traumatic panniculitis
    cold panniculitis
    injections including factitial panniculitis
    blunt trauma: sclerosing lipogranuloma

VIIID2. With Many Neutrophils

Neutrophilic inflammation diffusely involves the subcutis.

Necrotizing Fasciitis

CLINICAL SUMMARY.   Necrotizing fasciitis, like erysipelas, is caused by group A beta-hemolytic streptococci but also by a laundry list of other organisms, and it shows rapidly spreading erythema. However, the erythema is ill defined and progresses to painless ulceration and necrosis along fascial planes. Whereas erysipelas involves the more superficial layers of the skin, cellulitis extends more deeply into the subcutaneous tissues. Although virtually all cases of erysipelas are caused by beta-hemolytic streptococci, primarily group A, the differential diagnosis of cellulitis is much more extensive.

HISTOPATHOLOGY.   The histologic picture is characterized by acute and chronic inflammation with necrosis. Often there is thrombosis of blood vessels as the result of damage to vessel walls from the inflammatory process. The key feature in distinguishing necrotizing fasciitis from a less threatening superficial cellulitis is the location of the inflammation. In the former, the inflammation involves the subcutaneous fat, fascia, and muscle in addition to the dermis. A biopsy may be submitted at the time of surgical debridement for frozen section examination. In an appropriate setting, the presence of edema and neutrophils in these deep locations supports the diagnosis. Frank necrosis may not be demonstrable, and bacteria are frequently not evident in an initial biopsy.

Conditions to consider in the differential diagnosis:

    necrotizing fasciitis (bacterial infection)
    abscesses
    North American blastomycosis
    pyoderma gangrenosum (involves dermis also)
    ecthyma gangrenosum
    alpha-1-antitrypsin deficiency
    infection (cellulitis)
    dissecting cellulitis of the scalp (perifolliculitis
       abscedens et suffodiens)
    hidradenitis suppurativa
    ruptured follicles and cysts

VIIID3. With Many Eosinophils

Few to many eosinophils are present in subcutaneous lobules and septa.

Eosinophilic Fasciitis (Shulman's Syndrome)

CLINICAL SUMMARY.   Eosinophilic fasciitis (16) is a sclerodermalike disorder characterized by inflammation and thickening of the deep fascia. It has a rapid onset often after exercise, associated with pain, swelling, and progressive induration of the skin, leading to exaggerated deep grooving of the skin around superficial veins. This disorder is often accompanied by a peripheral eosinophilia and hypergammaglobulinemia and has been associated with aplastic anemia. Eosinophilic fasciitis often involves one or more extremities. In only a few cases are there lesions on the trunk, and the face is almost invariably spared. In nearly all reported cases, Raynaud's phenomenon and visceral lesions of scleroderma have been absent. The disorder has a varied course; some patients improve spontaneously, others improve with corticosteroids, whereas still others may have relapses and remissions. Eosinophilic fasciitis shares many features with generalized morphea; they both may show inflammation and fibrosis of the fascia and blood eosinophilia and hypergammaglobulinemia. Also, antinuclear antibodies are present in a significant number of cases. The term morphea profunda, analogous to lupus erythematosus profundus, has been applied to this disorder.

HISTOPATHOLOGY.   The fascia is markedly thickened, appears homogeneous, and is permeated by a mononuclear inflammatory infiltrate. In some instances the infiltrate in the fascia contains an admixture of eosinophils. The underlying skeletal muscle in some cases shows myofiber degeneration, severe inflammation with a component of eosinophils, and focal scarring; in other cases, however, it is not involved. In most cases, the fibrous septa separating deeply located fat lobules are thicker, paler staining, and more homogeneous and hyaline than normal subcutaneous connective tissue. In other cases, the collagen in the lower reticular dermis appears pale and homogeneous and the entire subcutaneous fat is replaced by horizontally oriented, thick, homogeneous

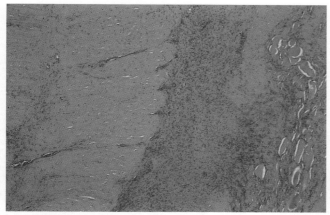

Fig. VIIID2.a

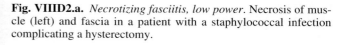

Fig. VIIID2.a. *Necrotizing fasciitis, low power.* Necrosis of muscle (left) and fascia in a patient with a staphylococcal infection complicating a hysterectomy.

Fig. VIIID2.b. *Necrotizing fasciitis, high power.* Necrotic muscle and fascia infiltrated by degenerating neutrophils.

Fig. VIIID2.c. *Necrotizing fasciitis, high power.* Fascia with focal edema and neutrophils. Presence of neutrophils in the fascia is compatible with this diagnosis in an appropriate clinical setting, even in the absence of necrosis in a particular biopsy specimen.

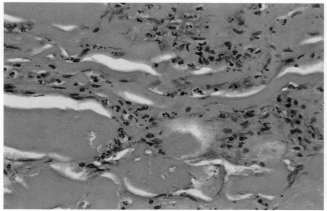

Fig. VIIID2.b

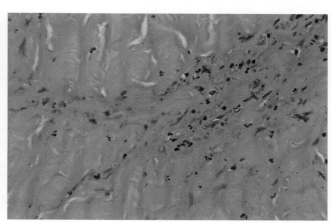

Fig. VIIID2.c

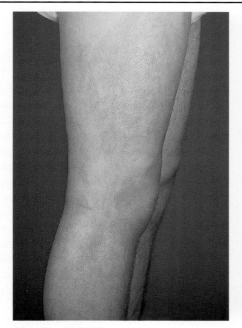

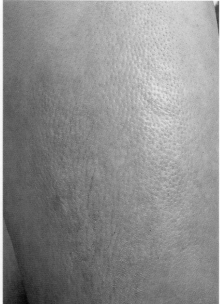

Clin. Fig. VIIID3.a   Clin. Fig. VIIID3.b

Clin. Fig. VIIID3.a. *Eosinophilic fasciitis.* The outer thigh skin is swollen and indurated.

Clin. Fig. VIIID3.b. *Eosinophilic fasciitis.* The skin appears sclerotic with surface dimpling. Morphea is in the differential diagnosis. *(continues)*

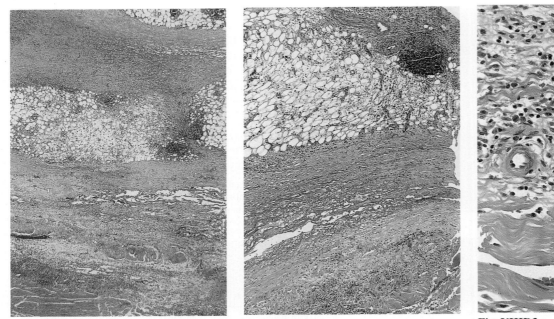

Fig. VIIID3.a   Fig. VIIID3.b   Fig. VIIID3.c

Fig. VIIID3.a. *Eosinophilic fasciitis, low power*. This deep biopsy shows subcutaneous fat in the upper portion of the photomicrograph and fascia in the lower half. The subcutaneous septum is markedly thickened and there is an associated predominantly septal inflammatory reaction that focally extends into the lobules.

Fig. VIIID3.b. *Eosinophilic fasciitis, medium power*. The subcutaneous septum shows fibrosis and inflammation with focal extension into the lobules.

Fig. VIIID3.c. *Eosinophilic fasciitis, high power*. Eosinophils are often not as numerous as in this example and in some cases may be rare or absent.

collagen containing only few fibroblasts and merging with the fascia.

Conditions to consider in the differential diagnosis:

eosinophilic fasciitis
eosinophilic panniculitis
arthropod bites
parasites

VIIID4. With Many Lymphocytes

Lymphocytic infiltrates diffusely involve the subcutis.

Subcutaneous Panniculitic or Lipotropic T-Cell Lymphoma

CLINICAL SUMMARY. Subcutaneous panniculitic or lipotropic T-cell lymphomas (17) may present with subcutaneous nodules, usually on the extremities. Some patients with this condition have associated hemophagocytic syndrome.

HISTOPATHOLOGY. The morphologic pattern overlaps with angiocentric lymphoma, as infiltration of vessel walls often accompanies subcutaneous infiltrates. Histopatho-

logic features include a dense subcutaneous infiltrate with a mixed septal and lobular distribution. The neoplastic cells have cytologic features similar to those of medium-sized or large-cell pleomorphic T-cell lymphoma, with irregularly shaped variably sized hyperchromatic nuclei, with small nucleoli; rarely, anaplastic large cells are prominent. In cases with hemophagocytic element, phagocytosis of erythrocytes by nonneoplastic macrophages is present in the subcutaneous infiltrate or the bone marrow. Foci of karyorrhexis and fat necrosis can occur and can be associated with a granulomatous inflammatory reaction. The neoplastic cells express a mature helper T-cell phenotype but can show loss of CD5 and CD7. Subcutaneous T-cell lymphomas resemble panniculitis at scanning magnification, and in the cases in which small pleomorphic T cells predominate, their infiltrates may not be obviously malignant, even under close scrutiny.

Conditions to consider in the differential diagnosis:

lupus panniculitis
chronic lymphocytic leukemia
subcutaneous T-cell lymphoma
histiocytic cytophagic panniculitis (early lesion)

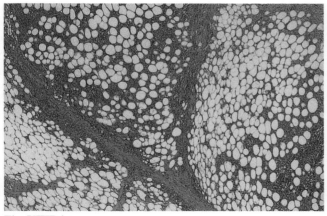

Fig. VIIID4.a

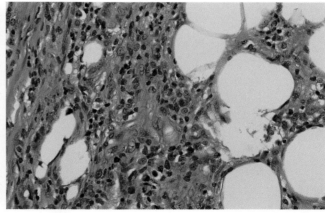

Fig. VIIID4.b

Fig. VIIID4.a. *Subcutaneous T-cell lymphoma, low power.* A septal and lobular infiltrate may mimic an inflammatory panniculitis, but the infiltrate is very dense. (P. Leboit and T. McCalmont)

Fig. VIIID4.b. *Subcutaneous T-cell lymphoma, high power.* Neoplastic lymphocytes are often inconspicuous in a heterogeneous infiltrate of macrophages, lymphocytes of varying sizes, and eosinophils. Genotypic analysis can be useful as an adjunct diagnostic tool in such instances. (P. Leboit and T. McCalmont)

VIIID5. With Cytophagic Histiocytes

Histiocytes with phagocytized erythrocytes diffusely infiltrate the subcutis. Rosai–Dorfman disease is a prototypic example (18).

Sinus Histiocytosis with Massive Lymphadenopathy (Rosai–Dorfman)

CLINICAL SUMMARY. Massive cervical lymphadenopathy, usually bilateral and painless, is the most common manifestation. This is generally a benign disorder despite a propensity to form large masses and to disseminate to both nodal and extranodal sites. In most patients the disease resolves spontaneously, others have persistent problems, and very few die. Skin is the most common extranodal site, with over 10% of patients having cutaneous involvement. The lesions are typically papules or nodules. A similar percentage has soft tissue involvement, usually of the subcutaneous tissue. Occasionally, the soft tissue lesion may present as a breast mass or panniculitis.

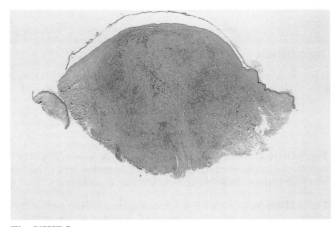

Fig. VIIID5.a

Fig. VIIID5.b

Fig. VIIID5.a. *Rosai–Dorfman disease, low power.* A nodular infiltrate spanning the dermis and entering the subcutis, with pale-staining cells centrally. (W. Burgdorf)

Fig. VIIID5.b. *Rosai–Dorfman disease, medium power.* Typical pattern of strands of pale sinus histiocytes admixed with darker-staining lymphocytes. (W. Burgdorf) (*continues*)

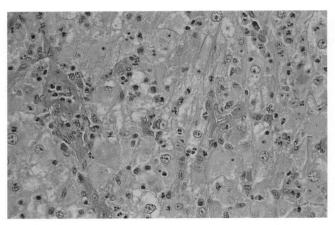

Fig. VIIID5.c. *Rosai–Dorfman disease, high power.* Numerous large histiocytes, some of which have ingested lymphocytes, demonstrating emperipolesis. (W. Burgdorf)

HISTOPATHOLOGY. The skin lesions contain a polymorphous infiltrate in which histiocytes with abundant cytoplasm are the most prominent element. Occasionally they may be multinucleated or have a foamy cytoplasm. How-

ever, the hallmark histologic feature is emperipolesis of lymphocytes. On occasion, red cells can also be taken up. In the lymph nodes, the sinuses are greatly dilated and crowded with inflammatory cells, particularly histiocytes. Here they tend to have an abundant foamy cytoplasm and also display emperipolesis. The histiocytes are S100-positive but CD1a-negative and do not contain Birbeck granules. About 50% are CD30-positive.

Conditions to consider in the differential diagnosis:

alpha-1-antitrypsin deficiency (late lesion)
histiocytic cytophagic panniculitis (late lesion)
Rosai–Dorfman disease (sinus histiocytosis with
    massive lymphadenopathy)

VIIID6. With Granulomas

There is granulomatous inflammation diffusely involving the subcutis.

Mycobacterial Panniculitis

Mycobacterial infection of the fat can produce a *mycobacterial panniculitis* that can mimic erythema nodosum and erythema induratum. Special stains for acid-fast bacteria and

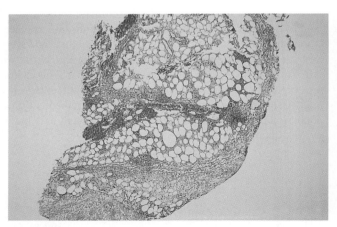

Fig. VIIID6.a

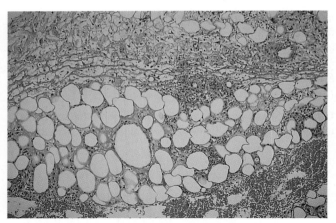

Fig. VIIID6.b

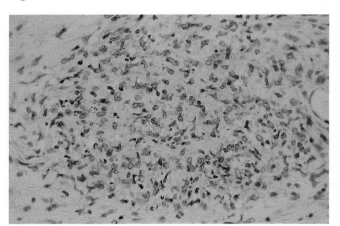

Fig. VIIID6.c

Fig. VIIID6.a. *Mycobacterial panniculitis, low power.* Direct mycobacterial infection of the fat has produced both a septal and lobular panniculitis. (N.S. McNutt, A. Moreno, F. Contreras)

Fig. VIIID6.b. *Mycobacterial panniculitis, medium power.* The infiltrate is mixed with collections of neutrophils, edema, and small granulomas. (N.S. McNutt, A. Moreno, F. Contreras)

Fig. VIIID6.c. *Mycobacterial panniculitis, high power.* Staining for mycobacteria shows that numerous red acid-fast bacilli are present in this example. (N.S. McNutt, A. Moreno, F. Contreras)

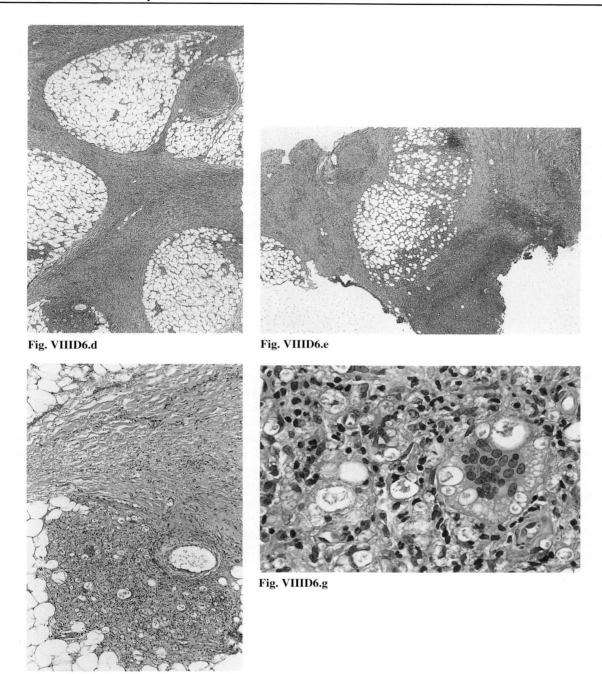

Fig. VIIID6.d

Fig. VIIID6.e

Fig. VIIID6.g

Fig. VIIID6.f

Fig. VIIID6.d. *Erythema nodosum leprosum, low power.* The architecture on scanning magnification may resemble erythema nodosum. Superiorly there is a large vessel within a fat lobule that is occluded and surrounded by a dense infiltrate.

Fig. VIIID6.e. *Erythema nodosum leprosum, low power.* This profile demonstrates dense inflammation within the septa and focally within the lobules. Vascular involvement is also evident.

Fig. VIIID6.f. *Erythema nodosum leprosum, medium power.* A granuloma composed of histiocytes and giant cells is present at the edge of a fat lobule. Clear spaces are identifiable within histiocytes.

Fig. VIIID6.g. *Erythema nodosum leprosum, high power.* Close inspection of the clear spaces within foamy macrophages and giant cells reveals numerous clumps of fragmented bacilli ("globi") within the foamy cells, which are known as lepra or Virchow cells. Neutrophils are scattered throughout this granuloma.

cultures are important for the identification of the mycobacteria that are responsible. Often, nontuberculous mycobacteria are involved in countries with a low incidence of tuberculosis and in immunodeficient subjects (19).

Erythema Nodosum Leprosum (Type 2 Leprosy Reaction)

CLINICAL SUMMARY.   Erythema nodosum leprosum occurs most commonly in lepromatous leprosy and less frequently in borderline lepromatous leprosy (20). It may be observed in patients under treatment or in untreated patients. Clinically, the reaction has a greater resemblance to erythema multiforme than to erythema nodosum. There is a widespread eruption accompanied by fever, malaise, arthralgia, and leukocytosis. On the skin there are tender red plaques and nodules together with areas of erythema and occasionally also purpura and vesicles. Ulceration, however, is rare.

HISTOPATHOLOGY.   The skin and subcutaneous lesions are foci of acute inflammation superimposed on chronic multibacillary leprosy. Polymorph neutrophils may be scanty or so abundant as to form a dermal abscess with ulceration. Whereas foamy macrophages containing fragmented bacilli are usual, in some patients no bacilli remain and macrophages have a granular pink hue on Wade–Fite staining, indicating mycobacterial debris. A necrotizing vasculitis affecting arterioles, venules, and capillaries occurs in some cases; these patients may have superficial ulceration.

Conditions to consider in the differential diagnosis:

    tuberculosis
    Crohn's disease
    gummatous tertiary syphilis
    erythema nodosum leprosum
    chronic erythema nodosum
    palisaded granulomas
    subcutaneous granuloma annulare/pseudorheumatoid
      nodule
    rheumatoid nodules
    mycobacterial panniculitis
    subcutaneous sarcoidosis

VIIIE. SUBCUTANEOUS ABSCESSES

There is a collection of neutrophils in the subcutis, usually surrounded by granulation tissue and fibrosis.

1. With Neutrophils

VIIIE1. With Neutrophils

The center of the abscess contains pus, which is viscous because of the presence of DNA fragments derived from neutrophils and dead organisms.

Phaeohyphomycotic Cyst

CLINICAL SUMMARY.   Phaeohyphomycosis (21) has been defined as a subcutaneous or systemic infection by dematiaceous mycelia-forming fungi, that is, those fungi having dark-walled hyphae. This is a histopathologic definition of a disease process that can be caused by many different organisms and that can have multiple different clinical presentations. Subcutaneous phaeohyphomycosis typically presents as a solitary abscess or nodule on the extremity of an adult male. A history of trauma or a splinter can sometimes be elicited.

HISTOPATHOLOGY.   Lesions of subcutaneous phaeohyphomycosis start as small often stellate foci of suppurative granulomatous inflammation. The area of inflammation gradually enlarges and usually forms a single large cavity with a surrounding fibrous capsule, the so-called phaeohyphomycotic cyst. The central space is filled with pus formed of polymorphonuclear leukocytes and fibrin. There is a surrounding granulomatous reaction composed of histiocytes, including epithelioid cells and multinucleated giant cells, lymphocytes, and plasma cells. Diligent search may identify an associated splinter in the tissue or liquid pus. The organisms are found within the cavity and at its edge, often within histiocytes. The hyphae often have irregularly placed branches and show constrictions around their septae. Mycelia, if present, are more loosely arranged than the compact masses of hyphae seen in eumycetoma. Pigment is not always obvious.

Conditions to consider in the differential diagnosis:

    acute or chronic bacterial abscesses
    deep fungal infections
    phaeohyphomycotic cyst
    North American blastomycosis
    chromoblastomycosis
    cutaneous alternariosis

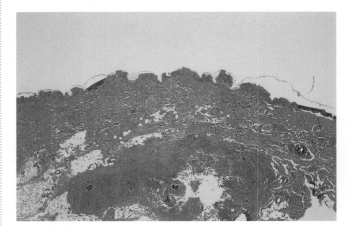

Fig. VIIIE1.a. *Phaeohyphomycotic cyst.* A subcutaneous nodule was comprised of sheets of neutrophils, with demonstrable fungal hyphae at higher magnification.

paracoccidioidomycosis
coccidioidomycosis
sporotrichosis
protothecosis
mycobacterial panniculitis

REFERENCES

1. Rademaker M, Lowe DG, Munro DD. Erythema induratum (Bazin's disease). *J Am Acad Dermatol* 1989;21:740.
2. Winkelmann RK, Forstrom L. New observations in the histopathology of erythema nodosum. *J Invest Dermatol* 1975; 65:441.
3. Rubin M, Lynch FW. Subcutaneous granuloma annulare. *Arch Dermatol Syphiligr* 1966;93:416.
4. Winkelmann RK. Panniculitis in connective tissue disease. *Arch Dermatol* 1983;119:336.
5. Tuffanelli DL. Lupus panniculitis. *Sem Dermatol* 1985;4:79.
6. Hytiroglou P, Phelps RG, Wattenberg DJ, Strauchen JA. Histiocytic cytophagic panniculitis: Molecular evidence for a clonal T-cell disorder. *J Am Acad Dermatol* 1992;27:333.
7. Ciclitira PJ, Wight DGD, Dick AP. Systemic Weber-Christian disease. *Br J Dermatol* 1980;103:685.
8. Norwood-Galloway A, Lebwohl M, Phelps RG, et al. Subcutaneous fat necrosis of the newborn with hypercalcemia. *J Am Acad Dermatol* 1987;16:435.
9. Hughes PSH, Apisarnthanarax P, Mullins JF. Subcutaneous fat necrosis associated with pancreatic disease. *Arch Dermatol* 1975;111:506.
10. Peters MS, Winkelmann RK. The histopathology of localized lipoatrophy. *Br J Dermatol* 1986;114:27.
11. Chartier S, Buzzanga JB, Paquin F. Partial lipodystrophy associated with a type 3 form of membranoproliferative glomerulonephritis. *J Am Acad Dermatol* 1987;16:201.
12. Alegre VA, Winkelmann RK, Aliaga A. Lipomembranous changes in chronic panniculitis. *J Am Acad Dermatol* 1988; 19:39.
13. Duncan WC, Freeman RG, Heaton CL. Cold panniculitis. *Arch Dermatol* 1966;94:722.
14. Winer LH, Steinberg TH, Lehman R, et al. Tissue reactions to injected silicone liquids. *Arch Dermatol* 1964;90:588.
15. Forstrom L, Winkelmann RK. Factitial panniculitis. *Arch Dermatol* 1974;110:747.
16. Helfman T, Falanga V. Eosinophilic fasciitis. *Clin Dermatol* 1994;12:449.
17. Perniciaro C, Zalla MJ, White JW Jr, Menke DM. Subcutaneous T-cell lymphoma: report of two additional cases and further observations. *Arch Dermatol* 1993;129:1171.
18. Perrin C, Michiels JF, Lacour JP, et al. Sinus histiocytosis (Rosai-Dorfman disease) clinically limited to the skin: an immunohistochemical and ultrastructural study. *J Cutan Pathol* 1993;20:368.
19. Inwald D, Nelson M, Cramp M, et al. Cutaneous manifestations of mycobacterial infection in patients with AIDS. *Br J Dermatol* 1994;130:111.
20. Hussain R, Lucas SB, Kifayet A, et al. Clinical and histological discrepancies in diagnosis of ENL reactions classified by assessment of acute phase proteins SAA and CRP. *Int J Lepr* 1995;63:222.
21. McGinnis MR. Chromoblastomycosis and phaeohyphomycosis: new concepts, diagnosis, and mycology. *J Am Acad Dermatol* 1983;8:1.

Alphabetical List of Diseases

Note: Page numbers in *italics* indicate figures.

A

Abscess, 200, 414, 418, 424
Acantholysis, intraspinous
    eosinophils, 146–150
    lymphocytes predominant, 146
    scant inflammatory cells, 143–146
Acantholytic actinic keratosis, 154, *155*
Acantholytic dermatosis, transient, 138,
    143–146, 152, *145*
Acantholytic dyskeratosis, 2
Acantholytic solar keratosis, 152
Acanthoma
    clear-cell, 21, *21–22*
    epidermolytic, 5
    large-cell, 5, 21
    pilar sheath, 298, 361, *300*
Acanthosis nigricans, 5, 36–37, 55, *38*
Accessory digit, 335, 336, *336*
Acne conglobata, 234, 381, 383–385
Acne fulminans, 381
Acne keloidalis, 385
    nuchae, 203
Acne rosacea, 175, 181
Acne varioliformis, 378
Acne vulgaris, 381
Acquired immunodeficiency syndrome
    (AIDS)
    Kaposi's sarcoma, 344–346, *345*
Acral lentiginous melanoma, 23–26, 34,
    395–396, *25–26, 396*
Acroangiodermatitis, 343–344, 353
Acrodermatitis, papular, 66, 84, 177
Acrodermatitis chronica atrophicans, 88,
    107, 208, 239
Acrodermatitis enteropathica, 95, 134
Acrokeratosis neoplastica, 9
Acroosteolysis, 239
Acropustulosis of infancy, 138
Actinic dermatitis, chronic, 84, 113
Actinic granuloma, 202, 222
Actinic keratosis, 16, 73, 103, 114, *17, 18,*
    103
    acantholytic, 154, *155*
    atrophic, 28, *29*

    hypertrophic, 55
    lichenoid, 107, 108, *110*
Actinic lentigo, 10, 27, 30–31, 37, *31*
Actinic prurigo, 55, 84
Actinomycosis, 230
Addison's disease, 10
Adenocarcinoma
    aggressive digital papillary, 296
    apocrine, 298
    eccrine, 296
    metastatic, 271, *272*
    primary, 271
Adenoid cystic eccrine carcinoma, 296
Adenoma
    aggressive digital papillary, 296
    apocrine tubular, 296–297, *297*
    papillary eccrine, 289
    sebaceous, 304–305, 306, *305*
Adenomatosis, erosive, 298
Adult mast cell disease, 82, *81–82*
Adult T cell lymphoma, 259
Aged skin, 88, *88*
Albinism, 13
Albright's hereditary osteodystrophy, 357,
    358
Alkaptonuric ochronosis, 252
Allergic contact dermatitis, 84, 139, 140,
    85
    acute, *85*
    chronic, 98–99, *99*
    subacute, *86*
Allergic granulomatous reaction, 193
    to chemical agents, 215
Allergic urticarial reaction, 71
Alopecia
    androgenetic, 368, *369*
    areata, 372, 378, *373–374*
    mucinosa, 378, *377*
    of secondary syphilis, 381
    syringolymphoid hyperplasia, 391
Alternariosis, cutaneous, 230, 424
Aluminum
    allergic granulomatous reaction, 215
    granuloma, 259

Amyloidosis, 81, 123, 195, 250
    lichen, 5, 13, *6*
    macular, 5, *5*
Androgenetic alopecia, 368, 372, *368–369*
Anetoderma, 242
Aneurysm
    cirsoid, 351
    fibrous histiocytoma, 332, 353
Angioedema, 179
Angioendotheliomatosis, reactive, 348
Angiofibroma, 326, 332, *327*
Angiohistocytoma, multinucleate cell, 353
Angioimmunoblastic lymphadenopathy,
    260
Angiokeratoma, 346, 348, *348*
Angioleiomyoma, 338, *338*
Angiolipoma, 353, 354, 357, *355*
Angiolymphoid hyperplasia with
    eosinophilia, 73, 179, 224–226, *225*
Angioma serpiginosum, 353
Angiomatosis, bacillary, 353
Angiomyolipoma, 353
Angiosarcoma
    cutaneous, 346, 353, *347*
    epithelioid, 321, 353
Anthrax, 234
Anticoagulant and anticardiolipin
    syndromes, 122–123
Antinuclear antibody, 130
Antiphospholipid syndromes, 122–123
alpha-1-Antitrypsin deficiency
    panniculitis, 411, 418, 422
Aplasia cutis, 241
Apocrine adenocarcinoma, 298
Apocrine adenoma, tubular, 296–297, *297*
Apocrine hidrocystoma, 364, 366, *365*
Apocrine nevus, 297
Areola, hyperkeratosis, 55
Argyria, 252, 389
Arrector pilae muscle tumors, 302
Arthritis, peripheral joints, 129
Arthropod bite reaction, 71, 73, 97, 107,
    108, 120, 185, 224, 391, 408, 420,
    392